DOSAGE
CALCULATIONS
A RATIO-PROPORTION APPROACH

FOURTH EDITION

Gloria D. Pickar, RN, EdD
Former Academic Dean and Professor of Nursing
Seminole State College of Florida
Sanford, Florida

Amy Pickar Abernethy, MD, PhD
Professor of Medicine and Nursing
Duke University
Durham, North Carolina

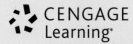

Australia • Brazil • Japan • Korea • Mexico • Singapore • Spain • United Kingdom • United States

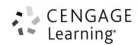
CENGAGE
Learning

Dosage Calculations: A Ratio-Proportion Approach, Fourth Edition

**Gloria D. Pickar, RN, EdD
and Amy Pickar Abernethy, MD, PhD**

Director, Development-Career and Computing: Marah Bellegarde

Senior Content Developer: Elisabeth Williams

Marketing Director: Michele McTighe

Marketing Manager: Jon Sheehan

Senior Production Director: Wendy Troeger

Production Manager: Andrew Crouth

Senior Content Project Manager: Kenneth McGrath

Senior Art Director: Jack Pendleton

For product information and technology assistance, contact us at
Cengage Learning Customer & Sales Support, 1-800-354-9706

For permission to use material from this text or product, submit all requests online at **www.cengage.com/permissions**
Further permissions questions can be e-mailed to
permissionrequest@cengage.com

Library of Congress Control Number: 2014931133

Book Only ISBN-13: 978-1-2854-2950-2

Package ISBN-13: 978-1-2854-2945-8

Cengage Learning
200 First Stamford Place, 4th Floor
Stamford, CT 06902
USA

Cengage Learning is a leading provider of customized learning solutions with office locations around the globe, including Singapore, the United Kingdom, Australia, Mexico, Brazil, and Japan. Locate your local office at: **www.cengage.com/global**

Cengage Learning products are represented in Canada by Nelson Education, Ltd.

To learn more about Cengage Learning, visit **www.cengage.com**

Purchase any of our products at your local college store or at our preferred online store **www.cengagebrain.com**

Notice to the Reader

Publisher does not warrant or guarantee any of the products described herein or perform any independent analysis in connection with any of the product information contained herein. Publisher does not assume, and expressly disclaims, any obligation to obtain and include information other than that provided to it by the manufacturer. The reader is expressly warned to consider and adopt all safety precautions that might be indicated by the activities described herein and to avoid all potential hazards. By following the instructions contained herein, the reader willingly assumes all risks in connection with such instructions. The publisher makes no representations or warranties of any kind, including but not limited to, the warranties of fitness for particular purpose or merchantability, nor are any such representations implied with respect to the material set forth herein, and the publisher takes no responsibility with respect to such material. The publisher shall not be liable for any special, consequential, or exemplary damages resulting, in whole or part, from the readers' use of, or reliance upon, this material.

Printed in the United States of America.
Print Number: 01   Print Year: 2014

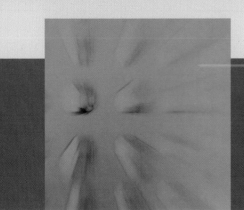

Contents

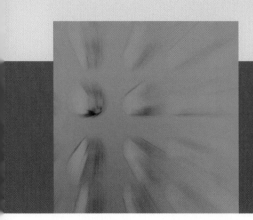

Preface

Introduction

Dosage Calculations: A Ratio-Proportion Approach, fourth edition, offers a clear and concise method of calculating drug dosages. The text is directed to students and professionals who want to increase their comfort level with mathematics and also to faculty members who prefer ratio and proportion for calculating dosages. Along with the companion text, *Dosage Calculations,* ninth edition, the content has been classroom tested and reviewed by well over 1 million faculty and students, who report that it has helped allay math anxiety and promote confidence in their ability to perform accurate calculations. As one reviewer noted, "I have looked at others [texts], and I don't feel they can compare."

The only math prerequisite is the ability to do basic arithmetic. For those who need a review, **Chapters 1** and **2** offer an overview of basic arithmetic calculations with extensive exercises for practice. The text teaches the learner to use a Three-Step Approach for calculating dosages.

1. Convert measurements to the same system and same size units.

2. Consider what dosage is reasonable.

3. Calculate using ratio and proportion.

Dosage Calculations: A Ratio-Proportion Approach, fourth edition, is based on feedback from users of the previous editions and users of other dosage calculations texts. The new edition also responds to changes in the health care field and includes the introduction of new drugs, replacement of outdated drugs, and discussion of new or refined methods of administering medications. The importance of avoiding medication errors is highlighted by the incorporation of applied critical thinking skills in clinical reasoning scenarios based on patient care situations, and a chapter on preventing medication errors. Clinical reasoning content has been expanded considering the Quality and Safety Education for Nurses (QSEN: www.qsen.org) competencies

that take into account the complexity of nursing work. Learners and faculty will find QSEN principles incorporated throughout: stacking, mindfulness, sensemaking, anticipating, memory aids, and work-arounds. To better prepare graduates for licensure examinations, test items patterned after NCLEX™-RN and NCLEX™-PN have been added for frequent practice.

Organization of Content

The text is organized in a natural progression of basic to more complex information. Learners gain self-confidence as they master content in small increments with ample review and reinforcement. Many learners claim that while using this text, they did not fear math for the very first time.

The seventeen chapters are divided into four sections.

Section 1 starts with a **Pretest** patterned after examinations often used by hospitals and health care agencies to evaluate the readiness of new graduates to prepare and administer medications. Learners can both evaluate their level of knowledge as they begin their study of dosage calculations and test their learning with the same examination as a posttest. This is followed by a mathematics diagnostic evaluation and a thorough mathematics review in **Chapters 1** and **2**. The **Mathematics Diagnostic Evaluation** allows learners to determine their computational strengths and weaknesses to guide them through the review of the **Section 1** chapters. **Chapters 1** and **2** provide a review of basic arithmetic skills, including fractions, decimals, ratios, percents, and simple equations, with numerous examples and practice problems to ensure that students can apply the procedures.

Section 2 includes **Chapters 3** through **9**. This section provides essential information that makes up the foundation for accurate dosage calculations and safe medication administration including medicine orders, labels, and equipment. **Chapters 3** and **4** introduce the three systems of measurement: metric, household, and apothecary. The metric system of measurement is emphasized because of its standardization in the health care field and the household system is included because of its implications for care at home. Apothecary measure and conversions can be found in ***Appendix B***, because the apothecary system is outdated and no longer recommended for use in health care. International or 24-hour time, and Fahrenheit and Celsius temperature conversions are presented in ***Chapter 5***.

In ***Chapter 6***, students learn to recognize and select appropriate equipment for the administration of medications based on the drug, dosage, and method of administration. Emphasis is placed on interpreting syringe calibrations to ensure that the dosage to be administered is accurate. All photos and drawings have been enhanced for improved clarity with updates from state-of-the-art technology and information systems.

Chapter 7 presents the common abbreviations used in health care so that learners can become proficient in interpreting medical orders. The content on computerized medication administration records has been updated and expanded for this edition.

It is essential that learners be able to read medication labels to calculate dosages accurately. This skill is developed by having readers interpret the medication labels provided beginning in ***Chapter 8***. These labels represent current commonly prescribed medications and are presented in full color and actual size (except in a few instances where the label is enlarged to improve readability). Some labels have been substituted with generic simulated labels to demonstrate critical calculations. This ensures that the entire range of medications seen in practice is presented, and gives the learners the experience with actual generic drugs. A full list of all labels in the text can be found in the ***Drug Label Index***.

Chapter 9 has been expanded and directs the learner's attention to the risks and responsibilities inherent in receiving medication prescriptions, transcribing orders, and administering medications. It provides the rationale for the patient's rights to safe medication administration and identifies the common causes of medication errors, including safe methods to prevent them. Throughout the text, care is taken to comply with standards and recommendations for medical notation available at the time of publication by The Joint Commission and The Institute for Safe Medication Practices. The *Official "Do Not Use" List* is emphasized. Learners are directed to stay abreast of these standards as they evolve to best ensure patient safety and prevent medication administration errors. More resources and tools for error prevention are presented, such as Tall Man letters to avoid mistaken identity of look-alike/sound-alike (LASA) drugs.

In ***Section 3***, students learn and practice the skill of dosage calculations applied to patients across the life span. The authors used QSEN quality and safety competencies as a guide for the development of realistic and challenging medication scenarios that simulate the complexity of various factors that challenge learners as they interpret, retrieve, prepare, calculate, and administer medications. These include obtaining pertinent drug information and making safe decisions for drug selection, preparation, dosage strength, equipment, and route for each patient. Various medication storage and retrieval systems are also demonstrated, such as unit-dose carts, automated dispensing cabinets (ADC) and ADC matrix drawers.

Safety competencies are incorporated to ensure learners carefully consider each aspect of the medication administration process for safe practice. Students learn to think through each problem logically for the right answer and then apply the ratio-proportion approach to double-check their thinking and verify their calculations. When this logical but unique system is applied every time to every problem, experience has shown that decreased math anxiety and increased accuracy result.

Chapters 10 and ***11*** guide the learner to apply all the skills mastered in previous chapters to achieve accurate oral and injectable drug dosage calculations. High-alert drugs, such as insulin and heparin, are thoroughly presented. Insulin types, species, and manufacturers have been updated with a description of insulin action time and the addition of U-500 insulin, including the difference between administering U-500 in the hospital and at home. The 70/30 and 50/50 insulins and the insulin pen are also thoroughly explained.

Chapter 12 introduces the concepts of solutions. Users learn the calculations associated with diluting solutions and reconstituting injectable drugs. This chapter provides a segue to intravenous calculations by fully describing the preparation of solutions. With the expanding role of the nurse and other health care workers in the home setting, clinical calculations for home care, such as nutritional feedings, are also emphasized.

Chapter 13 covers the calculation of pediatric and adult dosages and concentrates on the body weight method. Emphasis is placed on verifying safe dosages and applying concepts across the life span.

Chapter 14 introduces the formula and dimensional analysis methods of calculating dosages for faculty who may prefer these methods. Ample ***Review Sets*** and ***Practice Problems*** provide exposure to these methods, giving the learner an opportunity to sample other calculation methods and choose the one preferred.

Section 4 presents advanced clinical calculations applicable to both adults and children. Intravenous administration calculations are presented in ***Chapters 15*** through ***17***. Coverage reflects the greater application of IVs in drug therapy. Shortcut calculation methods are presented and explained fully. More electronic infusion devices are included. Heparin and saline locks, types of IV solutions, IV monitoring, IV administration records, and IV push drugs are included in **Chapter 15**. Pediatric IV calculations are presented in **Chapter 16**, and obstetric, heparin, insulin, and critical care IV calculations are covered in **Chapter 17**. Ample problems help students master the necessary calculations. Additional attention is directed to the clinical reasoning skills required to safely administer high-alert medications according to standard protocols, such as heparin and insulin.

Procedures in the text are introduced using **Rule** boxes and several **Examples**. Many examples use **Clinical Simulations** to guide learners through clinical reasoning and critical calculations. Examples and practice include finding and recording pertinent drug information from reputable drug resources. Key concepts are summarized and highlighted in **Quick Review** boxes before each set of **Review Problems** to give learners an opportunity to review major concepts prior to working through the problems. **Math Tips** provide memory joggers to assist learners in accurately solving problems. Learning is reinforced and evaluated by **Practice Problems** that conclude each chapter. The importance of calculation accuracy and patient safety is emphasized by patient scenarios that require careful and accurate consideration of every step of the medication administration process. **Clinical Reasoning Skills** scenarios allow learners to apply critical thinking to analyze and resolve medication administration errors at the end of each chapter beginning with **Section 2**. Additional scenarios accompany each chapter's **Practice Problems** to further emphasize accuracy and safety.

Information to be memorized is identified in **Remember** boxes, and **Caution** boxes alert learners to critical procedures and information.

Section Self-Evaluations found at the end of each section provide learners with an opportunity to test their mastery of chapter objectives prior to proceeding to the next section. Two **Posttests** at the conclusion of the text serve to evaluate the learner's overall skill in dosage calculations. The first **Posttest** refers the learner back to the new **Essential Skills Evaluation Pretest** from the beginning of the text, which covers essential skills commonly tested by employers. The second posttest, the **Comprehensive Skills Evaluation,** serves as a comprehensive examination covering all 17 chapters. Both are presented in a case study format to simulate actual clinical calculations.

An **Answer Key** at the back of the text provides all answers and solutions to selected problems in the **Pretest, Review Sets, Practice Problems, Section Self-Evaluations,** and **Posttests**. **Appendix A: Study Guide** is a new tool that provides essential abbreviations, equivalents, rules, and formulas from each clinical chapter, and **Appendix B: Apothecary System** describes apothecary conversions. Both a general content **Index** and a **Drug Label Index** conclude the text.

Features of the Fourth Edition

This text provides learners with the necessary knowledge and skills to accurately calculate dosages, safely prepare to administer medications, and carefully make decisions for error-free medication administration.

- Content is divided into four main sections to help learners better organize their studies.

- Measurable objectives at the beginning of each chapter emphasize the content to be mastered.

- More than 2,700 problems are included for learners to practice their skills and reinforce their learning, reflecting current drugs and protocols.

- **Clinical Reasoning Skills** scenarios apply critical thinking to real-life patient care situations to emphasize the importance of accurate dosage calculations and the avoidance of medication errors.

- Full color is used to make the text more user friendly, enhance presentation, and improve readability. Chapter elements, such as **Rules, Math Tips, Cautions, Remember** boxes, **Quick Reviews, Examples,** and **Summaries,** are color-coded for easy recognition and use. Color also highlights **Review Sets** and **Practice Problems**.

- Color has been added to selected syringe drawings throughout the text to *simulate a specific amount of medication,* as indicated in the example or problem. Because the color used may not correspond to the actual color of the medications named, *it must not be used as a reference for identifying medications.*

- Photos and drug labels are presented in full color. Special attention is given to visual clarity with some labels enlarged to ensure legibility.

- The **Math Review** brings learners up to the required level of basic math competence.

- SI conventional metric system notation is used (apothecary and household systems of measurement are introduced; apothecary measure can be found in **Appendix B**).

- **Rule** boxes draw the learner's attention to pertinent instructions.

- **Remember** boxes highlight information to be memorized.

- *Quick Review* boxes summarize critical information throughout the chapters before *Review Sets* are solved.

- *Caution* boxes alert learners to critical information.

- *Math Tips* serve to point out math shortcuts and reminders.

- Each new topic or skill presented is followed by *Review Sets* with end-of-chapter *Practice Problems* to assess understanding and skills and to reinforce learning.

- Many problems are included involving the interpretation of syringe scales to ensure that the proper dosage is administered. Once the dosage is calculated, the learner is directed to draw an arrow on a syringe at the proper value.

- Many more labels of current and commonly prescribed medications are presented, including a few simulated labels to help users learn how to select the proper information required to determine correct dosage. There are over 375 labels included.

- Hundreds of *Examples* are included to demonstrate the ratio-proportion, formula, or dimensional analysis methods of calculating dosages.

- The addition of the formula and dimensional analysis methods gives learners and instructors a choice of which method they prefer to use.

- Abbreviations, measurements, acronyms, and symbols follow The Joint Commission *Official "Do Not Use" List* and ISMP standards.

- Clear instructions are included for calculating IV medications administered in milligram per kilogram per minute.

- Clinical situations are simulated using actual medication labels, drug resource references, syringes, physician order forms, various medication storage and retrieval systems, and medication administration records.

- As requested by faculty and clinicians, the text has an enhanced emphasis on clinical decision making. While unit-dose preparations have eased calculation error rates, clinical complexity has increased them.

- The *Pretest, Section Evaluations, Chapter Practice Problems,* and *Posttests* include scenarios that simulate substantial aspects of real-world clinical calculation situations.

- An *Essential Skills Evaluation Pretest* and *Posttest* simulate exams commonly administered by employers for new hires, assess prior knowledge, and evaluate learning of essential calculation skills. A *Comprehensive Skills Evaluation* evaluates the learner's overall comprehension in preparation for a level or program assessment.

- *Appendix A: Study Guide* summarizes the most frequently used abbreviations, equivalents, and formulas from each chapter. Learners can refer to this valuable study tool for solving problems that will reinforce learning essential information and calculations.

- The general *Index* facilitates learner and instructor access to content and skills, and the *Drug Index* facilitates access to all labels used in the text.

New to the Fourth Edition

For more than 30 years, this text and its companion, *Dosage Calculations,* ninth edition, have guided health care students to learn the knowledge and skills necessary for safe and accurate dosage calculations and medication administration. Regular and frequent updates keep the information current and state-of-the-art. Here is what's new to this edition.

- *Quality and Safety in Nursing Education* (QSEN) principles and competencies have been adapted to reduce the risk of medication errors and improve patient safety.

- *Clinical simulations* provided in examples and test questions in *Chapters 10* through *13* develop clinical reasoning and calculation skills, beginning with seeking drug information from reputable resources, through the logic and safety precautions in the drug dosage calculation and administration process.

- Section Examinations include test items formatted like graduate licensure examinations, such as the *NCLEX-RN™ and NCLEX-PN™ exams*.

- A new *Pretest* and *Posttest* assess prior learning and evaluate skills commonly tested for new-hire graduates.

- Content on *high-alert drugs,* such as heparin and insulin, has been extensively augmented, including safety concerns with the increased use of *insulin pens* in hospitals. *U-500 insulin* content and calculations have been expanded, including conversions for preparation using both U-100 and 1 mL syringes.

- Administration protocols are expanded to include both insulin and heparin.

- New questions are added throughout to reflect current drugs and protocols.

- Computerized order and medication administration record systems have been updated to demonstrate a variety of drug retrieval systems, including Automated Dispensing Cabinets (ADC).

- Photographs of state-of-the-art equipment are replaced and updated, including the latest medication storage and retrieval systems.

- Practice has been added for the clinical reasoning essential to making correct choices when using different drug storage and retrieval systems.

- Apothecary calculations have been deleted within the text and evaluation items, consistent with current standards. Apothecary measure has been moved to **Appendix B**.

- Learners apply critical thinking to prevent medication errors in **Clinical Reasoning Skills** scenarios based on QSEN principles.

- Dosage calculations scenarios have been expanded to incorporate each step of safe and error-free medication administration: interpretation of order, acquisition of drug information, retrieval of drug, dosage calculation, dose measurement, preparation, and administration.

- Learners are purposely directed to be mindful of the seriousness of their clinical practice and the value of **safety alerts** to prevent errors.

- **Appendix A: Study Guide** summarizes essential rules, formulas, abbreviations, and equivalents to facilitate problem solving and reinforce learning.

- **Appendix B: Apothecary System** gives common units, abbreviations, and symbols of the original dosage measurement system, for faculty and students interested in comparing and converting between apothecary and metric measure.

- An exciting new **Premium Website** with **Practice Software** is available, offering a glossary review, chapter tutorials, interactive exercises, and hundreds of practice problems.

Learning Package for the Student
Premium Website
(ISBN 978-1-2854-2954-0)

The **Premium Website** can be accessed by users of the text at **www.CengageBrain.com**. Enter your passcode, found in the front of the book, and the Premium Website will be added to your bookshelf. Here you can access the engaging **Practice Software,** which includes:

- A user-friendly menu structure to immediately access the program's items.

- A bank of several hundred questions for practice and to reinforce the content presented in the text.

- A tutorial for each chapter outlining instructions and approaches to safe and accurate dosage calculation.

- **Quizzes, Pretest,** and **Posttest** that operate within a tutorial mode, which allows two tries before the correct answer is provided.

- Interactive exercises that ask you to fill a medicine cup or draw back a syringe to the correctly calculated dose.

- A comprehensive glossary of terms and drug names with definitions and pronunciations.

- Drop-down calculator available at a click of a button, as used on the NCLEX-RN™ and -PN examinations.

Teaching Package for the Instructor
(ISBN 978-1-2854-2955-7)

The **Instructor Companion Website to Accompany Dosage Calculations: A Ratio-Proportion Approach,** fourth edition, contains a variety of tools to help instructors successfully prepare lectures and teach within this subject area. The following components in the website are free to adopters of the text:

- A **Solutions Manual** includes answers and step-by-step solutions for every question in the **Pretest, Math Evaluation, Review Sets, Practice Problems, Section Evaluations,** and **Posttests** from the book.

- The **Computerized Test** Bank includes approximately 500 additional questions not found in the book for further assessment. The software also allows for the creation of test items and full tests, as well as coding for difficulty level.

- Lecture slides created in **PowerPoint**® offer a depiction of administration tools and include calculation tips helpful to classroom lecture of dosage calculations.

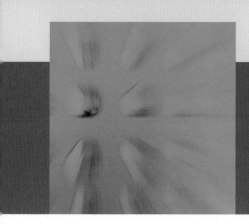

Acknowledgments

Contributor

Maureen D. Tremel, MSN, ARNP
Professor of Nursing
Seminole State College of Florida
Sanford, Florida

Reviewers

Michele Bach, MS
Mathematics Professor
Kansas City Kansas Community College
Kansas City, Kansas

Irene Coons, RN, MSN, CNE
Professor of Nursing
College of Southern Nevada
Henderson, Nevada

Melanie Moore, RN, MSN, PhD
Program Head, Practical Nursing
Associate Professor
Virginia Western Community College
Roanoke, Virginia

Accuracy Reviewers

Beverly Meyers, MEd, MAT
Professor, Mathematics and Science
Jefferson College
Hillsboro, Missouri

Julie E. Pickar
Freelance Copy Editor and Proofreader
Maitland, Florida

From the Authors

We wish to thank our many students and colleagues who have provided inspiration and made contributions to the production of the text. We are particularly grateful to Maureen Tremel for her careful attention to researching and updating information; to Julie Pickar and Beverly Meyers for their careful attention to accuracy; to Elisabeth Williams and Kenneth McGrath for their careful attention to deadlines and details; and to Roger Pickar and Steve Abernethy for their careful attention to us and our families.

Gloria D. Pickar, RN, EdD
Amy Pickar Abernethy, MD, PhD

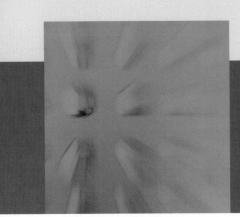

Introduction to the Learner

The accurate calculation of drug dosages is an essential skill in health care. Paracelsus (1493–1591), often referred to as the father of pharmacology, recognized that the difference between a poison, narcotic, hallucinogen, and medicine is dosage. Serious harm to the patient can result from inadequate knowledge, incorrect interpretation or transcription of a medication order, retrieving the wrong drug, or error during the calculation and subsequent administration of a drug dosage. It is the responsibility of those administering drugs to precisely and efficiently carry out medical orders and to recognize unsafe dosages, prescriptions, and practices.

Learning to calculate drug dosages need not be a difficult or burdensome process. *Dosage Calculations: A Ratio-Proportion Approach,* fourth edition, provides an uncomplicated, easy-to-learn, easy-to-recall Three-Step Approach to dosage calculations. Once you master this method, you will be able to consistently compute dosages with accuracy, ease, and confidence.

The text is a self-study guide that is divided into four main sections. The only mathematical prerequisite is the basic ability to add, subtract, multiply, and divide whole numbers. A review of fractions, decimals, percents, simple equations, ratios, and proportions is included. You are encouraged to work at your own pace and seek assistance from a qualified instructor as needed.

Each procedure in the text is introduced by several *Examples*. Key concepts are summarized and highlighted throughout each chapter, to give you an opportunity to review the concepts before working the problems. Ample *Review* and *Practice Problems* are given to reinforce your skill and confidence.

Before calculating the dosage, you are asked to consider the reasonableness of the computation. More often than not, the correct amount can be estimated in your head. Many errors can be avoided if you approach dosage calculation in this logical fashion. The mathematical computation can then be used to double-check your thinking. Answers to all problems and step-by-step solutions to select problems are included at the back of the text.

Many photos and drawings are included to demonstrate key concepts and equipment. Drug labels and measuring devices (for example, syringes) are included to give a simulated "hands-on" experience outside of the clinical setting or laboratory. *Clinical Reasoning Skills* emphasize the importance of dosage calculation accuracy, and medication administration scenarios provide opportunities to analyze pertinent information, make sound clinical decisions, calculate accurately, and prevent errors.

This text has helped hundreds of thousands of learners just like you to feel at ease about math and to master dosage calculations. I am interested in your feedback. Please write to me to share your reactions and success stories.

Gloria D. Pickar, RN, EdD
gpickar@cfl.rr.com

Dedicated to Julie,
in recognition of the importance of preventing errors.

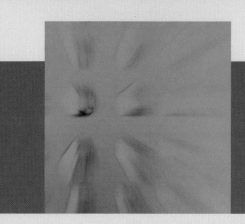

Using This Book

■ **Content** is presented from simple to complex, in small increments, followed by solved *Examples* and a *Quick Review. Review Sets* and *Practice Problems* provide opportunities for you to reinforce your learning.

3. Order: penicillin G potassium 1,000,000 units IV q.6h

05-4243-32-6

6505-00-958-3305

SEE ACCOMPANYING PRESCRIBING INFORMATION

RECOMMENDED STORAGE IN DRY FORM.

Store below 86°F (30°C).

Sterile solution may be kept in refrigerator for one (1) week without significant loss of potency.

NDC 0049-0520-83
Rx only

Buffered

Pfizerpen®
(penicillin G potassium)

For Injection

FIVE MILLION UNITS

Pfizer **Roerig**
Division of Pfizer Inc, NY, NY 10017

USUAL DOSAGE
Average single intramuscular injection: 200,000-400,000 units.
Intravenous: Additional information about the use of this product intravenously can be found in the package insert.

mL diluent added	Units per mL of solution
18.2 mL	250,000
8.2 mL	500,000
3.2 mL	1,000,000

Buffered with sodium citrate and citric acid to optimum pH.

PATIENT: _____

ROOM NO: _____

DATE DILUTED: _____

Describe the three concentrations, and calculate the amount to give for each of the supply dosage concentrations.

Reconstitute with _____ mL diluent for a concentration of _____ units/mL.

Give: _____ mL

Reconstitute with _____ mL diluent for a concentration of _____ units/mL.

Give: _____ mL

Reconstitute with _____ mL diluent for a concentration of _____ units/mL.

Give: _____ mL

Indicate the concentration you would choose, and explain the rationale for your selection.

Select _____ units/mL and give _____ mL. Rationale: _____

_____

■ **Measurable objectives** at the beginning of each chapter define learning outcomes.

OBJECTIVES

Upon mastery of Chapter 11, you will be able to apply clinical reasoning skills to prepare safe and accurate parenteral dosages of drugs. To accomplish this, you will also be able to:

■ Gather current information about the drug.

■ Retrieve the right drug in the correct supply dosage strength.

■ Apply the Three-Step Approach to dosage calculation: convert, think, and calculate using ratio-proportion.

■ Verify drug and dosage with a second nurse for high-alert medications and for wasting of controlled substances.

■ Measure correct dose amounts.

■ Collaborate with patients and families regarding their medications, including safe administration at home.

■ **Syringes** are drawn to full size, providing accurate scale renderings to help you master the reading of injectable dosages.

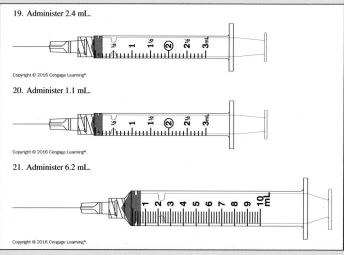

19. Administer 2.4 mL.

Copyright © 2016 Cengage Learning®.

20. Administer 1.1 mL.

Copyright © 2016 Cengage Learning®.

21. Administer 6.2 mL.

Copyright © 2016 Cengage Learning®.

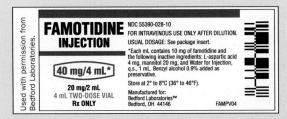

Used with permission from Bedford Laboratories.

FAMOTIDINE INJECTION

NDC 55390-028-10
FOR INTRAVENOUS USE ONLY AFTER DILUTION.
USUAL DOSAGE: See package insert.

*Each mL contains 10 mg of famotidine and the following inactive ingredients: L-aspartic acid 4 mg, mannitol 20 mg, and Water for Injection, q.s., 1 mL. Benzyl alcohol 0.9% added as preservative.

Store at 2° to 8°C (36° to 46°F).

Manufactured for:
Bedford Laboratories™
Bedford, OH 44146   FAMPV04

40 mg/4 mL*

20 mg/2 mL
4 mL TWO-DOSE VIAL
Rx ONLY

■ **Drug labels** and photos are presented in full color; actual size labels help prepare you to read and interpret content in its true-life format.

MATH TIP

Notice that to multiply 2 by 1,000, you are moving the decimal three places to the right. This is a shortcut. Sometimes to complete this operation, you add zeros to hold the places equal to the number of zeros in the equivalent. In this case, 1 g = 1,000 mg, so you add three zeros:

$2 \times 1,000 = 2.000. = 2,000$

■ *Math Tip* boxes provide you with clues to essential computations.

CAUTION

If any of the seven parts is missing or unclear, the order is considered incomplete and is therefore not a legal drug order.

■ *Caution* boxes alert you to critical information and safety concerns.

RULE

In a proportion, the ratio for a known equivalent equals the ratio for an unknown equivalent. To use ratio-proportion to convert from one unit to another, you need to follow these three steps.

1. Recall the equivalents.

2. Set up a proportion of two equivalent ratios.

3. Cross-multiply to solve for an unknown quantity, X.

■ *Rule* boxes highlight and draw your attention to important formulas and pertinent instructions.

REMEMBER

The Six Rights of safe and accurate medication administration are as follows:

The *right patient* must receive the *right drug* in the *right amount* by the *right route* at the *right time*, followed by the *right documentation*.

■ *Remember* boxes highlight information that you should memorize.

QUICK REVIEW

Look again at Steps 1 through 3 as a valuable dosage calculation checklist.

Step 1	Convert	Be sure that all measurements are in the same system and all units are the same size.
Step 2	Think	Carefully estimate the reasonable amount of the drug that you should administer.
Step 3	Calculate	$\dfrac{\text{Dosage on hand}}{\text{Amount on hand}} = \dfrac{\text{Dosage desired}}{\text{X Amount desired}}$

■ *Quick Review* boxes summarize critical information that you will need to know and understand to safely prepare and administer medications.

SUMMARY

At this point, you should be quite familiar with the equivalents for converting within the metric and household systems and from one system to another. From memory, you should be able to recall quickly and accurately the equivalents for conversions. If you are having difficulty understanding the concept of converting from one unit of measurement to another, review this chapter and seek additional help from your instructor.

Consider the two Clinical Reasoning Skills scenarios, and work the Practice Problems for Chapter 4. Concentrate on accuracy. One error can be a serious mistake when calculating the dosages of medicines or performing critical measurements of health status.

■ *Summary* boxes draw out key information from the chapter as a self-check and review tool.

EXAMPLE 4 ■

Convert: 0.15 kg to g

Equivalent: 1 kg = 1,000 g

$\dfrac{1 \text{ kg}}{1,000 \text{ g}} = \dfrac{0.15 \text{ kg}}{\text{X g}}$

$\dfrac{1 \text{ kg}}{1,000 \text{ g}} \diagup \dfrac{0.15 \text{ kg}}{\text{X g}}$ Cross-multiply

$\text{X} = 1,000 \times 0.15$ 0.150. Move the decimal 3 places to the right to multiply by 1,000. Add a zero to complete the operation.

$\text{X} = 150 \text{ g}$ Label the units to match the unknown X.

■ *Examples* walk you step-by-step through each calculation process, using different conversions, medications, and methods, to ensure that your mastery of the process is complete.

■ *Problems* illustrate questions that students will encounter in actual lab and clinical situations.

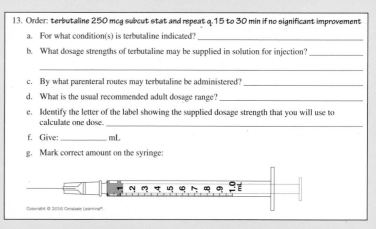

13. Order: *terbutaline 250 mcg subcut stat and repeat q.15 to 30 min if no significant improvement*

   a. For what condition(s) is terbutaline indicated? _____

   b. What dosage strengths of terbutaline may be supplied in solution for injection? _____

      _____

   c. By what parenteral routes may terbutaline be administered? _____

   d. What is the usual recommended adult dosage range? _____

   e. Identify the letter of the label showing the supplied dosage strength that you will use to calculate one dose. _____

   f. Give: _____ mL

   g. Mark correct amount on the syringe:

Copyright © 2016 Cengage Learning®.

■ *Illustrations* simulate critical dosage calculation and dose preparation skills.

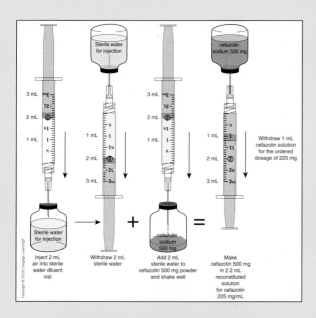

■ *Clinical Reasoning Skills* apply critical thinking to real-life patient care situations emphasizing the importance of accurate dosage calculations and the avoidance of medication errors. As an added benefit, clinical reasoning scenarios present prevention strategies so that you can learn how to avoid these errors in practice.

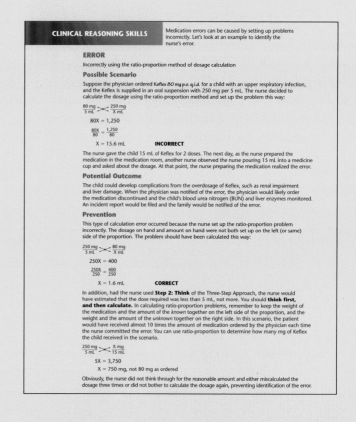

Review Set 13

Convert each of the following to the equivalent unit indicated.

1. 500 mL =	_____ L		16. 0.75 L =	_____ mL
2. 0.015 g =	_____ mg		17. 5,000 mL =	_____ L
3. 8 mg =	_____ g		18. 1 L =	_____ mL
4. 10 mg =	_____ g		19. 1 g =	_____ mg
5. 60 mg =	_____ g		20. 3,000 mL =	_____ L
6. 300 mg =	_____ g		21. 23 mcg =	_____ mg
7. 0.2 g =	_____ mg		22. 1.05 g =	_____ kg
8. 1.2 g =	_____ mg		23. 18 mcg =	_____ mg
9. 0.0025 kg =	_____ g		24. 0.4 mg =	_____ mcg
10. 0.065 g =	_____ mg		25. 2,625 g =	_____ kg
11. 0.005 L =	_____ mL		26. 50 cm =	_____ m
12. 1.5 L =	_____ mL		27. 10 L =	_____ mL
13. 100 mcg =	_____ mg		28. 450 mL =	_____ L
14. 250 mL =	_____ L		29. 5 mL =	_____ L
15. 2 kg =	_____ g		30. 30 mg =	_____ mcg

After completing these problems, see page 642 to check your answers.

■ *Review Sets* are inserted after each new topic, to encourage you to stop and check your understanding of the material just presented.

■ *Practice Problems* round out each chapter. This is your opportunity to put your skills to the test, to identify your areas of strength, and also to acknowledge those areas in which you need additional study.

PRACTICE PROBLEMS—CHAPTER 11

Calculate the amount you will prepare for 1 dose. Indicate the syringe you will select to measure the medication.

1. Order: hydromorphone (Dilaudid) 4 mg slow IV push (over 10 min) q.4h p.r.n., severe pain

   Supply: hydromorphone 10 mg/mL

   Give: _____ mL   Select: _____ syringe

2. Order: morphine sulfate 15 mg slow IV push (over 5 min) stat

   Supply: morphine sulfate 10 mg/mL

   Give: _____ mL   Select: _____ syringe

Mr. Smith is on restricted fluids. His IV order is: NS 1,500 mL IV q.24h c̄ 300,000 units penicillin G potassium IV PB in 100 mL NS q.4h over 30 min. The infusion set is calibrated at 60 gtt/mL.

38. Set Mr. Smith's regular IV at _____ gtt/min.

39. Set Mr. Smith's IV PB at _____ gtt/min.

Later during your shift, an electronic infusion pump becomes available. You decide to use it to regulate Mr. Smith's IVs.

40. Regulate Mr. Smith's regular IV at _____ mL/h.

41. Regulate Mr. Smith's IV PB at _____ mL/h.

■ *Essential Skills Pretest, Section Self-Evaluations, Posttest,* and *Comprehensive Skills Evaluation* test your mastery of concepts and critical calculation skills.

■ *Clinical Simulations* provide opportunities to practice your clinical reasoning combined with dosage calculation skills for safe and accurate medication administration.

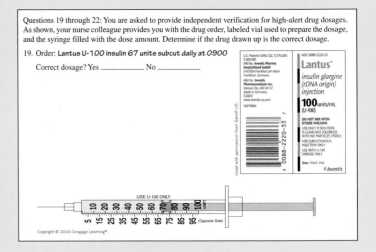

■ *NCLEX-RN™ and NCLEX-PN™* alternate test items give you an opportunity to practice answering questions formatted like these licensure examinations.

---

54. **NCLEX** *Drag-and-Drop / Ordered-Response* **Item**

Copy the tasks from the box onto the list in the proper sequence to *administer high-alert intravenous heparin by a standard weight-based protocol.*

Answer:

Check aPTT test results.
Start continuous infusion, if required.
Record weight in kilograms.
Administer bolus, if required.
Adjust infusion rate, if required.
Check aPTT test results.
Administer rebolus, if required.

_____
_____
_____
_____
_____
_____
_____

Dosage Calculations: Ratio-Proportion Method

$$\frac{\text{Dosage on hand}}{\text{Amount on hand}} = \frac{\text{Dosage desired}}{\text{X Amount desired}}$$

■ *Appendix A: Study Guide* summarizes equivalents, abbreviations, terms, and calculation methods.

■ *Appendix B: Apothecary System* describes the common units, symbols, and equivalent conversions of this measurement system.

Apothecary-Metric Approximate Equivalents

Volume		Weight	
oz mL	**min mL**	**gr mg**	**gr mg**
1 = 30	45 = 3	15 = 1,000	$\frac{1}{4}$ = 15
$\frac{1}{2}$ = 15	30 = 2	10 = 600	$\frac{1}{6}$ = 10
	15 = 1	$7\frac{1}{2}$ = 500	$\frac{1}{8}$ = 7.5
dr mL	12 = 0.75	5 = 300	$\frac{1}{10}$ = 6
$2\frac{1}{2}$ = 10	10 = 0.6	4 = 250	$\frac{1}{15}$ = 4
2 = 8	8 = 0.5	3 = 200	$\frac{1}{20}$ = 3
$1\frac{1}{4}$ = 5	5 = 0.3	$2\frac{1}{2}$ = 150	$\frac{1}{30}$ = 2
1 = 5	4 = 0.25	2 = 120	$\frac{1}{40}$ = 1.5
	3 = 0.2	$1\frac{1}{2}$ = 100	$\frac{1}{60}$ = 1
1 minim = 1 gtt	$1\frac{1}{2}$ = 0.1	1 = 60	$\frac{1}{100}$ = 0.6
	1 = 0.06	$\frac{3}{4}$ = 45	$\frac{1}{120}$ = 0.5
	$\frac{3}{4}$ = 0.05	$\frac{1}{2}$ = 30	$\frac{1}{150}$ = 0.4
	$\frac{1}{2}$ = 0.03	$\frac{1}{3}$ = 20	$\frac{1}{200}$ = 0.3
			$\frac{1}{250}$ = 0.25

■ *Drug Label Index* identifies each label in the text as a quick reference.

Drug Label Index

Boldface indicates generic drug name

A
acetaminophen, 250
acetaminophen (Tylenol), 610
acetaminophen and hydrocodone
   bitartrate (Lortab), 5, 168,
   177, 234
acetaminophen and oxycodone
   (Percocet), 168, 234, 262
acyclovir, 342, 361
albuterol sulfate, 244, 432, 459
Aldactone (spironolactone), 98,
   167, 262

B
Biaxin (clarithromycin), 170,
   217, 431
bumetanide injection, 176, 286
butorphanol tartrate injection, 7

C
Calan (verapamil), 4, 230
Carafate (sucralfate), 15, 160,
   216, 260
carbamazepine (Tegretol), 166,
   169, 231, 260, 424

codeine sulfate tablets, 459
Continu-Flo solution set, 494
Continu-Flo solution set with
   Duo-Vent spike, 18, 482, 495
Co-Trimoxazole (trimethoprim
   and sulfamethoxazole),
   407, 412
cytarabine injection, 369

D
Depakene (valproic acid), 244,
   424, 457

■ *Online Practice Software* is offered as your built-in learning tutor. As you study each chapter, be sure to also work with the online study tool. This valuable resource will help you verify your understanding of key rules and calculations.

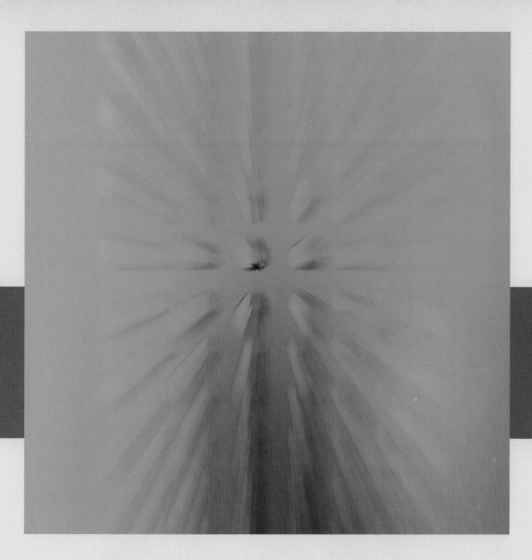

Pretest and Mathematics Review

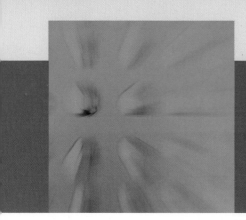

Essential Skills Evaluation: Pretest

Record your answers on the Essential Skills Evaluation: Pretest Answer Sheet on page 21. Do not record your answers on the test itself. You will refer back to this Essential Skills Evaluation as an essential skills posttest when you conclude your studies.

As you begin the study of safe dosage calculation, consider that you bring previous knowledge from life experiences. Perhaps you have worked or volunteered in a health care setting or administered medication to a family member or friend. This essential skills pretest will help you identify dosage calculation skills you already possess and highlight skills that you will learn and master as you work through the text. Take this pretest now, but do not be concerned if there are many questions you are unable to answer. That is to be expected. Use scrap paper to work the problems rather than writing on the test pages so that you can take this test again once you have completed this course of study. Separate answer sheets are provided following the pretest and again following Section 4 (as a posttest) for you to record your answers. Comparing your answers from the pretest with those of the posttest will allow you to measure your improvement and see what material you may need to revisit with your instructor.

The Essential Skills Evaluation is designed to be similar to the type of entry-level test given by hospitals and health care agencies during orientation for new graduates and new employees. It excludes the advanced calculation skills presented in Chapters 16 and 17. A more comprehensive skills evaluation will be available at the end of the text, to measure mastery of the full range of dosage calculation skills presented in all 17 chapters of the text.

Locate the Essential Skills Evaluation: Pretest Answer Sheet, gather some scratch paper, and let's get started!

Instructions for questions 1 through 19:

Throughout your assigned shift on a busy adult medical unit, you will give medications to a group of patients. The following labels represent the medications available on the medical unit to fill the orders given. Calculate the amount you will administer for one dose, and identify the frequency of administration of each dose. For solutions, mark an arrow on the syringe to indicate the correct volume. When multiple syringes are provided, choose the most appropriate one to mark.

1. Order: *verapamil 40 mg p.o. t.i.d.*

   Give: _____ tablet(s)   Frequency: _____

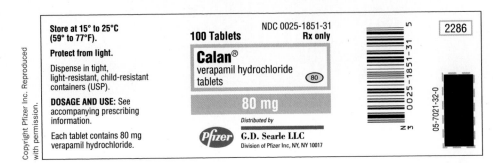

2. Order: *clonazepam 1.5 mg p.o. b.i.d.*

   Give: _____ tablet(s)   Frequency: _____

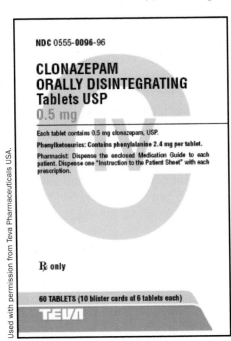

3. Order: *atomoxetine 20 mg p.o. daily*

   Choose: _____ mg capsules   Give: _____ capsule(s)   Frequency: _____

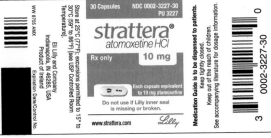

A

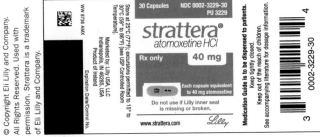

B

4. Order: **Lortab 2.5 mg p.o. q.3h, p.r.n., moderate pain** (ordered according to dose of hydrocodone)

   Give: _____ tablet(s)

   Frequency: _____

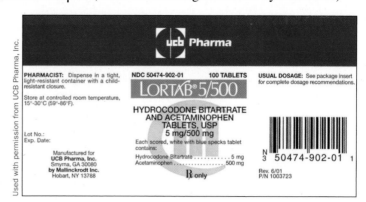

5. Order: **levothyroxine 0.3 mg p.o. q.AM**

   Give: _____ tablet(s)

   Frequency: _____

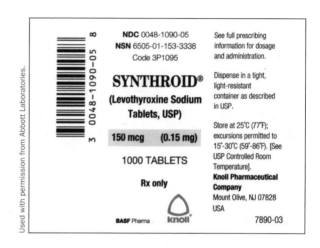

6. Order: **amoxicillin and clavulanate potassium 100 mg p.o. q.8h** (ordered according to dose of amoxicillin)

   Give: _____ mL   Frequency: _____

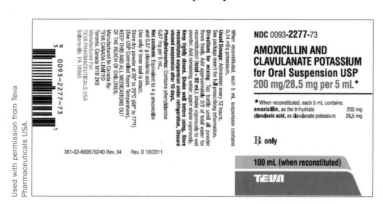

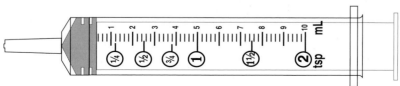

7. Order: promethazine 12.5 mg IV q.4h p.r.n., nausea

   Give: _____ mL (Use label A.)

   Frequency: _____

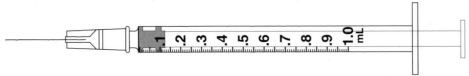

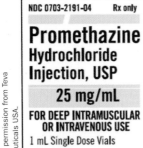

NDC 0703-2191-04 Rx only	Each mL contains: Promethazine hydrochloride 25 mg, edetate disodium 0.1 mg, calcium chloride 0.04 mg, sodium metabisulfite 0.25 mg and phenol 5 mg in water for injection. pH 4.0–5.5; buffered with acetic acid-sodium acetate. Sealed under nitrogen.
Promethazine Hydrochloride Injection, USP	**Usual Dosage:** See Package Insert. **PROTECT FROM LIGHT:** Keep covered in carton until time of use.
25 mg/mL FOR DEEP INTRAMUSCULAR OR INTRAVENOUS USE 1 mL Single Dose Vials 25 Vials	**Store at room temperature** 20°–25°C (68°–77°F) [See USP Controlled Room Temperature]. Teva Pharmaceuticals USA Sellersville, PA 18960 Rev. A 11/2011 Y10765

A

NDC 0703-2201-04 Rx only	Each mL contains: Promethazine hydrochloride 50 mg, edetate disodium 0.1 mg, calcium chloride 0.04 mg, sodium metabisulfite 0.25 mg and phenol 5 mg in water for injection. pH 4.0–5.5; buffered with acetic acid-sodium acetate. Sealed under nitrogen.
Promethazine Hydrochloride Injection, USP	**Usual Dosage:** See Package Insert. **PROTECT FROM LIGHT:** Keep covered in carton until time of use.
50 mg/mL FOR DEEP INTRAMUSCULAR USE ONLY 1 mL Single Dose Vials 25 Vials	**Store at room temperature** 20°–25°C (68°–77°F) [See USP Controlled Room Temperature]. Teva Pharmaceuticals USA Sellersville, PA 18960 Rev. A 11/2011 Y10766

B

8. Order: promethazine 40 mg IM stat

   Give: _____ mL (Use label B.)

   Frequency: _____

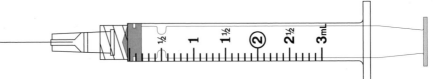

9. Order: **morphine sulfate 4 mg slow IV push q.4h p.r.n., severe pain**

   Give: _____ mL   Frequency: _____

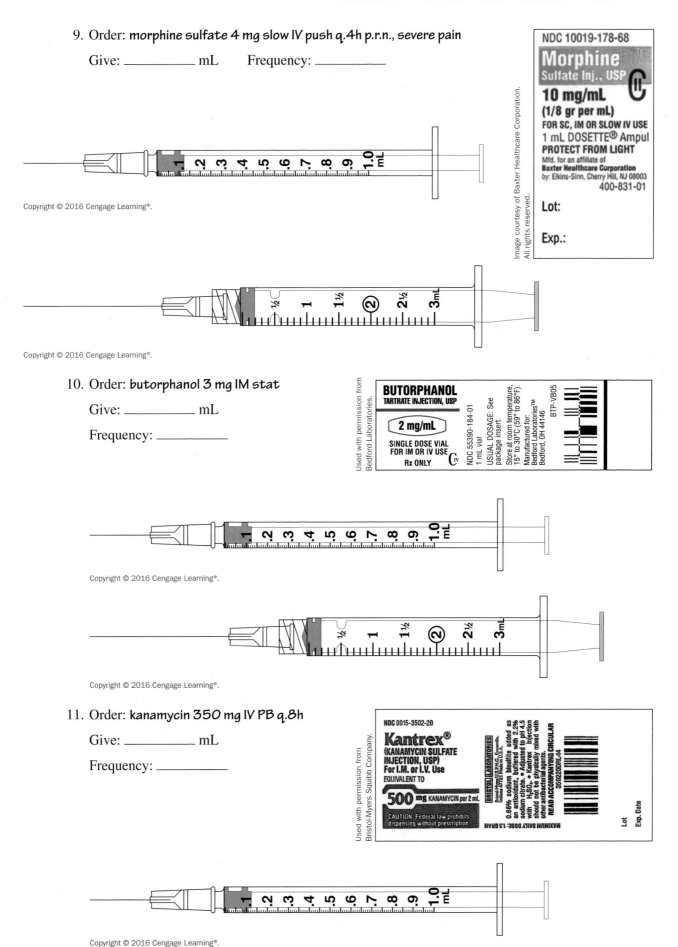

NDC 10019-178-68
Morphine
Sulfate Inj., USP
10 mg/mL
(1/8 gr per mL)
FOR SC, IM OR SLOW IV USE
1 mL DOSETTE® Ampul
PROTECT FROM LIGHT
Mfd. for an affiliate of
Baxter Healthcare Corporation
by: Elkins-Sinn, Cherry Hill, NJ 08003
400-831-01

Lot:

Exp.:

Copyright © 2016 Cengage Learning®.

Copyright © 2016 Cengage Learning®.

10. Order: **butorphanol 3 mg IM stat**

    Give: _____ mL

    Frequency: _____

BUTORPHANOL
TARTRATE INJECTION, USP

2 mg/mL

SINGLE DOSE VIAL
FOR IM OR IV USE

Rx ONLY   C ℞

NDC 55390-184-01
1 mL vial

USUAL DOSAGE: See
package insert.

Store at room temperature,
15° to 30°C (59° to 86°F).

Manufactured for:
Bedford Laboratories™
Bedford, OH 44146

BTP-VB05

Copyright © 2016 Cengage Learning®.

Copyright © 2016 Cengage Learning®.

11. Order: **kanamycin 350 mg IV PB q.8h**

    Give: _____ mL

    Frequency: _____

NDC 0015-3502-20
Kantrex®
(KANAMYCIN SULFATE
INJECTION, USP)
For I.M. or I.V. Use

BRISTOL LABORATORIES

EQUIVALENT TO

500 mg KANAMYCIN per 2 mL

CAUTION: Federal law prohibits
dispensing without prescription

0.66% sodium bisulfite added as
an antioxidant, buffered with 2.2%
sodium citrate. • Adjusted to pH 4.5
with H₂SO₄. • Kantrex Injection
should not be physically mixed with
other antibacterial agents.

READ ACCOMPANYING CIRCULAR

MAXIMUM DAILY DOSE: 1.5 GRAM

Lot

Exp. Date

Copyright © 2016 Cengage Learning®.

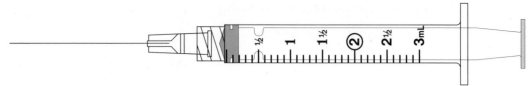

12. Order: *gentamicin 35 mg IM stat*

    Give: _____ mL

    Frequency: _____

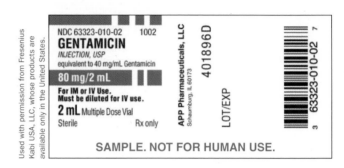

NDC 63323-010-02   1002

GENTAMICIN

INJECTION, USP

equivalent to 40 mg/mL Gentamicin

80 mg/2 mL

For IM or IV Use.
Must be diluted for IV use.

2 mL Multiple Dose Vial

Sterile   Rx only

APP Pharmaceuticals, LLC
Schaumburg, IL 60173

401896D

LOT/EXP

63323-010-02

SAMPLE. NOT FOR HUMAN USE.

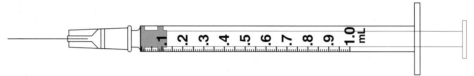

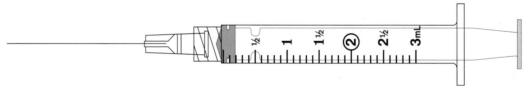

13. Order: *glycopyrrolate 200 mcg IV stat*

    Give: _____ mL

    Frequency: _____

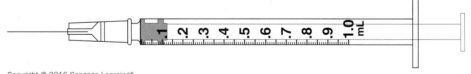

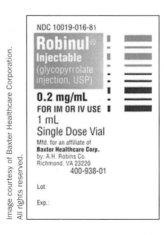

NDC 10019-016-81

Robinul®

Injectable

(glycopyrrolate
injection, USP)

0.2 mg/mL

FOR IM OR IV USE

1 mL

Single Dose Vial

Mfd. for an affiliate of
Baxter Healthcare Corp.
by: A.H. Robins Co.
Richmond, VA 23220

400-938-01

Lot:

Exp.:

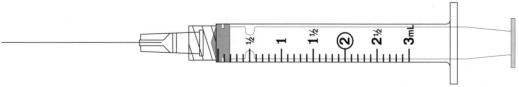

14. Order: *digoxin 0.125 mg IV q.AM*

Give: _____ mL

Frequency: _____

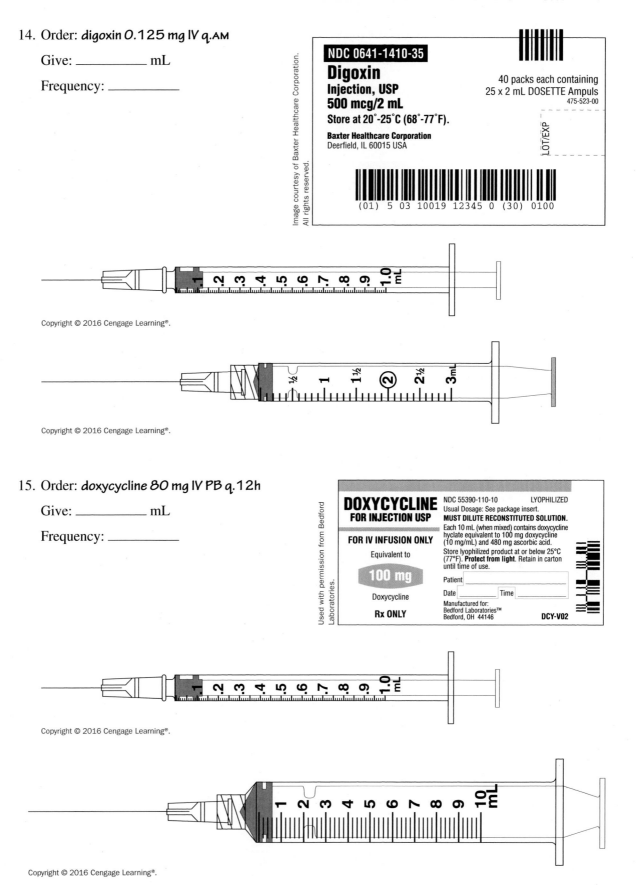

NDC 0641-1410-35

Digoxin
Injection, USP
500 mcg/2 mL
Store at 20°-25°C (68°-77°F).

Baxter Healthcare Corporation
Deerfield, IL 60015 USA

40 packs each containing
25 x 2 mL DOSETTE Ampuls
475-523-00

LOT/EXP

(01) 5 03 10019 12345 0 (30) 0100

Copyright © 2016 Cengage Learning®.

Copyright © 2016 Cengage Learning®.

15. Order: *doxycycline 80 mg IV PB q.12h*

Give: _____ mL

Frequency: _____

DOXYCYCLINE
FOR INJECTION USP

FOR IV INFUSION ONLY

Equivalent to

100 mg

Doxycycline

Rx ONLY

NDC 55390-110-10   LYOPHILIZED
Usual Dosage: See package insert.
MUST DILUTE RECONSTITUTED SOLUTION.
Each 10 mL (when mixed) contains doxycycline
hyclate equivalent to 100 mg doxycycline
(10 mg/mL) and 480 mg ascorbic acid.
Store lyophilized product at or below 25°C
(77°F). **Protect from light.** Retain in carton
until time of use.

Patient _____
Date _____ Time _____
Manufactured for:
Bedford Laboratories™
Bedford, OH 44146   **DCY-V02**

Copyright © 2016 Cengage Learning®.

Copyright © 2016 Cengage Learning®.

16. Order: **azithromycin 0.4 g IV PB q.12h**

   Give: _____ mL   Frequency: _____

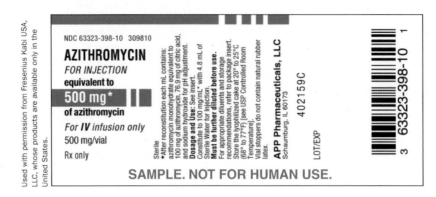

Copyright © 2016 Cengage Learning®.

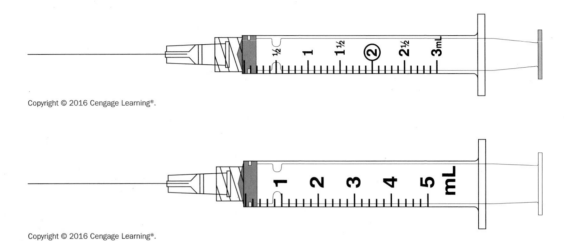

Copyright © 2016 Cengage Learning®.

17. Order: **phenytoin 50 mg IV push q.8h** (administer at the rate recommended on the label)

   Give: _____ mL at _____ mL/min, which equals _____ mL per 15 sec

   Frequency: _____

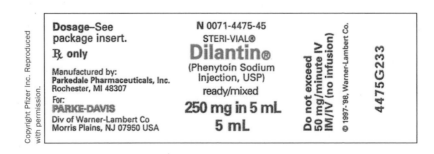

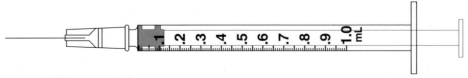

Copyright © 2016 Cengage Learning®.

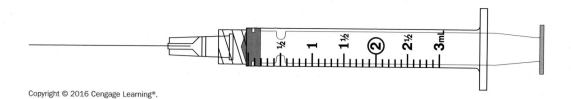

18. Order: **ranitidine 35 mg in 100 mL D$_5$W IV PB over 20 minutes q.6h**

    Add: _____ mL to the IV PB bag, and set the drip rate on the tubing to _____ gtt/min

    Frequency: _____

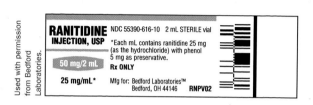

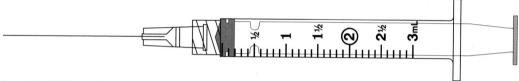

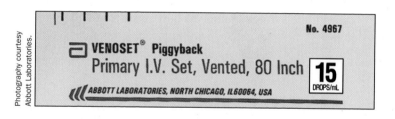

19. Order: **Novolin N NPH U-100 insulin 46 units c̄ Novolin R regular U-100 insulin 22 units subcut daily ā breakfast**

    You will give _____ units total. Frequency: _____

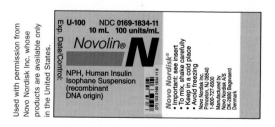

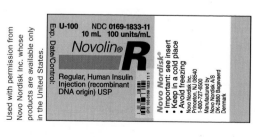

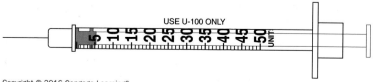

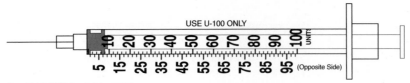

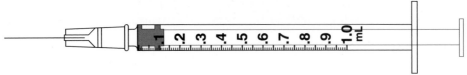

Refer to the following information to answer questions 20 through 24.

One of your assigned patients, Mrs. Betty Smedley, ID# 532729, with a history of osteoarthritis, is post-op following a total hip replacement. She received a bolus of morphine sulfate by the epidural route in the recovery room at 1000 hours and has medication orders for breakthrough pain and other comfort measures. Refer to the medication administration record (MAR) on page 13 to answer the questions regarding administration of medication to Mrs. Smedley.

20. At 2130, Mrs. Smedley complains of severe pain. How much ketorolac in the prefilled syringe will you give her now? Give _____ mL.

21. Mrs. Smedley is complaining of itching. What p.r.n. medication would you select, and how much will you administer? Select _____ and give _____ mL. Draw an arrow on the appropriate syringe to indicate how much you will give.

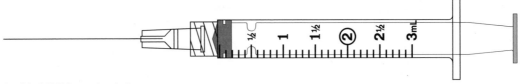

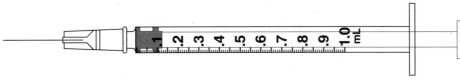

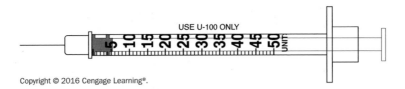

```
MEDICATION ADMINISTRATION RECORD                                    [_][□][x]
File  Edit  View  Window  Help
```

SMEDLEY, BETTY ID# 532729	┌ Schedule ───────────────────	┌ Start Time: ┐	┌ Stop Time: ┐
SSN = 100-02-5544	☑ Continuous ☑ On-Call	09/15 @ 0730 ▾	09/16 @ 0729 ▾
Height = 5'7", Weight = 154 lb	☑ PRN ☑ One-Time		
Location = MED SURG 217A			

Allergies: NO KNOWN ALLERGIES   ADRs: NO ADRS ON FILE

Active Medication	Dosage	Route	Admin Time	Last Action

KETOROLAC TROMETHAMINE INJ
  KETOROLAC TROMETHAMINE 60 MG/2 ML
  FOR BREAKTHROUGH PAIN X 1 DOSE
	60 MG X 1 DOSE	INTRAMUSCULAR	09/15 @ 1500	GIVEN

ACETAMINOPHEN TAB TYLENOL 325 MG	650 MG, PRN FOR TEMP GREATER THAN 101° F	ORAL	09/15 @ 2110	GIVEN

KETOROLAC TROMETHAMINE INJ
  KETOROLAC TROMETHAMINE 60 MG/2 ML
  FOR BREAKTHROUGH PAIN AFTER 60 MG
  DOSE
	30 MG, Q6H PRN	INTRAMUSCULAR		

DROPERIDOL INAPSINE 2.5 MG/ML	0.625 MG TO 1.25 MG, Q6H PRN NAUSEA	INTRAVENOUS		
DIPHENHYDRAMINE BENADRYL 50 MG/ML	35 MG, Q4H PRN, ITCHING	INTRAVENOUS		
NALOXONE NARCAN 0.4 MG/ML	0.4 MG, PRN FOR RR LESS THAN 8, AND IF PATIENT IS UNAROUSABLE	INTRAVENOUS		

Server Time: 9/15/xxxx 21:45

22. At 2400, Mrs. Smedley's respiratory rate (RR) is 7, and she is difficult to arouse. What medication is indicated? _____ Give _____ mL. Draw an arrow on the syringe to indicate how much of this medication you will give.

23. At 0215 on 09/15, Mrs. Smedley has a temperature of 39°C. Is Tylenol indicated? _____

    Explain: _____

    _____

24. How many tablets of Tylenol should she receive for each dose? _____ tablet(s)

Refer to the following information to answer questions 25 through 29.

Another one of your assigned patients, Mr. John Beck, ID# 768342, with a history of insulin-dependent diabetes, is admitted to the medical unit with asthma. Refer to the medication administration record (MAR) on page 16 and all labels provided to answer the questions regarding administration of medication to Mr. Beck.

25. Aminophylline is supplied in a solution strength of 25 mg/mL. How much aminophylline will you add to prepare the 50 mL piggyback bag? _____ mL

    Set the drip rate on the manually regulated IV tubing at _____ gtt/min.

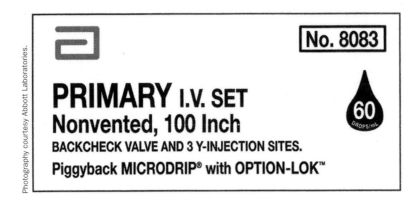

26. An infusion pump, calibrated in whole mL/h, becomes available, and you decide to use it for Mr. Beck's IV. To administer the aminophylline by infusion pump, set the pump at _____ mL/h.

27. Reconstitute the methylprednisolone with _____ mL diluent, and give _____ mL.

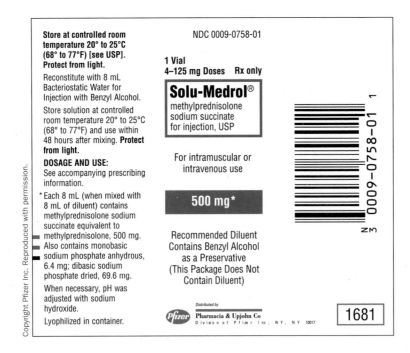

28. Mealtimes are 8 AM, 1 PM, and 6 PM. Using international time, give _____ tablet(s) of sucralfate per dose each day at _____, _____, and _____ hours.

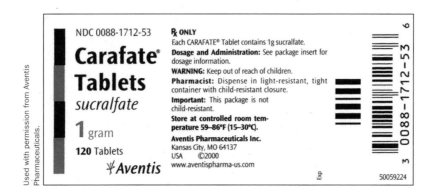

29. At 0730, Mr. Beck's blood sugar is 360. You will give him _____ units of insulin by the _____ route. Draw an arrow on the appropriate syringe to indicate the correct dosage.

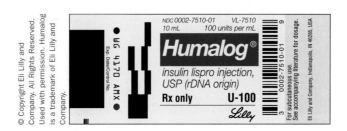

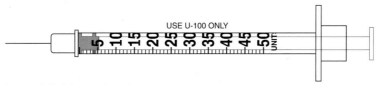

Copyright © 2016 Cengage Learning®.

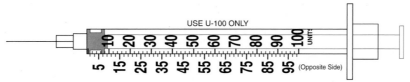

Copyright © 2016 Cengage Learning®.

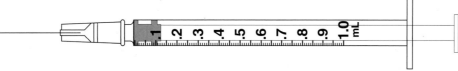

Copyright © 2016 Cengage Learning®.

PAGE __1__ of __1__

MEDICATION ADMINISTRATION RECORD

ORIGINAL ORDER DATE	DATE STARTED / RENEWED	MEDICATION - DOSAGE	ROUTE	SCHEDULE 11-7	SCHEDULE 7-3	SCHEDULE 3-11	DATE 3/10/xx 11-7	DATE 3/10/xx 7-3	DATE 3/10/xx 3-11	DATE 3/11/xx 11-7	DATE 3/11/xx 7-3	DATE 3/11/xx 3-11	DATE 3/12/xx 11-7	DATE 3/12/xx 7-3	DATE 3/12/xx 3-11	DATE 3/13/xx 11-7	DATE 3/13/xx 7-3	DATE 3/13/xx 3-11
3-10-xx	3-10	aminophylline 100 mg in 50 mL D₅W x 30 min q.6h	IV PB	12 6	12	6		GP 12	MS 6	JJ12 JJ6								
3-10-xx	3-10	methylprednisolone 125 mg q.6h	IV	12 6	12	6		GP 12	MS 6	JJ12 JJ6								
3-10-xx	3-10	sucralfate 1 g 60 min ac	PO		7 12	5		GP7 GP12	MS5									
3-10-xx	3-10	Humalog U-100 insulin 30 min ac	Sub-cut		7:30 11:30	5:30		GP7:30 GP11:30	MS5:30									
		per sliding scale: Blood sugar Units																
		0-150 0 units																
		151-250 8 units																
		251-350 13 units																
		351-400 18 units																
		greater than 400 Call M.D.																

INJECTION SITES

B - RIGHT ARM	D - RIGHT ANTERIOR THIGH	H - LEFT ABDOMEN	L - LEFT BUTTOCKS
C - RIGHT ABDOMEN	G - LEFT ARM	J - LEFT ANTERIOR THIGH	M - RIGHT BUTTOCKS

DATE GIVEN	TIME	INT.	ONE - TIME MEDICATION - DOSAGE	RT.	11-7	7-3	3-11	11-7	7-3	3-11	11-7	7-3	3-11	11-7	7-3	3-11
					SCHEDULE			DATE			DATE			DATE		

SIGNATURE OF NURSE ADMINISTERING MEDICATIONS

- 11-7 JJJ. Jones, LPN
- 7-3   GP G.Pickar, RN
- 3-11 MS M.Smith, RN

DATE GIVEN	TIME	INT.	MEDICATION-DOSAGE-CONT.	RT.

RECOPIED BY:

CHECKED BY:

Beck, John
ID #768342

ALLERGIES:
None Known

Refer to the following information to answer questions 30 through 32.

You are working in the health department pediatric clinic. Your first patient, Jimmy Bryan, a 22 lb child, is brought to the clinic by his mother and diagnosed with otitis media, an ear infection. Answer the following questions to determine the safe dosage, and administer the correct dose amount.

30. The nurse practitioner orders **amoxicillin 100 mg p.o. q.8h** for Jimmy. To reconstitute the amoxicillin, add _____ mL water.

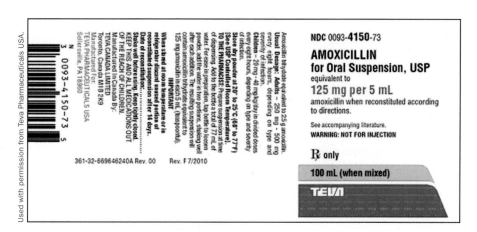

31. Is Jimmy's amoxicillin order safe and reasonable? _____ Explain: _____

_____

32. The nurse practitioner asks you to give Jimmy 1 dose of the amoxicillin stat. You will give Jimmy _____ mL.

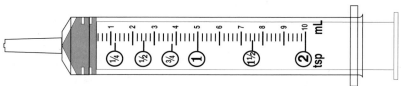

Copyright © 2016 Cengage Learning®.

Refer to the following information to answer questions 33 and 34.

Your next patient, Marcus Williams, is a 4-year-old, 40 lb preschooler being treated for an upper respiratory infection. The nurse practitioner prescribes **amoxicillin clavulanate 240 mg p.o. q.8h** based on the amoxicillin dose of the combination medication. (The supply on hand is shown on the next page.)

33. According to a drug reference, the recommended dosage of amoxicillin is 40 mg/kg/day in divided doses q.8h. Will the ordered dosage provide the recommended dosage for Marcus? _____
Explain: _____

34. If the order is the correct recommended dosage, how much would you administer for 1 dose?

Give: _____ mL

If it is not the recommended dose, what would you do next?

_____

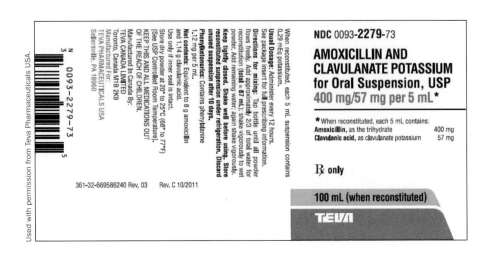

Refer to the following information to answer questions 35 through 37.

Your third patient seen at the pediatric clinic is Alexandra Martin, a 6-year-old, 62 lb school-age child with a fever of 39.6°C. The nurse practitioner orders **acetaminophen 300 mg p.o. stat.** For hyperthermia in children, the recommended dosage of acetaminophen is 10 to 15 mg/kg p.o. q.4h, not to exceed 5 doses per day.

35. Alexandra's mother is not familiar with Celsius measurements and asks what the temperature is in Fahrenheit. What will you tell her? _____ °F

36. What is the safe single dosage range of acetaminophen for Alexandra? _____ mg/dose to _____ mg/dose

37. Acetaminophen is available in the clinic supply as a suspension of 80 mg per 2.5 mL. How many mL will you administer for this dose? _____ mL

Refer to the following information to answer questions 38 through 41.

Your patient, Jill Jones, a 16-year-old, 110 lb adolescent, is admitted to the medical unit. She has a history of a duodenal ulcer, and her current problem is abdominal pain. Answer the following questions regarding a safe ordered dose of IV medication, infusion rate, and intake and output.

38. The physician orders **cimetidine 250 mg IV q.6h.** According to a drug reference, the recommended dosage range of cimetidine is 20 to 30 mg/kg/day in 4 divided doses. What is the recommended single dosage range for Jill? _____ mg/dose to _____ mg/dose. Will the order provide the recommended dosage? _____

39. The pharmacy has supplied a vial of cimetidine 300 mg per 2 mL and a D_5W 50 mL IV PB bag, with instructions to infuse over 20 min. Add _____ mL of cimetidine to the IV PB bag, and set the manual drip rate at _____ gtt/min.

CLEARLINK System   **2C8541s**

CONTINU-FLO Solution Set with DUO-VENT Spike
105" (2.7 m)
3 Luer Activated Valves
Male Luer Lock Adapter

10
10 drops/mL
Approx.

40. Jill is on strict intake and output measurements. Calculate the 8-hour total fluid intake for documentation in the metric system.

Time	Oral Intake	Time	IV Intake
0800	Gelatin 4 fl oz, Water 3 fl oz	0800	50 mL
1000	Water 3 fl oz		
1300	Apple juice 16 fl oz		
		1400	50 mL

What is her total fluid intake for the 8-hour shift? _____ mL

41. The following day the physician orders **washed, packed red blood cells 2 units (600 mL) IV to infuse in 4 hours.** The manually regulated IV tubing has a drop factor of 10 gtt/mL. You will set the IV drip rate to _____ gtt/min.

Refer to the following information to answer questions 42 through 49.

Mr. Ralph Callahan, a 52-year-old man, has just returned to the surgical unit, following abdominal surgery, with a patient-controlled analgesic (PCA) pump started at 1430. The medication cartridge in the pump contains morphine sulfate 50 mg per 50 mL, set for patient administration at **1 mg q.10 min p.r.n.**

42. Mr. Callahan may self-administer _____ mL every 10 minutes.

43. If he attempts and receives 5 doses this hour, he would receive a total of _____ mg per _____ mL of morphine.

44. Based on the amount of morphine in the syringe in the PCA pump, how many total doses can Mr. Callahan receive? _____ dose(s)

45. If he receives 5 doses every hour, at what time would he finish receiving his morphine dosage? _____ hours or _____ in traditional AM/PM time.

46. Post-op orders for Mr. Callahan include **ceftriaxone 0.5 g IV q.8h.**

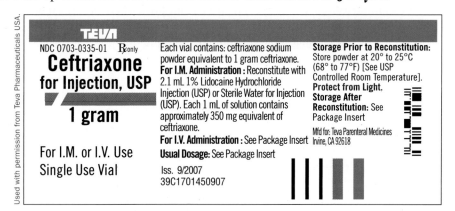

The supplied medication needs to be reconstituted prior to use. Administration instructions include:

Intravenous Administration

Ceftriaxone for injection, USP should be administered intravenously by infusion over a period of 30 minutes. Concentrations between 10 mg/mL and 40 mg/mL are recommended; however, lower concentrations may be used if desired. Reconstitute vials with an appropriate IV diluent (see **COMPATIBILITY AND STABILITY**).

Vial Dosage Size	Amount of Diluent to be Added
250 mg	2.4 mL
500 mg	4.8 mL
1 g	9.6 mL
2 g	19.2 mL

After reconstitution, each 1 mL of solution contains approximately 100 mg equivalent of ceftriaxone. Withdraw entire contents and dilute to the desired concentration with the appropriate IV diluent.

The total volume of the ceftriaxone after reconstitution is _____ mL.

47. The resulting dosage strength of ceftriaxone is _____ mg per _____ mL.

48. Give _____ mL of ceftriaxone.

49. You reconstituted the drug at 1500 on 1/30/xx. The package insert for ceftriaxone states: "Reconstituted solution is stable at room temperature for 24 hours and refrigerated for 3 days." Prepare a reconstitution label for the ceftriaxone.

50. Describe the clinical reasoning you would use to prevent this medication error.

Possible Scenario

Order: *dexamethasone 4 mg IV q.6h*

Day 1 Supply: dexamethasone 4 mg/mL

Student nurse prepared and administered 1 mL.

Day 2 Supply: dexamethasone 10 mg/mL

Student nurse prepared 1 mL.

Potential Outcome

On Day 2, the student's instructor asked the student to recheck the order, think about the action, check the calculation, and provide the rationale for the amount prepared. The student was alarmed at the possibility of administering two-and-a-half times the prescribed dosage. The student insisted that the pharmacy should consistently supply the same unit dosage. The instructor advised the student of the possibility that different pharmacy technicians could be involved or possibly the original supply dosage was not available.

Prevention

_____

_____

After completing these problems, see pages 627–634 to check your answers. Give yourself 2 points for each correct question.

Perfect score = 100   My score = _____

Minimum mastery score = 90 (45 correct)

Essential Skills Evaluation: Pretest Answer Sheet

1. Give: _____ tablet(s)   Frequency: _____

2. Give: _____ tablet(s)   Frequency: _____

3. Choose: _____ mg capsules   Give: _____ capsule(s)   Frequency: _____

4. Give: _____ tablet(s)   Frequency: _____

5. Give: _____ tablet(s)   Frequency: _____

6. Give: _____ mL   Frequency: _____

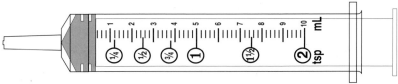

7. Give: _____ mL   Frequency: _____

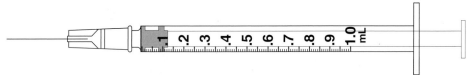

8. Give: _____ mL   Frequency: _____

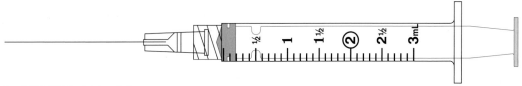

9. Give: _____ mL   Frequency: _____

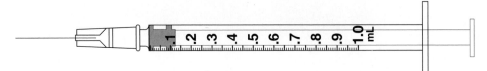

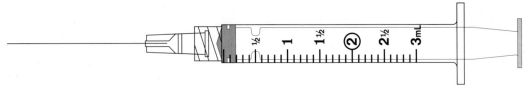

10. Give: _____ mL   Frequency: _____

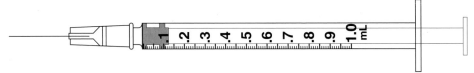

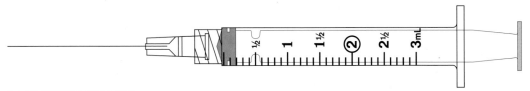

11. Give: _____ mL   Frequency: _____

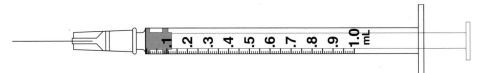

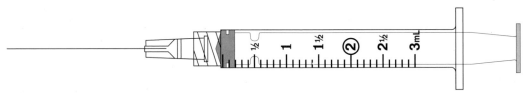

12. Give: _____ mL   Frequency: _____

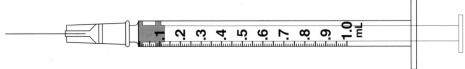

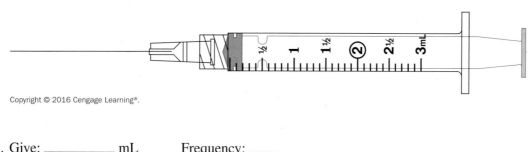

13. Give: _____ mL　　　Frequency: _____

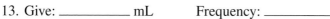

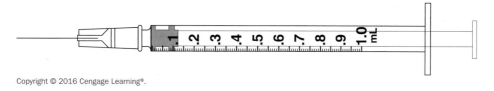

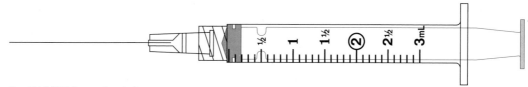

14. Give: _____ mL　　　Frequency: _____

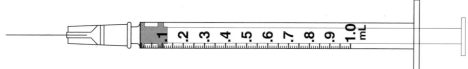

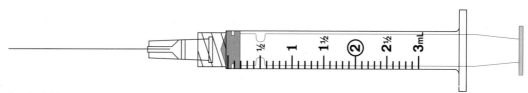

15. Give: _____ mL　　　Frequency: _____

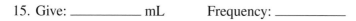

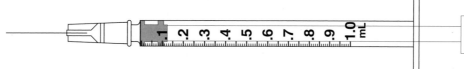

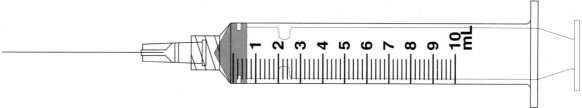

16. Give: _____ mL   Frequency: _____

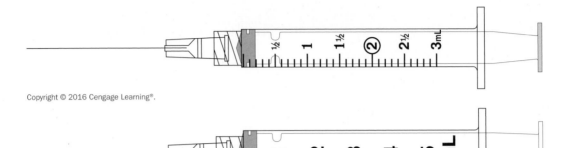

17. Give: _____ mL at _____ mL/min, which equals _____ mL per 15 sec

    Frequency: _____

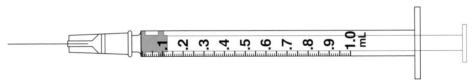

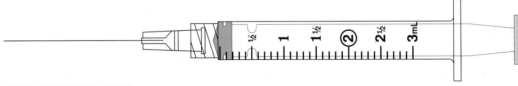

18. Add: _____ mL to the IV PB bag, and set the drip rate on the tubing to _____ gtt/min

    Frequency: _____

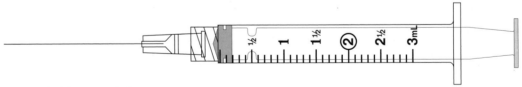

19. You will give _____ units total.   Frequency: _____

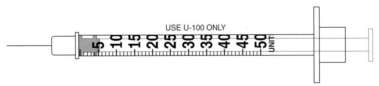

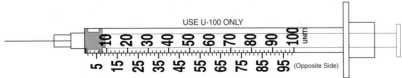

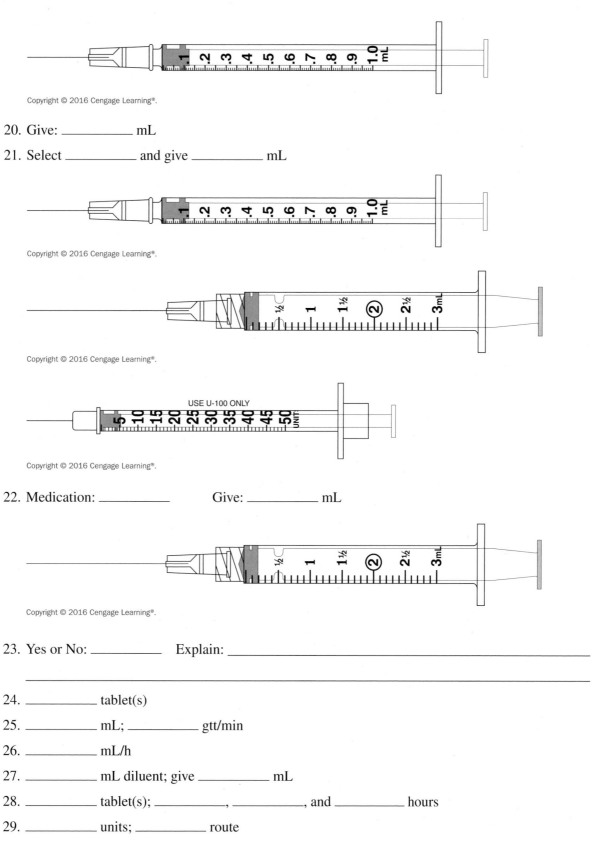

20. Give: _____ mL

21. Select _____ and give _____ mL

22. Medication: _____   Give: _____ mL

23. Yes or No: _____   Explain: _____

_____

24. _____ tablet(s)

25. _____ mL; _____ gtt/min

26. _____ mL/h

27. _____ mL diluent; give _____ mL

28. _____ tablet(s); _____, _____, and _____ hours

29. _____ units; _____ route

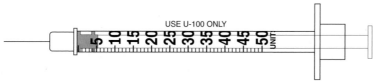

USE U-100 ONLY

10 20 30 40 50 60 70 80 90 100 UNITS

5 15 25 35 45 55 65 75 85 95 (Opposite Side)

.1 .2 .3 .4 .5 .6 .7 .8 .9 1.0 mL

30. _____ mL

31. Yes or No: _____   Explain: _____

_____

32. _____ mL

33. Yes or No: _____   Explain: _____

_____

34. _____ mL   Next action: _____

35. _____ °F

36. _____ mg/dose to _____ mg/dose

37. _____ mL

38. _____ mg/dose to _____ mg/dose; Yes or No: _____

39. _____ mL; _____ gtt/min

40. _____ mL

41. _____ gtt/min

42. _____ mL

43. _____ mg; _____ mL

44. _____ dose(s)

45. _____ hours; _____ (AM/PM)

46. _____ mL

47. _____ mg per _____ mL

48. _____ mL

49.

50. **Prevention:** _____

_____

After completing these problems, see pages 627–634 to check your answers. Give yourself 2 points for each correct answer.

Perfect score = 100   My score = _____

Minimum mastery score = 90 (45 correct)

MATHEMATICS DIAGNOSTIC EVALUATION

As a prerequisite objective, *Dosage Calculations* takes into account that you can add, subtract, multiply, and divide whole numbers. You should have a working knowledge of fractions, decimals, ratios, percents, and basic problem solving as well. This text reviews these important mathematical operations, which support all dosage calculations in health care.

Set aside $1\frac{1}{2}$ hours in a quiet place to complete the 50 items in the following diagnostic evaluation. You will need scratch paper and a pencil to work the problems.

Use your results to determine your computational strengths and weaknesses to guide your review. A minimum score of 86 is recommended as an indicator of readiness for dosage calculations. If you achieve that score, you may proceed to Chapter 3. However, note any problems that you answered incorrectly, and use the related review materials in Chapters 1 and 2 to refresh your skills.

This mathematics diagnostic evaluation and the review that follows are provided to enhance your confidence and proficiency in arithmetic skills, thereby helping you to avoid careless mistakes when you perform dosage calculations.

Good luck!

Directions

1. Carry answers to three decimal places and round to two places.

   (Examples: 5.175 = 5.18; 5.174 = 5.17)

2. Express fractions in lowest terms.

   (Example: $\frac{6}{10} = \frac{3}{5}$)

Mathematics Diagnostic Evaluation

1. $1{,}517 + 0.63 =$ _____

2. Express the value of $0.7 + 0.035 + 20.006$ rounded to two decimal places. _____

3. $9.5 + 17.06 + 32 + 41.11 + 0.99 =$ _____

4. $\$19.69 + \$304.03 =$ _____

5. $93.2 - 47.09 =$ _____

6. $1{,}005 - 250.5 =$ _____

7. Express the value of $17.156 - 0.25$ rounded to two decimal places. _____

8. $509 \times 38.3 =$ _____

9. $\$4.12 \times 42 =$ _____

10. $17.16 \times 23.5 =$ _____

11. $972 \div 27 =$ _____

12. $2.5 \div 0.001 =$ _____

13. Express the value of $\frac{1}{4} \div \frac{3}{8}$ as a fraction reduced to lowest terms. _____

14. Express $\frac{1{,}500}{240}$ as a decimal. _____

15. Express 0.8 as a fraction. _____

16. Express $\frac{2}{5}$ as a percent. _____

17. Express 0.004 as a percent.

18. Express 5% as a decimal.

19. Express $33\frac{1}{3}\%$ as a ratio in lowest terms.

20. Express 1:50 as a decimal.

21. $\frac{1}{2} + \frac{3}{4} =$

22. $1\frac{2}{3} + 4\frac{7}{8} =$

23. $1\frac{5}{6} - \frac{2}{9} =$

24. Express the value of $\frac{1}{100} \times 60$ as a fraction.

25. Express the value of $4\frac{1}{4} \times 3\frac{1}{2}$ as a mixed number.

26. Identify the fraction with the greatest value: $\frac{1}{150}, \frac{1}{200}, \frac{1}{100}.$

27. Identify the decimal with the least value: 0.009, 0.19, 0.9.

28. $\frac{6.4}{0.02} =$

29. $\frac{0.02 + 0.16}{0.4 - 0.34} =$

30. Express the value of $\frac{3}{12 + 3} \times 0.25$ as a decimal.

31. 8% of 50 =

32. $\frac{1}{2}\%$ of 18 =

33. 0.9% of 24 =

For questions 34 through 40, find the value of X. Express your answer as a decimal.

34. $\frac{1:1,000}{1:100} \times 250 = X$

35. $\frac{300}{150} \times 2 = X$

36. $\frac{2.5}{5} \times 1.5 = X$

37. $\frac{1,000,000}{250,000} \times X = 12$

38. $\frac{0.51}{1.7} \times X = 150$

39. $X = (82.4 - 52)\frac{3}{5}$

40. $\dfrac{\frac{1}{150}}{\frac{1}{300}} \times 1.2 = X$

41. Express 2:10 as a fraction in lowest terms.

42. Express 2% as a ratio in lowest terms.

43. If five equal medication containers contain a total of 25 tablets, how many tablets are in each container?

44. A person is receiving 0.5 milligrams of a medication four times a day. What is the total amount of milligrams of this medication received each day?

45. If 1 kilogram equals 2.2 pounds, how many kilograms does a 66 pound child weigh?

46. If 1 kilogram equals 2.2 pounds, how many pounds are in 1.5 kilograms? (Express your answer as a decimal.)

47. If 1 centimeter equals $\frac{3}{8}$ inch, how many centimeters are in $2\frac{1}{2}$ inches? (Express your answer as a decimal.)   _____

48. If 2.5 centimeters equal 1 inch, how long in centimeters is a 3-inch wound?   _____

49. This diagnostic test has a total of 50 problems. If you incorrectly answer 5 problems, what percentage will you have answered correctly?   _____

50. For every 5 female student nurses in a nursing class, there is 1 male student nurse. What is the ratio of female to male student nurses?   _____

After completing these problems, see pages 634–635 to check your answers. Give yourself 2 points for each correct answer.

Perfect score = 100   My score = _____

Minimum readiness score = 86 (43 correct)

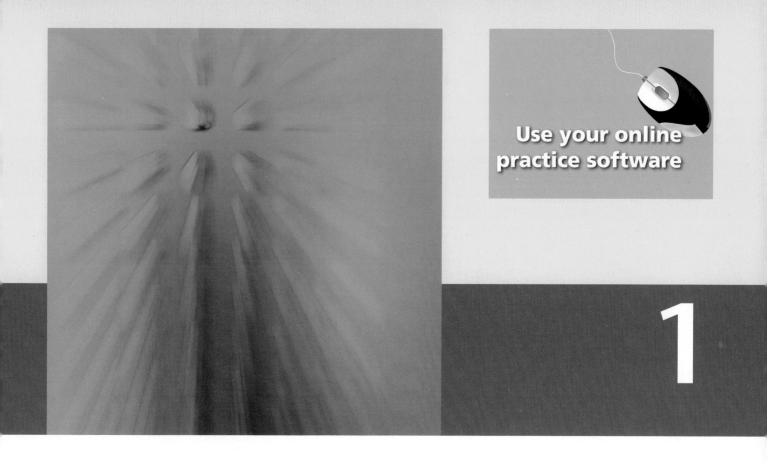

Fractions and Decimals

OBJECTIVES

Upon mastery of Chapter 1, you will be able to perform basic mathematical computations essential for clinical calculations that involve fractions and decimals. Specifically, you will be able to:

- Compare the values of fractions and decimals.
- Convert between mixed numbers and improper fractions, and between reduced and equivalent forms of fractions.
- Add, subtract, multiply, and divide fractions and decimals.
- Round a decimal to a given place value.
- Read and write out the values of decimal numbers.

Health care professionals need to understand fractions and decimals to be able to interpret and act on medical orders, read prescriptions, and understand patient records and information in health care literature. The most common system of measurement used in prescription, dosage calculation, and administration of medications is the metric system. The metric system is international, and it is the most precise system of measurement. Metric measure is based on decimals. Occasionally, you will see fractions used in apothecary and household measures in dosage calculations. The method of solving dosage problems in this book relies on expressing relationships in fractional form. Therefore, proficiency with fractions and decimals will add to your success with a variety of medical applications.

FRACTIONS

A *fraction* indicates a portion of a whole number. There are two types of fractions: *common fractions,* such as $\frac{1}{2}$ (usually referred to simply as *fractions*) and *decimal fractions,* such as 0.5 (usually referred to simply as *decimals*).

A fraction is an expression of division, with one number placed over another number $\left(\frac{1}{4}, \frac{2}{3}, \frac{4}{5}\right)$. The bottom number, or *denominator,* indicates the total number of equal-sized parts into which the whole is divided. The top number, or *numerator,* indicates how many of those parts are considered. The fraction may also be read as *the numerator divided by the denominator.*

EXAMPLE ■

$\frac{1}{4}$ numerator
      denominator

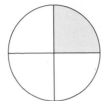

The whole is divided into four equal parts (denominator), and one part (numerator) is considered.

Copyright © 2016 Cengage Learning®.

$\frac{1}{4} = 1$ part of 4 parts, or $\frac{1}{4}$ of the whole.

The fraction $\frac{1}{4}$ may also be read as *1 divided by 4.*

MATH TIP
The *d*enominator begins with *d* and is *d*own below the line in a fraction.

Types of Fractions

There are four types of fractions: proper, improper, mixed numbers, and complex.

Proper Fractions

Proper fractions are fractions in which the value of the numerator is less than the value of the denominator. The value of the proper fraction is less than 1.

RULE
Whenever the numerator is less than the denominator, the value of the fraction must be less than 1.

EXAMPLE ■

$\frac{5}{8}$ is less than 1.

Improper Fractions

Improper fractions are fractions in which the value of the numerator is greater than or equal to the value of the denominator. The value of the improper fraction is greater than or equal to 1.

RULE
Whenever the numerator is greater than the denominator, the value of the fraction must be greater than 1.

EXAMPLE ▪

$\frac{8}{5}$ is greater than 1.

RULE

Whenever the numerator and denominator are equal, the value of the improper fraction is always equal to 1; a nonzero number divided by itself is equal to 1.

EXAMPLE ▪

$\frac{5}{5} = 1$

Mixed Numbers

When a whole number and a proper fraction are combined, the result is referred to as a *mixed number*. The value of the mixed number is always greater than 1.

EXAMPLE ▪

$1\frac{5}{8} = 1 + \frac{5}{8}$ $1\frac{5}{8}$ is greater than 1.

Complex Fractions

Complex fractions include fractions in which the numerator, the denominator, or both contain a fraction, decimal, or mixed number. The value may be less than, greater than, or equal to 1.

EXAMPLES ▪

$\dfrac{\frac{5}{8}}{\frac{1}{2}}$ is greater than 1. $\dfrac{\frac{5}{8}}{2}$ is less than 1. $\dfrac{1\frac{5}{8}}{\frac{1}{5}}$ is greater than 1. $\dfrac{\frac{1}{2}}{\frac{2}{4}} = 1$

To perform dosage calculations that involve fractions, you must be able to convert among these different types of fractions and reduce them to lowest terms. You must also be able to add, subtract, multiply, and divide fractions. Review these simple rules of working with fractions. Continue to practice until the concepts are crystal clear and automatic.

Equivalent Fractions

The value of a fraction can be expressed in several ways. This is called *finding an equivalent fraction*. In finding an equivalent fraction, both terms of the fraction (numerator and denominator) are either multiplied or divided by the same nonzero number.

MATH TIP

In an equivalent fraction, the form of the fraction is changed, but the value of the fraction remains the same.

EXAMPLES ▪

$\frac{2}{4} = \frac{2 \div 2}{4 \div 2} = \frac{1}{2}$ $\frac{1}{3} = \frac{1 \times 3}{3 \times 3} = \frac{3}{9}$

Reducing Fractions to Lowest Terms

When calculating dosages, it is usually easier to work with fractions using the smallest possible numbers. Finding these equivalent fractions is called *reducing the fraction to the lowest terms* or *simplifying the fraction.*

RULE
To reduce a fraction to lowest terms, divide both the numerator and denominator by the largest nonzero whole number that will go evenly into both the numerator and the denominator.

EXAMPLE ▪

Reduce $\frac{6}{12}$ to lowest terms.

6 is the largest number that will divide evenly into both 6 (numerator) and 12 (denominator).

$\frac{6}{12} = \frac{6 \div 6}{12 \div 6} = \frac{1}{2}$ in lowest terms

Sometimes this reduction can be done in several steps. Always check a fraction to see if it can be reduced further.

EXAMPLE ▪

$\frac{5,000}{20,000} = \frac{5,000 \div 1,000}{20,000 \div 1,000} = \frac{5}{20}$ (not in lowest terms)

$\frac{5}{20} = \frac{5 \div 5}{20 \div 5} = \frac{1}{4}$ (in lowest terms)

MATH TIP
If neither the numerator nor the denominator can be divided evenly by a nonzero number other than 1, then the fraction is already in lowest terms.

Enlarging Fractions

RULE
To find an equivalent fraction in which both terms are larger, multiply both the numerator and the denominator by the same nonzero number.

EXAMPLE ▪

Enlarge $\frac{3}{5}$ to the equivalent fraction in tenths.

$\frac{3}{5} = \frac{3 \times 2}{5 \times 2} = \frac{6}{10}$

Conversion

It is important to be able to convert among different types of fractions. Conversion allows you to perform various calculations with greater ease and permits you to express answers in simplest terms.

Converting Mixed Numbers to Improper Fractions

RULE
To change or convert a mixed number to an improper fraction with the same denominator, multiply the whole number by the denominator and add the numerator. This value becomes the numerator, while the denominator remains the same as it was in the fraction of the initial mixed number.

EXAMPLE ▪

$$2\frac{5}{8} = \frac{(2 \times 8) + 5}{8} = \frac{16 + 5}{8} = \frac{21}{8}$$

Converting Improper Fractions to Mixed Numbers

RULE
To change or convert an improper fraction to an equivalent mixed number or whole number, divide the numerator by the denominator. Any remainder becomes the numerator of a proper fraction that should be reduced to lowest terms.

EXAMPLES ▪

$$\frac{8}{5} = 8 \div 5 = 1\frac{3}{5}$$

$$\frac{10}{4} = 10 \div 4 = 2\frac{2}{4} = 2\frac{1}{2}$$

Comparing Fractions

In calculating some drug dosages, it is helpful to know when the value of one fraction is greater or less than another. The relative sizes of fractions can be determined by comparing the numerators when the denominators are the same or comparing the denominators if the numerators are the same.

RULE
If the denominators are the same, the fraction with the smaller numerator has the lesser value.

EXAMPLE ▪

Compare $\frac{2}{5}$ and $\frac{3}{5}$.

Denominators are both 5.

Numerators: 2 is less than 3.

$\frac{2}{5}$ has a lesser value.

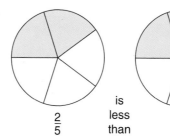

$\frac{2}{5}$ is less than $\frac{3}{5}$

RULE
If the numerators are the same, the fraction with the smaller denominator has the greater value.

EXAMPLE ▪

Compare $\frac{1}{2}$ and $\frac{1}{4}$.

Numerators are both 1.

Denominators: 2 is less than 4.

$\frac{1}{2}$ has a greater value.

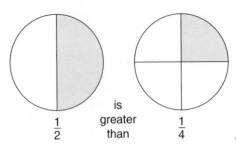

$\frac{1}{2}$ is greater than $\frac{1}{4}$

Note: A smaller denominator means the whole has been divided into fewer pieces, so each piece is larger.

QUICK REVIEW

- Proper fraction: numerator is less than denominator; value is less than 1. Example: $\frac{1}{2}$

- Improper fraction: numerator is greater than denominator; value is greater than 1.

   Example: $\frac{4}{3}$

   Or numerator = denominator; value = 1. Example: $\frac{5}{5}$

- Mixed number: whole number + a fraction; value is greater than 1. Example: $1\frac{1}{2}$

- Complex fraction: numerator and/or denominator are composed of a fraction, decimal, or mixed number; value is less than, greater than, or equal to 1.

   Example: $\dfrac{\frac{1}{2}}{\frac{1}{50}}$

- Any nonzero number divided by itself = 1. Example: $\frac{3}{3} = 1$

- To reduce a fraction to lowest terms, divide both terms by the largest nonzero whole number that will divide both the numerator and denominator evenly. Value remains the same.

   Example: $\frac{6}{10} = \frac{6 \div 2}{10 \div 2} = \frac{3}{5}$

- To enlarge a fraction, multiply both terms by the same nonzero number. Value remains the same.

   Example: $\frac{1}{12} = \frac{1 \times 2}{12 \times 2} = \frac{2}{24}$

- To convert a mixed number to an improper fraction, multiply the whole number by the denominator and add the numerator; use the original denominator in the fractional part.

   Example: $1\frac{1}{3} = \frac{(1 \times 3) + 1}{3} = \frac{3 + 1}{3} = \frac{4}{3}$

- To convert an improper fraction to a mixed number, divide the numerator by the denominator. Express any remainder as the numerator of a proper fraction reduced to lowest terms.

   Example: $\frac{21}{9} = 21 \div 9 = 2\frac{3}{9} = 2\frac{1}{3}$

- When numerators are equal, the fraction with the smaller denominator is greater.

   Example: $\frac{1}{2}$ is greater than $\frac{1}{3}$

- When denominators are equal, the fraction with the larger numerator is greater.

   Example: $\frac{2}{3}$ is greater than $\frac{1}{3}$

Review Set 1

1. Circle the *improper* fraction(s).

$$\frac{2}{3} \qquad 1\frac{3}{4} \qquad \frac{6}{6} \qquad \frac{7}{5} \qquad \frac{16}{17} \qquad \frac{\frac{1}{9}}{\frac{2}{3}}$$

2. Circle the *complex* fraction(s).

$$\frac{4}{5} \qquad 3\frac{7}{8} \qquad \frac{2}{2} \qquad \frac{9}{8} \qquad \frac{8}{9} \qquad \frac{\frac{1}{100}}{\frac{1}{150}}$$

3. Circle the *proper* fraction(s).

$$\frac{1}{4} \qquad \frac{1}{14} \qquad \frac{14}{1} \qquad \frac{14}{14} \qquad \frac{144}{14}$$

4. Circle the *mixed* number(s) *reduced to the lowest terms.*

$$3\frac{4}{8} \qquad \frac{2}{3} \qquad 1\frac{2}{9} \qquad \frac{1}{3} \qquad 1\frac{1}{4} \qquad 5\frac{7}{8}$$

5. Circle the pair(s) of *equivalent* fractions.

$$\frac{3}{4} = \frac{6}{8} \qquad \frac{1}{5} = \frac{2}{10} \qquad \frac{3}{9} = \frac{1}{3} \qquad \frac{3}{4} = \frac{4}{3} \qquad 1\frac{4}{9} = 1\frac{2}{3}$$

Change the following mixed numbers to improper fractions.

6. $6\frac{1}{2} =$ _____   9. $7\frac{5}{6} =$ _____

7. $1\frac{1}{5} =$ _____   10. $102\frac{3}{4} =$ _____

8. $10\frac{2}{3} =$ _____

Change the following improper fractions to whole numbers or mixed numbers; reduce to lowest terms.

11. $\frac{24}{12} =$ _____   14. $\frac{100}{75} =$ _____

12. $\frac{8}{8} =$ _____   15. $\frac{44}{16} =$ _____

13. $\frac{30}{9} =$ _____

Enlarge the following fractions to the number of parts indicated.

16. $\frac{3}{4}$ to eighths   _____   19. $\frac{2}{5}$ to tenths   _____

17. $\frac{1}{4}$ to sixteenths   _____   20. $\frac{2}{3}$ to ninths   _____

18. $\frac{2}{3}$ to twelfths   _____

Circle the correct answer.

21. Which is larger? $\frac{1}{150}$ or $\frac{1}{100}$

22. Which is smaller? $\frac{1}{1,000}$ or $\frac{1}{10,000}$

23. Which is larger? $\frac{2}{9}$ or $\frac{5}{9}$

24. Which is smaller? $\frac{3}{10}$ or $\frac{5}{10}$

25. A patient is supposed to drink a bottle containing 10 fluid ounces of magnesium citrate prior to his X-ray study. He has been able to drink 6 fluid ounces. What portion of the liquid remains? (Express your answer as a fraction reduced to lowest terms.) _____

26. If 1 medicine bottle contains 12 doses, how many full and fractional bottles of medicine are required for 18 doses? (Express your answer as a fraction reduced to lowest terms.) _____

27. A respiratory therapy class consists of 24 men and 36 women. What fraction of the students in the class are men? (Express your answer as a fraction reduced to lowest terms.) _____

28. A nursing student answers 18 out of 20 questions correctly on a test. Write a proper fraction (reduced to lowest terms) to represent the portion of the test questions that were answered correctly.

_____

29. A typical dose of Children's Tylenol contains 160 milligrams of medication per teaspoonful. Each 80 milligrams is what part of a typical dose? _____

30. In question 29, how many teaspoons of Children's Tylenol would you need to give a dosage of 80 milligrams? _____

After completing these problems, see page 635 to check your answers.

If you answered question 30 correctly, you can already calculate a dosage! However, there are many factors to consider when accurately calculating dosages. This text will cover the additional steps necessary to ensure patient safety.

Addition and Subtraction of Fractions

To add or subtract fractions, all the denominators must be the same. You can determine the least common denominator by finding the smallest whole number into which all denominators will divide evenly. Once the least common denominator is determined, convert the fractions to equivalent fractions with the least common denominator. This operation involves *enlarging the fractions,* which we examined in the last section. Let's look at an example of this important operation.

EXAMPLE ■

Find the equivalent fractions with the least common denominator for $\frac{3}{8}$ and $\frac{1}{3}$.

1. Find the smallest whole number into which the denominators 8 and 3 will divide evenly. The least common denominator is 24.

2. Convert the fractions to equivalent fractions with 24 as the denominator.

$$\frac{3}{8} = \frac{3 \times 3}{8 \times 3} = \frac{9}{24} \qquad \frac{1}{3} = \frac{1 \times 8}{3 \times 8} = \frac{8}{24}$$

You have enlarged $\frac{3}{8}$ to $\frac{9}{24}$ and $\frac{1}{3}$ to $\frac{8}{24}$. Now both fractions have the same denominator. Finding the least common denominator is the first step in adding or subtracting fractions.

RULE

To add or subtract fractions:

1. Convert all fractions to equivalent fractions with the least common denominator.

2. Add or subtract the numerators, place that value in the numerator, and use the least common denominator as the denominator.

3. Convert to a mixed number and/or reduce the fraction to lowest terms, if possible.

MATH TIP

To add or subtract fractions, no calculations are performed on the denominators once they are all converted to equivalent fractions with the least common denominators. Perform the mathematical operation (addition or subtraction) on the *numerators* only, and use the least common denominator as the denominator of the answer. Never add or subtract denominators.

Adding Fractions

EXAMPLE 1 ▪

$\frac{3}{4} + \frac{1}{4} + \frac{2}{4}$

1. Find the least common denominator. This step is not necessary in this example, because the fractions already have the same denominator.

2. Add the numerators, and use the common denominator: $\frac{3 + 1 + 2}{4} = \frac{6}{4}$

3. Convert to a mixed number, and reduce to lowest terms: $\frac{6}{4} = 1\frac{2}{4} = 1\frac{1}{2}$

EXAMPLE 2 ▪

$\frac{1}{3} + \frac{3}{4} + \frac{1}{6}$

1. Find the least common denominator: 12. The number 12 is the smallest number that 3, 4, and 6 will all equally divide into.

    Convert to equivalent fractions in twelfths. This is the same as enlarging the fractions.

    $\frac{1}{3} = \frac{1 \times 4}{3 \times 4} = \frac{4}{12}$

    $\frac{3}{4} = \frac{3 \times 3}{4 \times 3} = \frac{9}{12}$

    $\frac{1}{6} = \frac{1 \times 2}{6 \times 2} = \frac{2}{12}$

2. Add the numerators, and use the common denominator: $\frac{4 + 9 + 2}{12} = \frac{15}{12}$

3. Convert to a mixed number, and reduce to lowest terms: $\frac{15}{12} = 1\frac{3}{12} = 1\frac{1}{4}$

Subtracting Fractions

EXAMPLE 1 ▪

$\frac{15}{18} - \frac{8}{18}$

1. Find the least common denominator. This is not necessary in this example, because the denominators are the same.

2. Subtract the numerators, and use the common denominator: $\frac{15 - 8}{18} = \frac{7}{18}$

3. Reduce to lowest terms. This is not necessary here, because no further reduction is possible.

EXAMPLE 2 ▪

$1\frac{1}{10} - \frac{3}{5}$

1. Find the least common denominator: 10. The number 10 is the smallest number that both 10 and 5 will equally divide into.

   Convert to equivalent fractions in tenths:

   $1\frac{1}{10} = \frac{11}{10}$ Note: First convert mixed numbers into improper fractions for computations.

   $\frac{3}{5} = \frac{3 \times 2}{5 \times 2} = \frac{6}{10}$

2. Subtract the numerators, and use the common denominator: $\frac{11 - 6}{10} = \frac{5}{10}$

3. Reduce to lowest terms: $\frac{5}{10} = \frac{1}{2}$

   Let's review one more time how to add and subtract fractions.

QUICK REVIEW

To add or subtract fractions:

▪ Convert to equivalent fractions with the least common denominator.

▪ Add or subtract the numerators; place that value in the numerator. Use the least common denominator as the denominator of the answer.

▪ Convert the answer to a mixed number and/or reduce to lowest terms, if possible.

Review Set 2

Add, and reduce the answers to lowest terms.

1. $7\frac{4}{5} + \frac{2}{3} =$ _____

2. $\frac{3}{4} + \frac{2}{3} =$ _____

3. $4\frac{2}{3} + 5\frac{1}{24} + 7\frac{1}{2} =$ _____

4. $\frac{3}{4} + \frac{1}{8} + \frac{1}{6} =$ _____

5. $12\frac{1}{2} + 20\frac{1}{3} =$ _____

6. $\frac{1}{4} + 5\frac{1}{3} =$ _____

7. $\frac{1}{7} + \frac{2}{3} + \frac{11}{21} =$ _____

8. $\frac{4}{9} + \frac{5}{8} + 4\frac{2}{3} =$ _____

9. $34\frac{1}{2} + 8\frac{1}{2} =$ _____

10. $\frac{12}{17} + 5\frac{2}{7} =$ _____

11. $\frac{6}{5} + 1\frac{1}{3} =$ _____

12. $\frac{1}{4} + \frac{5}{33} =$ _____

Subtract, and reduce the answers to lowest terms.

13. $\frac{3}{4} - \frac{1}{4} =$ _____

14. $8\frac{1}{12} - 3\frac{1}{4} =$ _____

15. $\frac{1}{8} - \frac{1}{12} =$ _____

16. $100 - 36\frac{1}{3} =$ _____

17. $355\frac{1}{5} - 55\frac{2}{5} =$ _____

18. $\frac{1}{3} - \frac{1}{6} =$ _____

19. $2\frac{3}{5} - 1\frac{1}{5} =$ _____

20. $14\frac{3}{16} - 7\frac{1}{8} =$ _____

21. $25 - 17\frac{7}{9} =$ _____

22. $4\frac{7}{10} - 3\frac{9}{20} =$ _____

23. $48\frac{6}{11} - 24 =$ _____

24. $1\frac{2}{3} - 1\frac{1}{12} =$ _____

25. A patient weighs 50 pounds on admission and 48 pounds on day 3 of his hospital stay. Write a fraction, reduced to lowest terms, to express the fraction of his original weight that he has lost.

   _____

26. A patient is on strict recording of fluid intake and output, including measurement of liquids used to prepare medications. A nursing student mixed the 8 AM medication with $2\frac{1}{2}$ fluid ounces of juice and the 8 PM medication with $3\frac{1}{3}$ fluid ounces of water. What is the total amount of liquid the patient consumed with medications? _____

27. An infant has grown $\frac{1}{2}$ inch during his first month of life, $\frac{1}{4}$ inch during his second month, and $\frac{3}{8}$ inch during his third month. How much did he grow during his first 3 months? _____

28. The required margins for your term paper are $1\frac{1}{2}$ inches at the top and bottom of a paper that has 11 inches of vertical length. How long is the vertical area available for typed information?

   _____

29. A stock clerk finds that there are $34\frac{1}{2}$ pints of hydrogen peroxide on the shelf. If the fully stocked shelf held 56 pints of hydrogen peroxide, how many pints were used?

   _____

30. Your 1-year-old patient weighs $20\frac{1}{2}$ pounds. At birth, she weighed $7\frac{1}{4}$ pounds. How much weight has she gained in 1 year? _____

After completing these problems, see pages 635–636 to check your answers.

Multiplication of Fractions

To multiply fractions, multiply numerators (for the numerator of the answer) and multiply denominators (for the denominator of the answer) to arrive at the *product,* or result.

   When possible, *cancellation of terms* simplifies and shortens the process of multiplication of fractions. Cancellation (like reducing to lowest terms) is based on the fact that the division of both the numerator and denominator by the same nonzero whole number does not change the value of the resulting number. In fact, it makes the calculation simpler, because you are working with smaller numbers.

EXAMPLE ▪

$\frac{1}{3} \times \frac{250}{500}$ (numerator and denominator of $\frac{250}{500}$ are both divisible by 250)

$= \frac{1}{3} \times \frac{\overset{1}{\cancel{250}}}{\underset{2}{\cancel{500}}} = \frac{1}{3} \times \frac{1}{2} = \frac{1}{6}$

   Also, a numerator and a denominator of any of the fractions involved in the multiplication may be cancelled when they can be divided by the same number. This is called *cross-cancellation.*

EXAMPLE ▪

$$\frac{1}{8} \times \frac{8}{9} = \frac{1}{\overset{8}{\underset{1}{\cancel{8}}}} \times \overset{1}{\cancel{8}} = \frac{1}{1} \times \frac{1}{9} = \frac{1}{9}$$

RULE

To multiply fractions:

1. Cancel terms, if possible.

2. Multiply numerators for the numerator of the answer, and multiply denominators for the denominator of the answer.

3. Reduce the result *(product)* to lowest terms, if possible.

EXAMPLE 1 ▪

$$\frac{3}{4} \times \frac{2}{6}$$

1. Cancel terms: Divide 2 and 6 by 2.

$$\frac{3}{4} \times \frac{\overset{1}{\cancel{2}}}{\underset{3}{\cancel{6}}} = \frac{3}{4} \times \frac{1}{3}$$

Divide 3 and 3 by 3.

$$\frac{\overset{1}{\cancel{3}}}{4} \times \frac{1}{\underset{1}{\cancel{3}}} = \frac{1}{4} \times \frac{1}{1}$$

2. Multiply numerators and denominators:

$$\frac{1}{4} \times \frac{1}{1} = \frac{1}{4}$$

3. Reduce to lowest terms. This is not necessary here, because no further reduction is possible.

EXAMPLE 2 ▪

$$\frac{15}{30} \times \frac{2}{5}$$

1. Cancel terms: Divide 15 and 30 by 15.

$$\frac{\overset{1}{\cancel{15}}}{\underset{2}{\cancel{30}}} \times \frac{2}{5} = \frac{1}{2} \times \frac{2}{5}$$

Divide 2 and 2 by 2.

$$\frac{1}{\underset{1}{\cancel{2}}} \times \frac{\overset{1}{\cancel{2}}}{5} = \frac{1}{1} \times \frac{1}{5}$$

2. Multiply numerators and denominators:

$$\frac{1}{1} \times \frac{1}{5} = \frac{1}{5}$$

3. Reduce to lowest terms. This is not necessary here, because no further reduction is possible.

MATH TIP

When multiplying a fraction by a nonzero whole number, first convert the whole number to a fraction with a denominator of 1; the value of the number remains the same.

EXAMPLE 3 ■

$\frac{2}{3} \times 4$

1. No terms to cancel. (You cannot cancel 2 and 4, because both are numerators. To do so would change the value.) Convert the whole number to a fraction.

$$\frac{2}{3} \times 4 = \frac{2}{3} \times \frac{4}{1}$$

2. Multiply numerators and denominators:

$$\frac{2}{3} \times \frac{4}{1} = \frac{8}{3}$$

3. Convert to a mixed number.

$$\frac{8}{3} = 8 \div 3 = 2\frac{2}{3}$$

MATH TIP

To multiply mixed numbers, first convert them to improper fractions, and then multiply.

EXAMPLE 4 ■

$3\frac{1}{2} \times 4\frac{1}{3}$

1. Convert: $3\frac{1}{2} = \frac{7}{2}$

$$4\frac{1}{3} = \frac{13}{3}$$

Therefore, $3\frac{1}{2} \times 4\frac{1}{3} = \frac{7}{2} \times \frac{13}{3}$

2. Cancel: not necessary. No numbers can be cancelled.

3. Multiply: $\frac{7}{2} \times \frac{13}{3} = \frac{91}{6}$

4. Convert to a mixed number: $\frac{91}{6} = 15\frac{1}{6}$

Division of Fractions

The division of fractions uses three terms: *dividend, divisor,* and *quotient.* The *dividend* is the fraction being divided, or the first number. The *divisor,* the number to the right of the division sign, is the fraction by which the dividend is divided. The *quotient* is the result of the division. To divide fractions, the divisor is inverted and the operation is changed to multiplication. Once inverted, the calculation is the same as for multiplication of fractions.

EXAMPLE ■

$$\frac{1}{4} \div \frac{2}{7} = \frac{1}{4} \times \frac{7}{2} = \frac{7}{8}$$

↑　　　↑　　　　　↑　　　↑　　　↑

Dividend　**Divisor**　　　**÷ Changed**　**Inverted**　**Quotient**
　　　　　　　　　　　　to ×　　**Divisor**

RULE

To divide fractions:

1. Invert the terms of the divisor; change ÷ to ×.

2. Cancel terms, if possible.

3. Multiply the resulting fractions.

4. Convert the result (quotient) to a mixed number, and/or reduce to lowest terms, if possible.

EXAMPLE 1 ■

$\frac{3}{4} \div \frac{1}{3}$

1. Invert divisor, and change ÷ to ×: $\frac{3}{4} \div \frac{1}{3} = \frac{3}{4} \times \frac{3}{1}$

2. Cancel: not necessary. No numbers can be cancelled.

3. Multiply: $\frac{3}{4} \times \frac{3}{1} = \frac{9}{4}$

4. Convert to mixed number: $\frac{9}{4} = 2\frac{1}{4}$

EXAMPLE 2 ■

$\frac{2}{3} \div 4$

1. Invert divisor, and change ÷ to ×: $\frac{2}{3} \div \frac{4}{1} = \frac{2}{3} \times \frac{1}{4}$

2. Cancel terms: $\frac{\overset{1}{\cancel{2}}}{3} \times \frac{1}{\underset{2}{\cancel{4}}} = \frac{1}{3} \times \frac{1}{2}$

3. Multiply: $\frac{1}{3} \times \frac{1}{2} = \frac{1}{6}$

4. Reduce: not necessary; already reduced to lowest terms.

MATH TIP

To divide mixed numbers, first convert them to improper fractions.

EXAMPLE 3 ■

$1\frac{1}{2} \div \frac{3}{4}$

1. Convert: $\frac{3}{2} \div \frac{3}{4}$

2. Invert divisor, and change ÷ to ×: $\frac{3}{2} \times \frac{4}{3}$

3. Cancel: $\frac{\overset{1}{\cancel{3}}}{\underset{1}{\cancel{2}}} \times \frac{\overset{2}{\cancel{4}}}{\underset{1}{\cancel{3}}} = \frac{1}{1} \times \frac{2}{1}$

4. Multiply: $\frac{1}{1} \times \frac{2}{1} = \frac{2}{1}$

5. Simplify: $\frac{2}{1} = 2$

MATH TIP

Multiplying complex fractions also involves the division of fractions.

In the next example the divisor is the same as the denominator, so you will invert the denominator and multiply. Multiplying complex fractions can be confusing—take your time and study this carefully.

EXAMPLE 4 ■

$$\frac{\frac{1}{150}}{\frac{1}{100}} \times 2$$

1. Convert: Express 2 as a fraction. $\dfrac{\frac{1}{150}}{\frac{1}{100}} \times \frac{2}{1}$

2. Rewrite complex fraction as division: $\frac{1}{150} \div \frac{1}{100} \times \frac{2}{1}$

3. Invert divisor, and change ÷ to ×: $\frac{1}{150} \times \frac{100}{1} \times \frac{2}{1}$

4. Cancel: $\frac{1}{\underset{3}{\cancel{150}}} \times \frac{\overset{2}{\cancel{100}}}{1} \times \frac{2}{1} = \frac{1}{3} \times \frac{2}{1} \times \frac{2}{1}$

5. Multiply: $\frac{1}{3} \times \frac{2}{1} \times \frac{2}{1} = \frac{4}{3}$

6. Convert to mixed number: $\frac{4}{3} = 1\frac{1}{3}$

This example appears difficult at first, but when solved logically, one step at a time, it is just like the others.

QUICK REVIEW

- To *multiply* fractions, cancel terms, multiply numerators, and multiply denominators.
- To *divide* fractions, invert the divisor, cancel terms, and multiply.
- Convert results to a mixed number and/or reduce to lowest terms, if possible.

Review Set 3

Multiply, and reduce the answers to lowest terms.

1. $\frac{3}{10} \times \frac{1}{12} =$ _____

2. $\frac{12}{25} \times \frac{3}{5} =$ _____

3. $\frac{5}{8} \times 1\frac{1}{6} =$ _____

4. $\frac{1}{100} \times 3 =$ _____

5. $\dfrac{\frac{1}{6}}{\frac{1}{4}} \times \dfrac{\frac{3}{2}}{\frac{2}{3}} =$ _____

9. $\frac{3}{4} \times \frac{2}{3} =$ _____

6. $\dfrac{\frac{1}{150}}{\frac{1}{100}} \times 2\frac{1}{2} =$ _____

10. $4\frac{2}{3} \times 5\frac{1}{24} =$ _____

7. $\frac{30}{75} \times 2 =$ _____

11. $\frac{3}{4} \times \frac{1}{8} =$ _____

8. $9\frac{4}{5} \times \frac{2}{3} =$ _____

12. $12\frac{1}{2} \times 20\frac{1}{3} =$ _____

Divide, and reduce the answers to lowest terms.

13. $\frac{3}{4} \div \frac{1}{4} =$ _____

19. $2\frac{1}{2} \div \frac{3}{4} =$ _____

14. $6\frac{1}{12} \div 3\frac{1}{4} =$ _____

20. $\dfrac{\frac{1}{20}}{\frac{1}{3}} =$ _____

15. $\frac{1}{8} \div \frac{7}{12} =$ _____

21. $\frac{1}{150} \div \frac{1}{50} =$ _____

16. $\frac{1}{33} \div \frac{1}{3} =$ _____

22. $\frac{7}{8} \div 1\frac{1}{2} =$ _____

17. $5\frac{1}{4} \div 10\frac{1}{2} =$ _____

23. $\dfrac{\frac{3}{5}}{\frac{3}{4}} \div \dfrac{\frac{4}{5}}{1\frac{1}{9}} =$ _____

18. $\frac{1}{60} \div \frac{1}{2} =$ _____

24. The nurse is maintaining calorie counts (or counting calories) for a patient who is not eating well. The patient ate $\frac{3}{4}$ of a large apple. If one large apple contains 80 calories, how many calories were consumed? _____

25. How many seconds are there in $9\frac{1}{3}$ minutes? _____

26. A bottle of Children's Tylenol contains 20 teaspoons of liquid. If each dose for a 2-year-old child is $\frac{1}{2}$ teaspoon, how many doses for a 2 year old are available in this bottle? _____

27. The patient needs to take $1\frac{1}{2}$ tablets of medication 3 times per day for 7 days. Over the 7 days, how many tablets will the patient take? _____

28. The nurse aide observes that the patient's water pitcher is $\frac{1}{3}$ full. If the patient drank 850 milliliters of water, how many milliliters does the pitcher hold? (Hint: The 850 milliliters does not represent $\frac{1}{3}$ of the pitcher.) _____

29. A pharmacist weighs a tube of antibiotic eye ointment and documents that it weighs $\frac{7}{10}$ of an ounce. How much would 75 tubes weigh? _____

30. A patient is taking a liquid antacid from a bottle that contains 16 fluid ounces. If the patient takes $\frac{1}{2}$ fluid ounce every 4 hours while awake beginning at 7 AM and ending with a final dose at 11 PM, how many full days would this bottle last? (Hint: First, draw a clock.) _____

After completing these problems, see page 636 to check your answers.

DECIMALS

Decimal Fractions and Decimal Numbers

Decimal fractions are fractions with a denominator of 10, 100, 1,000, or any power of 10. At first glance, they appear to be whole numbers because of the way they are written. But the numeric value of a decimal fraction is always less than 1.

EXAMPLES ▪

$0.1 \quad = \frac{1}{10}$

$0.01 \quad = \frac{1}{100}$

$0.001 \ = \frac{1}{1,000}$

     Decimal numbers are numeric values that include a whole number, a decimal point, and a decimal fraction. Generally, decimal fractions and decimal numbers are referred to simply as *decimals*.

EXAMPLES ▪

4.67 and 23.956

     Nurses and other health care professionals must have an understanding of decimals to be competent at dosage calculations. Medication orders and other measurements in health care primarily use metric measure, which is based on the decimal system. Decimals are a special shorthand for designating fractional values. They are simpler to read and faster to use when performing mathematical computations.

MATH TIP

When dealing with decimals, think of the decimal point as the center that separates whole and fractional amounts. The position of the numbers in relation to the decimal point indicates the place value of the numbers.

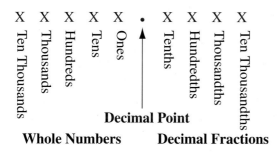

MATH TIP

The words for all decimal fractions end in *th(s)*.

EXAMPLES ▪

0.001 = one thousand*th*

0.02 = two hundred*ths*

0.7 = seven ten*ths*

RULE

The decimal number is read by stating the whole number first, the decimal point as *and,* and then the decimal fraction by naming the value of the last decimal place.

EXAMPLE ■

Look carefully at the decimal number 4.125. The last decimal place is thousandths. Therefore, the number is read as *four and one hundred twenty-five thousandths.*

4 . 1 2 5

Ones | Tenths | Hundredths | Thousandths

EXAMPLES ■

The number 6.2 is read as *six and two tenths.*

The number 10.03 is read as *ten and three hundredths.*

MATH TIP

Given a decimal fraction (whose value is less than 1), the decimal number is read alone, without stating the zero. However, the zero is written to emphasize the decimal point. In fact, since 2005, this has been a requirement by the accrediting body for health care organizations, The Joint Commission (2013), when writing decimal fractions in medical notation.

EXAMPLE ■

0.125 is read as *one hundred twenty-five thousandths.*

A set of rules governs the decimal system of notation.

RULE

The whole number value is controlled by its position to the left of the decimal point.

EXAMPLES ■

10.1 = ten and one tenth. The whole number is *10.*

1.01 = one and one hundredth. The whole number is *1.*

Notice that the decimal point's position completely changes the numeric value.

RULE

The decimal fraction value is controlled by its position to the right of the decimal point.

EXAMPLES ■

25.1 = twenty-five and one tenth. The decimal fraction is *one tenth.*

25.01 = twenty-five and one hundredth. The decimal fraction is *one hundredth.*

MATH TIP
Each decimal place is counted off as a power of 10 to tell you which denominator is expected.

EXAMPLE 1 ▪

437.5 = four hundred thirty-seven and **five tenths** $\left(437 + \frac{5}{10}\right)$

One decimal place indicates *tenths*.

EXAMPLE 2 ▪

43.75 = forty-three and **seventy-five hundredths** $\left(43 + \frac{75}{100}\right)$

Two decimal places indicate *hundredths*.

EXAMPLE 3 ▪

4.375 = four and **three hundred seventy-five thousandths** $\left(4 + \frac{375}{1,000}\right)$

Three decimal places indicate *thousandths*.

RULE
Zeros added after the last digit of a decimal fraction do not change its value and are not necessary, except when a zero is required to demonstrate the level of precision of the value being reported, such as for laboratory results.

EXAMPLE ▪
0.25 = 0.25**0**

Twenty-five hundredths equals two hundred fifty thousandths.

CAUTION
When writing decimals, eliminate unnecessary zeros at the end of the number to avoid confusion. The Joint Commission (2013) forbids the use of trailing zeros for medication orders or other medication-related documentation and cautions that, in such cases, the decimal point may be missed when an unnecessary zero is written. This is part of The Joint Commission's *Official "Do Not Use" List* for medical notation, which will be discussed again in Chapters 3 and 9.

Because the last zero does not change the value of the decimal, it is not necessary. For example, the required notation is 0.25 rather than 0.250 and 10 not 10.0, which can be misinterpreted as 250 and 100, respectively, if the decimal point is not clear.

RULE
Zeros added before or after the decimal point of a decimal number *may* change its value.

EXAMPLES ▪
0.125 ≠ (is not equal to) 0.**0**125

1.025 ≠ **10**.025

However, .6 = **0**.6 and 12 = 12.**0**, but you should write 0.6 (with a leading zero) and 12 (without a trailing zero).

Comparing Decimals

It is important to be able to compare decimal amounts, noting which has a greater or lesser value.

CAUTION
A common error in comparing decimals is to overlook the exact placement of the decimal point and then misinterpret the value of the number.

MATH TIP
You can accurately compare decimal amounts by aligning the decimal points and adding zeros so that the numbers to be compared have the same number of decimal places. Remember that adding zeros at the end of a decimal fraction for the purposes of comparison does not change the original value.

EXAMPLE 1 ■

Compare 0.125, 0.05, and 0.2 to find which decimal fraction is largest.

Align decimal points and add zeros.

$0.125 = \frac{125}{1,000}$ or one hundred twenty-five thousandths

$0.05\mathbf{0} = \frac{50}{1,000}$ or fifty thousandths

$0.2\mathbf{00} = \frac{200}{1,000}$ or two hundred thousandths

Now it is easy to see that 0.2 is the greatest amount and 0.05 is the least. But at first glance, you might have been tricked into thinking that 0.2 was the least amount and 0.125 was the greatest amount. This kind of error can have dire consequences in dosage calculations and health care.

EXAMPLE 2 ■

Suppose 0.5 microgram of a drug has been ordered. The recommended maximum dosage of the drug is 0.25 microgram, and the minimum recommended dosage is 0.125 microgram. Comparing decimals, you can see that the ordered dosage is not within the recommended range.

0.125 microgram (recommended minimum dosage)

0.25**0** microgram (recommended maximum dosage)

0.5**00** microgram (ordered dosage)

Now you can see that 0.5 microgram is outside the allowable limits of the recommended dosage range of 0.125 to 0.25 microgram for this medication. In fact, it is twice the recommended maximum dosage.

CAUTION
It is important to eliminate possible confusion and avoid errors in dosage calculation. To avoid overlooking a decimal point in a decimal fraction and thereby reading the numeric value as a whole number, always place a zero to the left of the decimal point to emphasize that the number has a value less than 1. This is another of The Joint Commission's requirements. The Joint Commission's *Official "Do Not Use" List* (2013) prohibits writing a decimal fraction that is less than 1 without a leading zero. This important concept will be emphasized again in Chapters 3 and 9.

EXAMPLES ■

0.425, **0**.01, or **0**.005

Conversion Between Fractions and Decimals

For dosage calculations, you may need to convert decimals to fractions and vice versa.

RULE

To convert a fraction to a decimal, divide the numerator by the denominator.

MATH TIP

Make sure the numerator is inside the division sign and the denominator is outside. You will avoid reversing the numerator and the denominator in division if you write down the number you read first and put the division sign around that number, with the second number written outside the division sign. This will work regardless of whether it is written as a fraction or as a division problem (such as $\frac{1}{2}$ or $1 \div 2$).

EXAMPLE 1 ■

Convert $\frac{1}{4}$ to a decimal.

$$\frac{1}{4} = 4)\overline{\begin{array}{l} .25 \\ 1.00 \\ \underline{8} \\ 20 \\ \underline{20} \end{array}} = 0.25$$

EXAMPLE 2 ■

Convert $\frac{2}{5}$ to a decimal.

$$\frac{2}{5} = 5)\overline{\begin{array}{l} .4 \\ 2.0 \\ \underline{2.0} \end{array}} = 0.4$$

RULE

To convert a decimal to a fraction:

1. Express the decimal number as a whole number in the numerator of the fraction.

2. Express the denominator of the fraction as the number 1 followed by as many zeros as there are places to the right of the decimal point.

3. Reduce the resulting fraction to lowest terms.

EXAMPLE 1 ■

Convert 0.125 to a fraction.

1. Numerator: 125

2. Denominator: 1 followed by 3 zeros = 1,000

3. Reduce: $\frac{125}{1,000} = \frac{1}{8}$

EXAMPLE 2 ■

Convert 0.65 to a fraction.

1. Numerator: 65

2. Denominator: 1 followed by 2 zeros = 100

3. Reduce: $\frac{65}{100} = \frac{13}{20}$

MATH TIP

State the complete name of the decimal, and write the fraction that has the same name.

$0.65 = $ sixty-five hundredths $= \frac{65}{100}$

QUICK REVIEW

- In a decimal number, whole number values are to the left of the decimal point and fractional values are to the right.

- Zeros added to a decimal fraction before the decimal point of a decimal number less than 1 or at the end of the decimal fraction do not change the value. (Example: .5 = **0**.5 = 0.5**0**) A trailing zero should not be used (0.5**0**) except when a zero is required to demonstrate the level of precision of the reported value. However, using the leading zero (**0**.5) is an acceptable and recommended notation, including medication orders.

- In a decimal number, zeros added before or after the decimal point *may* change the value.
  Example: 1.5 ≠ 1.**05** and 1.5 ≠ **1**0.5.

- To avoid overlooking the decimal point in a decimal fraction, *always* place a zero to the left of the decimal point.
  Example:
  .5 ← Avoid writing a decimal fraction this way; it could be mistaken for the whole number 5.

  Example:
  0.5 ← This is the required method of writing a decimal fraction with a value less than 1.

- The number of places in a decimal fraction indicates the power of 10.
  Examples:
  0.5 = five tenths
  0.05 = five hundredths
  0.005 = five thousandths

- Compare decimals by aligning decimal points and adding zeros at the end.
  Example:
  Compare 0.5, 0.05, and 0.005.
  0.500 = five hundred thousandths (greatest)
  0.050 = fifty thousandths
  0.005 = five thousandths (least)

- To convert a fraction to a decimal, divide the numerator by the denominator.

- To convert a decimal to a fraction, express the decimal number as a whole number in the numerator and the denominator as the correct power of 10. Reduce the fraction to lowest terms.
  Example:

$$0.04 = \frac{4 \text{ (numerator is a whole number)}}{100 \text{ (denominator is 1 followed by 2 zeros)}} = \frac{\overset{1}{\cancel{4}}}{\underset{25}{\cancel{100}}} = \frac{1}{25}$$

Review Set 4

Complete the following table of equivalent fractions and decimals. Reduce fractions to lowest terms.

Fraction	Decimal	The decimal number is read as:
1. $\frac{1}{5}$	_____	_____
2. _____	_____	eighty-five hundredths

Fraction	Decimal	The decimal number is read as:
3. _____	1.05	_____
4. _____	0.006	_____
5. $10\frac{3}{200}$	_____	_____
6. _____	1.9	_____
7. _____	_____	five and one tenth
8. $\frac{4}{5}$	_____	_____
9. _____	250.5	_____
10. $33\frac{3}{100}$	_____	_____
11. _____	0.95	_____
12. $2\frac{3}{4}$	_____	_____
13. _____	_____	seven and five thousandths
14. $\frac{21}{250}$	_____	_____
15. _____	12.125	_____
16. _____	20.09	_____
17. _____	_____	twenty-two and twenty-two thousandths
18. _____	0.15	_____
19. $1,000\frac{1}{200}$	_____	_____
20. _____	_____	four thousand eighty-five and seventy-five thousandths

21. Change 0.017 to a four-place decimal. _____

22. Change 0.2500 to a two-place decimal. _____

23. Convert $\frac{75}{100}$ to a decimal. _____

24. Convert 0.045 to a fraction reduced to lowest terms. _____

Circle the correct answer.

25. Which is largest?	0.012	0.12	0.021
26. Which is smallest?	0.635	0.6	0.063
27. True or False?	0.375 = 0.0375		
28. True or False?	2.2 grams = 2.02 grams		
29. True or False?	6.5 ounces = 6.500 ounces		

30. For a certain medication, the safe dosage should be greater than or equal to 0.5 gram but less than or equal to 2 grams. Circle each dosage that falls within this range.

    0.8 gram   0.25 gram   2.5 grams   1.25 grams

After completing these problems, see page 637 to check your answers.

Addition and Subtraction of Decimals

The addition and subtraction of decimals is similar to the addition and subtraction of whole numbers. There are two simple but essential rules that are different. Health care professionals must use these two rules to perform accurate dosage calculations for some medications.

RULE
To add and subtract decimals, line up the decimal points.

CAUTION
In final answers, eliminate unnecessary zeros at the end of a decimal to avoid confusion.

EXAMPLE 1 ■
$$1.25 + 1.75 = \begin{array}{r} 1.25 \\ +\ 1.75 \\ \hline 3.00 \end{array} = 3$$

EXAMPLE 2 ■
$$1.25 - 0.13 = \begin{array}{r} 1.25 \\ -\ 0.13 \\ \hline 1.12 \end{array}$$

EXAMPLE 3 ■
$$3.54 + 1.26 = \begin{array}{r} 3.54 \\ +\ 1.26 \\ \hline 4.80 \end{array} = 4.8$$

EXAMPLE 4 ■
$$2.54 - 1.04 = \begin{array}{r} 2.54 \\ -\ 1.04 \\ \hline 1.50 \end{array} = 1.5$$

RULE
To add and subtract decimals, add zeros at the end of decimal fractions if necessary to make all decimal numbers of equal length.

EXAMPLE 1 ■
$$3.75 - 2.1 = \begin{array}{r} 3.75 \\ -\ 2.10 \\ \hline 1.65 \end{array}$$

EXAMPLE 2 ■
Add 0.9, 0.65, 0.27, 4.712
$$\begin{array}{r} 0.900 \\ 0.650 \\ 0.270 \\ +\ 4.712 \\ \hline 6.532 \end{array}$$

EXAMPLE 3 ■
$$5.25 - 3.6 = \begin{array}{r} 5.25 \\ -\ 3.60 \\ \hline 1.65 \end{array}$$

EXAMPLE 4 ■
$$66.96 + 32 = \begin{array}{r} 66.96 \\ +\ 32.00 \\ \hline 98.96 \end{array}$$

QUICK REVIEW
- To add or subtract decimals, align the decimal points and add zeros at the end of the decimal fraction, making all decimals of equal length. Eliminate unnecessary zeros at the end in the final answer.

EXAMPLES ∎

$$1.5 + 0.05 = 1.50$$
$$\underline{+\ 0.05}$$
$$1.55$$

$$7.8 + 1.12 = 7.80$$
$$\underline{+\ 1.12}$$
$$8.92$$

$$0.725 - 0.5 = 0.725$$
$$\underline{-\ 0.500}$$
$$0.225$$

$$12.5 - 1.5 = 12.5$$
$$\underline{-\ 1.5}$$
$$11.0 = 11$$

Review Set 5

Find the results of the following problems.

1. $0.16 + 5.375 + 1.05 + 16 =$ _____

2. $7.517 + 3.2 + 0.16 + 33.3 =$ _____

3. $13.009 - 0.7 =$ _____

4. $5.125 + 6.025 + 0.15 =$ _____

5. $175.1 + 0.099 =$ _____

6. $25.2 - 0.193 =$ _____

7. $0.58 - 0.062 =$ _____

8. $\$10.10 - \$0.62 =$ _____

9. $\$19 - \$0.09 =$ _____

10. $\$5.05 + \$0.17 + \$17.49 =$ _____

11. $4 + 1.98 + 0.42 + 0.003 =$ _____

12. $0.3 - 0.03 =$ _____

13. $16.3 - 12.15 =$ _____

14. $2.5 - 0.99 =$ _____

15. $5 + 2.5 + 0.05 + 0.15 + 2.55 =$ _____

16. $0.03 + 0.16 + 2.327 =$ _____

17. $700 - 325.65 =$ _____

18. $645.32 - 40.9 =$ _____

19. $18 + 2.35 + 7.006 + 0.093 =$ _____

20. $13.529 + 10.09 =$ _____

21. A dietitian calculates the sodium in a patient's breakfast: raisin bran cereal = 0.1 gram, 1 cup 2% milk = 0.125 gram, 6 ounces orange juice = 0.001 gram, 1 corn muffin = 0.35 gram, and butter = 0.121 gram. How many grams of sodium did the patient consume? _____

22. In a 24-hour period, a premature infant drank 7.5 milliliters, 15 milliliters, 10 milliliters, 15 milliliters, 6.25 milliliters, and 12.5 milliliters of formula. How many milliliters did the infant drink in 24 hours?

_____

23. A patient has a hospital bill for $16,709.43. Her insurance company pays $14,651.37. What is her balance due? _____

24. A patient's hemoglobin was 14.8 grams before surgery. During surgery, the hemoglobin dropped 4.5 grams. What was the hemoglobin value after it dropped? _____

25. A home health nurse accounts for her day of work. If she spent 3 hours and 20 minutes at the office, 40 minutes traveling, $3\frac{1}{2}$ hours caring for patients, 24 minutes for lunch, and 12 minutes on break, what is her total number of hours including all of her activities? Express your answer as a decimal. (Hint: First convert each time to hours and minutes.) _____

After completing these problems, see page 637 to check your answers.

Multiplying Decimals

The procedure for multiplication of decimals is similar to that used for whole numbers. The only difference is the decimal point, which must be properly placed in the product or answer. Use the following simple rule.

RULE

To multiply decimals:

1. Multiply the decimals without concern for decimal point placement.

2. Count off the total number of decimal places in both of the decimals multiplied.

3. Move the decimal point in the product by moving it to the left the number of places counted.

EXAMPLE 1 ▪

$1.5 \times 0.5 = $ 1.5   (1 decimal place)

      $\times\ 0.5$ (1 decimal place)

      0.75   (The decimal point is located 2 places to the left, because a total of 2 decimal places are counted in the numbers that are multiplied.)

EXAMPLE 2 ▪

$1.72 \times 0.9 = $ 1.72   (2 decimal places)

      $\times\ 0.9$ (1 decimal place)

      1.548   (The decimal point is located 3 places to the left, because a total of 3 decimal places are counted.)

EXAMPLE 3 ▪

$5.06 \times 1.3 = $ 5.06   (2 decimal places)

      $\times\ 1.3$ (1 decimal place)

      1518

      506

      6.578   (The decimal point is located 3 places to the left, because a total of 3 decimal places are counted.)

EXAMPLE 4 ▪

$1.8 \times 0.05 = $ 1.8   (1 decimal place)

      $\times\ 0.05$ (2 decimal places)

      0.090   (The decimal point is located 3 places to the left. Notice that a zero has to be inserted between the decimal point and the 9 to allow for enough decimal places.)

   $0.090 = 0.09$ (Eliminate unnecessary zero.)

RULE
When multiplying a decimal by a power of 10, move the decimal point as many places to the right as there are zeros in the multiplier.

EXAMPLE 1 ▪

1.25×10

The multiplier 10 has 1 zero; move the decimal point 1 place to the right.

$1.25 \times 10 = 1\underset{\smile}{.2}5 = 12.5$

EXAMPLE 2 ▪

2.3×100

The multiplier 100 has 2 zeros; move the decimal point 2 places to the right. (Note: Add zeros as necessary to complete the operation.)

$2.3 \times 100 = 2\underset{\smile}{.30.} = 230$

EXAMPLE 3 ▪

$0.001 \times 1,000$

The multiplier 1,000 has 3 zeros; move the decimal point 3 places to the right.
$0.001 \times 1,000 = 0\underset{\smile}{.001.} = 1$

Dividing Decimals

When dividing decimals, set up the problem the same as for the division of whole numbers. Follow the same procedure for dividing whole numbers after you apply the following rule.

RULE
To divide decimals:

1. Move the decimal point in the *divisor* (number divided by) and the *dividend* (number divided) the number of places needed to make the *divisor* a *whole number*.

2. Place the decimal point in the *quotient* (answer) above the *new* decimal point place in the *dividend.*

EXAMPLE 1 ▪

$$
100.75 \div 2.5 = 2.5\overline{)100.7\,5} = 40.3
$$

(dividend) (divisor)   40.3 (quotient)

$$
\begin{array}{r}
40.3 \\
100 \\
\overline{07} \\
00 \\
\overline{75} \\
75 \\
\hline
\end{array}
$$

EXAMPLE 2 ▪

$$
56.5 \div 0.02 = 0.02\overline{)56.50} = 2,825
$$

2,825.

$$
\begin{array}{r}
2,825. \\
4 \\
\overline{16} \\
16 \\
\overline{5} \\
4 \\
\overline{10} \\
10 \\
\hline
\end{array}
$$

MATH TIP

Recall that adding a zero at the end of a decimal number does not change its value (56.5 = 56.50). Adding a zero was necessary in the last example to complete the operation.

RULE

When dividing a decimal by a power of 10, move the decimal point to the left as many places as there are zeros in the divisor.

EXAMPLE 1 ■

$0.65 \div 10$

The divisor 10 has 1 zero; move the decimal point 1 place to the left.

$0.65 \div 10 = .0.65 = 0.065$

(Note: Place a zero to the left of the decimal point to avoid confusion and to emphasize that this is a decimal.)

EXAMPLE 2 ■

$7.3 \div 100$

The divisor 100 has 2 zeros; move the decimal point 2 places to the left.

$7.3 \div 100 = .07.3 = 0.073$

(Note: Add zeros as necessary to complete the operation.)

EXAMPLE 3 ■

$0.5 \div 1,000$

The divisor 1,000 has 3 zeros; move the decimal point 3 places to the left.

$0.5 \div 1,000 = .000.5 = 0.0005$

Rounding Decimals

For many dosage calculations, it will be necessary to compute decimal calculations to *thousandths* (*three* decimal places) and round back to *hundredths* (*two* places) for the final answer. For example, pediatric care and critical care require this degree of accuracy. At other times, you will need to round to *tenths* (*one* place). Let's look closely at this important math skill.

RULE

To round a decimal to hundredths, drop the number in thousandths place, and

1. Do not change the number in hundredths place if the number in thousandths place was 4 or less.

2. Increase the number in hundredths place by 1 if the number in thousandths place was 5 or more.

EXAMPLES ■

All rounded to hundredths (2 places)

0 . 1 2 3   = 0.12

1 . 7 4 4   = 1.74

5 . 3 2 5   = 5.33

0 . 6 6 6   = 0.67

0 . 3 0   = 0.3   (When this is rounded to hundredths, the final zero should be dropped. It is not needed to clarify the number and is potentially confusing.)

RULE

To round a decimal to tenths, drop the number in hundredths place, and

1. Do not change the number in tenths place if the number in hundredths place was 4 or less.

2. Increase the number in tenths place by 1 if the number in hundredths place was 5 or more.

EXAMPLES ■

All rounded to tenths (1 place)

0 . 1 3   = 0.1

5 . 6 4   = 5.6

0 . 7 5   = 0.8

1 . 6 6   = 1.7

0 . 9 5   = 1.0 = 1   (The zero at the end of this decimal number is dropped, because it is unnecessary and potentially confusing.)

QUICK REVIEW

■ To multiply decimals, place the decimal point in the product to the left as many total decimal places as there are in the two decimals multiplied.
Example:
$0.25 \times 0.2 = 0.050 = 0.05$ (Zero at the end of the decimal is unnecessary and potentially confusing.)

■ To divide decimals, move the decimal point in the divisor and dividend the number of decimal places that will make the divisor a whole number and align it in the quotient.

Example: $24 \div 1.2$

$$
\begin{array}{r}
2\,0. \\
1.2\overline{)24.0}
\end{array}
$$

■ To multiply or divide decimals by a power of 10, move the decimal point to the right (to multiply) or to the left (to divide) the same number of decimal places as there are zeros in the power of 10.

Examples:
$5.06 \times 10 = 5.0\underset{\frown}{.}6 = 50.6$

$2.1 \div 100 = .0\underset{\frown}{2}.1 = 0.021$

- When rounding decimals, add 1 to the place value considered if the next decimal place is 5 or greater.

Examples:
Rounded to hundredths: $3.054 = 3.05$; $0.566 = 0.57$

Rounded to tenths: $3.05 = 3.1$; $0.54 = 0.5$

Review Set 6

Multiply, and round your answers to two decimal places.

1. $1.16 \times 5.03 =$ _____

2. $0.314 \times 7 =$ _____

3. $1.71 \times 25 =$ _____

4. $3.002 \times 0.05 =$ _____

5. $16.1 \times 25.04 =$ _____

6. $75.1 \times 1,000.01 =$ _____

7. $16.03 \times 2.05 =$ _____

8. $55.5 \times 0.05 =$ _____

9. $23.2 \times 15.025 =$ _____

10. $1.14 \times 0.014 =$ _____

Divide, and round your answers to two decimal places.

11. $16 \div 0.04 =$ _____

12. $25.3 \div 6.76 =$ _____

13. $0.02 \div 0.004 =$ _____

14. $45.5 \div 15.25 =$ _____

15. $515 \div 0.125 =$ _____

16. $73 \div 13.40 =$ _____

17. $16.36 \div 0.06 =$ _____

18. $0.375 \div 0.25 =$ _____

19. $100.04 \div 0.002 =$ _____

20. $45 \div 0.15 =$ _____

Multiply or divide by the power of 10 indicated. Draw an arrow to demonstrate movement of the decimal point. Do not round answers.

21. $562.5 \times 100 =$ _____

22. $16 \times 10 =$ _____

23. $25 \div 1,000 =$ _____

24. $32.005 \div 1,000 =$ _____

25. $0.125 \div 100 =$ _____

26. $23.25 \times 10 =$ _____

27. $717.717 \div 10 =$ _____

28. $83.16 \times 10 =$ _____

29. $0.33 \times 100 =$ _____

30. $14.106 \times 1,000 =$ _____

After completing these problems, see page 637 to check your answers.

PRACTICE PROBLEMS—CHAPTER 1

1. Convert 0.35 to a fraction in lowest terms. _____

2. Convert $\frac{3}{8}$ to a decimal. _____

Find the least common denominator for the following pairs of fractions.

3. $\frac{5}{7}$; $\frac{2}{3}$ _____   5. $\frac{4}{9}$; $\frac{5}{6}$ _____

4. $\frac{1}{5}$; $\frac{4}{11}$ _____   6. $\frac{1}{3}$; $\frac{3}{5}$ _____

Perform the indicated operation, and reduce fractions to lowest terms.

7. $1\frac{2}{3} + \frac{9}{5} =$ _____

8. $4\frac{5}{12} + 3\frac{1}{15} =$ _____

9. $\frac{7}{9} - \frac{5}{18} =$ _____

10. $5\frac{1}{6} - 2\frac{7}{8} =$ _____

11. $\frac{4}{9} \times \frac{7}{12} =$ _____

12. $1\frac{1}{2} \times 6\frac{3}{4} =$ _____

13. $7\frac{1}{5} \div 1\frac{7}{10} =$ _____

14. $\frac{3}{16} + \frac{3}{10} =$ _____

15. $8\frac{4}{11} \div 1\frac{2}{3} =$ _____

16. $\dfrac{9\frac{1}{2}}{1\frac{4}{5}} =$ _____

17. $\dfrac{13\frac{1}{3}}{4\frac{6}{13}} =$ _____

18. $\dfrac{\frac{1}{10}}{\frac{2}{3}} =$ _____

19. $\frac{1}{125} \times \frac{1}{25} =$ _____

20. $\dfrac{\frac{7}{8}}{\frac{1}{3}} \div \dfrac{3\frac{1}{2}}{\frac{1}{3}} =$ _____

21. $\frac{20}{35} \times 3 =$ _____

22. $2\frac{1}{4} \times 7\frac{1}{8} =$ _____

Perform the indicated operations, and round the answers to two decimal places.

23. $11.33 + 29.16 + 19.78 =$ _____

24. $93.712 - 26.97 =$ _____

25. $43.69 - 0.7083 =$ _____

26. $66.4 \times 72.8 =$ _____

27. $360 \times 0.53 =$ _____

28. $268.4 \div 14 =$ _____

29. $10.10 - 0.62 =$ _____

30. $5 + 2.5 + 0.05 + 0.15 =$ _____

31. $1.71 \times 25 =$ _____

32. $45 \div 0.15 =$ _____

33. $2{,}974 \div 0.23 =$ _____

34. $51.21 \div 0.016 =$ _____

35. $0.74 \div 0.37 =$ _____

36. $1.5 + 146.73 + 1.9 + 0.832 =$ _____

Multiply or divide by the power of 10 indicated. Draw an arrow to demonstrate movement of the decimal point. Do not round answers.

37. $9.716 \times 1{,}000 =$ _____

38. $50.25 \div 100 =$ _____

39. $0.25 \times 100 =$ _____

40. $5.75 \times 1{,}000 =$ _____

41. $0.25 \div 10 =$ _____

42. $11.525 \times 10 =$ _____

43. A 1-month-old infant drinks $3\frac{1}{2}$ fluid ounces of formula every 4 hours day and night. How many fluid ounces will the infant drink in 1 week on this schedule? _____

44. There are 368 people employed at Riverview Clinic. If $\frac{3}{8}$ of the employees are nurses, $\frac{1}{8}$ are maintenance personnel/cleaners, $\frac{1}{4}$ are technicians, and $\frac{1}{4}$ are all other employees, calculate the number of employees that each fraction represents. _____

45. True or False? A specific gravity of urine of $1\frac{1}{16}$ falls within the normal range of 1.01 to 1.025 for an adult patient. _____

46. Last week, a nurse earning \$32.66 per hour gross pay worked 40 hours plus 6.5 hours overtime, which is paid at twice the hourly rate. What is the total regular and overtime gross pay for last week? _____

47. The instructional assistant is ordering supplies for the nursing skills laboratory. A single box of 12 urinary catheters costs \$98.76. A case of 12 boxes containing 12 catheters per box costs \$975. Calculate the savings per catheter when a case is purchased. _____

48. If each ounce of a liquid laxative contains 0.065 gram of a drug, how many grams of the drug would be contained in 4.75 ounces? (Round answer to the nearest hundredth.) _____

49. A patient is to receive 1,200 milliliters of fluid in a 24-hour period. How many milliliters should the patient drink between the hours of 7:00 AM and 7:00 PM if he is to receive $\frac{2}{3}$ of the total amount during that time? _____

50. A baby weighed 3.7 kilograms at birth. The baby now weighs 6.65 kilograms. How many kilograms did the baby gain? _____

After completing these problems, see page 638 to check your answers.

Be sure to use the online software for additional practice!

REFERENCE

The Joint Commission. (2013). Facts about the *Official "Do Not Use" List*. Retrieved from http://www.jointcommission.org/assets/1/18/Do_Not_Use_List.pdf

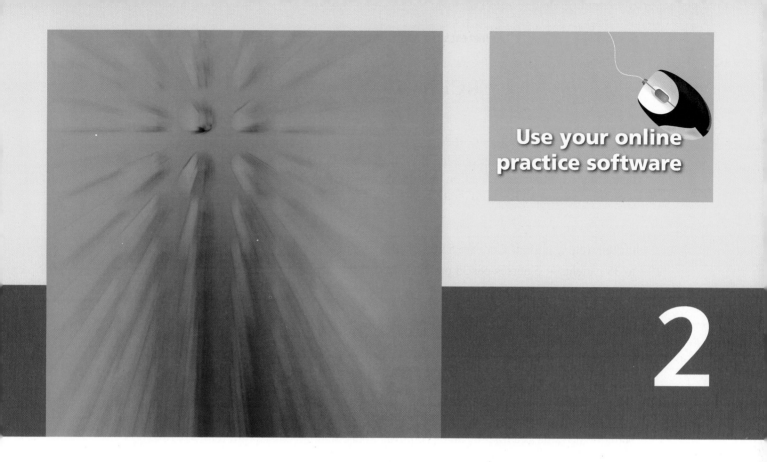

2

Ratios, Percents, Simple Equations, and Ratio-Proportion

OBJECTIVES

Upon mastery of Chapter 2, you will be able to perform basic mathematical computations that involve ratios, percents, simple equations, and proportions. Specifically, you will be able to:

- Interpret values expressed in ratios.
- Convert among fractions, decimals, ratios, and percents.
- Compare the size of fractions, decimals, ratios, and percents.
- Determine the value of X in simple equations.
- Set up proportions for solving problems.
- Cross-multiply to find the value of X in a proportion.
- Calculate the percentage of a quantity.

Health care professionals need to understand ratios and percents to be able to accurately interpret, prepare, and administer a variety of medications and treatments. Let's take a look at each of these important ways of expressing ratios and percents and how they are related to fractions and decimals. It is important for you to be able to convert equivalent ratios, percents, decimals, and fractions quickly and accurately.

RATIOS AND PERCENTS

Ratios

Like a fraction, a *ratio* is used to indicate the relationship of one part of a quantity to the whole. The two quantities are written as a fraction or separated by a colon (:). The use of the colon is a traditional way to write the division sign within a ratio.

EXAMPLE ▪

On an evening shift, if there are 5 nurses and 35 patients, what is the ratio of nurses to patients? 5 nurses to 35 patients = 5 nurses per 35 patients = $\frac{5}{35}$ = $\frac{1}{7}$. This is the same as a ratio of 5:35 or 1:7.

MATH TIP
The terms of a ratio are the numerator (always to the left of the colon) and the denominator (always to the right of the colon) of a fraction. Like fractions, ratios should be stated in lowest terms.

If you think back to the discussion of fractions and parts of a whole, it is easy to see that a ratio is actually the same as a fraction and its equivalent decimal. It is just a different way of expressing the same quantity. Recall from Chapter 1 that to convert a fraction to a decimal, you simply divide the numerator by the denominator.

EXAMPLE ▪

Adrenalin 1:1,000 for injection = 1 part Adrenalin to 1,000 total parts of solution. It is a fact that 1:1,000 is the same as $\frac{1}{1,000}$.

In some drug solutions, such as Adrenalin 1:1,000, the ratio is used to indicate the drug's concentration. This will be covered in more detail later.

Percents

A percent is a type of ratio. *Percent* comes from the Latin phrase *per centum,* translated *per hundred.* This means per hundred parts or hundredth part.

MATH TIP
To remember the value of a given percent, replace the % symbol with "/" for *per* and "100" for *cent.* THINK: percent (%) means "/100" or "*per hundred.*"

EXAMPLE ▪

3% = 3 percent = 3/100 = $\frac{3}{100}$ = 0.03

Converting Among Ratios, Percents, Fractions, and Decimals

When you understand the relationship of ratios, percents, fractions, and decimals, you can readily convert from one to the other. Let's begin by converting a percent to a fraction.

RULE

To convert a percent to a fraction:

1. Delete the % sign.

2. Write the remaining number as the numerator.

3. Write 100 as the denominator.

4. Reduce the result to lowest terms.

EXAMPLE ■

$5\% = \frac{5}{100} = \frac{1}{20}$

It is also easy to express a percent as a ratio.

RULE

To convert a percent to a ratio:

1. Delete the % sign.

2. Write the remaining number as the numerator.

3. Write 100 as the denominator.

4. Reduce the result to lowest terms.

5. Express the fraction as a ratio.

EXAMPLE ■

$25\% = \frac{25}{100} = \frac{1}{4} = 1{:}4$

Because the denominator of a percent is always 100, it is easy to find the equivalent decimal. Recall that to divide by 100, you move the decimal point two places to the left, the number of places equal to the number of zeros in the denominator.

RULE

To convert a percent to a decimal:

1. Delete the % sign.

2. Divide the remaining number by 100, which is the same as moving the decimal point two places to the left.

EXAMPLE ■

$25\% = \frac{25}{100} = 25 \div 100 = .25. = 0.25$

Conversely, it is easy to change a decimal to a percent.

RULE

To convert a decimal to a percent:

1. Multiply the decimal number by 100, which is the same as moving the decimal point two places to the right.

2. Add the % sign.

EXAMPLE ■

$0.25 \times 100 = 0.25. = 25\%$

MATH TIP

When converting a decimal to a percent, always move the decimal point two places to the right and add the % sign. This will result in a number that may appear to be larger, but actually has the same value as its decimal counterpart.

Now you know all the steps to change a ratio to the equivalent percent.

RULE

To convert a ratio to a percent:

1. Convert the ratio to a fraction.
2. Convert the fraction to a decimal.
3. Convert the decimal to a percent.

EXAMPLE ■

Convert 1 : 1,000 Adrenalin solution to the equivalent concentration expressed as a percent.

1. $1 : 1,000 = \frac{1}{1,000}$ (ratio converted to fraction)
2. $\frac{1}{1,000} = .001. = 0.001$ (fraction converted to decimal)
3. $0.001 = 0.00.1 = 0.1\%$ (decimal converted to percent)

Thus, 1 : 1,000 Adrenalin solution = 0.1% Adrenalin solution.

Review the preceding example again slowly until it is clear. Ask your instructor for assistance as needed. If you go over this one step at a time, you can master these important calculations. You need never fear fractions, decimals, ratios, and percents again.

Comparing Percents and Ratios

Nurses and other health care professionals frequently administer solutions with the concentration expressed as a percent or ratio. Consider two intravenous (which means given directly into a person's vein) solutions: one that is 0.9%, the other 5%. It is important to be clear that 0.9% is *less* than 5%. A 0.9% solution means that there are 0.9 parts of the solid per 100 total parts (0.9 parts is less than one whole part, so it is less than 1%). Compare this to the 5% solution, with 5 parts of the solid (or more than five times 0.9 parts) per 100 total parts. Therefore, the 5% solution is much more concentrated, or stronger, than the 0.9% solution. A misunderstanding of these numbers and the quantities they represent can have dire consequences.

Likewise, you may see a solution concentration expressed as $\frac{1}{3}\%$ and another expressed as 0.45%. Convert these amounts to equivalent decimals to clarify values and compare concentrations.

EXAMPLE 1 ■

$$\frac{1}{3}\% = \frac{\frac{1}{3}}{100} = \frac{1}{3} \div \frac{100}{1} = \frac{1}{3} \times \frac{1}{100} = \frac{1}{300} = 0.003\overline{3}$$

EXAMPLE 2 ■

$0.45\% = \frac{0.45}{100} = 0.0045$ (greater value, stronger concentration)

MATH TIP

In the last set of examples, the line over the last 3 in the decimal fraction $0.003\overline{3}$ indicates that the number 3 repeats itself indefinitely.

Compare solution concentrations expressed as a ratio, such as $1:1,000$ and $1:100$.

EXAMPLE 1 ■

$1:1,000 = \frac{1}{1,000} = 0.001$

EXAMPLE 2 ■

$1:100 = \frac{1}{100} = 0.01$ or 0.010 (add zero for comparison); $1:100$ is a stronger concentration.

QUICK REVIEW

- Fractions, decimals, ratios, and percents are related equivalents.

  Example: $1:2 = \frac{1}{2} = 0.5 = 50\%$

- Like fractions, ratios should be reduced to lowest terms.

  Example: $2:4 = 1:2$

- To express a ratio as a fraction, the number to the left of the colon becomes the numerator and the number to the right of the colon becomes the denominator. The colon in a ratio is equivalent to the division sign in a fraction.

  Example: $2:3 = \frac{2}{3}$

- To change a ratio to a decimal, convert the ratio to a fraction and divide the numerator by the denominator.

  Example: $1:4 = \frac{1}{4} = 1 \div 4 = 0.25$

- To change a percent to a fraction, drop the % sign and place the remaining number as the numerator over the denominator 100. Reduce the fraction to lowest terms. THINK: per (/) cent (100).

  Example: $75\% = \frac{75}{100} = \frac{3}{4}$

- To change a percent to a ratio, first convert the percent to a fraction in lowest terms. Then, place the numerator to the left of a colon and the denominator to the right of that colon.

  Example: $35\% = \frac{35}{100} = \frac{7}{20} = 7:20$

- To change a percent to a decimal, drop the % sign and divide by 100.

  Example: $4\% = .04. = 0.04$

- To change a decimal to a percent, multiply by 100 and add the % sign.

  Example: $0.5 = 0.50. = 50\%$

- To change a ratio to a percent, first convert the ratio to a fraction. Convert the resulting fraction to a decimal and then to a percent.

  Example: $1:2 = \frac{1}{2} = 1 \div 2 = 0.5 = 0.50. = 50\%$

Review Set 7

Change the following ratios to fractions that are reduced to lowest terms.

1. $3:150 =$ _____   4. $4:7 =$ _____

2. $6:10 =$ _____   5. $6:8 =$ _____

3. $0.05:0.15 =$ _____

Change the following ratios to decimals; round to two decimal places, if needed.

6. 20:40 = _____   9. 0.3:4.5 = _____

7. $\frac{1}{1,000} : \frac{1}{150}$ = _____   10. $1\frac{1}{2} : 6\frac{2}{9}$ = _____

8. 0.12:0.88 = _____

Change the following ratios to percents; round to two decimal places, if needed.

11. 12:48 = _____   14. 7:10 = _____

12. 2:5 = _____   15. 50:100 = _____

13. 0.08:0.64 = _____

Change the following percents to fractions that are reduced to lowest terms.

16. 45% = _____   19. 1% = _____

17. 60% = _____   20. $66\frac{2}{3}$% = _____

18. 0.5% = _____

Change the following percents to decimals; round to two decimal places, if needed.

21. 2.94% = _____   24. 33% = _____

22. 4.5% = _____   25. 0.9% = _____

23. 6.32% = _____

Change the following percents to ratios that are reduced to lowest terms.

26. 16% = _____   29. 45% = _____

27. 25% = _____   30. 6% = _____

28. 50% = _____

Which of the following is largest? Circle your answer.

31. 0.9%   0.9   1:9 $\frac{1}{90}$ 34. $\frac{1}{150}$ $\frac{1}{300}$ 0.5 $\frac{2}{3}$%

32. 0.05 $\frac{1}{5}$ 0.025   1:25   35. 1:1,000   0.0001 $\frac{1}{100}$ 0.1%

33. 0.0125%   0.25%   0.1%   0.02%

After completing these problems, see page 638 to check your answers.

SOLVING SIMPLE EQUATIONS FOR X

You can set up and solve dosage calculations in different ways. One way is to use a simple equation form. The following examples demonstrate the various forms of this equation. Learn to express your answers in decimal form, because decimals will be used most often in dosage calculations and administration.

MATH TIP
Round decimals to hundredths or to two places. For most dosage calculations, you will round to no more than two decimal places.

MATH TIP
The unknown quantity is represented by X.

EXAMPLE 1 ■

$$\frac{100}{200} \times 1 = X$$

MATH TIP

You can drop the 1, because a number multiplied by 1 is the same number.

$\frac{100}{200} \times 1 = X$ is the same as $\frac{100}{200} = X$.

1. Reduce to lowest terms: $\frac{100}{200} = \frac{\overset{1}{\cancel{100}}}{\underset{2}{\cancel{200}}} = \frac{1}{2} = X$

2. Convert to decimal form: $\frac{1}{2} = 0.5 = X$

3. You have your answer. $X = 0.5$

EXAMPLE 2 ■

$$\frac{3}{5} \times 2 = X$$

MATH TIP

Dividing a number by 1 does not change its value.

1. Convert: Express 2 as a fraction: $\frac{3}{5} \times \frac{2}{1} = X$

2. Multiply fractions: $\frac{3}{5} \times \frac{2}{1} = \frac{6}{5} = X$

3. Convert to a mixed number: $\frac{6}{5} = 1\frac{1}{5} = X$

4. Convert to decimal form: $1\frac{1}{5} = 1.2 = X$

5. You have your answer. $X = 1.2$

EXAMPLE 3 ■

$$\frac{\frac{1}{6}}{\frac{1}{4}} \times 5 = X$$

1. Convert: Express 5 as a fraction: $\frac{\frac{1}{6}}{\frac{1}{4}} \times \frac{5}{1} = X$

2. Divide fractions: $\frac{1}{6} \div \frac{1}{4} \times \frac{5}{1} = X$

3. Invert the divisor, and multiply: $\frac{1}{6} \times \frac{4}{1} \times \frac{5}{1} = X$

4. Cancel terms: $\frac{1}{\underset{3}{\cancel{6}}} \times \frac{\overset{2}{\cancel{4}}}{1} \times \frac{5}{1} = \frac{1}{3} \times \frac{2}{1} \times \frac{5}{1} = \frac{10}{3} = X$

5. Convert to a mixed number: $\frac{10}{3} = 3\frac{1}{3} = X$

6. Convert to decimal form: $3\frac{1}{3} = 3.33\overline{3} = X$

7. Round to hundredths place: $3.33\overline{3} = 3.33 = X$

8. It is easy, when you take it one step at a time. $X = 3.33$

EXAMPLE 4 ■

$$\frac{\frac{1}{10}}{\frac{1}{15}} \times 2.2 = X$$

1. Convert: Express 2.2 in fraction form: $\dfrac{\frac{1}{10}}{\frac{1}{15}} \times \dfrac{2.2}{1} = X$

2. Divide fractions: $\dfrac{1}{10} \div \dfrac{1}{15} \times \dfrac{2.2}{1} = X$

3. Invert the divisor, and multiply: $\dfrac{1}{10} \times \dfrac{15}{1} \times \dfrac{2.2}{1} = X$

4. Cancel terms: $\dfrac{1}{\cancel{10}_2} \times \dfrac{\cancel{15}^3}{1} \times \dfrac{2.2}{1} = \dfrac{1}{\cancel{2}_1} \times \dfrac{3}{1} \times \dfrac{\cancel{2.2}^{1.1}}{1} = \dfrac{1}{1} \times \dfrac{3}{1} \times \dfrac{1.1}{1} = X$

5. Multiply: $\dfrac{1}{1} \times \dfrac{3}{1} \times \dfrac{1.1}{1} = \dfrac{3.3}{1} = 3.3 = X$

6. That's it! X = 3.3

EXAMPLE 5 ■

$$\frac{0.125}{0.25} \times 1.5 = X$$

1. Convert: Express 1.5 in fraction form: $\dfrac{0.125}{0.25} \times \dfrac{1.5}{1} = X$

2. Convert: For easier comparison, add a zero to thousandths place for 0.25: $\dfrac{0.125}{0.250} \times \dfrac{1.5}{1} = X$

3. Cancel terms: $\dfrac{\cancel{0.125}^1}{\cancel{0.250}_2} \times \dfrac{1.5}{1} = \dfrac{1}{2} \times \dfrac{1.5}{1} = X$

4. Multiply: $\dfrac{1}{2} \times \dfrac{1.5}{1} = \dfrac{1.5}{2} = X$

5. Divide: $\dfrac{1.5}{2} = 0.75 = X$

6. You've got it! X = 0.75

MATH TIP
It may be easier to work with whole numbers than decimals. If you had difficulty with Step 3, try multiplying the numerator and denominator by 1,000 to eliminate the decimal fractions.

$$\frac{0.125}{0.250} \times \frac{1,000}{1,000} = \frac{125}{250} = \frac{1}{2}$$

Example 5 can also be solved by computing with fractions instead of decimals.

Try this: $\dfrac{0.125}{0.25} \times 1.5 = X$

1. Convert: Express 1.5 in fraction form: $\dfrac{0.125}{0.25} \times \dfrac{1.5}{1} = X$

2. Convert: Add zeros for easier comparison, making *both* decimals of equal length: $\dfrac{0.125}{0.250} \times \dfrac{1.5}{1.0} = X$

3. Cancel terms: $\frac{\overset{1}{0.\cancel{125}}}{\underset{2}{0.\cancel{250}}} \times \frac{\overset{3}{\cancel{1.5}}}{\underset{2}{\cancel{1.0}}} = \frac{1}{2} \times \frac{3}{2}$ (It is easier to work with whole numbers.)

4. Multiply: $\frac{1}{2} \times \frac{3}{2} = \frac{3}{4} = X$

5. Convert: $\frac{3}{4} = 0.75 = X$

6. You've got it again! X = 0.75

Which way do you find easier?

EXAMPLE 6 ■

$\frac{3}{4} \times 45\% = X$

1. Convert: Express 45% as a fraction reduced to lowest terms: $45\% = \frac{45}{100} = \frac{9}{20}$

2. Multiply fractions: $\frac{3}{4} \times \frac{9}{20} = X$

    $\frac{27}{80} = X$

3. Divide: $\frac{27}{80} = 0.337 = X$

4. Round to hundredths place: 0.34 = X

5. You have your answer. X = 0.34

QUICK REVIEW

■ To solve simple equations, perform the mathematical operations indicated to find the value of the unknown X.

■ Express the result (value of X) in decimal form.

Review Set 8

Solve the following problems for X. Express answers as decimals rounded to two places.

1. $\frac{75}{125} \times 5 = X$ _____

2. $\frac{\frac{3}{4}}{\frac{1}{2}} \times 2.2 = X$ _____

3. $\frac{150}{300} \times 2.5 = X$ _____

4. $\frac{40\%}{60\%} \times 8 = X$ _____

5. $\frac{0.35}{2.5} \times 4 = X$ _____

6. $\frac{0.15}{0.1} \times 1.2 = X$ _____

7. $\frac{0.4}{2.5} \times 4 = X$ _____

8. $\frac{1,200,000}{400,000} \times 4.2 = X$ _____

9. $\frac{\frac{2}{3}}{\frac{1}{6}} \times 10 = X$ _____

10. $\frac{30}{50} \times 0.8 = X$ _____

11. $\frac{200,000}{300,000} \times 1.5 = X$ _____

12. $\frac{0.08}{0.1} \times 1.2 = X$ _____

13. $\frac{7.5}{5} \times 3 = X$ _____

14. $\frac{250,000}{2,000,000} \times 7.5 = X$ _____

15. $\frac{600}{150} \times 2.5 = X$ _____   18. $\frac{0.25}{0.125} \times 5 = X$ _____

16. $\frac{600{,}000}{750{,}000} \times 0.5 = X$ _____   19. $\frac{1{,}000{,}000}{250{,}000} \times 5 = X$ _____

17. $\frac{75\%}{60\%} \times 1.2 = X$ _____   20. $\dfrac{\frac{1}{100}}{\frac{1}{150}} \times 1.2 = X$ _____

After completing these problems, see pages 638–639 to check your answers.

RATIO-PROPORTION: CROSS-MULTIPLYING TO SOLVE FOR X

A *proportion* is two ratios that are equal or an equation between two equal ratios.

MATH TIP
A proportion is written as two ratios separated by an equal sign, such as 5:10 = 10:20. More commonly, the ratios may be expressed as fractions, such as $\frac{5}{10} = \frac{10}{20}$.

Some of the calculations you will perform will have the unknown X as a different term in the equation. To determine the value of the unknown X, you must apply the rule for cross-multiplying used in a proportion.

RULE
In a proportion, the product of the means (the two inside numbers) equals the product of the extremes (the two outside numbers). Finding the product of the means and the extremes is called *cross-multiplying*.

EXAMPLE ■

Extremes
5:10   =   10:20
Means

$5 \times 20 = 10 \times 10$

$100 = 100$

Because ratios are the same as fractions, the same proportion can be expressed like this: $\frac{5}{10} = \frac{10}{20}$. The fractions are *equivalent,* or equal. The numerator of the first fraction and the denominator of the second fraction are the *extremes,* and the denominator of the first fraction and the numerator of the second fraction are the *means*.

EXAMPLE ■

Extreme $\frac{5}{10}$ ⤬ $\frac{10}{20}$ Mean
Mean   Extreme

Cross-multiply to find the equal products of the means and extremes.

RULE

If two fractions are equivalent, or equal, their cross-products are also equal.

EXAMPLE ■

$$\frac{5}{10} \diagdown\diagup \frac{10}{20}$$

$$5 \times 20 = 10 \times 10$$

$$100 = 100$$

When one of the quantities in a proportion is unknown, a letter, such as X, may be substituted for this unknown quantity. You would solve the equation to find the value of X. In addition to cross-multiplying, there is one more rule you need to know to solve for X in a proportion.

RULE

Dividing or multiplying each side (member) of an equation by the same nonzero number produces an equivalent equation.

MATH TIP

Dividing each side of an equation by the same nonzero whole number is the same as reducing or simplifying the equation. Multiplying each side by the same nonzero whole number enlarges the equation.

Let's examine how to simplify an equation.

EXAMPLE ■

$25X = 100$ ($25X$ means $25 \times X$)

Simplify the equation to find X. Divide both sides by 25, the number before X. Reduce to lowest terms.

$$\frac{\overset{1}{25X}}{\underset{1}{25}} = \frac{\overset{4}{100}}{\underset{1}{25}}$$

$\frac{1X}{1} = \frac{4}{1}$ (Dividing or multiplying a number by 1 does not change its value. 1X is understood to be simply X.)

$X = 4$

Replace X with 4 in the same equation, and you can prove that the calculations are correct.

$25 \times 4 = 100$

Now you are ready to apply the concepts of cross-multiplying and simplifying an equation to solve for X in a proportion.

EXAMPLE 1 ▪

$$\frac{90}{2} = \frac{45}{X}$$

You have a proportion with an unknown quantity X in the denominator of the second fraction. Find the value of X.

1. Cross-multiply: $\frac{90}{2} \diagdown\!\!\!\!\diagup \frac{45}{X}$

2. Multiply terms: $90 \times X = 2 \times 45$

$$90X = 90 \ (90X \text{ means } 90 \times X)$$

3. Simplify the equation: Divide both sides of the equation by the number before the unknown X. You are equally reducing the terms on both sides of the equation.

$$\frac{\overset{1}{\cancel{90}}X}{\underset{1}{\cancel{90}}} = \frac{\overset{1}{\cancel{90}}}{\underset{1}{\cancel{90}}}$$

$$X = 1$$

Try another one. You will use a proportion to solve this equation.

EXAMPLE 2 ▪

$$\frac{80}{X} \times 60 = 20$$

1. Convert: Express 60 as a fraction.

$$\frac{80}{X} \times \frac{60}{1} = 20$$

2. Multiply fractions: $\frac{80}{X} \times \frac{60}{1} = 20$

$$\frac{4,800}{X} = 20$$

3. Convert: Express 20 as a fraction.

$$\frac{4,800}{X} = \frac{20}{1}$$

You now have a proportion.

4. Cross-multiply: $\frac{4,800}{X} \diagdown\!\!\!\!\diagup \frac{20}{1}$

$$20X = 4,800$$

5. Simplify: Divide both sides of the equation by the number before the unknown X.

$$\frac{\overset{1}{\cancel{20}}X}{\underset{1}{\cancel{20}}} = \frac{\overset{240}{\cancel{4,800}}}{\underset{1}{\cancel{20}}}$$

$$X = 240$$

EXAMPLE 3 ▪

$$\frac{X}{160} = \frac{2.5}{80}$$

1. Cross-multiply: $\frac{X}{160} \diagdown\!\!\!\!\diagup \frac{2.5}{80}$

$$80 \times X = 2.5 \times 160$$

$$80X = 400$$

2. Simplify: $\frac{\overset{1}{\cancel{80}X}}{\underset{1}{\cancel{80}}} = \frac{\overset{5}{\cancel{400}}}{\underset{1}{\cancel{80}}}$

   $X = 5$

EXAMPLE 4 ■

$\frac{40}{100} = \frac{X}{2}$

1. Cross-multiply: $\frac{40}{100} \diagdown\!\!\!\!\!\diagup \frac{X}{2}$

2. Multiply terms: $100 \times X = 40 \times 2$

   $100X = 80$

3. Simplify the equation: $\frac{\overset{1}{\cancel{100}X}}{\underset{1}{\cancel{100}}} = \frac{\overset{}{\cancel{80}}}{\cancel{100}}$

   $X = 0.8$

Calculations that result in an amount less than 1 should be expressed as a decimal. Most medications are ordered and supplied in metric measure. Metric measure is a decimal-based system.

QUICK REVIEW

■ A *proportion* is an equation of two equal ratios. The ratios may be expressed as fractions.

   Example: $1 : 4 = X : 8$ or $\frac{1}{4} = \frac{X}{8}$

■ In a proportion, the product of the means equals the product of the extremes.

   Extremes

   Example: $1{:}4 \quad = \quad X{:}8$ Therefore, $4 \times X = 1 \times 8$

   Means

■ If two fractions are equal, their cross-products are equal. This operation is referred to as *cross-multiplying*.

   Example: $\frac{1}{4} \diagdown\!\!\!\!\!\diagup \frac{X}{8}$ Therefore, $4 \times X = 1 \times 8$, or $4X = 8$

■ Dividing each side of an equation by the same number produces an equivalent equation. This operation is referred to as *simplifying the equation*.

   Example: If $4X = 8$, then $\frac{4X}{4} = \frac{8}{4}$, and $X = 2$

Review Set 9

Find the value of X. Express answers as decimals rounded to two places.

1. $\frac{1,000}{2} = \frac{125}{X}$ _____

2. $\frac{500}{2} = \frac{250}{X}$ _____

3. $\frac{500}{1} = \frac{280}{X}$ _____

4. $\frac{0.5}{2} = \frac{250}{X}$ _____

5. $\frac{75}{1.5} = \frac{35}{X}$ _____

6. $\frac{40}{X} \times 12 = 60$ _____

7. $\frac{10}{X} \times 60 = 28$ _____

8. $\frac{2}{2,000} \times X = 0.5$ _____

9. $\frac{15}{500} \times X = 6$ _____

16. $\frac{60}{15} = \frac{125}{X}$ _____

10. $\frac{5}{X} = \frac{10}{21}$ _____

17. $\frac{60}{10} = \frac{100}{X}$ _____

11. $\frac{250}{1} = \frac{750}{X}$ _____

18. $\frac{80}{X} \times 60 = 20$ _____

12. $\frac{80}{5} = \frac{10}{X}$ _____

19. $\frac{X}{0.5} = \frac{6}{4}$ _____

13. $\frac{5}{20} = \frac{X}{40}$ _____

20. $\frac{5}{2.2} = \frac{X}{1}$ _____

14. $\frac{\frac{1}{100}}{1} = \frac{\frac{1}{150}}{X}$ _____

21. $\frac{\frac{1}{4}}{15} = \frac{X}{60}$ _____

15. $\frac{2.2}{X} = \frac{8.8}{5}$ _____

22. $\frac{25\%}{30\%} = \frac{5}{X}$ _____

23. In any group of 100 nurses, you would expect to find 45 nurses who will specialize in a particular field of nursing. In a class of 240 graduating nurses, how many would you expect to specialize? _____

24. Low-fat cheese has 48 calories per ounce. A client who is having his caloric intake measured has eaten $1\frac{1}{2}$ ounces of low-fat cheese. How many calories has he eaten? _____

25. If a patient receives 450 milligrams of a medication given evenly over 5.5 hours, how many milligrams does the patient receive per hour? _____

After completing these problems, see page 639 to check your answers.

FINDING THE PERCENTAGE OF A QUANTITY

An important computation that health care professionals use for dosage calculations is to find a given percentage or part of a quantity. *Percentage* is a term that describes a *part* of a whole quantity. A *known percent* determines the part in question. Said another way, the percentage (or part in question) is equal to some known percent multiplied by the whole quantity.

RULE

Percentage (Part) = Percent × Whole Quantity
To find a percentage or part of a whole quantity:

1. Change the percent to a decimal.

2. Multiply the decimal by the whole quantity.

EXAMPLE ■

A patient reports that he drank 75% of his 8 fluid ounce cup of coffee for breakfast. To record in his chart the amount he actually drank, you must determine what amount is 75% of 8 fluid ounces.

MATH TIP

In a mathematical expression, the word *"of"* means *"times"* and indicates that you should multiply.

To continue with the example:

Percentage (Part) = Percent × Whole Quantity

Let X represent the unknown.

1. Change 75% to a decimal: $75\% = \frac{75}{100} = .75. = 0.75$

2. Multiply 0.75 × 8 fluid ounces: X = 0.75 × 8 fluid ounces = 6 fluid ounces

Therefore, 75% of 8 fluid ounces is 6 fluid ounces.

QUICK REVIEW
- Percentage (Part) = Percent × Whole Quantity

  Example: What is 12% of 48? X = 12% × 48 = 0.12 × 48 = 5.76

Review Set 10

Perform the indicated operation; round decimals to hundredths place.

1. What is 0.25% of 520? _____

2. What is 5% of 95? _____

3. What is 40% of 140? _____

4. What is 0.7% of 62? _____

5. What is 3% of 889? _____

6. What is 20% of 75? _____

7. What is 4% of 20? _____

8. What is 7% of 34? _____

9. What is 15% of 250? _____

10. What is 75% of 150? _____

11. A patient has an order for an anti-infective in the amount of 500 milligrams by mouth twice a day for 10 days to treat pneumonia. He received a bottle of 20 pills. How many pills has this patient taken if he has used 40% of the 20 pills? _____

12. The patient is on oral fluid restrictions of 1,200 milliliters for a 24-hour period. For breakfast and lunch he has consumed 60% of the total fluid allowance. How many milliliters has he had? _____

13. A patient's hospital bill for surgery is $17,651.07. Her insurance company pays 80%. How much will the patient owe? _____

14. Table salt (sodium chloride) is 40% sodium by weight. If a box of salt weighs 18 ounces, how many ounces of sodium is in the box of salt? _____

15. A patient has an average daily intake of 3,500 calories. At breakfast she eats 20% of the total daily caloric allowance. How many calories did she ingest? _____

After completing these problems, see pages 639–640 to check your answers.

PRACTICE PROBLEMS—CHAPTER 2

Find the equivalent decimal, fraction, percent, and ratio forms. Reduce fractions and ratios to lowest terms; round decimals to hundredths and percents to the nearest whole number.

Decimal	Fraction	Percent	Ratio
1. _____	$\frac{2}{5}$	_____	_____
2. 0.05	_____	_____	_____
3. _____	_____	17%	_____
4. _____	_____	_____	1:4
5. _____	_____	6%	_____
6. _____	$\frac{1}{6}$	_____	_____
7. _____	_____	50%	_____
8. _____	_____	_____	1:100
9. 0.09	_____	_____	_____
10. _____	$\frac{3}{8}$	_____	_____
11. _____	_____	_____	2:3
12. _____	$\frac{1}{3}$	_____	_____
13. 0.52	_____	_____	_____
14. _____	_____	_____	9:20
15. _____	$\frac{6}{7}$	_____	_____
16. _____	_____	_____	3:10
17. _____	$\frac{1}{50}$	_____	_____
18. 0.6	_____	_____	_____
19. 0.04	_____	_____	_____
20. _____	_____	10%	_____

Convert as indicated.

21. 1:25 to a decimal _____

22. $\frac{10}{400}$ to a ratio _____

23. 0.075 to a percent _____

24. 17:34 to a fraction _____

25. 75% to a ratio _____

Perform the indicated operation. Round decimals to hundredths.

26. What is 35% of 750? _____

27. What is 7% of 52? _____

28. What is 8.2% of 24? _____

Identify the strongest solution in each of the following groups:

29. 1:40   1:400   1:4   _____

30. 1:10   1:200   1:50

Find the value of X in the following equations. Express your answers as decimals rounded to the nearest hundredth.

31. $\frac{20}{400} = \frac{X}{1,680}$ _____

32. $\frac{75}{X} = \frac{\frac{1}{300}}{4}$ _____

33. $\frac{X}{5} = \frac{3}{15}$ _____

34. $\frac{500}{250} = \frac{2.2}{X}$ _____

35. $\frac{0.6}{1.2} = \frac{X}{200}$ _____

36. $\frac{3}{9} = \frac{X}{117}$ _____

37. $\frac{\frac{1}{8}}{\frac{1}{3}} \times 2 = X$ _____

38. $\frac{X}{7} = \frac{12}{4}$ _____

39. $\frac{X}{8} = \frac{9}{0.6}$ _____

40. $\frac{0.4}{0.1} \times 22.5 = X$ _____

41. A portion of meat totaling 125 grams contains 20% protein and 5% fat. How many grams each of protein and fat does the meat contain? _____ protein _____ fat

42. The total points for a course in a nursing program is 308. A nursing student needs to achieve 75% of the total points to pass the semester. How many points are required to pass? _____

43. To work off 90 calories, Angie must walk for 27 minutes. How many minutes would she need to walk to work off 200 calories? _____

44. The doctor orders a record of the patient's fluid intake and output. The patient drinks 25% of a bowl of broth. How many milliliters of intake will be recorded if the bowl holds 200 milliliters?
_____

45. The recommended daily allowance (RDA) of a particular vitamin is 60 milligrams. If a multivitamin tablet claims to provide 45% of the RDA, how many milligrams of the particular vitamin would a patient receive from the multivitamin tablet? _____

46. A label on a dinner roll wrapper reads, "2.7 grams of fiber per $\frac{3}{4}$ ounce serving." If you eat $1\frac{1}{2}$ ounces of dinner rolls, how many grams of fiber will you consume? _____

47. A patient received an intravenous medication at a rate of 6.75 milligrams per minute. After 42 minutes, how much medication had she received? _____

48. A person weighed 130 pounds at his last doctor's office visit. At this visit the patient has lost 5% of his weight. How many pounds has the patient lost? _____

49. The cost of a certain medication is expected to decrease by 17% next year. If the cost is $12.56 now, how much would you expect it to cost at this time next year? _____

50. A patient is to be started on 150 milligrams of a medication that is then decreased by 10% of the original dose for each dose until he is receiving 75 milligrams. When he takes his 75 milligram dose, how many total doses will he have taken? HINT: Be sure to count his first (150 milligrams) and last (75 milligrams) doses. _____

After completing these problems, see page 640 to check your answers.

📝 Be sure to use the online software for additional practice!

SECTION 1 SELF-EVALUATION

Directions

1. Round decimals to two places, as needed.

2. Express fractions in lowest terms.

Section 1 Mathematics Review for Dosage Calculations

Multiply or divide by the power of 10 indicated. Draw an arrow to demonstrate movement of the decimal point.

1. $30.5 \div 10 =$ _____

2. $40.025 \times 100 =$ _____

3. $63 \div 100 =$ _____

4. $72.327 \times 10 =$ _____

Identify the least common denominator for the following sets of numbers.

5. $\frac{1}{6}, \frac{2}{3}, \frac{3}{4}$ _____

6. $\frac{2}{5}, \frac{3}{10}, \frac{3}{11}$ _____

Complete the operations indicated.

7. $\frac{1}{4} + \frac{2}{3} =$ _____

8. $\frac{6}{7} - \frac{1}{9} =$ _____

9. $1\frac{3}{5} \times \frac{5}{8} =$ _____

10. $\frac{3}{8} \div \frac{3}{4} =$ _____

11. $13.2 + 32.55 + 0.029 =$ _____

12. 20% of $0.09 =$ _____

13. $80.3 - 21.06 =$ _____

14. $0.3 \times 0.3 =$ _____

15. $1.5 \div 0.125 =$ _____

16. $\frac{1}{150} \div \frac{1}{100} =$ _____

Arrange in order from smallest to largest.

17. $\frac{1}{3}$ $\frac{1}{2}$ $\frac{1}{6}$ $\frac{1}{10}$ $\frac{1}{5}$ _____

18. $\frac{3}{4}$ $\frac{7}{8}$ $\frac{5}{6}$ $\frac{2}{3}$ $\frac{9}{10}$ _____

19. 0.25 0.125 0.3 0.009 0.1909 _____

20. 0.9% $\frac{1}{2}\%$ 50% 500% 100% _____

21. Identify the strongest solution of the following: $1:3$, $1:60$, $1:6$ _____

22. Identify the weakest solution of the following: $1:75$, $1:600$, $1:60$ _____

Convert as indicated.

23. $1:100$ to a decimal _____

24. 0.009 to a percent _____

25. $33\frac{1}{3}\%$ to a fraction _____

26. $\frac{5}{9}$ to a ratio _____

27. 0.05 to a fraction _____

28. $\frac{1}{2}\%$ to a ratio _____

29. $2:3$ to a fraction _____

30. $3:4$ to a percent _____

31. $\frac{2}{5}$ to a percent _____

32. $\frac{1}{6}$ to a decimal _____

Find the value of X in the following equations. Express your answers as decimals; round to the nearest hundredth.

33. $\frac{0.35}{1.3} \times 4.5 = X$ _____

34. $\frac{0.3}{2.6} = \frac{0.15}{X}$ _____

35. $\frac{1,500,000}{500,000} \times X = 7.5$ _____

36. $\frac{1:100}{1:4} \times 2,500 = X$ _____

37. $\frac{0.25}{0.125} \times 2 = X$ _____

38. $\frac{1,000,000}{600,000} \times 5 = X$ _____

39. In a drug study, it was determined that 4% of the participants developed the headache side effect. If there were 600 participants in the study, how many developed headaches? _____

40. You are employed in a health care clinic where each employee must work 25% of 8 major holidays. How many holidays will you expect to work?

41. If the cost of 1 roll of gauze is $0.69, what is the cost of $3\frac{1}{2}$ rolls? _____

42. To prepare a nutritional formula from frozen concentrate, you mix 3 cans of water to every 1 can of concentrate. How many cans of water will you need to prepare formula from 4 cans of concentrate? _____

43. If 1 centimeter equals $\frac{3}{8}$ inch, how many centimeters is a laceration that measures 3 inches? _____

Section 1 Board Examination Practice

To obtain licensure, you will be required to pass a board examination. The following problems represent a simulated version of the various types of computerized items on the NCLEX-RN (National Council Licensure Examination for Registered Nurses) and NCLEX-PN (National Council Licensure Examination for Practical Nurses) computerized exams. Whether you will be taking one of these board examinations or one from another licensure board, alternate test items such as these are good practice. The board examination may not utilize every alternate format question to evaluate dosage calculation skills, but items such as these help you to prepare for other content areas, too. For additional practice, go to the online practice software that accompanies this text to respond to more interactive test items, including those using the calculator tool.

44. NCLEX *Fill-in-the-Blank* Item

You are recording intake and output for your patient who is on fluid restrictions of 1,000 milliliters per day. During the last 24 hours, the patient has consumed $3\frac{1}{2}$ fluid ounces milk, 725 milliliters intravenous fluid, and 4 fluid ounces of juice with the potassium supplement. If 1 fluid ounce is equivalent to 30 milliliters, how many milliliters of liquids did the patient consume in 24 hours?

Answer: _____

45. NCLEX *Multiple-Choice One-Response* Item

An infant requires 3.5 fluid ounces of formula per day for each kilogram of body weight. The infant weighs 6.6 kilograms. How much formula does the infant need? (Express the answer rounded to one decimal place. Place a check mark beside the correct answer.)

Answer:

a. 23 fluid ounces _____

b. 23.1 fluid ounces _____

c. 26.4 fluid ounces _____

d. 35 fluid ounces _____

e. 42 fluid ounces _____

46. NCLEX *Fill-in-the-Blank* Item

A child weighs 39 pounds. If each kilogram is equivalent to 2.2 pounds, what is the child's weight in kilograms? (Express the answer rounded to one decimal place.)

Answer: _____ kilograms

47. NCLEX *Exhibit* Item

Use the information in the table to determine which is the largest amount of fluid. (Place a check mark beside the correct answer.)

Answer:

a. Strawberry gelatin _____

b. Orange juice _____

c. Intravenous fluid _____

d. Milk _____

Fluid	Milliliters
Orange juice	25.25
Strawberry gelatin	30
Milk	120
Intravenous fluid	25.5

48. NCLEX *Drag-and-Drop / Ordered-Response* Item

Simulate the drag-and-drop computer response by copying the amounts from the box onto the list in ascending order from smallest to largest.

Answer:

0.05
5
2.5
2.25
5.075
0.175
0.049

_____
_____
_____
_____
_____
_____
_____

49. NCLEX *Multiple-Response* Item

Which of the following amounts are greater than 2.05? (Place a check mark beside all that apply.)

a. 0.26 _____   d. 2.06 _____

b. 2.104 _____   e. 2.4 _____

c. 2.006 _____

50. NCLEX *Hot Box* Item

Place an X in the box that contains the amount that is written using safe decimal notation.

.913	0.913
0.9130	9.130

After completing these problems, see page 641 to check your answers. Give yourself 2 points for each correct answer.

Perfect score = 100   My score = _____

Minimum mastery score = 86 (43 correct)

For more practice, go back to the beginning of this section and repeat the Mathematics Diagnostic Evaluation.

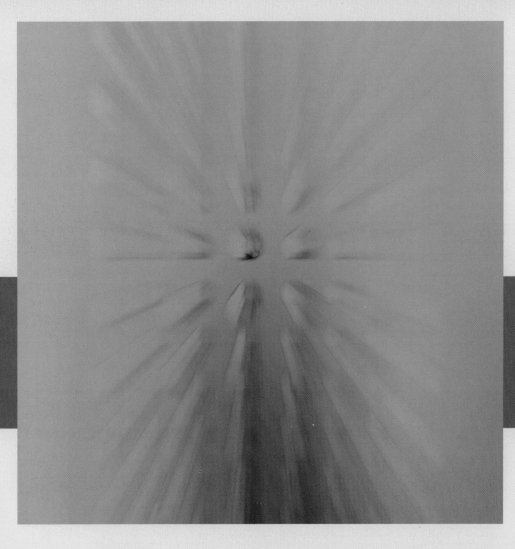

Measurement Systems, Drug Orders, and Drug Labels

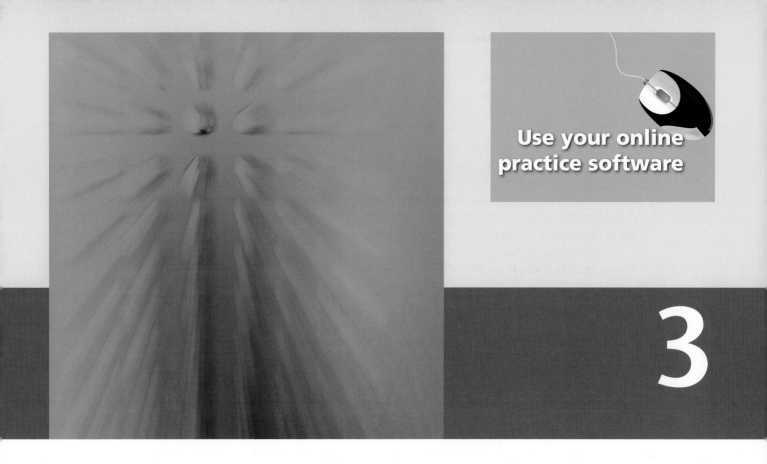

3

Systems of Measurement

OBJECTIVES

Upon mastery of Chapter 3, you will be able to recognize and express the basic systems of measurement used to calculate dosages. To accomplish this, you will also be able to:

- Differentiate metric, apothecary, and household systems of measurement.
- Recall metric and household notation and equivalents.
- Explain the use of milliequivalent (mEq), international unit, unit, and milliunit in dosage calculation.

To administer the correct amount of the prescribed medication to the patient, you must have a thorough knowledge of the measurement systems used to prescribe, measure, and administer medications. Metric is the preferred system of measurement in health care. The household system is still in use in home care. Because metric measure is the universal and international system, let's first concentrate on the metric system.

METRIC SYSTEM

All prescriptions should be written in the metric system, and all U.S. Food and Drug Administration (FDA) approved prescription drug labels provide metric dosage. The metric system was first adopted in 1799 in France. It is the most widely used system of measurement in the world. It is preferred for prescribing, measuring, and recording the administration of medications because, as a decimal system, it is the most precise. It is based on powers of 10 with three base units: gram, liter, and meter.

Three essential parameters of measurement are associated with the prescription and administration of medications: weight, volume, and length. Weight is the most utilized parameter. It is important as a dosage unit. The metric base unit of weight is the *gram* (g).

Think of capacity or how much a container holds as you contemplate volume, which is the next most important parameter. Volume usually refers to liquids. Volume also adds two additional parameters to dosage calculations: quantity and concentration. Quantity defines the amount, and concentration describes the strength, of a solution. The *liter* (L) is the metric base unit for volume, and the *milliliter* (mL) is the most common metric volume unit for dosage calculations.

Length is the least utilized parameter for dosage calculations, but linear measurement is still important in health care. A person's height, the circumference of an infant's head, body surface area, length of an amount of ointment, and the size of lacerations and tumors are examples of important length measurements. The metric length base unit is the *meter* (m). Most length measurements in health care are *millimeters* (mm) and *centimeters* (cm).

In the metric system, prefixes are used to show which portion of the base unit is being considered. It is important that you learn the most commonly used prefixes for health care.

REMEMBER

Metric Prefixes

micro	=	one millionth or 0.000001 or $\frac{1}{1,000,000}$ of the base unit
milli	=	one thousandth or 0.001 or $\frac{1}{1,000}$ of the base unit
centi	=	one hundredth or 0.01 or $\frac{1}{100}$ of the base unit
deci	=	one tenth or 0.1 or $\frac{1}{10}$ of the base unit
kilo	=	one thousand or 1,000 times the base unit

Figure 3-1 demonstrates the relationship of metric units. Notice that the values of most of the common prefixes used in health care and the ones applied in this text are highlighted in red: **kilo-, base, milli-,** and **micro-.** These units are three places away from the next place. Often you can either multiply or divide by 1,000 to calculate an equivalent quantity. The only exception is **centi-,** which is also highlighted. Centi- is easy to remember, though, if you think of the relationship between one cent and one U.S. dollar as a clue to the relationship of centi- to the base, $\frac{1}{100}$. **Deci-** is one-tenth $\left(\frac{1}{10}\right)$ of the base. See Chapter 1 to review the rules of multiplying and dividing decimals by a power of 10.

MATH TIP

Try this to remember the order of six of the metric units—**k**ilo-, **h**ecto-, **d**eca-, (BASE), **d**eci-, **c**enti-, and **m**illi-: "**K**ing **H**enry **D**ied from a **D**isease **C**alled **M**umps."

			gram			
			liter			
			meter			
kilo	hecto	deca	BASE	deci	centi	milli
K	**H**	**D**	**Δ**	**D**	**C**	**M**
"King	Henry	Died	from a	Disease	Called	Mumps."

The international standardization of metric units was adopted throughout much of the world in 1960 with the International System of Units, or SI (from the French *Système International*). The abbreviations of this system of metric notation are the most widely accepted. The metric units of measurement and the SI abbreviations most often used for dosage calculations and measurements of health status are given in the following units of weight, volume, and length. This text uses SI standardized abbreviations throughout. Learn and practice these notations.

FIGURE 3-1 Relationship and value of metric units, with comparison of common metric units used in health care

Prefix	Kilo-	Hecto-	Deca-	BASE	Deci-	Centi-	Milli-	Decimilli-	Centimilli-	Micro-
Weight	kilogram			gram			milligram			microgram
Volume				liter	deciliter		milliliter			
Length				meter		centimeter	millimeter			
Value to Base	1,000	100	10	1	0.1	0.01	0.001	0.0001	0.00001	0.000001

REMEMBER

SI METRIC SYSTEM

	Unit	Abbreviation	Equivalents
Weight	**gram** (base unit)	g	**1 g** = 1,000 mg = 1,000,000 mcg
	milligram	mg	0.001 g = **1 mg** = 1,000 mcg
	microgram	mcg	0.000001 g = 0.001 mg = **1 mcg**
	kilogram	kg	**1 kg** = 1,000 g
Volume	**liter** (base unit)	L	**1 L** = 1,000 mL
	deciliter	dL	0.1 L = **1 dL**
	milliliter	mL	0.001 L = **1 mL**
Length	**meter** (base unit)	m	**1 m** = 100 cm =1,000 mm
	centimeter	cm	0.01 m = **1 cm** = 10 mm
	millimeter	mm	0.001 m = 0.1 cm = **1 mm**

CAUTION

You may see gram abbreviated as Gm or gm, liter as lowercase l, milliliter as ml, or microgram as µg. These abbreviations are considered obsolete or too easily misinterpreted, and should be avoided. You should only use the standardized SI abbreviations. Use g for gram, L for liter, and mL for milliliter. Further, the unit of measurement *cubic centimeter*, abbreviated cc, has been used interchangeably with mL. The use of cc for mL is now prohibited by many health care organizations because cc can be mistaken for zeros (00) or units (U). The abbreviation U is also now prohibited and must be spelled out (unit).

CAUTION

The SI abbreviations for milligram (mg) and milliliter (mL) appear to be somewhat similar, but in fact mg is a weight unit and mL is a volume unit. Confusing these two units can have dire consequences in dosage calculations. Learn now to clearly differentiate them.

In addition to learning the metric units, their equivalent values, and their abbreviations, it is important to use the following rules of metric notation.

RULES

The following 10 critical rules will help to ensure that you accurately write and interpret metric notation.

1. The unit or abbreviation always follows the amount. Example: *5 g* NOT *g 5*

2. Do not put a period after the unit abbreviation, because it may be mistaken for the number 1 if poorly written. Example: *20 mg* NOT *20 mg.*

3. Do not add an s to make the unit plural, because it may be misread for another unit. Example: *5 mL* NOT *5 mLs*

4. Separate the amount from the unit so the number and unit of measure do not run together, because the unit can be mistaken as zero or zeros, risking a 10-fold to 100-fold overdose. Example: *20 mg* NOT *20mg*

5. Place commas for amounts at or above 1,000. Example: *10,000 mcg* NOT *10000 mcg*

6. Decimals are used to designate fractional amounts. Example: *1.5 mL* NOT *1½ mL*

7. Use a leading zero to emphasize the decimal point for fractional amounts less than 1. Without the zero, the amount may be interpreted as a whole number, resulting in serious overdosing. Example: *0.5 mg* NOT *.5 mg*

8. Omit unnecessary or trailing zeros that can be misread as part of the amount if the decimal point is not seen. Example: *1.5 mg* NOT *1.50 mg*

9. Do not use the abbreviation *μg* for microgram, because it might be mistaken for mg, which is 1,000 times the intended amount. Example: *150 mcg* NOT *150 μg*

10. Do not use the abbreviation cc for mL, because the unit can be mistaken for zeros. Example: *500 mL* NOT *500 cc*

Always ask the writer to clarify if you are not sure of the abbreviation or notation used. Never guess!

The metric system is the most common and the only standardized system of measurement in health care. Take a few minutes to review the following essential points.

QUICK REVIEW

- The metric base units are gram (g), liter (L), and meter (m).

- Subunits are designated by the appropriate prefix and the base unit (such as milligram) and standard abbreviations (such as mg).

- There are 10 critical rules for ensuring that units and amounts are accurately interpreted. Review them again now, and learn to rigorously adhere to them.

- Never guess as to the meaning of metric notation. When in doubt about the exact amount or the abbreviation used, ask the writer to clarify.

Review Set 11

1. The system of measurement most commonly used for prescribing and administering medications is the _____ system.

2. Liter and milliliter are metric units that measure _____.

3. Gram and milligram are metric units that measure _____.

4. Meter and millimeter are metric units that measure _____.

5. 1 mg is _____ of a g.

6. There are _____ mL in a liter.

7. Which is smaller—milligram or microgram? _____

8. Which is the largest—kilogram, gram, or milligram? _____

9. Which is the smallest—kilogram, gram, or milligram? _____

10. 1 liter = _____ mL

11. 1,000 mcg = _____ mg

12. 1 kg = _____ g

13. 1 cm = _____ mm

Select the correctly written metric notation.

14. .3 g, 0.3 Gm, 0.3 g, .3 Gm, 0.30 g   _____

15. $1\frac{1}{3}$ mL, 1.33 mL, 1.33 ML, $1\frac{1}{3}$ ML, 1.330 mL   _____

16. 5 Kg, 5.0 kg, kg 05, 5 kg, 5 kG   _____

17. 1.5 mm, $1\frac{1}{2}$ mm, 1.5 Mm, 1.50 MM, $1\frac{1}{2}$ MM   _____

18. mg 10, 10 mG, 10.0 mg, 10 mg, 10 MG   _____

Interpret these metric abbreviations.

19. mcg   _____   23. mm   _____

20. mL   _____   24. kg   _____

21. mg   _____   25. cm   _____

22. g   _____

After completing these problems, see page 641 to check your answers.

APOTHECARY AND HOUSEHOLD SYSTEMS

Apothecary and household measures are most prevalent in home care settings but began to disappear from hospitals and other health care organizations in the 1950s. The historic interconnection between these systems is interesting. The ancient apothecary system was the first system of medication measurement used by apothecaries (pharmacists) and physicians. It originated in Greece and made its way to Europe. The English used it during the late 1600s, and the colonists brought it to America. A modified system of measurement for everyday use evolved; it is now recognized as the household system. Large liquid volumes were based on familiar trading measurements—such as pints, quarts, and gallons—which originated as apothecary measurements. Vessels to accommodate each measurement were made by craftspersons and widely circulated in colonial America. Likewise, units of weight (such as grain, ounce, and pound) are rooted in apothecary. The grain originated as the standard weight of a single grain of wheat.

The Institute for Safe Medication Practices (2013) discourages the use of apothecary units and symbols, such as minims (♍), drams (℥), ounces (℥), and grains (gr). But remnants of this system are still evident in health care. After more than 100 years as the world's most popular pill, 5 grains of aspirin is now labeled in the metric equivalent of 325 milligrams. Drams and ounces still appear on some disposable medicine cups along with the metric equivalent, and some 3 mL syringes still show minims (see Chapter 6). Further, it was customary to express apothecary amounts using lowercase Roman numerals and to write the amount after the unit of measure. Oddly, the lowercase Roman numeral also had a horizontal line over it. Some physicians continue to write amounts using apothecary notation, as in the following examples.

EXAMPLES ■

give iii *tablets*   Meaning: "Give 3 tablets"

give grains v̄ *aspirin*   Meaning: "Give a 5 grain aspirin tablet"

While measurement in grains is disappearing from medication labels and physician orders, some medication labels may still include both apothecary and metric measure. Let's compare an older label for morphine sulfate (Figure 3-2) that includes both the apothecary measure in *grains* and metric measure in *milligrams* with a current label for the same drug measured in *milligrams* only (Figure 3-3).

FIGURE 3-2 Morphine sulfate 10 mg/mL (1/8 gr/mL)

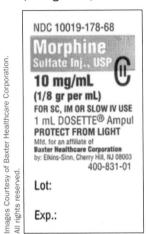

FIGURE 3-3 Morphine sulfate 10 mg/mL

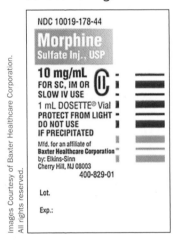

FIGURE 3-4 Nitrostat 0.4 mg (1/150 gr)

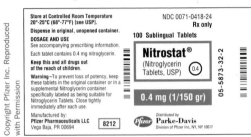

And notice the apothecary measure on the Nitrostat (nitroglycerin) label (Figure 3-4). The information on the label also tells you that $\frac{1}{150}$ gr is equivalent to *0.4 mg*. You can see how the grain abbreviation can easily be misread and confused with gram. It is apparent why The Institute for Safe Medication Practices (2013) strongly discourages the use of apothecary measure, to prevent medication errors. It is the metric measurement on these labels that you will need to identify for dosage calculations.

CAUTION

The following apothecary units and symbols may appear on some labels, syringes, and medicine cups, or may be written as shorthand by older practitioners. Because they are considered obsolete, do not use these symbols, and be careful to differentiate them from acceptable units of measure. They are provided here for recognition purposes only, but they can easily be misinterpreted and lead to a medication error. **If you receive a written order using one of these symbols or abbreviations, be safe and ask for clarification.**

DO NOT USE THESE SYMBOLS OR ABBREVIATIONS:

gr   **grain**: apothecary unit of weight, approximately 60 mg; easily confused with metric *gram*

ɱ   **minim**: apothecary drop, approximately 16 minims per mL

ʒ   **dram**: apothecary symbol for amount that is slightly less than a teaspoon, approximately 4 mL

℥   **ounce**: apothecary symbol for fluid ounce, approximately 30 mL

ss   **one-half**: apothecary symbol for $\frac{1}{2}$

See Appendix B for a comparison of apothecary units and their metric equivalents.

The following household units are likely to be used by the patient at home where metric measuring devices may not be available. They are important for discharge teaching when advising patients and their families about take-home prescriptions. We will consider the metric equivalents of these units in Chapter 4. Unlike the more precise metric system, fractional amounts in the household system are expressed as common fractions (rather than decimals), such as $\frac{1}{2}$ or $\frac{3}{4}$.

REMEMBER

HOUSEHOLD SYSTEM

Unit	Abbreviation	Equivalents
teaspoon	t (or tsp)	
tablespoon	T (or tbs)	1 T = 3 t
ounce (fluid)	fl oz	1 fl oz = 2 T
cup	cup	1 cup = 8 fl oz
pint	pt	1 pt = 2 cups = 16 fl oz
quart	qt	1 qt = 2 pt = 4 cups = 32 fl oz
ounce (weight)	oz	16 oz = 1 lb
pound	lb	

MATH TIP

When comparing the tablespoon and the teaspoon, the tablespoon is the larger unit, and its abbreviation is expressed with a capital, or "large," T. The teaspoon is the smaller unit, and its abbreviation is expressed with a lowercase, or "small," t.

CAUTION

Although some households may use metric measure, many do not, especially in the United States. There can be a wide variation in household measuring devices, such as in tableware teaspoons, which can constitute a safety risk. Talking to your patients and their families about administering medications at home is an excellent teaching opportunity. Determine their familiarity with metric units, such as milliliters, and ask what kind of medicine measuring devices they use at home. It is best to advise your patients and their families to use the measuring devices packaged with the medication or provided by the pharmacy.

OTHER COMMON DRUG MEASUREMENTS: UNITS AND MILLIEQUIVALENTS

Four other measurements may be used to indicate the quantity of medicine prescribed: international unit, unit, milliunit, and milliequivalent (mEq). The quantity is expressed in Arabic numbers with the unit of measure following. The *international unit* represents a unit of potency used to measure such things as vitamins and chemicals. The *unit* is a standardized amount needed to produce a desired effect. Medications such as penicillin, heparin, and insulin have their own meaning and numeric value related to the type of unit. One thousandth $\left(\frac{1}{1,000}\right)$ of a unit is a *milliunit*. The equivalent of 1 unit is 1,000 milliunits. Oxytocin is a drug measured in milliunits. The *milliequivalent* (mEq) is one thousandth $\left(\frac{1}{1,000}\right)$ of an equivalent weight of a chemical. The mEq is the unit used when referring to the concentration of serum electrolytes, such as calcium, magnesium, potassium, and sodium.

CAUTION

The abbreviations *U* and *IU* are included on the *Official "Do Not Use" List* published by The Joint Commission (2013). The written words *unit* and *international unit* should be used instead, because the abbreviations are considered obsolete and too easily misinterpreted for safe practice. See Chapter 9 for the full *Official "Do Not Use" List*.

It is not necessary to learn conversions for the international unit, unit, or milliequivalent, because medications prescribed in these measurements are also prepared and administered in the same system.

EXAMPLE 1 ▪

Heparin *800* units is ordered, and *heparin 1,000 units per 1 mL* is the stock drug.

Because there is no standard metric equivalent for units, when a medication is ordered in units (such as heparin), the stock drug should be supplied in units.

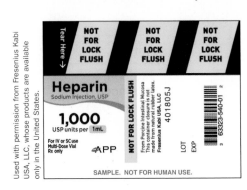

EXAMPLE 2 ▪

Potassium chloride *10* mEq is ordered, and *potassium chloride 20 mEq per 15 mL* is the stock drug.

Because there is no standard metric equivalent for mEq, when a medication is ordered in mEq (such as potassium chloride), the stock drug should be supplied in mEq.

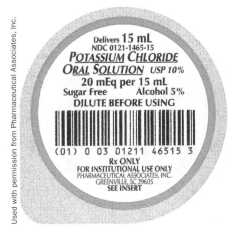

EXAMPLE 3 ▪

Oxytocin *2* milliunits (*0.002* USP units) intravenous per minute is ordered, and *oxytocin 10 usp units per 1 mL* to be added to 1,000 mL intravenous solution is available. Very small doses of a medication (such as oxytocin) may be ordered in milliunits. Remember, the prefix milli- means one thousandth. Sometimes converting from units to milliunits is necessary.

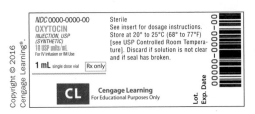

QUICK REVIEW

- Some symbols and abbreviations are obsolete or can lead to medication errors. If you come across these symbols, ask the writer to clarify. Do not use: gr, ɱ, ʒ, ʒ, I, ml, cc, U, or IU.

- Household measurement was developed from the ancient apothecary system. Household units are most frequently used in home care: **t**, T, fl oz, cup, pt, qt, and lb.

- Fractional amounts in the household system are expressed as common fractions.

- No conversion is necessary for unit, international unit, and mEq, because the ordered dosage and supply dosage are in the same system.

- 1 unit = 1,000 milliunits

Review Set 12

Interpret the following notations.

1. 3 qt _____

2. 10 lb _____

3. 10 mEq _____

4. $2\frac{1}{2}$ lb _____

5. 10 T _____

Express the following using medical notation.

6. seventy-five pounds   _____

7. thirty milliequivalents   _____

8. five tablespoons   _____

9. one and one-half teaspoons   _____

10. fourteen units   _____

11. True or False? The household system of measurement is commonly used in hospital dosage calculations. _____

12. True or False? 1,000 mcg = 1 g _____

13. True or False? 1 kg = 1,000 g _____

14. Drugs such as heparin and insulin are commonly measured in _____.

15. 1 T =   _____ t

16. 1 fl oz =   _____ T

17. 16 oz =   _____ lb

18. 2 pt =   _____ qt

19. 8 fl oz =   _____ cup

20. The unit used to measure the concentration of serum electrolytes (such as calcium, magnesium, potassium, and sodium) is the _____ and is abbreviated _____.

After completing these problems, see page 641 to check your answers.

CLINICAL REASONING SKILLS

The importance of the placement of the decimal point cannot be overemphasized. Let's look at some examples of potential medication errors related to placement of the decimal point.

ERROR

Not placing a zero before a decimal point in medication orders

Possible Scenario

An emergency room physician wrote an order for the bronchodilator terbutaline for a patient with asthma. The order was written as follows.

Incorrectly Written

Terbutaline .5 mg subcutaneously now, repeat dose in 30 minutes if no improvement

Suppose the nurse, not noticing the faint decimal point, administered 5 mg of terbutaline subcutaneously instead of 0.5 mg. The patient would receive ten times the dose intended by the physician.

Potential Outcome

Within minutes of receiving the injection, the patient would likely complain of headache and develop tachycardia, nausea, and vomiting. The patient's hospital stay would be lengthened because of the need to recover from the overdose.

Prevention

This type of medication error is avoided by remembering the rule to place a 0 in front of a decimal to avoid confusion regarding the dosage: **0**.5 mg. Further, remember to question orders that are unclear or seem unsafe or impractical.

Correctly Written

Terbutaline 0.5 mg subcutaneously now, repeat dose in 30 minutes if no improvement

CLINICAL REASONING SKILLS

Many medication errors occur by confusing mg and mL. Remember that mg is the weight of the medication and mL is the volume of the medication preparation.

ERROR

Confusing mg and mL

Possible Scenario

Suppose a physician ordered the steroid prednisolone syrup 15 mg by mouth twice a day for a patient with cancer. Prednisolone syrup is supplied in a concentration of 15 mg in 5 mL. The pharmacist supplied a bottle of prednisolone containing a total volume of 240 mL with 15 mg of prednisolone in every 5 mL. The nurse, in a rush to give her medications on time, misread the order as 15 mL and gave the patient 15 mL of prednisolone instead of 5 mL. Therefore, the patient received 45 mg of prednisolone, or three times the correct dosage.

Potential Outcome

The patient could develop a number of complications related to a high dosage of steroids: gastrointestinal bleeding, hyperglycemia, hypertension, agitation, and severe mood disturbances, to name a few.

Prevention

The mg is the weight of a medication, and mL is the volume you prepare. Do not allow yourself to get rushed or distracted so that you confuse milligrams with milliliters. When you know you are distracted or stressed, have another nurse double-check the calculation of the dose.

PRACTICE PROBLEMS—CHAPTER 3

Give the metric prefix for the following parts of the base units.

1. 0.001 _____   3. 0.01 _____

2. 0.000001 _____   4. 1,000 _____

Identify the equivalent unit with a value of 1 that is indicated by the following amounts (such as 1 unit = 1,000 milliunits).

5. 0.001 gram   _____   7. 0.001 milligram _____

6. 1,000 grams   _____   8. 0.01 meter   _____

Identify the metric base unit for the following.

9. length   _____   11. volume   _____

10. weight   _____

Interpret the following notations.

12. fl oz   _____   21. pt   _____

13. oz   _____   22. T   _____

14. mg   _____   23. mm   _____

15. mcg   _____   24. g   _____

16. lb   _____   25. cm   _____

17. mEq   _____   26. L   _____

18. t   _____   27. m   _____

19. qt   _____   28. kg   _____

20. mL   _____   29. lb   _____

Express the following amounts in proper notation.

30. three hundred and twenty-five micrograms   _____

31. one-half teaspoon   _____

32. two teaspoons   _____

33. one-third fluid ounce   _____

34. five million units   _____

35. one-half liter   _____

36. five hundredths of a milligram   _____

37. six hundred milliliters   _____

38. two and five-tenths centimeters   _____

39. eight hundredths of a milliliter   _____

40. five and five-tenths kilograms   _____

Express the following numeric amounts in words.

41. $8\frac{1}{4}$ fl oz   _____

42. 375 g   _____

43. 0.5 kg   _____

44. 2.6 mL   _____

45. 20 mEq   _____

46. 0.4 L   _____

47. 3.05 mcg   _____

48. 0.17 mg   _____

49. $14\frac{1}{2}$ lb   _____

50. Describe the clinical reasoning that you would use to prevent the medication error.

Possible Scenario

Suppose a physician ordered oral Coumadin (warfarin), an anticoagulant, for a patient with a history of deep vein thrombosis. The physician wrote an order for 10 mg but while writing the order placed a decimal point after the 10 and added a 0:

Incorrectly Written

Coumadin 10.0 mg orally once per day

Coumadin 10.0 mg was transcribed on the medication record as Coumadin 100 mg. The patient received ten times the correct dosage.

Potential Outcome

The patient would likely begin hemorrhaging. An antidote, such as vitamin K, would be necessary to reverse the effects of the overdose. However, it is important to remember that not all drugs have antidotes.

Prevention

_____

_____

51. **BONUS:** Describe the strategy that would prevent this medication error.

Possible Scenario

Suppose a physician ordered oral codeine, a narcotic analgesic, for an adult patient recovering from nasal surgery. The physician wrote the following order for one grain of codeine (approximately equivalent to 60 mg). The gr smeared, and the abbreviation of i gr is now unclear. Is it *grains* or *grams*?

Physician's Apothecary Order

Codeine i gr orally every 4 hours as needed for pain

Codeine 1 gram was transcribed on the medication record. Because 1 gram is equivalent to 1,000 mg or about 15 grains, this erroneous dosage is about 15 times more than the intended amount.

Potential Outcome

The maximum dosage of codeine is 60 mg every 4 to 6 hours, not to exceed 360 mg per day. If the nurse had administered the transcribed dosage, the patient could have experienced acute intoxication resulting in violent GI tract symptoms, abdominal pain, burning of the throat, rapid and weak pulse, CNS depression, respiratory paralysis, and even death, depending on the fragility of the patient's prior status.

Prevention

_____

_____

_____

After completing these problems, see pages 641–642 to check your answers.

Be sure to use the online software for additional practice!

REFERENCES

The Institute for Safe Medication Practices. (2013). Medication safety alert February 2013 issue. Retrieved from http://www.ismp.org/newsletters/ambulatory/archives/201302.asp

The Joint Commission. (2013). Facts about the *Official "Do Not Use" List*. Retrieved from http://www.jointcommission.org/assets/1/18/Do_Not_Use_List.pdf

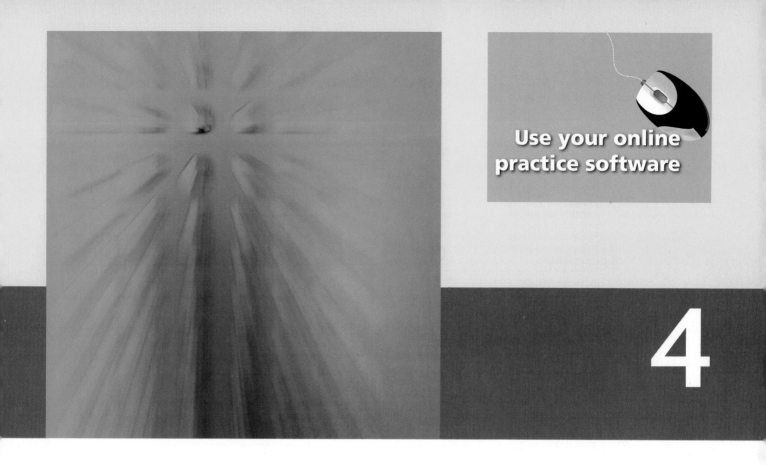

4

Conversions: Metric and Household Systems

OBJECTIVES

Upon mastery of Chapter 4, you will be able to complete Step 1, Conversion, in the Three-Step Approach to dosage calculations. To accomplish this, you will also be able to:

■ Recall from memory the metric and household approximate equivalents.

■ Convert among units of measurement within the same system.

■ Convert units of measurement from one system to another.

Medications are usually prescribed or ordered in a unit of weight measurement such as grams or milligrams. The nurse must interpret this order and administer the correct number of tablets, capsules, teaspoons, milliliters, or some other unit of volume or capacity measurement to deliver the prescribed amount of medication.

EXAMPLE 1 ■

A prescription notation may read:

Aldactone 100 mg to be given orally twice a day

The nurse has on hand a 100 tablet bottle of *Aldactone* labeled *50 mg in each tablet*. To administer the correct amount of the drug, the nurse must calculate the prescribed weight of 100 mg to the correct number of tablets. In this case, the nurse gives the patient two of the 50 mg tablets, which equals *100 mg of Aldactone.* To give the prescribed dosage, the nurse must be able to calculate the order in weight to the correct number of tablets of the drug on hand or in stock. THINK: if one tablet equals 50 mg, then two tablets equal 100 mg.

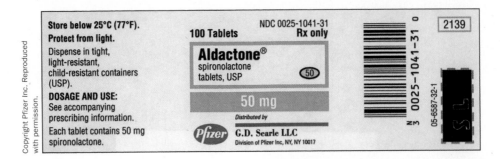

EXAMPLE 2 ■

A prescription notation may read:

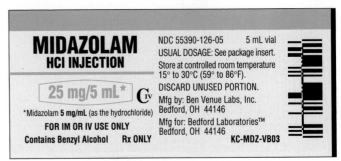

Used with permission from Bedford Laboratories.

midazolam HCl 2.5 mg by intravenous injection immediately

The nurse has on hand a vial of *midazolam HCl* labeled *25 mg per 5 mL* or *5 mg/mL*. To administer the correct amount of the drug, the nurse must be able to fill the injection syringe with the correct number of milliliters. As the nurse, how many milliliters would you give? THINK: if 5 mg = 1 mL, then 2.5 mg = 0.5 mL. Therefore, 0.5 mL should be administered.

IDENTIFYING NEED FOR UNIT CONVERSION

Sometimes a drug order may be written in a unit of measurement that is different from the supply of drugs the nurse has on hand. Usually this will be an order for a medicine that is written in one size of metric unit (such as milligrams) but where the medicine is supplied in another metric unit (such as grams). You will occasionally encounter a medicine ordered in household or apothecary measure (such as fluid ounces). However, the drug will be supplied in metric measure (such as milliliters). The Institute for Safe Medication Practices (2013) discourages the use of apothecary measure; but until it is prohibited, you may still see it in use. Therefore, we will consider examples of conversion within the metric system and between other systems. Converting a unit of measure does not change the amount of the ordered dosage of medication, but provides an equal but alternate expression of the dosage. Let's look at examples of medicines ordered and supplied in both different size units and different systems of measurement.

EXAMPLE 1 ■

Medication order: triazolam 250 mcg orally at bedtime

Supply on hand: Halcion 0.25 mg tablets

The drug order is written in micrograms, but the drug is supplied in milligrams.

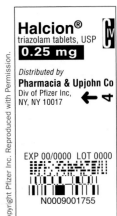

EXAMPLE 2 ■

Medication order: Antacid Plus $\frac{1}{2}$ fl oz after meals

Supply on hand: Antacid Plus 1 fl oz (30 mL)

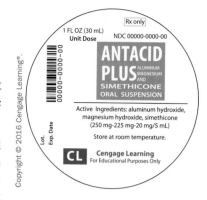

The drug order is written in fluid ounces (household measure), but the drug is supplied in a form that measures both milliliters (metric measure) and fluid ounces (household measure).

   In the first example, the prescribed quantity must be converted into the unit of measure as supplied. The nurse or other health care professional can then calculate the correct dosage to prepare and administer to the patient. But in this second example, the nurse must take care to select the correct unit of measure from the two options provided on the label before calculating the ordered dose. Thus, determining the need for and calculating unit conversions are the first steps in dosage calculations.

CONVERTING FROM ONE UNIT TO ANOTHER USING RATIO-PROPORTION

After learning the systems of measurement common for dosage calculations and their equivalents (Chapter 3), the next step is to learn how to use them. First, you must be able to convert or change from one unit to another within the same measurement system. A method of performing conversions is to set up a proportion of two ratios expressed as fractions. Refer to Chapter 2 to review ratio-proportion, if needed.

RULE

In a proportion, the ratio for a known equivalent equals the ratio for an unknown equivalent. To use ratio-proportion to convert from one unit to another, you need to follow these three steps.

1. Recall the equivalents.

2. Set up a proportion of two equivalent ratios.

3. Cross-multiply to solve for an unknown quantity, X.

   Each ratio in a proportion must have the same relationship and follow the same sequence. A proportion compares like things to like things. Be sure the units in the numerators match and the units in the denominators match. Label the units in each ratio.

   Let's look at how this works with units already familiar to you.

EXAMPLE 1 ■

How many cups are in 3 quarts?

1. What is the known equivalent that applies to this problem? You know it is 1 qt = 4 cups.

2. Now you are ready to set up a proportion of two equivalent ratios. The first ratio of the proportion contains the *known equivalent,* that is 1 quart : 4 cups. The second ratio contains the *desired unit of measure* and the *unknown equivalent* expressed as X, that is 3 quarts : X cups. Express the ratios as fractions. The proportion now looks like this.

$$\frac{1 \text{ qt}}{4 \text{ cups}} = \frac{3 \text{ qt}}{\text{X cups}}$$

CAUTION

Notice that the ratios follow the same sequence. **THIS IS ESSENTIAL.** The proportion is set up so that like units are across from each other. The units in the numerators match (qt) and the units in the denominators match (cups).

3. Cross-multiply to solve the proportion for X. Refer to Chapter 2 to review this skill, if needed.

$$\frac{1 \text{ qt}}{4 \text{ cups}} \diagtimes \frac{3 \text{ qt}}{X \text{ cups}}$$ Cross-multiply

$$1 \times X = 4 \times 3$$

$$1X = 12$$

$$\frac{1X}{1} = \frac{12}{1}$$ Simplify: Divide both sides of the equation by the number before the unknown X.

$$X = 12 \text{ cups}$$ Label the units to match the unknown X.

You know the answer is in cups, because cups is the unknown equivalent. Therefore, 3 qt = 12 cups.

MATH TIP

Multiplying or dividing a number by 1 does not change its value. It is the same number.

Therefore in the previous example, it is not necessary to simplify, because $1X = X$. You can shorten the calculation. Look again at the math.

$$\frac{1 \text{ qt}}{4 \text{ cups}} \diagtimes \frac{3 \text{ qt}}{X \text{ cups}}$$ Cross-multiply

$$X = 4 \times 3$$

$$X = 12 \text{ cups}$$

In the next example the unknown X is in the numerator. It does not matter, as long as the sequence is the same (numerator units match and denominator units match). Remember, a proportion must compare like things to like things. In the first example, the unknown was cups. In the second example the unknown is quarts.

EXAMPLE 2 ▪

How many quarts are in 8 cups?

To solve this you also use the ratio-proportion rule.

1. Recall the known equivalent (1 qt = 4 cups).

2. Set up a proportion of two equivalent ratios.

3. Cross-multiply to solve for X.

$$\frac{1 \text{ qt}}{4 \text{ cups}} = \frac{X \text{ qt}}{8 \text{ cups}}$$

$$\frac{1 \text{ qt}}{4 \text{ cups}} \diagtimes \frac{X \text{ qt}}{8 \text{ cups}}$$ Cross-multiply

$$4X = 8$$

$$\frac{4X}{4} = \frac{8}{4}$$ Simplify: Divide both sides of the equation by the number before the unknown X.

$$X = 2 \text{ qt}$$ Label the units to match the unknown X.

CONVERTING WITHIN THE METRIC SYSTEM

The most common conversions in dosage calculations and health care are within the metric system. As you recall from Chapter 3, most metric conversions are simply derived by multiplying or dividing by 1,000. Recall from Chapter 1 that multiplying by 1,000 is the same as moving the decimal point three places to the right. Notice that in the following examples you are asked to find the equivalent amount of the smaller unit. It makes sense that the resulting number of smaller units would be greater than the original number of larger units. In this first example, you are converting grams to milligrams. Notice that the unknown X is in the denominator.

EXAMPLE 1 ■

Convert 2 grams to the equivalent number of milligrams.

1. Recall the known equivalent: 1 g = 1,000 mg.

2. Set up a proportion of two equivalent ratios.

3. Cross-multiply to solve for X.

$$\frac{1\ g}{1,000\ mg} = \frac{2\ g}{X\ mg}$$

$$\frac{1\ g}{1,000\ mg} \times \frac{2\ g}{X\ mg} \qquad \text{Cross-multiply}$$

$$X = 1,000 \times 2$$

$$X = 2,000\ mg \qquad \text{Label the units to match the unknown X.}$$

Thus, you know that a medicine container labeled 2 grams per tablet means the same as 2,000 milligrams per tablet.

MATH TIP

Notice that to multiply 2 by 1,000, you are moving the decimal three places to the right. This is a shortcut. Sometimes to complete this operation, you add zeros to hold the places equal to the number of zeros in the equivalent. In this case, 1 g = 1,000 mg, so you add three zeros: 2 × 1,000 = 2.000. = 2,000

EXAMPLE 2 ■

Convert: 0.3 mg to mcg

Equivalent: 1 mg = 1,000 mcg

$$\frac{1\ mg}{1,000\ mcg} = \frac{0.3\ mg}{X\ mcg}$$

$$\frac{1\ mg}{1,000\ mcg} \times \frac{0.3\ mg}{X\ mcg} \qquad \text{Cross-multiply}$$

$$X = 1,000 \times 0.3 \qquad \text{0.300. Move the decimal 3 places to the right to multiply by 1,000. Add zeros to complete the operation.}$$

$$X = 300\ mcg \qquad \text{Label the units to match the unknown X.}$$

EXAMPLE 3 ■

Convert: 2.5 g to mg

Equivalent: 1 g = 1,000 mg

$$\frac{1\ g}{1,000\ mg} = \frac{2.5\ g}{X\ mg}$$

$$\frac{1\ g}{1,000\ mg} \diagdown \frac{2.5\ g}{X\ mg}$$ Cross-multiply

$$X = 1,000 \times 2.5$$ 2.500. Move the decimal 3 places to the right to multiply by 1,000. Add zeros to complete the operation.

$$X = 2,500\ mg$$ Label the units to match the unknown X.

EXAMPLE 4 ■

Convert: 0.15 kg to g

Equivalent: 1 kg = 1,000 g

$$\frac{1\ kg}{1,000\ g} = \frac{0.15\ kg}{X\ g}$$

$$\frac{1\ kg}{1,000\ g} \diagdown \frac{0.15\ kg}{X\ g}$$ Cross-multiply

$$X = 1,000 \times 0.15$$ 0.150. Move the decimal 3 places to the right to multiply by 1,000. Add a zero to complete the operation.

$$X = 150\ g$$ Label the units to match the unknown X.

EXAMPLE 5 ■

Convert: 0.04 L to mL

Equivalent: 1 L = 1,000 mL

$$\frac{1\ L}{1,000\ mL} = \frac{0.04\ L}{X\ mL}$$

$$\frac{1\ L}{1,000\ mL} \diagdown \frac{0.04\ L}{X\ mL}$$ Cross-multiply

$$X = 1,000 \times 0.04$$ 0.040. Move the decimal 3 places to the right to multiply by 1,000. (1 zero is added to complete the operation.)

$$X = 40\ mL$$ Label the units to match the unknown X.

EXAMPLE 6 ■

Knowing how to do unit conversions is also helpful when conducting physical assessment. An infant's head circumference is 40.5 cm. How many millimeters does that equal?

Convert: 40.5 cm to mm

Equivalent: 1 cm = 10 mm

Notice the ratio is now 1:10, not 1:1,000. In this example you are multiplying by 10 (not 1,000), so you will move the decimal point 1 place to the right.

$$\frac{1 \text{ cm}}{10 \text{ mm}} = \frac{40.5 \text{ cm}}{X \text{ mm}}$$

$$\frac{1 \text{ cm}}{10 \text{ mm}} \diagdown\!\!\!\!\diagup \frac{40.5 \text{ cm}}{X \text{ mm}}$$ Cross-multiply

$$X = 10 \times 40.5$$ 40.5 Move the decimal 1 place to the right to multiply by 10.

$$X = 405 \text{ mm}$$ Label the units to match the unknown X.

Now let's consider conversions that go the opposite way—from a smaller unit (such as mL) to a larger unit (such as L). It makes sense that the resulting number of larger units will now be less than the original number of smaller units. In the next set of examples, notice that the unknown X is now in the numerator.

EXAMPLE 1 ▪

Convert: 5,000 mL to L

Equivalent: 1 L = 1,000 mL

$$\frac{1 \text{ L}}{1,000 \text{ mL}} = \frac{X \text{ L}}{5,000 \text{ mL}}$$

$$\frac{1 \text{ L}}{1,000 \text{ mL}} \diagdown\!\!\!\!\diagup \frac{X \text{ L}}{5,000 \text{ mL}}$$ Cross-multiply

$$1,000X = 5,000$$

$$\frac{1,000X}{1,000} = \frac{5,000}{1,000}$$ Simplify: Divide both sides of the equation by the number before the unknown X. The zeros cancel.

$$X = 5 \text{ L}$$ Label the units to match the unknown X.

MATH TIP
Let's look at the shortcut for dividing 5,000 by 1,000. Now you are moving the decimal three places to the left, and then eliminating unnecessary zeros. 5,000 ÷ 1,000 = 5.000. = 5

CAUTION
Leaving unnecessary zeros may lead to confusion and misinterpretation. For safety, the unnecessary zeros must be eliminated. Likewise, use a leading zero for emphasis of a decimal point when a decimal number is less than 1. Both of these cautions are demonstrated in the next example.

EXAMPLE 2 ▪

Convert: 500 mcg to mg

Equivalent: 1 mg = 1,000 mcg

$$\frac{1 \text{ mg}}{1{,}000 \text{ mcg}} = \frac{X \text{ mg}}{500 \text{ mcg}}$$

$$\frac{1 \text{ mg}}{1{,}000 \text{ mcg}} \diagdown \diagup \frac{X \text{ mg}}{500 \text{ mcg}}$$ Cross-multiply

$$1{,}000X = 500$$

$$\frac{1{,}000X}{1{,}000} = \frac{500}{1{,}000}$$ Simplify: Divide both sides of the equation by the number before the unknown X.

$$X = 0.5$$ 0.500. Move the decimal 3 places to the left to divide by 1,000. Eliminate unnecessary zeros. Because the amount is less than 1, use a leading zero for emphasis of the decimal point.

$$X = 0.5 \text{ mg}$$ Label the units to match the unknown X.

MATH TIP

Sometimes, to complete the operation, you must add zeros equal to the number of zeros in the equivalent to hold the places, as shown in Examples 3 and 4.

EXAMPLE 3 ▪

Convert: 20 mg to g

Equivalent: 1 g = 1,000 mg

$$\frac{1 \text{ g}}{1{,}000 \text{ mg}} = \frac{X \text{ g}}{20 \text{ mg}}$$

$$\frac{1 \text{ g}}{1{,}000 \text{ mg}} \diagdown \diagup \frac{X \text{ g}}{20 \text{ mg}}$$ Cross-multiply

$$1{,}000X = 20$$

$$\frac{1{,}000X}{1{,}000} = \frac{20}{1{,}000}$$ Simplify: Divide both sides of the equation by the number before the unknown X.

$$X = 0.02$$ 0.020. Move the decimal 3 places to the left to divide by 1,000. First you must add a zero to complete the operation. Then eliminate the unnecessary zero and use a leading zero for emphasis in your final answer.

$$X = 0.02 \text{ g}$$ Label the units to match the unknown X.

EXAMPLE 4 ▪

Convert: 5 g to kg

Equivalent: 1 kg = 1,000 g

$$\frac{1 \text{ kg}}{1,000 \text{ g}} = \frac{X \text{ kg}}{5 \text{ g}}$$

$$\frac{1 \text{ kg}}{1,000 \text{ g}} \bowtie \frac{X \text{ kg}}{5 \text{ g}}$$ Cross-multiply

$$1,000X = 5$$

$$\frac{1,000X}{1,000} = \frac{5}{1,000}$$ Simplify: Divide both sides of the equation by the number before the unknown X.

$$X = 0.005$$ 0.005. Move the decimal 3 places to the left after adding zeros to complete the operation. Use a leading zero for emphasis.

$$X = 0.005 \text{ kg}$$ Label the units to match the unknown X.

EXAMPLE 5 ▪

A patient's wound measures 31 millimeters. What does it measure in centimeters?

Convert: 31 mm to cm

Equivalent: 1 cm = 10 mm

Notice the ratio is 1:10, not 1:1,000. In this example you are dividing by 10 (not 1,000), so you will move the decimal point 1 place to the left.

$$\frac{1 \text{ cm}}{10 \text{ mm}} = \frac{X \text{ cm}}{31 \text{ mm}}$$

$$\frac{1 \text{ cm}}{10 \text{ mm}} \bowtie \frac{X \text{ cm}}{31 \text{ mm}}$$ Cross-multiply

$$10X = 31$$

$$\frac{10X}{10} = \frac{31}{10}$$

$$X = 3.1$$ 3.1. Move the decimal 1 place to the left to divide by 10.

$$X = 3.1 \text{ cm}$$ Label the units to match the unknown X.

REMEMBER

When converting from a larger to a smaller unit of measure, the resulting number of smaller units should be greater than the original number of larger units. Conversely, when converting from a smaller to a larger unit of measure, the resulting number of larger units should be less than the original number of smaller units. After all calculations, ask yourself, "Does this answer make sense?" If it does not, stop and check for your mistake.

MATH TIP

Remember this diagram when converting within the metric system.

Move the decimal point three places to the left for each step.

◄────────────────────────────────

kg   g   mg   mcg

────────────────────────────────►

Move the decimal point three places to the right for each step.

EXAMPLES ■

1 mcg = 0.001 mg (moved decimal point to the left 3 places)

2 g = 2,000 mg (moved decimal point to the right 3 places)

2 g = 2,000,000 mcg (moved decimal point to the right 6 places, because the conversion required two steps)

    In time, you will probably do these calculations in your head with little difficulty. If you feel you do not understand the concept of conversions within the metric system, review again the decimal section in Chapter 1 and the metric section in Chapter 3. Also get help from your instructor before proceeding further.

QUICK REVIEW

To use the ratio-proportion method to convert from one unit of measurement to another:

1. Recall the metric equivalents.

2. Set up a proportion of two equivalent ratios.

3. Cross-multiply to solve for an unknown quantity, X.

Review Set 13

Convert each of the following to the equivalent unit indicated.

1. 500 mL =	_____ L		16. 0.75 L =	_____ mL
2. 0.015 g =	_____ mg		17. 5,000 mL =	_____ L
3. 8 mg =	_____ g		18. 1 L =	_____ mL
4. 10 mg =	_____ g		19. 1 g =	_____ mg
5. 60 mg =	_____ g		20. 3,000 mL =	_____ L
6. 300 mg =	_____ g		21. 23 mcg =	_____ mg
7. 0.2 g =	_____ mg		22. 1.05 g =	_____ kg
8. 1.2 g =	_____ mg		23. 18 mcg =	_____ mg
9. 0.0025 kg =	_____ g		24. 0.4 mg =	_____ mcg
10. 0.065 g =	_____ mg		25. 2,625 g =	_____ kg
11. 0.005 L =	_____ mL		26. 50 cm =	_____ m
12. 1.5 L =	_____ mL		27. 10 L =	_____ mL
13. 100 mcg =	_____ mg		28. 450 mL =	_____ L
14. 250 mL =	_____ L		29. 5 mL =	_____ L
15. 2 kg =	_____ g		30. 30 mg =	_____ mcg

After completing these problems, see page 642 to check your answers.

APPROXIMATE EQUIVALENTS

Fortunately, the use of the apothecary and household systems is infrequent and may soon become completely obsolete in health care to prevent medication errors. These systems are most often still used in the home care setting. Conversions between the apothecary and household units still in use are based on approximate equivalents. More exact equivalents are not practical and, therefore, rarely used by health care workers. For example, a more exact equivalent of 1 U.S. fluid ounce as measured in milliliters is 29.5735296875 milliliters, or approximately 30 milliliters; but in the U.K. 1 fluid ounce is 28.4130625 milliliters. There are 32 fluid ounces per 1 U.S. quart, and this is generally accepted to be approximately 1 liter; but the more exact equivalent is 946.35295 milliliters. This is further complicated by the relationship of pints, quarts, and fluid ounces, all of which explains why these systems are discouraged by The Institute for Safe Medication Practices (2013) and are becoming obsolete in traditional health care settings.

The approximate equivalents in the following Remember box are the ones you need to learn so that you can convert from one system to another. Other obsolete approximate equivalents are included in Appendix B: *drams* (volume measure that is still evident on some disposable medicine cups along with teaspoons, tablespoons, fluid ounces, and milliliters), *minims* (volume measure which is still evident on some hypodermic syringes along with the metric equivalent), and *grains* (weight measure, still evident on labels of some older medications along with the metric equivalent). Memorize these approximate equivalents.

 REMEMBER

Approximate Equivalents

$$1\ t = 5\ mL$$
$$1\ T = 3\ t = 15\ mL = \tfrac{1}{2}\ fl\ oz$$
$$1\ fl\ oz = 30\ mL = 6\ t$$
$$1\ L = 1\ qt = 32\ fl\ oz = 2\ pt = 4\ cups$$
$$1\ pt = 16\ fl\ oz = 2\ cups$$
$$1\ cup = 8\ fl\ oz = 240\ mL$$
$$1\ kg = 2.2\ lb$$
$$1\ in = 2.5\ cm$$

CONVERTING BETWEEN SYSTEMS OF MEASUREMENT

Now let's convert between systems of measurement using approximate equivalents. In the first three examples we will convert from a larger to a smaller unit of measure. Remember, the resulting number of smaller units should be greater than the original number of larger units.

EXAMPLE 1 ■

Convert: 2 fl oz to mL

Approximate equivalent: 1 fl oz = 30 mL

$$\frac{1\ fl\ oz}{30\ mL} \diagdown \diagup \frac{2\ fl\ oz}{X\ mL}$$
$$X = 30 \times 2$$
$$X = 60\ mL$$

EXAMPLE 2 ▪

Convert: 75 in to cm

Approximate equivalent: 1 in = 2.5 cm

$$\frac{1 \text{ in}}{2.5 \text{ cm}} \diagdown\kern-1em\diagup \frac{75 \text{ in}}{X \text{ cm}}$$

$$X = 75 \times 2.5$$
$$X = 187.5 \text{ cm}$$

EXAMPLE 3 ▪

The hospital scale weighs a child at 40 kg. The mother wants to know her child's weight in pounds.

Convert: 40 kg to lb

Approximate equivalent: 1 kg = 2.2 lb

$$\frac{1 \text{ kg}}{2.2 \text{ lb}} \diagdown\kern-1em\diagup \frac{40 \text{ kg}}{X \text{ lb}}$$

$$X = 2.2 \times 40$$
$$X = 88 \text{ lb}$$

Use the same method to convert from a smaller to a larger unit of measure. Now the resulting number of larger units will be less than the original number of smaller units. Notice that the unknown is in the numerator. Remember to keep like units across from each other.

EXAMPLE 1 ▪

Convert: 45 mL to t

Approximate equivalent: 1 t = 5 mL

$$\frac{1 \text{ t}}{5 \text{ mL}} \diagdown\kern-1em\diagup \frac{X \text{ t}}{45 \text{ mL}}$$

$$5X = 45$$
$$\frac{5X}{5} = \frac{45}{5}$$
$$X = 9 \text{ t}$$

EXAMPLE 2 ▪

Convert 66 lb to kg.

Approximate equivalent: 1 kg = 2.2 lb

$$\frac{1 \text{ kg}}{2.2 \text{ lb}} \diagdown\kern-1em\diagup \frac{X \text{ kg}}{66 \text{ lb}}$$

$$2.2X = 66$$
$$\frac{2.2X}{2.2} = \frac{66}{2.2}$$
$$X = 30 \text{ kg}$$

EXAMPLE 3 ■

Convert 40 cm to in (inches).

Approximate equivalent: 1 in = 2.5 cm

$$\frac{1 \text{ in}}{2.5 \text{ cm}} \diagup\!\!\!\diagdown \frac{X \text{ in}}{40 \text{ cm}}$$

$$2.5X = 40$$

$$\frac{2.5X}{2.5} = \frac{40}{2.5}$$

$$X = 16 \text{ in}$$

MATH TIP

A clue for remembering the approximate equivalent 1 kg = 2.2 lb is to realize that there are about 2 pounds for every kilogram, so the number of kilograms you weigh is about half the number of pounds you weigh. (This could make getting on a metric scale pleasant.)

Try this: Convert your weight in pounds to kilograms rounded to hundredths, or two decimal places. Now check your answer. Is your weight in kilograms approximately $\frac{1}{2}$ your weight in pounds? Then you are correct!

QUICK REVIEW

To use the ratio-proportion method to convert from one unit to another or between systems of measurement:

- Recall the equivalent.

- Set up a proportion: Ratio for known equivalent equals ratio for unknown equivalent.

- Label the units and match the units in the numerators and denominators.

- Cross-multiply to find the value of the unknown X equivalent.

- Label the units in the answer to match the unknown X.

Review Set 14

Convert each of the following amounts to the unit indicated. Indicate the approximate equivalent(s) used in the conversion. If rounding is necessary, round decimals to two places (hundredths).

Approximate Equivalent

1. 48 fl oz = _____ cups   _____

2. 13 t = _____ mL   _____

3. 15 mL = _____ fl oz   _____

4. $2\frac{1}{2}$ fl oz = _____ mL   _____

5. 750 mL = _____ qt   _____

6. 20 mL = _____ t   _____

7. 4 T = _____ mL   _____

8. 9 kg = _____ lb   _____

9. 250 lb = _____ kg   _____

10. 3 L = _____ qt   _____

11. 55 kg = _____ lb   _____

12. 12 in = _____ cm   _____

13. 2 qt = _____ L   _____

14. 3 t = _____ mL   _____

15. 99 lb = _____ kg   _____

16. 1 pt = _____ mL   _____

17. $1\frac{1}{2}$ cups = _____ mL   _____

18. 1.5 m = _____ ft   _____

19. 30 cm = _____ in   _____

20. 60 mL = _____ fl oz   _____

21. 32 in = _____ cm   _____

22. 350 mm = _____ in   _____

23. 7.5 cm = _____ in   _____

24. 2 in = _____ mm   _____

25. 40 kg = _____ lb   _____

26. 7.16 kg = _____ lb   _____

27. 110 lb = _____ kg   _____

28. 3.5 kg = _____ lb   _____

29. 63 lb = _____ kg   _____

30. A newborn infant is $21\frac{1}{2}$ inches long. Her length is _____ cm.

31. The label for a granular medicine recommends mixing it with at least 120 mL of water or juice. At the time of discharge, the nurse should advise the patient to mix the medicine with _____ fluid ounce(s) or _____ cup(s) of water or juice.

32. A patient who weighs 250 lb starts a weight-loss program with a goal of losing 10 lb before the next doctor's appointment. At the next office visit, the patient is weighed at 108 kg. Has the patient met the weight-loss goal? _____

33. Calculate the total fluid intake in mL for 24 hours.

Breakfast	8 fl oz milk	
	6 fl oz orange juice	
	4 fl oz water with medication	
Lunch	8 fl oz iced tea	
Snack	10 fl oz coffee	
	4 fl oz gelatin dessert	
Dinner	8 fl oz water	
	6 fl oz tomato juice	
	6 fl oz beef broth	
Snack	5 fl oz pudding	
	12 fl oz diet soda	
	4 fl oz water with medication	Total = _____ mL

34. A child who weighs 55 lb is to receive 0.05 mg of a drug per kg of body weight per dose. How much of the drug should the child receive for each dose? _____ mg

35. A child is taking 12 mL of a medication 4 times per day. If the full bottle contains 16 fluid ounces of the medication, how many days will the bottle last? _____ day(s)

36. A doctor prescribes 10 mL of Betadine concentrate in 480 mL of warm water as a soak for a finger infection. Using measures commonly found in the home, how would you instruct the patient to prepare the solution?

_____

37. A patient is to receive 10 mL of a drug. How many teaspoonsful should the patient take?

_____ t

38. An infant is taking a ready-to-feed formula. The formula comes in quart containers. If the infant usually takes 4 fluid ounces of formula every 3 hours during the day and night, how many quarts of formula should the mother buy for a 3-day supply? _____ qt

39. An infant's head circumference is 40 cm. The parents ask for the equivalent in inches. You tell the parents their infant's head circumference is _____ in.

40. A patient tells you he was weighed in the physician's office and was told he weighs 206 pounds. What is his weight in kilograms? _____ kg

After completing these problems, see pages 642–643 to check your answers.

SUMMARY

At this point, you should be quite familiar with the equivalents for converting within the metric and household systems and from one system to another. From memory, you should be able to recall quickly and accurately the equivalents for conversions. If you are having difficulty understanding the concept of converting from one unit of measurement to another, review this chapter and seek additional help from your instructor.

Consider the two Clinical Reasoning Skills scenarios, and work the Practice Problems for Chapter 4. Concentrate on accuracy. One error can be a serious mistake when calculating the dosages of medicines or performing critical measurements of health status.

CLINICAL REASONING SKILLS

ERROR

Incorrectly interpreting an apothecary symbol

Possible Scenario

To prevent hypokalemia (lowered potassium), a physician ordered ℥ $\frac{1}{2}$ *potassium gluconate 20 mEq elixir three times a day*, for a hospitalized patient who was also receiving digitalis and diuretic therapy. The nursing student did not recognize the fluid ounce symbol and interpreted the order as $\frac{1}{2}$ of the 20 mEq amount. The potassium gluconate was supplied as 20 mEq per 15 mL, and the physician intended for the patient to receive 15 mL three times a day; instead, the student nurse prepared 7.5 mL or $1\frac{1}{2}$ t of the elixir in a medicine cup. The nursing instructor asked the student nurse to explain how she determined the amount to give, and the student explained that the order is for $\frac{1}{2}$ of the 20 mEq per 15 mL amount, so $\frac{1}{2}$ of 15 mL is 7.5 mL, or $1\frac{1}{2}$ t. The instructor pointed to the ℥ symbol and asked if the student understood its meaning.

Potential Outcome

The approximate equivalent of the apothecary ℥ (fl oz) is 1 fl oz = 30 mL; therefore, $\frac{1}{2}$ fl oz = 15 mL. If the student nurse had given over several days the dose amount she prepared, the patient would have received only 50% of the intended dosage of the potassium gluconate and could potentially have developed digitalis toxicity leading to confusion, vomiting, diarrhea, blurred vision, irregular pulse, and palpitations.

Prevention

This type of medication error is avoided by clarifying all drug orders that are confusing or that include unfamiliar symbols. If you are not sure: stop, think, and ask. In this case, the physician should have been contacted to clarify the order. Ideally, the hospital would discourage the use of apothecary units and symbols because they are too easily misinterpreted.

CLINICAL REASONING SKILLS

ERROR

Not moving the correct number of decimal spaces when using the shortcut method to multiply by a power of 10

Possible Scenario

A physician ordered 125 *mcg of digoxin p.o. once daily* for a patient treated for congestive heart failure. Supplied were scored tablets in individual packages labeled 0.25 mg per tablet. The conversion needed was mg to mcg, a larger unit to a smaller unit. The nurse knew that 1,000 mcg = 1 mg, so she set up a ratio-proportion to figure out how many 0.25 mg tablets she should administer:

$$\frac{1,000 \text{ mcg}}{1 \text{ mg}} \times \frac{\text{X mcg}}{0.25 \text{ mg}}$$

$$\text{X} = 1,000 \times 0.25$$

The nurse remembered that to multiply by 1,000 you should simply move the decimal 3 places to the right. But, in her haste, the nurse forgot to add a zero to create the correct number of decimal spaces and incorrectly figured the problem this way:

$$1,000 \times 0.25 = 0.25. = 25 \text{ mcg} \qquad\qquad \textbf{INCORRECT}$$

The nurse then reasoned, "If the physician's order was 125 mcg, then with 25 mcg tablets on hand, the patient must need 5 tablets because 5 × 25 equals 125 mcg." The nurse started to administer the 5 tablets, but hesitated because it seemed like a large number of tablets. She then asked a fellow nurse to double-check her calculation. The second nurse found the error and correctly figured the problem this way:

$$1,000 \times 0.25 = 0.250. = 250 \text{ mcg} \qquad\qquad \textbf{CORRECT}$$

The tablets are 250 mcg each, not 25 mcg each. The patient should receive $\frac{1}{2}$ tablet, not 5 tablets.

Potential Outcome

Digoxin is a high-alert cardiac medication that may lead to serious adverse reactions at toxic levels. If the nurse had proceeded with the incorrect amount, the patient would have received 10 times the normal dose and very likely would have had serious complications, such as severe bradycardia or cardiac arrhythmias.

Prevention

Fortunately, the error was caught and the patient was given the correct amount, which was $\frac{1}{2}$ tablet. A medication administration error was prevented because the nurse stopped to consider, "Does this make sense?" After every dosage calculation, ask if the answer makes sense. If still in doubt, especially with high-alert medications, ask another nurse to double-check your thinking and the calculation.

PRACTICE PROBLEMS—CHAPTER 4

Give the following equivalents without consulting conversion tables. If rounding is necessary, round decimals to two places (hundredths).

1. 0.5 g = _____ mg
2. 0.01 g = _____ mg
3. 7.5 mL = _____ L
4. 3 qt = _____ L
5. 4 mg = _____ mcg
6. 500 mL = _____ L
7. 250 mL = _____ pt
8. 300 g = _____ kg
9. 28 in = _____ cm
10. 68 kg = _____ lb
11. 2,025 g = _____ lb
12. $3\frac{1}{2}$ fl oz = _____ mL
13. 5 lb 4 oz = _____ kg
14. 16 cm = _____ in
15. 4 T = _____ fl oz
16. 65 in = _____ m
17. $70\frac{1}{2}$ lb = _____ kg
18. 3,634 g = _____ lb
19. 8 mL = _____ L
20. 450 mg = _____ g
21. 237.5 cm = _____ in
22. 0.5 g = _____ mg
23. 0.6 mg = _____ mcg
24. 4,050 mL = _____ L
25. 150 lb = _____ kg
26. 7.5 L = _____ qt
27. 22 lb = _____ kg
28. 2 cups = _____ mL
29. 6 t = _____ T
30. 90 mL = _____ fl oz
31. 375 mcg = _____ mg
32. 2 T = _____ mL
33. 2.2 lb = _____ kg
34. 5 mL = _____ t
35. 1,000 mL = _____ L
36. 1.5 g = _____ mg
37. $1\frac{1}{2}$ fl oz = _____ mL
38. 1,500 mL = _____ qt
39. 2 kg = _____ lb
40. 25 mg = _____ g
41. 4.3 kg = _____ g
42. 60 mg = _____ g
43. 0.015 g = _____ mg
44. 45 mL = _____ T
45. 0.25 mg = _____ mcg

46. As a camp nurse for 9- to 12-year-old children, you are administering $2\frac{1}{2}$ teaspoons of oral liquid Children's Tylenol to 6 feverish campers every 4 hours for oral temperatures above 100°F. You have on hand a 4 fluid ounce bottle of liquid Children's Tylenol. How many complete, or full, doses are available from this bottle? _____ full doses

47. At this same camp, the standard dosage of Pepto-Bismol for 9- to 12-year-old children is 1 tablespoon. How many full doses are available in a 120 mL bottle? _____ full doses

48. Calculate the total fluid intake in mL of this clear liquid lunch:

apple juice	4 fluid ounces
chicken broth	8 fluid ounces
gelatin dessert	6 fluid ounces
hot tea	10 fluid ounces
TOTAL =	_____ mL

49. A newborn weighs 5,250 g. Her weight is approximately equivalent to _____ lb.

50. Describe the strategy to prevent this medication error.

Possible Scenario

An attending physician ordered *cefotaxime 2 g intravenously immediately* for a patient with a leg abscess. The supply dosage available is *1,000 mg per 10 mL*. The nurse was in a rush to give the medication and calculated the dose this way:

If: 1 g = 1,000 mg

then: 2 g = 1,000 ÷ 2 = 500 mg per 5 mL   **INCORRECT**

Then the nurse administered 5 mL of the available cefotaxime.

Potential Outcome

The patient received only $\frac{1}{4}$, or 25%, of the dosage ordered. The patient should have received 2,000 mg, or 20 mL, of cefotaxime. The leg abscess could progress to osteomyelitis (a severe bone infection) or septicemia (a blood infection) because of underdosage.

Prevention

_____

_____

After completing these problems, see pages 643–644 to check your answers.

⬛ Be sure to use the online software for additional practice!

REFERENCE

The Institute for Safe Medication Practices. (2013). Medication safety alert. Retrieved from http://www.ismp.org/newsletters/ambulatory/archives/201302.asp

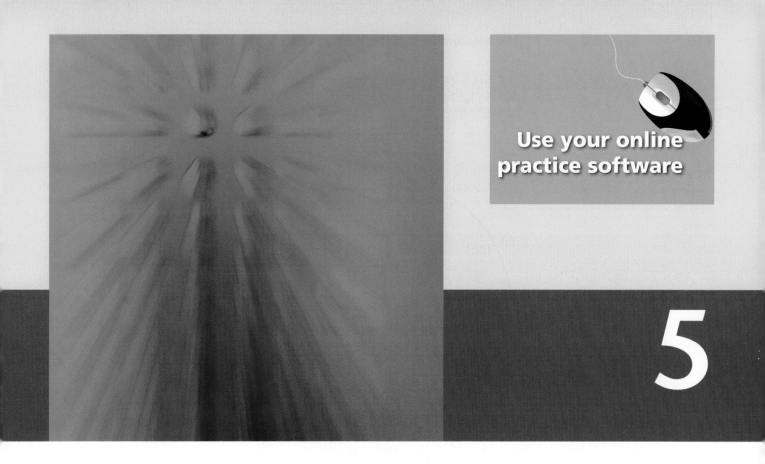

5

Conversions for Other Clinical Applications: Time and Temperature

OBJECTIVES

Upon mastery of Chapter 5, you will be able to:

- Convert between traditional and international time.
- Convert between Celsius and Fahrenheit temperature.

This chapter focuses on two other conversions applied in health care. *Time* is an essential part of the drug order. *Temperature* is an important measurement of health status.

CONVERTING BETWEEN TRADITIONAL AND INTERNATIONAL TIME

It is becoming increasingly popular in health care settings to keep time with a system more straightforward than traditional time, using the 24-hour clock. In use around the world and in the U.S. military for many years, this system is known as *international time* or *military time*.

Look at the 24-hour clock (Figure 5-1). Each time designation is comprised of a unique four-digit number. Notice that there are two circles of numbers (an inner and an outer circle) that identify the hours from 0100 to 2400. The inside numbers correlate to traditional AM time (midnight to 11:59 AM)—time periods that are ante meridian, or before noon. The outside numbers correlate to traditional PM time (noon to 11:59 PM)—time periods that are post meridian, or after noon.

FIGURE 5-1   24-hour clock depicting 0015 (12:15 AM) and 1215 (12:15 PM)

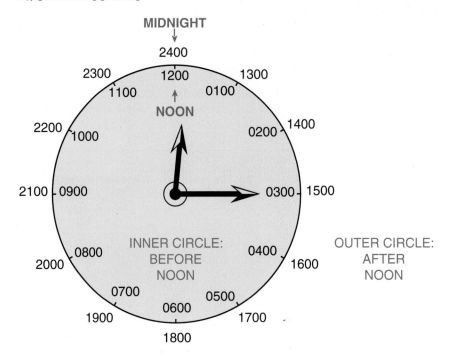

Hours on the 24-hour clock after 0059 minutes (zero-zero fifty-nine) are stated in hundreds, and the word **zero** precedes hours under ten hundred (single-digit hours in traditional time).

EXAMPLE 1 ▪

0400 is stated as *zero four hundred.*

EXAMPLE 2 ▪

1600 is stated as *sixteen hundred.*

Between each hour, the time is read simply as the hour and the number of minutes, preceded by *zero* as needed.

EXAMPLE 1 ▪

0421 is stated as *zero four twenty-one.*

EXAMPLE 2 ▪

1659 is stated as *sixteen fifty-nine.*

The minutes between 2400 (midnight) and 0100 (1:00 AM) are written as 0001, 0002, 0003 . . . 0058, 0059. Each zero is stated before the number of minutes.

EXAMPLE 1 ▪

0009 is stated as *zero-zero-zero nine.*

EXAMPLE 2 ▪

0014 is stated as *zero-zero fourteen.*

Midnight can be written two different ways in international time:

▪ 2400 and read as *twenty-four hundred,* or

▪ 0000 (used by the military) and read as *zero hundred.*

Use of the 24-hour clock decreases the possibility for error in administering medications and documenting time, because no two times are expressed by the same number. There is less chance for misinterpreting time using the 24-hour clock.

EXAMPLE 1 ▪

13 minutes after 1 AM is written *0113.*

EXAMPLE 2 ▪

13 minutes after 1 PM is written *1313.*

The same cannot be said for traditional time. The AM or PM notations are the only things that differentiate traditional times.

EXAMPLE 1 ■

13 minutes after 1 AM is written *1:13 AM.*

EXAMPLE 2 ■

13 minutes after 1 PM is written *1:13 PM.*

Careless notation in a medical order or in patient records can create misinterpretation about when a therapy is due or actually occurred. Figure 5-2 shows the comparison of traditional and international time. Notice that international time is less ambiguous.

FIGURE 5-2 Comparison of traditional and international time

AM	Int'l Time	PM	Int'l Time
12:00 midnight	2400	12:00 noon	1200
1:00	0100	1:00	1300
2:00	0200	2:00	1400
3:00	0300	3:00	1500
4:00	0400	4:00	1600
5:00	0500	5:00	1700
6:00	0600	6:00	1800
7:00	0700	7:00	1900
8:00	0800	8:00	2000
9:00	0900	9:00	2100
10:00	1000	10:00	2200
11:00	1100	11:00	2300

Copyright © 2016 Cengage Learning®.

RULES

1. Traditional time and international time have similar numbering from 1:00 AM (0100) through 12:59 PM (1259).

2. Minutes after 12:00 AM (midnight) and before 1:00 AM are 0001 through 0059 in international time.

3. Hours from 1:00 PM through 12:00 AM (midnight) are 1200 hours greater in international time (1300 through 2400).

4. International time is designated by a unique four-digit number.

5. The hour(s) and minute(s) are separated by a colon in traditional time, but no colon is typically used in international time. However, you may see international time represented with a colon, such as 14:00 for 1400 (for 2:00 PM) and so forth.

MATH TIP

For the hours between 1:00 PM (1300) and 12:00 AM (2400), add 1200 to traditional time to find equivalent international time; subtract 1200 from international time to convert to equivalent traditional time.

Let's apply these rules to convert between the two time systems.

EXAMPLE 1 ■

3:00 PM = 300 + 1200 = 1500

EXAMPLE 2 ■

2212 = 2212 − 1200 = 10:12 PM

EXAMPLE 3 ■

12:45 AM = 0045

EXAMPLE 4 ■

0004 = 12:04 AM

EXAMPLE 5 ■   EXAMPLE 6 ■
0130 = 1:30 AM   11:00 AM = 1100

QUICK REVIEW

■ International time is designated by 0001 through 1259 for 12:01 AM through 12:59 PM and 1300 through 2400 for 1:00 PM through 12:00 midnight.

■ The hours from 1:00 PM through 12:00 midnight in traditional time are 1200 hours greater in international time (1300 through 2400).

Review Set 15

Convert international time to traditional AM/PM time.

1. 0032 = _____	6. 1215 = _____	
2. 0730 = _____	7. 0220 = _____	
3. 1640 = _____	8. 1010 = _____	
4. 2121 = _____	9. 1315 = _____	
5. 2359 = _____	10. 1825 = _____	

Convert traditional to international time.

11. 1:30 PM = _____	16. 3:45 AM = _____	
12. 12:04 AM = _____	17. 12:00 midnight = _____	
13. 9:45 PM = _____	18. 3:30 PM = _____	
14. 12:00 noon = _____	19. 6:20 AM = _____	
15. 11:15 PM = _____	20. 5:45 PM = _____	

Fill in the blanks by writing out in words the times indicated.

21. In 24-hour time, 0623 is stated _____.

22. In 24-hour time, 0041 is stated _____.

23. In 24-hour time, 1903 is stated _____.

24. In 24-hour time, 2311 is stated _____.

25. In 24-hour time, 0300 is stated _____.

After completing these problems, see page 644 to check your answers.

CONVERTING BETWEEN CELSIUS AND FAHRENHEIT TEMPERATURES

Another important conversion in health care involves Celsius and Fahrenheit temperatures. Simple formulas are used for converting between the two temperature scales. It is easier to remember the formulas when you understand how they are related. The Fahrenheit (F) scale establishes the freezing point of pure water at 32° and the boiling point of pure water at 212°. The Celsius (C) scale establishes the freezing point of pure water at 0° and the boiling point of pure water at 100°.

FIGURE 5-3 Comparison of Celsius and Fahrenheit temperature scales
Copyright © 2016 Cengage Learning®.

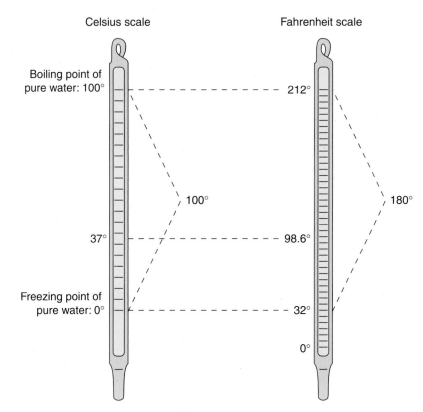

FIGURE 5-4 Comparison of Celsius and Fahrenheit body temperature scales. Bold type indicates normal body temperature.

°C	°F
40.6	105.1
40.4	104.7
40.2	104.4
40.0	104.0
39.8	103.6
39.6	103.3
39.4	102.9
39.2	102.6
39.0	102.2
38.8	101.8
38.6	101.5
38.4	101.1
38.2	100.8
38.0	100.4
37.8	100.0
37.6	99.7
37.4	99.3
37.2	99.0
37.0	**98.6**
36.0	96.8
35.0	95.0
34.0	93.2
33.0	91.4

Copyright © 2016 Cengage Learning®.

Look at Figure 5-3. Note that there is 180° difference between the boiling and freezing points on the Fahrenheit thermometer and 100° between the boiling and freezing points on the Celsius thermometer. The ratio of the difference between the Fahrenheit and Celsius scales can be expressed as 180:100 or $\frac{180}{100}$. When reduced, this ratio is equivalent to 1.8. You will use this constant in temperature conversions.

The glass thermometers pictured in Figure 5-3 are for demonstration purposes. Electronic digital temperature devices are more commonly used in health care settings. Most electronic devices can instantly convert between the two scales, freeing the health care provider from doing the actual calculations. However, the health care provider's ability to understand the difference between Celsius and Fahrenheit remains important.

The range of body temperatures seen in health care situations is usually limited to those that are compatible with life, so it is practical to keep a chart handy that lists potential equivalent temperatures (Figure 5-4). You will find it helpful to memorize Celsius and Fahrenheit normal body temperature and some other commonly reported ones (as highlighted on the body temperature chart) for quick conversions.

To convert between Fahrenheit and Celsius temperature, formulas have been developed based on the differences between the freezing and boiling points on each scale.

RULE

To convert a given Fahrenheit temperature to Celsius, first subtract 32 and then divide the result by 1.8.

$$°C = \frac{°F - 32}{1.8}$$

EXAMPLE ▪

Convert 98.6°F to °C.

$$°C = \frac{98.6 - 32}{1.8}$$

$$°C = \frac{66.6}{1.8}$$

$$°C = 37°$$

RULE

To convert Celsius temperature to Fahrenheit, multiply by 1.8 and add 32.

$$°F = 1.8°C + 32$$

EXAMPLE ▪

Convert 35°C to °F.

$$°F = 1.8 \times 35 + 32$$

$$°F = 63 + 32$$

$$°F = 95°$$

QUICK REVIEW

Use these formulas to convert between Fahrenheit and Celsius temperatures:

▪ $°C = \frac{°F - 32}{1.8}$

▪ $°F = 1.8°C + 32$

Review Set 16

Convert these temperatures as indicated. Round your answers to tenths.

1. 100.4°F = _____ °C   3. 36.2°C = _____ °F

2. 38.4°C = _____ °F   4. 32°C = _____ °F

5. 98.6°F = _____ °C   11. 100°F = _____ °C

6. 99°F = _____ °C   12. 39°C = _____ °F

7. 103.6°F = _____ °C   13. 37.4°C = _____ °F

8. 40°C = _____ °F   14. 94.2°F = _____ °C

9. 38.9°C = _____ °F   15. 102.8°F = _____ °C

10. 36.4°C = _____ °F

For each of the following statements, convert the given temperature in °F or °C to its corresponding equivalent in °C or °F.

16. An infant has a body temperature of 95.5°F.   _____ °C

17. Store the vaccine serum at 7°C.   _____ °F

18. Do not expose medication to temperatures greater than 88°F.   _____ °C

19. Normal body temperature is 37°C.   _____ °F

20. If Mr. Rose's temperature is greater than 103.5°F, call MD.   _____ °C

After completing these problems, see pages 644–645 to check your answers.

CLINICAL REASONING SKILLS

ERROR

Incorrect interpretation of an order because of a misunderstanding of traditional time

Possible Scenario

A physician ordered a mild sedative for an anxious patient who is scheduled for a sigmoidoscopy in the morning. The order read Valium 5 mg orally at 6:00 × 1 dose. The evening nurse interpreted that single-dose order to be scheduled for 6 o'clock PM along with the enema and other preparations to be given to the patient. The doctor meant for the Valium to be given at 6 o'clock AM to help the patient relax prior to the test.

Potential Outcome

Valium would help the patient relax during the enema and make the patient sleepy. But it is not desirable for the patient to be drowsy or sedated during the evening preparations. Because of the omission of the AM designation, the patient would not benefit from this mild sedative at the intended time, just before the test. The patient would have likely experienced unnecessary anxiety both before and during the test.

Prevention

This scenario emphasizes the benefit of the 24-hour clock. If international time had been in use at this facility, the order would have been written as Valium 5 mg orally at 0600 × 1 dose, clearly indicating the exact time of administration. *Be careful to verify AM and PM times if your facility uses traditional time.*

PRACTICE PROBLEMS—CHAPTER 5

Give the following time equivalents as indicated.

AM/PM Clock	**24-Hour Clock**	**AM/PM Clock**	**24-Hour Clock**
1. _____	0257	11. 7:31 PM	_____
2. 3:10 AM	_____	12. 12:00 midnight	_____
3. 4:22 PM	_____	13. 6:45 AM	_____
4. _____	2001	14. _____	0915
5. _____	1102	15. _____	2107
6. 12:33 AM	_____	16. _____	1823
7. 2:16 AM	_____	17. _____	0540
8. _____	1642	18. 11:55 AM	_____
9. _____	2356	19. 10:12 PM	_____
10. 4:20 AM	_____	20. 9:06 PM	_____

Find the length of each time interval in hours and minutes for questions 21 through 30.

21. 0200 to 0600 _____
22. 1100 to 1800 _____
23. 1500 to 2330 _____
24. 0935 to 2150 _____
25. 0003 to 1453 _____

26. 2316 to 0328 _____
27. 8:22 AM to 1:10 PM _____
28. 4:35 PM to 8:16 PM _____
29. 1:00 AM to 7:30 AM _____

30. 10:05 AM Friday to 2:43 AM Saturday _____

31. True or False? The 24-hour clock is imprecise and not suited to health care. _____

32. Indicate whether these international times would be AM or PM when converted to traditional time.

    a. 1030 _____
    b. 1920 _____
    c. 0158 _____
    d. 1230 _____

Give the following temperature equivalents as indicated.

33. 99.6°F _____ °C
34. 36.5°C _____ °F
35. 39.2°C _____ °F
36. 100.2°F _____ °C
37. 98°F _____ °C
38. 37.4°C _____ °F
39. 38.2°C _____ °F
40. 104°F _____ °C

41. 97.8°F _____ °C
42. 35.4°C _____ °F
43. 103.5°F _____ °C
44. 39°C _____ °F
45. 36.9°C _____ °F
46. 101.4°F _____ °C
47. 97.2°F _____ °C

48. Four temperature readings in °C for Mrs. Baskin are 37.6, 35.5, 38.1, and 37.6. Find her average (or mean) °C temperature and convert it to °F. Average: _____ °C = _____ °F

49. True or False? The freezing and boiling points of pure water on the Fahrenheit and Celsius temperature scales were used to develop the conversion formulas. _____

50. Describe the clinical reasoning you would use to prevent this conversion error.

   Possible Scenario

   A student nurse takes a child's temperature and finds that it is 38.2°C. The child's mother asks what that equates to in Fahrenheit temperature. The student nurse does a quick calculation in her head and multiplies 38° by 2 and adds 32, because she recalls that the conversion constant is 1.8 and thinks 2 is close enough. The student nurse tells the mother, "Well, about 108°." The mother replies, "I hope not" and smiles.

   Potential Outcome

   The student nurse immediately recognizes that she has made an error and feels embarrassed. The mother could have become alarmed and experienced undue anxiety and a loss of confidence in the student nurse. The correct temperature measurement is 100.8°F. Fever-reducing medical orders often vary the dosage depending on the severity of the elevated temperature. An incorrect conversion could result in over- or undermedication of the child.

   Prevention

   _____

   _____

After completing these problems, see page 645 to check your answers.

⬛ Be sure to use the online software for additional practice!

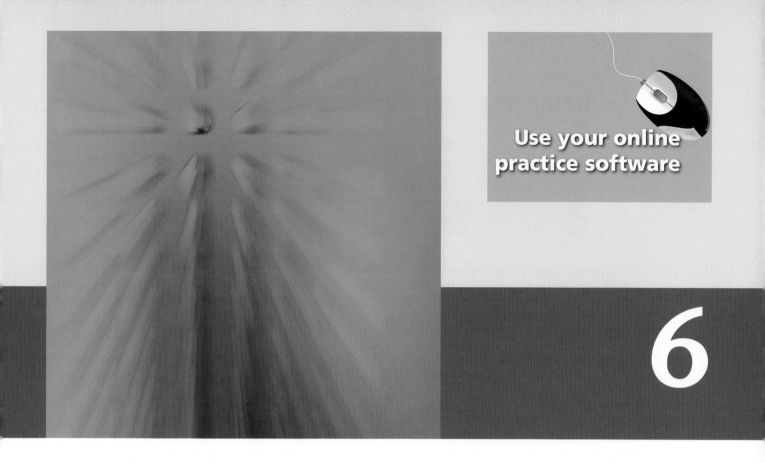

Equipment Used in Dosage Measurement

OBJECTIVES

Upon mastery of Chapter 6, you will be able to correctly measure the prescribed dosages that you calculate. To accomplish this, you will also be able to:

- Recognize and select the appropriate equipment for the medication, dosage, and method of administration ordered.
- Read and interpret the calibrations of each utensil presented.

Now that you are familiar with the systems of measurement used in the calculation of dosages, let's take a look at the common measuring utensils. In this chapter, you will learn to recognize and read the calibrations of devices used in both oral and parenteral (other than gastrointestinal) administration. The oral utensils include the medicine cup, pediatric oral devices, and calibrated droppers. The parenteral devices include the 3 mL syringe, the prefilled syringe, a variety of insulin syringes, the 1 mL syringe, and special safety and intravenous syringes.

ORAL ADMINISTRATION

Medicine Cup

Figure 6-1 shows three side views of the 30-milliliter 1-fluid-ounce medicine cup that is used to measure most liquids for oral administration. Three views are presented to show all of the scales. Notice that the approximate equivalents of the metric, apothecary, and household systems of measurement are indicated

FIGURE 6-1   Medicine cup (three views) with approximate equivalent measures

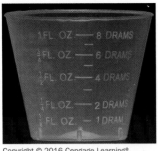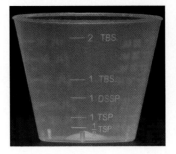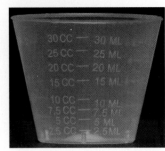

Copyright © 2016 Cengage Learning®.

on the cup. The medicine cup can serve as a great study aid to help you learn the volume equivalents of the three systems of measurement. Look at the calibrations for milliliters, teaspoons, tablespoons, fluid ounces, and drams. As you fill the cup, you can see that 30 milliliters equal 1 fluid ounce, 5 milliliters equal 1 teaspoon, and so forth. Dram, a unit of measurement in the apothecary system, is no longer used but may still appear on medicine cups. Cubic centimeters (cc), formerly used interchangeably with milliliters (mL) in clinical situations, may still be noted on measuring devices. The correct unit to use is milliliter (mL). For volumes less than 2.5 mL, a smaller, more accurate device should be used (see Figures 6-2, 6-3, and 6-4).

Calibrated Dropper

Figure 6-2 shows the calibrated dropper, which is used to administer some small quantities. A dropper is used when giving medicine to children and the elderly and when adding small amounts of liquid to water or juice. Eye and ear medications are also dispensed from a medicine dropper or squeeze drop bottle.

The amount of the drop, abbreviated gtt, varies according to the diameter of the hole at the tip of the dropper. For this reason, a properly calibrated dropper usually accompanies the medicine (Figure 6-3). It is calibrated according to the way in which that drug is prescribed. The calibrations are usually given in milliliters or drops.

FIGURE 6-2   Calibrated dropper

FIGURE 6-3   Furosemide Oral Solution label

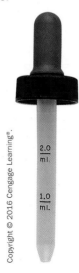

Copyright © 2016 Cengage Learning®.

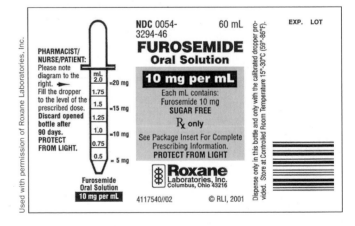

Used with permission of Roxane Laboratories, Inc.

CAUTION

To be safe, never exchange packaged droppers between medications, because drop size varies from one dropper to another.

Pediatric Oral Devices

Various types of calibrated equipment are available to administer oral medications to children. Two devices intended only for oral use are shown in Figure 6-4. Parents and child caregivers should be taught to always use calibrated devices when administering medications to children. Household spoons vary in size and are not reliable for accurate dosing.

FIGURE 6-4   Devices for administering oral medications

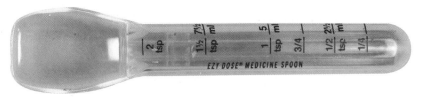

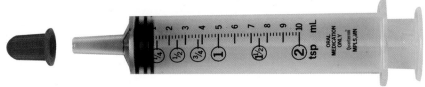

CAUTION

To be safe, do not use syringes intended for injections in the administration of oral medications. Confusion about the route of administration may occur.

You can distinguish oral from parenteral syringes in two ways. Syringes intended for oral use typically do not have a luerlock hub (see Figures 6-5 and 6-6). They also usually have a cap on the tip, which must be removed before administering the medication. Syringes intended for parenteral use have a luerlock hub that allows a needle to be secured tightly.

PARENTERAL ADMINISTRATION

The term *parenteral* interpreted literally designates routes of administration other than gastrointestinal. However, in this text, as well as most clinical settings, parenteral means injection routes.

3 mL Syringe

Figure 6-5 shows a 3 mL syringe assembled with needle unit. The parts of the syringe are identified in Figure 6-6. Notice that the black rubber tip of the suction plunger is visible. The nurse pulls back on the plunger to withdraw the medicine from the storage container. *The calibrations are read from the top (needle end) black ring, NOT the raised middle section and NOT the bottom (plunger end) ring.* Look closely at the metric scale in Figure 6-5, which is calibrated in milliliters (mL) for each tenth (0.1) of a milliliter. Each 0.5 (or $\frac{1}{2}$) milliliter is marked up to the maximum volume of 3 milliliters.

Standardized to the syringe calibrations, standard drug dosages of 1 mL or greater can be rounded to the nearest tenth (0.1) of a mL and measured on the mL scale. Refer to Chapter 1 to review the rules of decimal rounding. For example, 1.45 mL is rounded to 1.5 mL. Notice that the volume of the colored liquid in Figure 6-5 is 1.5 mL, which is also illustrated in Figure 6-6.

FIGURE 6-5 3 mL syringe with needle unit measuring 1.5 mL

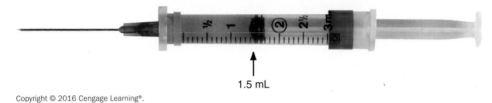

1.5 mL

Copyright © 2016 Cengage Learning®.

FIGURE 6-6 Illustration of 3 mL syringe with needle unit measuring 1.5 mL

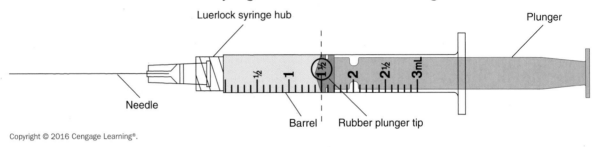

Luerlock syringe hub

Plunger

Needle

Barrel   Rubber plunger tip

Copyright © 2016 Cengage Learning®.

Prefilled Single-Dose Syringe

Figure 6-7 is an example of a *prefilled single-dose syringe*. Such syringes contain the usual single dose of a medication and are to be used only once. The syringe is discarded after the single use.

If you are to give *less* than the full single dose of a drug provided in a prefilled single-dose syringe, you should discard the extra amount *before* injecting the patient.

EXAMPLE ■

The drug order prescribes 100 mg of medroxyprogesterone acetate to be administered to a patient. You have a prefilled single-dose syringe containing 150 mg per mL of solution (as in Figure 6-7). You would discard 50 mg of the drug solution; then 100 mg would remain in the syringe. You will learn more about calculating drug dosages beginning in Chapter 10. (Some medications, such as controlled substances, require another nurse to observe the discarding of the unused portion.)

FIGURE 6-7 Prefilled single-dose syringe

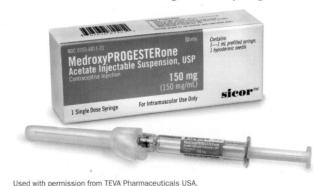

Used with permission from TEVA Pharmaceuticals USA.

Insulin Syringe

Figure 6-8(a) shows both sides of a standard U-100 insulin syringe. This syringe is to be used for the measurement and administration of U-100 insulin *only*. It must not be used to measure other medications that are measured in units.

CAUTION

U-100 insulin should only be measured in a U-100 insulin syringe. U-100 insulin concentration is 100 units of insulin per mL.

Notice that Figure 6-8(a) pictures one side of the insulin syringe calibrated in odd-number two-unit increments and the other side calibrated in even-number two-unit increments. The plunger in Figure 6-9(a) simulates the measurement of 70 units of U-100 insulin. It is important to note that for U-100 insulin, 100 units equal 1 mL.

Figure 6-8(b) shows two Lo-Dose U-100 insulin syringes. The enlarged scale is easier to read and is calibrated for each 1 unit up to 50 units per 0.5 mL, or 30 units per 0.3 mL. Every unit is marked, with the scale designating corresponding numbers by fives. The 30 unit syringe is commonly used for pediatric administration of insulin. The plunger in Figure 6-9(b) simulates the measurement of 19 units of U-100 insulin.

FIGURE 6-8 Insulin syringes with safety covers removed for easy viewing of calibrations: (a) Front and back of a standard U-100 insulin syringe; (b) Lo-Dose U-100 insulin syringes, 50 and 30 units

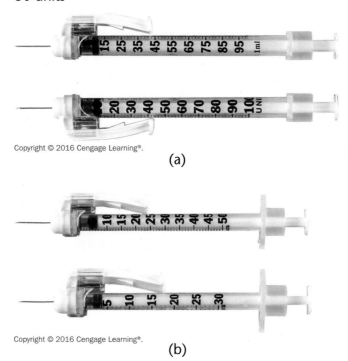

Copyright © 2016 Cengage Learning®.

(a)

Copyright © 2016 Cengage Learning®.

(b)

FIGURE 6-9   (a) Standard U-100 insulin syringe measuring 70 units of U-100 insulin; (b) Lo-Dose U-100 insulin syringe measuring 19 units of U-100 insulin; all with safety covers removed for easy viewing of calibrations

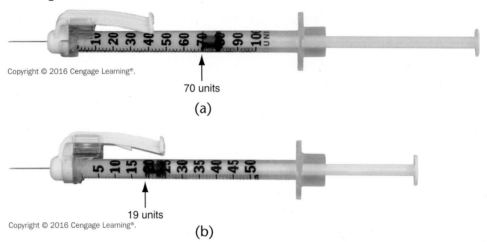

70 units

(a)

19 units

(b)

Copyright © 2016 Cengage Learning®.

CAUTION

Be careful to measure the insulin dose by reading the units at the top of the black rubber stopper at the end of the plunger, not the bottom. A common error is to incorrectly read the dose by looking at the bottom of the stopper. Look again at Figure 6-9 to see that the insulin syringes demonstrate doses of 70 and 19 units, respectively.

All insulin doses should be double-checked by another nurse before administration to the patient.

1 mL Syringe

Figure 6-10 shows the 1 mL syringe. This syringe is also referred to as the *tuberculin*, or *TB, syringe*. It is used when a small dose of a drug must be measured, such as an allergen extract, vaccine, or child's medication. Notice that the 1 mL syringe is calibrated in hundredths (0.01) of a milliliter, with each one tenth (0.1) milliliter labeled on the metric scale. Pediatric and critical care doses of less than 1 mL can be rounded to hundredths and measured in the 1 mL syringe. It is preferable to measure all amounts less than 0.5 mL in a 1 mL syringe.

EXAMPLE ▪

The amount 0.366 mL would be rounded to 0.37 mL and measured in the 1 mL syringe (Figure 6-10).

FIGURE 6-10   1 mL syringe

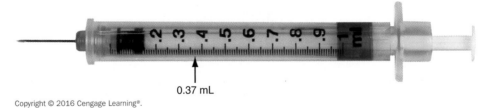

0.37 mL

Copyright © 2016 Cengage Learning®.

Safety Syringe

Figures 6-10 and 6-11 show 3 mL, 1 mL, and insulin safety syringes. Notice that the needles may be protected by shields after administration of an injectable medication, to prevent accidental needlestick injury to the nurse.

FIGURE 6-11   Safety syringes: **(a)** 3 mL; **(b)** 1 mL; **(c)** Lo-Dose U-100 insulin; **(d)** Standard U-100 insulin

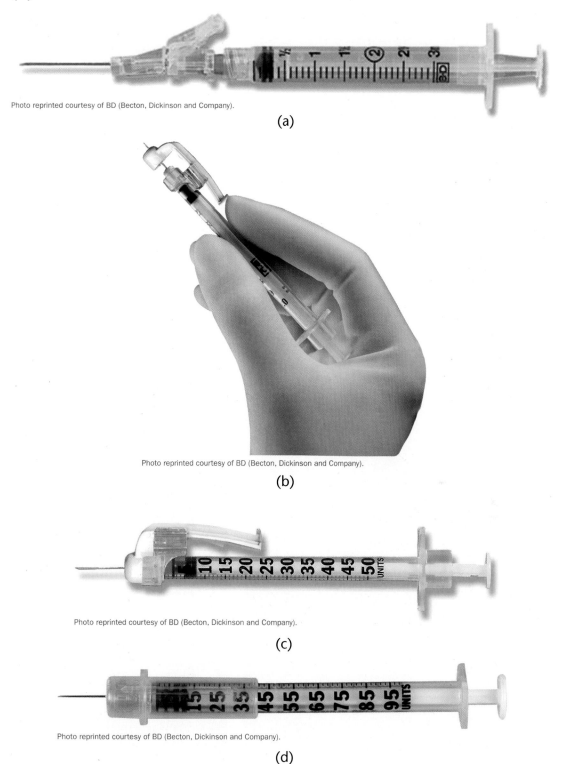

Photo reprinted courtesy of BD (Becton, Dickinson and Company).

(a)

Photo reprinted courtesy of BD (Becton, Dickinson and Company).

(b)

Photo reprinted courtesy of BD (Becton, Dickinson and Company).

(c)

Photo reprinted courtesy of BD (Becton, Dickinson and Company).

(d)

Intravenous Syringe

Figure 6-12 shows large syringes commonly used to prepare medications for intravenous administration. The volume and calibration of these syringes vary. To be safe, examine the calibrations of the syringes, and select the one best suited for the volume to be administered.

FIGURE 6-12 Intravenous syringes: (a) 5 mL; (b) 10 mL; (c) 30 mL; (d) 60 mL

FIGURE 6-12   Intravenous syringes: **(a)** 5 mL; **(b)** 10 mL; **(c)** 30 mL; **(d)** 60 mL

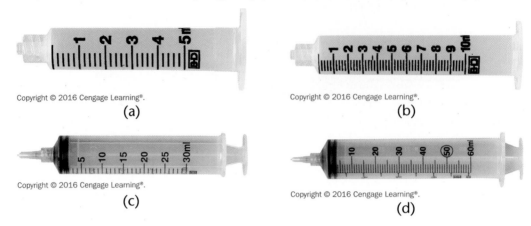

(a)

(b)

(c)

(d)

Needleless Syringe

Figure 6-13 pictures a needleless syringe system designed to prevent accidental needlesticks during intravenous administration.

FIGURE 6-13   Example of a needleless syringe system

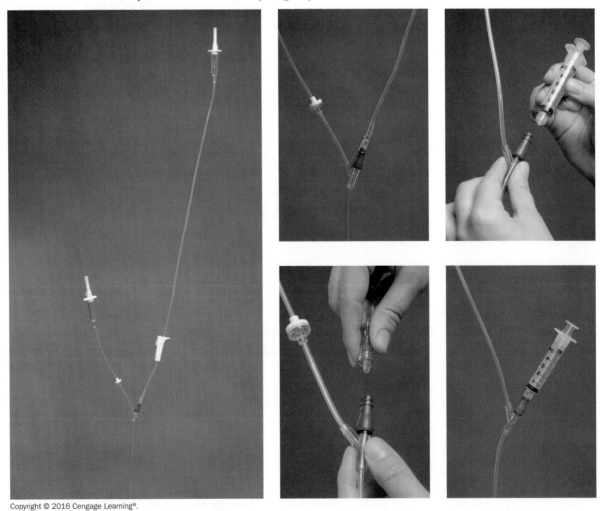

QUICK REVIEW

- The medicine cup has a 1 fluid ounce, or 30 milliliter, capacity for oral liquids. It is also calibrated to measure teaspoons, tablespoons, and drams. The apothecary measurement dram is no longer used. Oral dosages less than 2.5 milliliters should be measured in a smaller device, such as an oral syringe.

- The calibrated dropper measures small amounts of oral liquids. The size of the drop varies according to the diameter of the tip of the dropper. Drop is abbreviated as gtt.

- The standard 3 mL syringe is used to measure most injectable drugs. It is calibrated in tenths of a mL.

- The prefilled single-dose syringe cartridge is to be used once and then discarded.

- The standard U-100 insulin syringe is only used to measure U-100 insulin. It is calibrated for a total of 100 units per 1 mL.

- The Lo-Dose U-100 insulin syringe is used for measuring small amounts of U-100 insulin. It is calibrated for a total of 50 units per 0.5 mL or 30 units per 0.3 mL. The smaller syringe is commonly used for administering small amounts of insulin.

- The 1 mL syringe is used to measure small or critical amounts of injectable drugs. It is calibrated in hundredths of a mL.

- Safety and needleless syringes prevent needlestick injuries.

- Syringes intended for injections should never be used to measure or administer oral medications.

Review Set 17

1. In which syringe should 0.25 mL of a drug solution be measured? _____

2. How can 1.25 mL be measured in the regular 3 mL syringe? _____

   _____

3. Should insulin be measured in a 1 mL syringe? _____

4. Fifty (50) units of U-100 insulin equal how many milliliters? _____

5. a. True or False? The gtt is considered a consistent quantity for comparisons between different droppers. _____

   b. Why? _____

6. Can you measure 3 mL in a medicine cup? _____

7. How would you measure 3 mL of oral liquid to be administered to a child? _____

   _____

8. The medicine cup indicates that each teaspoon is the equivalent of _____ mL.

9. Describe your action if you are to administer less than the full amount of a drug supplied in a prefilled single-dose syringe. _____

   _____

10. What is the primary purpose of the safety and needleless syringes? _____

    _____

Draw an arrow to point to the calibration that corresponds to the dose to be administered.

11. Administer 0.75 mL.

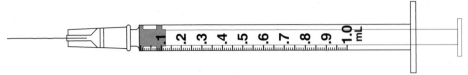

12. Administer 1.33 mL.

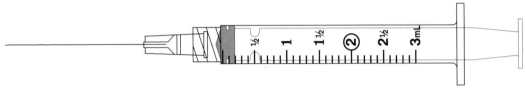

13. Administer 2.2 mL.

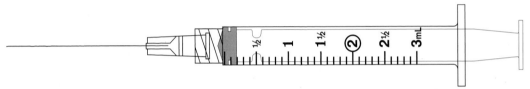

14. Administer 1.3 mL.

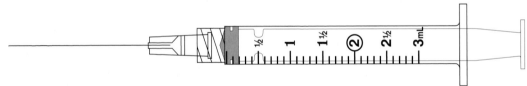

15. Administer 0.33 mL.

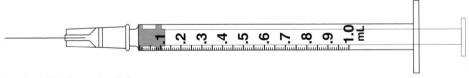

16. Administer 65 units of U-100 insulin.

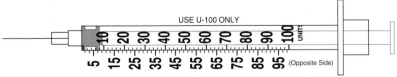

17. Administer 27 units of U-100 insulin.

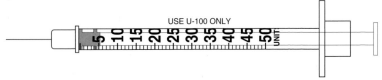

18. Administer 75 units of U-100 insulin.

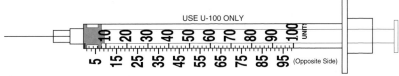

19. Administer 4.4 mL.

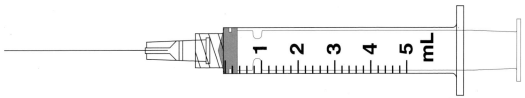

20. Administer 16 mL.

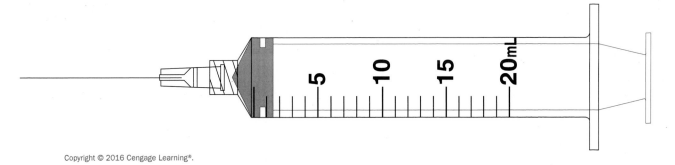

21. On the 5 mL syringe, each calibration is equal to _____. (Express the answer as a decimal.)

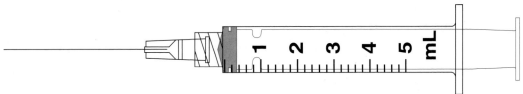

22. On the 20 mL syringe, each calibration is equal to _____.

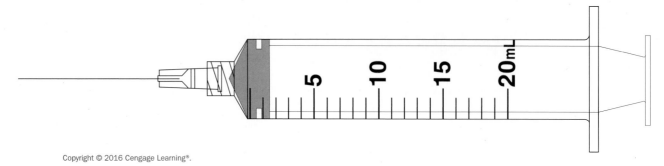

23. On the 10 mL syringe, each calibration is equal to _____. (Express the answer as a decimal.)

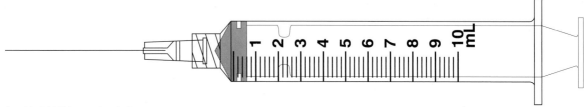

After completing these problems, see pages 645–647 to check your answers.

CLINICAL REASONING SKILLS

Select correct equipment to prepare medications. In the following situation, the correct dosage was not given, because an incorrect measuring device was used.

ERROR

Using an inaccurate measuring device for oral medications

Possible Scenario

Suppose a pediatrician ordered *Amoxil suspension (250 mg per 5 mL) 1 teaspoon orally every 8 hours* to be given to a child. The child should receive the medication for 10 days for otitis media, an ear infection. The pharmacy dispensed the medication in a bottle containing 150 mL, or a 10-day supply. The nurse did not clarify for the mother how to measure and administer the medication. The child returned to the clinic in 10 days for routine follow-up. The nurse asked whether the child had taken all the prescribed Amoxil. The child's mother stated, "No, we have almost half of the bottle left." When the nurse asked how the medication had been given, the mother described small plastic disposable teaspoons she had obtained from the grocery store. The nurse measured the spoon's capacity and found it to be less than 3 mL (remember, 1 t = 5 mL). The child would have received only $\frac{3}{5}$, or 60%, of the correct dose.

Potential Outcome

The child did not receive a therapeutic dosage of the medication and was actually underdosed. The child could develop a resistant infection, which could lead to a more severe illness such as meningitis.

Prevention

Teach family members (and patients, as appropriate) to use calibrated measuring spoons or specially designed oral syringes to measure the correct dosage of medication. The volumes of spoons can vary considerably, as this situation illustrates.

CLINICAL REASONING SKILLS

Recognize variations in syringes used to measure insulin. In the following situation, the nurse administered the incorrect dose of insulin because the nurse did not understand the design of the insulin syringe and the relationship of the rubber stopper at the end of the plunger as the measuring device for the insulin dose.

ERROR

Incorrectly reading the dose of insulin in an insulin syringe

Possible Scenario

The physician ordered *25 units of U-100 Regular Humulin insulin* for a patient with diabetes. In a hurry, the nurse prepared and administered the incorrect insulin dose as shown.

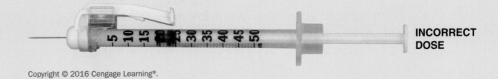

INCORRECT DOSE

Copyright © 2016 Cengage Learning®.

Potential Outcome

The patient received only 19 units of insulin, which is a significant underdosage of almost 25% less than the prescribed dosage. The patient would likely develop symptoms of hyperglycemia. If the nurse continued to incorrectly measure each insulin dose, the patient could progress into a diabetic coma.

Prevention

The nurse needs to review the proper measurement of injectable medications in syringes. Inaccurate measurement of insulin is a common and extremely serious medication error with dire consequences. The insulin syringe above showing the incorrect dose measures 19 units of insulin. The top of the rubber stopper is the correct part of the syringe for determining the amount of insulin and the proper dose. Notice the difference between the correct and incorrect dose as shown. Further, each insulin dose should be double-checked by another nurse before administration.

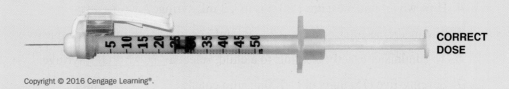

CORRECT DOSE

Copyright © 2016 Cengage Learning®.

CLINICAL REASONING SKILLS

Precisely measure doses in 1 mL and 3 mL syringes. In the following situation, an incorrect dose was administered because the computed volume was not rounded properly.

ERROR

Rounding more decimal places than are necessary and selecting the wrong-size syringe

Possible Scenario

A newborn infant was ordered to receive *gentamicin sulfate 7.5 mg intravenously every 24 hours.* Using the 2 mL vial supplied with 10 mg/mL of gentamicin, the nurse calculated the volume needed as 0.75 mL. This volume may be administered precisely using a 1 mL syringe. No rounding is needed. In this case, the nurse rounded 0.75 to the whole number 1 and administered 1 mL of medication using a 3 mL syringe. The infant was given 0.25 mL, or 2.5 mg, additional medication. If the nurse continued to care for this infant on subsequent days, the error might continue, with serious overdosage implications.

Potential Outcome

Gentamicin sulfate, an aminoglycoside, is a high-alert drug with serious potential adverse effects. One adverse effect associated with high doses is ototoxicity, leading to irreversible hearing loss. Blood levels are monitored during therapy to ensure that safe doses are ordered. By administering this higher dose, the nurse may have placed this infant at an increased risk for ototoxicity.

Prevention

It is important to know the correct size of syringe to use and the number of decimal places to round for computed dose volumes. Syringes with a total volume of 1 mL are calibrated in hundredths (2 decimal places), and 3 mL syringes are calibrated in tenths (1 decimal place). Volumes of less than 1 mL should be measured as precisely as possible in a 1 mL syringe, especially when administering high-alert medications.

PRACTICE PROBLEMS—CHAPTER 6

1. In the U-100 insulin syringe, 100 units = _____ mL.

2. The 1 mL syringe is calibrated in _____ of a mL.

3. Can you measure 1.25 mL in a single tuberculin syringe? _____ Explain. _____

    _____

    _____

4. How would you measure 1.33 mL in a 3 mL syringe? _____

5. The medicine cup has a _____ mL, or _____ fl oz, capacity.

6. To administer exactly 0.52 mL to a child, select a _____ syringe.

7. Seventy-five (75) units of U-100 insulin equals _____ mL.

8. True or False? All droppers are calibrated to deliver standardized drops of equal amounts regardless of the dropper used. _____

9. True or False? The prefilled syringe is a multiple-dose system. _____

10. True or False? Insulin should only be measured in an insulin syringe. _____

11. The purpose of needleless syringes is _____.

12. Medications are measured in syringes by aligning the calibrations with the _____ of the black rubber tip of the plunger (top ring, raised middle, or bottom ring).

13. The medicine cup calibrations indicate that 2 teaspoons are approximately _____ milliliters.

14. True or False? Safety syringes are designed to protect the patient. _____

15. The _____ syringe(s) is (are) intended to measure parenteral doses of medications. (3 mL, 1 mL, or insulin)

Draw an arrow to indicate the calibration that corresponds to the dose to be administered.

16. Administer 0.45 mL.

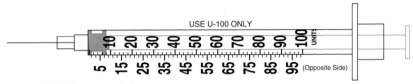

17. Administer 80 units of U-100 insulin.

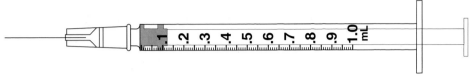

18. Administer $\frac{1}{2}$ fluid ounce.

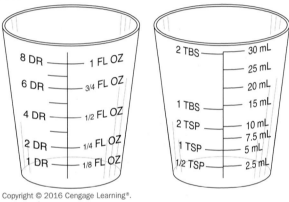

19. Administer 2.4 mL.

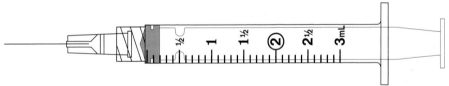

20. Administer 1.1 mL.

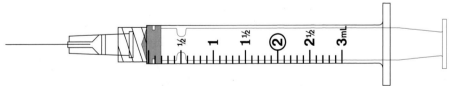

21. Administer 6.2 mL.

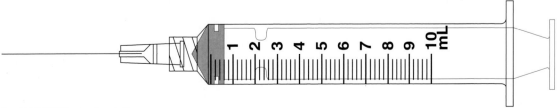

22. Administer 3.6 mL.

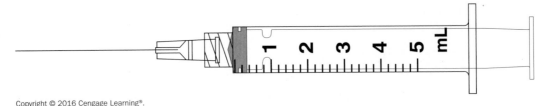

23. Administer 4.8 mL.

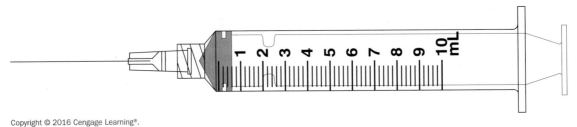

24. Administer 12 mL.

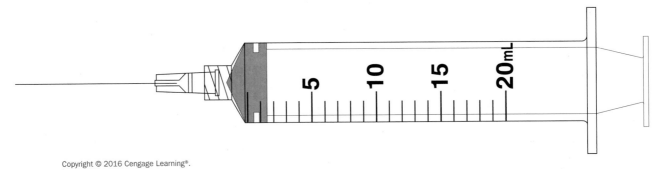

25. Describe the clinical reasoning you would use to prevent this medication error.

Possible Scenario

Suppose a patient with cancer has oral Compazine (prochlorperazine) liquid ordered for nausea. Because the patient has had difficulty taking the medication, the nurse decided to draw up the Compazine in a syringe without a needle to facilitate giving the medication. The nurse found this to be quite helpful and prepared several doses in syringes without the needles. A nurse from another unit covered for the nurse during lunch, and when the patient complained of nausea, the nurse assumed that the Compazine prepared in an injection syringe was to be given via injection. The nurse attached a needle and injected the oral medication.

Potential Outcome

The oral preparation may not be sterile and, if absorbed systemically, could lead to a bloodstream infection. Also, oral preparations have different preparative agents that likely should not be injected (such as glucose, which is traumatic to veins).

Prevention

_____

_____

26. Describe the strategy that would prevent this medication administration error.

Possible Scenario

A child with ear infections is to receive cefaclor oral liquid as an anti-infective. The medication is received in oral syringes for administration. The nurse fails to remove the cap on the tip of the syringe and attempts to administer the medication.

Potential Outcome

The nurse would exert enough pressure on the syringe plunger that the protective cap could pop off in the child's mouth and possibly cause the child to choke.

Prevention

_____

_____

After completing these problems, see pages 647–648 to check your answers.

Be sure to use the online software for additional practice!

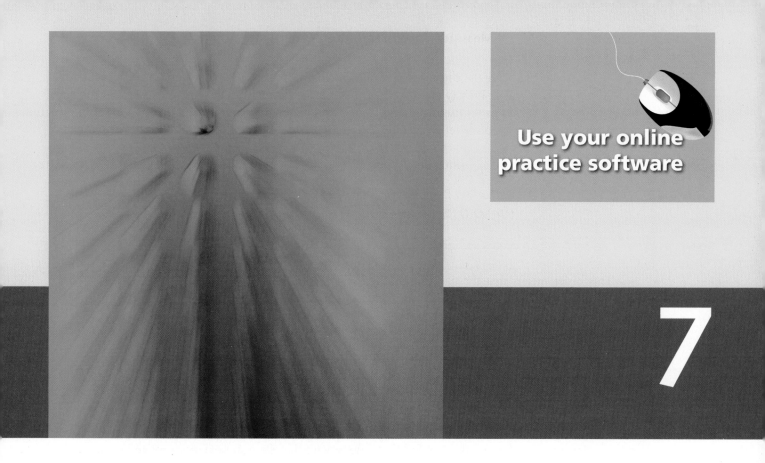

7

Interpreting Drug Orders

OBJECTIVES

Upon mastery of Chapter 7, you will be able to interpret drug orders. To accomplish this, you will also be able to:

- Read and write correct medical notation.
- Write the standard medical abbreviation from a list of common terminology.
- Interpret medicine orders of physicians and other prescribing practitioners.
- Interpret medication administration records.

The prescription, or medication order, conveys the therapeutic drug plan for the patient. It is the responsibility of the nurse to:

- Interpret the order.
- Gather information about the drug.
- Select and prepare the exact dosage of the prescribed drug.
- Identify the patient.
- Administer the proper dosage by the prescribed route, at the prescribed time intervals.
- Educate the patient regarding the medication.
- Record the administration of the prescribed drug.
- Monitor the patient's response for desired (therapeutic) and adverse effects.

Before you can prepare the correct dosage of the prescribed drug, you must learn to interpret, or read, the written drug order. For brevity and speed, the health care professions have adopted certain standards and common abbreviations for use in notation. You should learn to recognize and interpret the abbreviations from memory. As you practice reading drug orders, you will find that this skill becomes second nature to you.

An example of a typical written drug order is:

9/4/XX 0730 Amoxil 500 mg p.o. q.i.d. p.c. et bedtime
J. Physician, M.D.

This order means that the patient should receive 500 milligrams of an antibiotic named Amoxil (or amoxicillin) orally 4 times a day after meals and at bedtime. You can see that the medical notation shortens the written-out order considerably.

MEDICAL ABBREVIATIONS

The following table lists common medical abbreviations used in writing drug orders. The abbreviations are grouped according to the route (or method) of administration, the frequency (time interval), and other general terms. Commit these to memory, along with the other abbreviations related to systems of measurement presented in Chapter 3.

REMEMBER
Common Medical Abbreviations

Abbreviation	Interpretation	Abbreviation	Interpretation
Route:		**Frequency:**	
IM	intramuscular	h	hour
IV	intravenous	q.h	every hour
IV PB	intravenous piggyback	q.2h	every 2 hours
Subcut	subcutaneous	q.3h	every 3 hours
SL	sublingual, under the tongue	q.4h	every 4 hours
ID	intradermal	q.6h	every 6 hours
GT	gastrostomy tube	q.8h	every 8 hours
NG	nasogastric tube	q.12h	every 12 hours
NJ	nasojejunal tube	**General:**	
p.o.	by mouth, orally	$\bar{a}$	before
p.r.	per rectum, rectally	$\bar{p}$	after
Frequency:		$\bar{c}$	with
a.c.	before meals	$\bar{s}$	without
p.c.	after meals	q	every
ad. lib.	as desired, freely	qs	quantity sufficient
p.r.n.	when necessary	aq	water
stat	immediately, at once	NPO	nothing by mouth
asap	as soon as possible	gtt	drop
b.i.d.	twice a day	tab	tablet
t.i.d.	3 times a day	cap	capsule
q.i.d.	4 times a day	et	and
min	minute	noct	night

THE DRUG ORDER

The drug order consists of seven parts:

1. Name of the *patient*

2. Name of the *drug* to be administered

3. *Dosage* of the drug

4. *Route* by which the drug is to be administered

5. *Frequency,* time, and special instructions related to administration

6. *Date and time* when the order was written

7. *Signature and licensure* of the person writing the order

CAUTION

If any of the seven parts is missing or unclear, the order is considered incomplete and is therefore not a legal drug order.

Parts one through five of the drug order are known as the original Five Rights of safe medication administration. They are essential, and each one must be faithfully checked every time a medication is prepared and administered. After safe administration of the medication, the nurse or health care practitioner must accurately document the drug administration. Combining accurate documentation with the original Five Rights, the patient is entitled to *Six Rights* of safe and accurate medication administration and documentation with each and every dose.

REMEMBER

The Six Rights of safe and accurate medication administration are as follows:

The *right patient* must receive the *right drug* in the *right amount* by the *right route* at the *right time,* followed by the *right documentation.*

Each drug order should follow a specific sequence. The name of the drug is written first, followed by the dosage, route, and frequency. When correctly written, the brand (or trade) name of the drug begins with a capital, or uppercase, letter. The generic name begins with a lowercase letter.

EXAMPLE ▪

Procanbid 500 mg p.o. b.i.d.

1. **Procanbid** is the brand name of the drug.

2. **500 mg** is the dosage.

3. **p.o.** is the route.

4. **b.i.d.** is the frequency.

This order means: *Give 500 milligrams of Procanbid orally twice a day.*

CAUTION

If the nurse has difficulty understanding and interpreting the drug order, the nurse must clarify the order with the writer. Usually this person is the physician or another authorized practitioner, such as an advanced registered nurse practitioner.

Let's practice reading and interpreting drug orders.

EXAMPLE 1 ■

phenytoin 100 mg p.o. t.i.d.

This order means: *Give 100 milligrams of phenytoin orally 3 times a day.*

EXAMPLE 2 ■

procaine penicillin G 400,000 units IV q.6h

This order means: *Give 400,000 units of procaine penicillin G intravenously every 6 hours.*

EXAMPLE 3 ■

hydromorphone 2 mg IM q.4h p.r.n., moderate to severe pain

This order means: *Give 2 milligrams of hydromorphone intramuscularly every 4 hours when necessary for moderate to severe pain.*

CAUTION

The p.r.n. frequency designates the minimum time allowed between doses. There is no maximum time other than automatic stops as defined by hospital or agency policy.

EXAMPLE 4 ■

Humulin R regular U-100 insulin 5 units subcut stat

This order means: *Give 5 units of Humulin R regular U-100 insulin subcutaneously immediately.*

EXAMPLE 5 ■

cefazolin 1 g IV PB q.6h

This order means: *Give 1 gram of cefazolin by intravenous piggyback every 6 hours.*

The administration times are designated by hospital policy. For example, t.i.d. administration times may be 0900 or 9 AM, 1300 or 1 PM, and 1700 or 5 PM. This is different than q.8h administration times, which may be 0600, 1400, and 2200. Administration times for b.i.d., t.i.d., and q.i.d. are typically during waking hours.

QUICK REVIEW

■ The *right patient* must receive the *right drug* in the *right amount* by the *right route* at the *right time* followed by the *right documentation*.

■ Understanding drug orders requires interpreting common medical abbreviations.

■ The drug order must contain (in this sequence): drug name, dosage, route, and frequency.

■ All parts of the drug order must be stated clearly for accurate, exact interpretation.

■ If you are ever in doubt as to the meaning of any part of a drug order, ask the writer to clarify before proceeding.

Review Set 18

For questions 1 through 13, interpret the following medication (drug) orders:

1. naproxen 250 mg p.o. b.i.d. _____

   _____

2. Humulin N NPH insulin 30 units subcut daily 30 min ā breakfast _____

   _____

3. cefaclor 500 mg p.o. stat, then 250 mg q.8h _____

_____

4. Synthroid 25 mcg p.o. daily _____

_____

5. Ativan 10 mg IM q.4h p.r.n., agitation _____

_____

6. furosemide 20 mg slow IV stat _____

_____

7. Mylanta 10 mL p.o. p.c. et bedtime _____

_____

8. atropine sulfate ophthalmic 1% 2 gtt right eye q.15 min X 4 _____

_____

9. morphine sulfate 15 mg IM q.3h p.r.n., pain _____

_____

10. digoxin 0.25 mg p.o. daily _____

_____

11. tetracycline 250 mg p.o. q.i.d. _____

_____

12. nitroglycerin 150 mcg SL stat _____

_____

13. Cortisporin otic suspension 2 gtt each ear t.i.d. et bedtime _____

_____

14. Compare and contrast *t.i.d.* and *q.8h* administration times. Include sample administration times for each in your explanation. _____

_____

15. Describe your action if no method of administration is written. _____

_____

16. Do q.i.d. and q.4h have the same meaning? _____ Explain. _____

_____

17. Who determines the medication administration times? _____

_____

18. Name the seven parts of a written medication prescription. _____

_____

19. Which parts of the written medication prescription/order are included in the original Five Rights of medication administration? _____

_____

20. State the Six Rights of safe and accurate medication administration. _____

_____

After completing these problems, see page 649 to check your answers.

MEDICATION ORDER AND ADMINISTRATION FORMS

Hospitals have a special form for recording drug orders. As hospitals transition to electronic medical records, handwritten forms will be replaced by electronic order entry. Figure 7-1 shows a sample written physician's order form. Find and name each of the seven parts of the drug orders listed. Notice that the nurse or other health care professional must verify and initial each order, ensuring that each of the seven parts is accurate. In some facilities, the pharmacist may be responsible for verifying the order as part of the computerized record.

FIGURE 7-1 Paper-based physician's order form

	ENTERED	FILLED	CHECKED	VERIFIED

Physician's Order Form

Parts list (left side):
1. Patient
2. Drug
3. Dosage
4. Route
5. Frequency and special instructions
6. Date and time
7. Signature

DATE	TIME WRITTEN	ORDER	DISPENSE AS WRITTEN	TIME NOTED	NURSE'S SIGNATURE
11/3/xx	0815	cephalexin 250 mg p.o. q.6h	✓		
		Humulin N NPH Insulin 40 units subcut c̄ breakfast	✓	0830	G. Pickar, R.N.
		hydromorphone 2 mg IV q. 3h p.r.n., severe pain	✓		
		codeine 30 mg p.o. q.4h p.r.n., mild-mod pain	✓		
		Tylenol 650 mg p.o. q.4h p.r.n., fever greater than 101°F	✓		
		furosemide 40 mg p.o. daily	✓		
		K-Dur 10 mEq p.o. b.i.d.	✓		
		J. Physician, M.D.			
11/3/xx	2200	furosemide 80 mg IV stat	✓		
		J. Physician, M.D.		2210	M. Smith, R.N.

AUTO STOP ORDERS: UNLESS REORDERED, FOLLOWING WILL BE D/C^D AT 0800 ON:

DATE	ORDER		
		☐ CONT	PHYSICIAN SIGNATURE
		☐ D/C	
		☐ CONT	PHYSICIAN SIGNATURE
		☐ D/C	
		☐ CONT	PHYSICIAN SIGNATURE
		☐ D/C	

INDICATE IF ANTIBIOTICS ORDERED ☐ Prophylactic ☐ Empiric ☐ Therapeutic

PATIENT DIAGNOSIS
Diabetes

PATIENT ALLERGIES
None Known

PATIENT HEIGHT 5' 5"   PATIENT WEIGHT 130 lb

① Patient, Mary Q.
#3-11316-7

If traditional handwritten records are still in use, the drug orders from the physician's order form are transcribed to a medication administration record (MAR) and the administration times are scheduled (Figure 7-2). The nurse or other health care professional uses this record as a guide to:

- Check the drug order.
- Prepare the correct dosage.
- Record the drug administered and time.

These three checkpoints help to ensure accurate medication administration.

FIGURE 7-2   Paper-based medication administration record

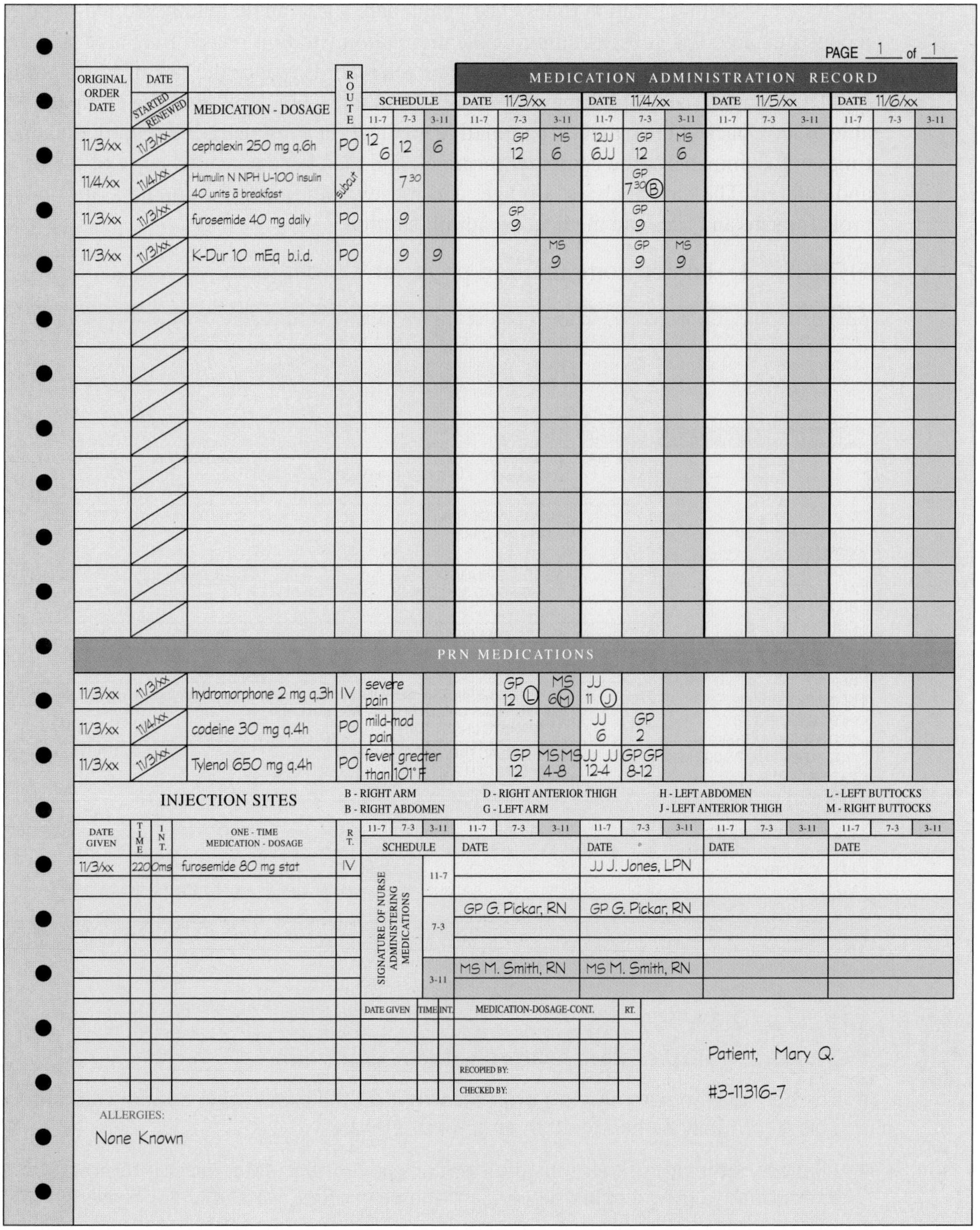

PAGE 1 of 1

MEDICATION ADMINISTRATION RECORD

ORIGINAL ORDER DATE	DATE STARTED/RENEWED	MEDICATION - DOSAGE	ROUTE	SCHEDULE 11-7	7-3	3-11	11/3/xx 11-7	7-3	3-11	11/4/xx 11-7	7-3	3-11	11/5/xx 11-7	7-3	3-11	11/6/xx 11-7	7-3	3-11
11/3/xx	11/3/xx	cephalexin 250 mg q.6h	PO	12 6	12	6		GP 12	MS 6	12JJ 6JJ	GP 12	MS 6						
11/4/xx	11/4/xx	Humulin N NPH U-100 insulin 40 units ā breakfast	SubQ		7³⁰						GP 7³⁰ Ⓑ							
11/3/xx	11/3/xx	furosemide 40 mg daily	PO		9			GP 9			GP 9							
11/3/xx	11/3/xx	K-Dur 10 mEq b.i.d.	PO		9	9			MS 9		GP 9	MS 9						

PRN MEDICATIONS

11/3/xx	11/3/xx	hydromorphone 2 mg q.3h	IV	severe pain			GP 12 Ⓛ	MS 6 Ⓜ	JJ 11 Ⓙ									
11/3/xx	11/4/xx	codeine 30 mg q.4h	PO	mild-mod pain						JJ 6	GP 2							
11/3/xx	11/3/xx	Tylenol 650 mg q.4h	PO	fever greater than 101° F			GP 12	MSMS 4-8	JJ JJ 12-4	GPGP 8-12								

INJECTION SITES   B - RIGHT ARM   B - RIGHT ABDOMEN   D - RIGHT ANTERIOR THIGH   G - LEFT ARM   H - LEFT ABDOMEN   J - LEFT ANTERIOR THIGH   L - LEFT BUTTOCKS   M - RIGHT BUTTOCKS

DATE GIVEN	TIME	INT.	ONE - TIME MEDICATION - DOSAGE	RT.	SCHEDULE 11-7	7-3	3-11	DATE 11-7	7-3	3-11	DATE 11-7	7-3	3-11	DATE 11-7	7-3	3-11	DATE
11/3/xx	2200	ms	furosemide 80 mg stat	IV													

SIGNATURE OF NURSE ADMINISTERING MEDICATIONS

	11-7	JJ J. Jones, LPN
	7-3	GP G. Pickar, RN GP G. Pickar, RN
	3-11	MS M. Smith, RN MS M. Smith, RN

DATE GIVEN	TIME	INT.	MEDICATION-DOSAGE-CONT.	RT.

RECOPIED BY:

CHECKED BY:

Patient, Mary Q.

#3-11316-7

ALLERGIES:
None Known

COMPUTERIZED MEDICATION ADMINISTRATION SYSTEMS

Most health care facilities now use computers for processing drug orders. The Health Information Technology for Economic and Clinical Health Act (HITECH) of 2009 calls for electronic medical records for all patients by 2014. To earn stimulus incentives, physicians and hospitals must demonstrate meaningful use of a certified electronic health record (EHR) solution. Starting in 2015, doctors and hospitals that do not use EHRs may receive financial penalties under Medicare. Drug orders are either electronically transmitted or manually entered into the computer from an order form, such as Figure 7-3. Through the computer, the nurse or other health care professional can transmit the order within seconds to the pharmacy for filling. The computer can keep track of drug stock and usage patterns and even notify the business office to post charges to the patient's account. Most importantly, it can scan for information previously entered, such as drug incompatibilities, drug allergies, safe dosage ranges, doses already given, or recommended administration times. The health care staff can be readily alerted to potential problems or inconsistencies. The corresponding medication administration record may also be printed directly from the computer as in Figure 7-4. Such computerized records reduce the risk of misinterpreting handwriting.

The computerized MAR may be viewed from a printed copy or at the computer. The nurse may be able to look back at the patient's cumulative medication administration record, document administration times and comments at the computer terminal, and then keep a printed copy of the information obtained and entered. The data analysis, storage, and retrieval abilities of computers are making them essential tools for safe and accurate medication administration.

FIGURE 7-3 Printed computerized physician's order form

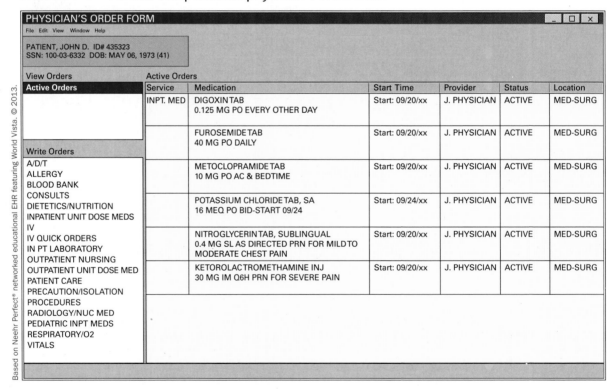

Based on Neehr Perfect® networked educational EHR featuring World Vista. © 2013.

PHYSICIAN'S ORDER FORM

File Edit View Window Help

PATIENT, JOHN D. ID# 435323
SSN: 100-03-6332 DOB: MAY 06, 1973 (41)

View Orders   Active Orders

Active Orders

Write Orders

A/D/T
ALLERGY
BLOOD BANK
CONSULTS
DIETETICS/NUTRITION
INPATIENT UNIT DOSE MEDS
IV
IV QUICK ORDERS
IN PT LABORATORY
OUTPATIENT NURSING
OUTPATIENT UNIT DOSE MED
PATIENT CARE
PRECAUTION/ISOLATION
PROCEDURES
RADIOLOGY/NUC MED
PEDIATRIC INPT MEDS
RESPIRATORY/O2
VITALS

Service	Medication	Start Time	Provider	Status	Location
INPT. MED	DIGOXIN TAB 0.125 MG PO EVERY OTHER DAY	Start: 09/20/xx	J. PHYSICIAN	ACTIVE	MED-SURG
	FUROSEMIDE TAB 40 MG PO DAILY	Start: 09/20/xx	J. PHYSICIAN	ACTIVE	MED-SURG
	METOCLOPRAMIDE TAB 10 MG PO AC & BEDTIME	Start: 09/20/xx	J. PHYSICIAN	ACTIVE	MED-SURG
	POTASSIUM CHLORIDE TAB, SA 16 MEQ PO BID-START 09/24	Start: 09/24/xx	J. PHYSICIAN	ACTIVE	MED-SURG
	NITROGLYCERIN TAB, SUBLINGUAL 0.4 MG SL AS DIRECTED PRN FOR MILD TO MODERATE CHEST PAIN	Start: 09/20/xx	J. PHYSICIAN	ACTIVE	MED-SURG
	KETOROLAC TROMETHAMINE INJ 30 MG IM Q6H PRN FOR SEVERE PAIN	Start: 09/20/xx	J. PHYSICIAN	ACTIVE	MED-SURG

QUICK REVIEW

- Drug orders are prescribed on the physician's order form.

- The person who administers a drug records it on the medication administration record (MAR). This record may be handwritten or computerized.

- All parts of the drug order must be stated clearly for accurate, exact interpretation. If you are ever in doubt as to the meaning of any part of a drug order, ask the writer to clarify.

FIGURE 7-4   Printed computerized medication administration record

MEDICATION ADMINISTRATION RECORD					— □ ×

File Edit View Window Help

PATIENT, JOHN D. ID# 435323
SSN = 100-03-6332
DOB = 05/06/1973 (41)
Height = 5'10'', Weight = 165 lb
Location = MED-SURG

Schedule
☑ Continuous   ☑ On-Call
☑ PRN   ☑ One-Time

Start Time: 09/23@2000 ▼   Stop Time: 09/24@1300 ▼

Allergies: NO KNOWN ALLERGIES   ADRs: NO ADRS ON FILE

Active Medication	Dosage	Route	Admin Time	Last Action
METOCLOPRAMIDE TAB REGLAN 10 MG	10 MG, AC & BEDTIME	ORAL	09/23@2200	GIVEN
METOCLOPRAMIDE TAB REGLAN 10 MG	10 MG, AC & BEDTIME	ORAL	09/24@0730	GIVEN
DIGOXIN TAB LANOXIN, 0.125 MG	0.125 MG, EVERY OTHER DAY	ORAL	09/24@0900	GIVEN
FUROSEMIDE TAB FUROSEMIDE 40 MG	40 MG, DAILY	ORAL	09/24@0900	GIVEN
POTASSIUM CHLORIDE TAB, SA POTASSIUM CHLORIDE 20 MEQ START 09/24	16 MEQ, BID	ORAL	09/24@0900	GIVEN
METOCLOPRAMIDE TAB REGLAN 10 MG	10 MG, AC & BEDTIME	ORAL	09/24@1130	GIVEN
METOCLOPRAMIDE TAB REGLAN 10 MG	10 MG, AC & BEDTIME	ORAL	09/24@1630	
POTASSIUM CHLORIDE TAB, SA POTASSIUM CHLORIDE 20 MEQ START 09/24	16 MEQ, BID	ORAL	09/24@1700	
METOCLOPRAMIDE TAB REGLAN 10 MG	10 MG, AC & BEDTIME	ORAL	09/24@2200	
NITROGLYCERIN TAB, SUBLINGUAL NITROGLYCERIN 0.4 MG FOR MILD TO MODERATE CHEST PAIN	0.4 MG, AS DIRECTED PRN	SUBLINGUAL		
KETOROLAC TROMETHAMINE INJ KETOROLAC TROMETHAMINE 60 MG/2 ML FOR SEVERE PAIN	30 MG, Q6H PRN	INTRAMUSCULAR		

Server Time: 9/24/xxxx 01:35

Review Set 19

Refer to the computerized MAR, Figure 7-4, to answer questions 1 through 10. Convert the scheduled international time to traditional AM/PM time.

1. What is the ordered route for digoxin? _____

2. What are the scheduled times for administering digoxin? _____

3. What are the scheduled times for administering metoclopramide? _____

4. What is the next time potassium chloride should be administered? _____

5. How often should the ketorolac tromethamine be given? _____

6. When is the next date and time digoxin should be given? _____

7. What is the ordered route of administration for the nitroglycerin? _____

8. How many times a day is furosemide ordered? _____

9. The equivalent dosage of digoxin is _____ mcg.

10. Which drugs are ordered to be administered "as necessary"? _____

Refer to the paper-based MAR (Figure 7-2) on page 149 to answer questions 11 through 21.

11. What is the route of administration for the insulin? _____

12. How many times in a 24-hour period should furosemide be administered? _____

13. What is the only medication ordered to be given routinely at noon? _____

14. At what time of day should the insulin be administered? _____

15. A dosage of 10 mEq of K-Dur is ordered. What does mEq mean? _____

16. You work 3 PM to 11 PM on November 5. Which routine medications should you administer to Mary Q. Patient during your shift? _____

17. Mary Q. Patient has a fever of 101.4°F. What medication should you administer? _____

18. How many times in a 24-hour period should K-Dur be administered? _____

19. What is the equivalent of the scheduled administration time(s) for the K-Dur as converted to international time?

_____

20. What is the equivalent of the scheduled administration time(s) for the cephalexin as converted to international time? _____

21. Identify the place on the MAR where the stat IV furosemide was charted. _____

After completing these problems, see page 649 to check your answers.

CLINICAL REASONING SKILLS

It is the responsibility of the nurse to clarify any drug order that is incomplete—that is, an order that does not contain the essential seven parts discussed in this chapter. Let's look at an example in which an error resulted from not clarifying an incomplete order.

ERROR

Failing to clarify incomplete orders

Possible Scenario

Suppose a physician ordered *omeprazole capsules p.o. ā bedtime* for a patient with an active duodenal ulcer. You will note that there is no dosage listed. The nurse thought the medication came in only one dosage strength, added 20 mg to the order, and sent it to the pharmacy. The pharmacist prepared the dosage written on the physician's order sheet. Two days later, during rounds, the physician noted that the patient had not responded well to the medication. When asked about this, the nurse explained that the patient had received 20 mg at bedtime. The physician informed the nurse that the patient should have received the 40 mg dosage for high acid suppression.

Potential Outcome

Potentially, the delay in correct dosage could result in gastrointestinal bleeding or delayed healing of the ulcer.

Prevention

This medication error could have been avoided simply by the physician writing the strength of the medication. Because it was omitted, the nurse should have checked the dosage before sending the order to the pharmacy. When you add to an incomplete order, you are essentially practicing medicine without a license, which is illegal and potentially dangerous.

CLINICAL REASONING SKILLS

Read the entire medication record to ensure that the planned administration times are scheduled correctly according to the medication order. In the following situation, two doses of a medication were omitted each day until an observant nurse picked up on the transcription error.

ERROR

Omitting medication due to incorrect scheduling of doses

Possible Scenario

An order was written for *ampicillin 500 mg IV PB q.4h*, which was handwritten on the medication administration record (MAR). The registered nurse was distracted while verifying the order and writing in the scheduled times of administration. The nurse saw the number 4 and instead of scheduling the medication every 4 hours, scheduled the medication to be given 4 times a day—at 0600, 1200, 1800, and 2400. For 2 days, the shift nurses each checked to see what medications needed to be given on their scheduled shifts but did not take the time to compare the ordered frequency to the scheduled times. Eventually, a nurse did look over the entire medication record and noticed the error. The medication times were corrected and the doctor was notified. A medication variance form was completed, documenting the error, and it was submitted to the hospital risk management department.

Potential Outcome

Over the course of 2 days the patient missed 4 doses, for a total of 2 grams of ampicillin. This could have led to a prolonged illness as a result of the persistent infection, increased patient discomfort, and a prolonged hospitalization.

Prevention

At the beginning of each shift, read the entire medication administration record. Verify that the times scheduled for medications to be administered on your shift comply with the ordered frequency. Also review medications scheduled for other shifts, to consider any potential drug interactions or inconsistencies. This practice might also prevent others from making a medication error.

PRACTICE PROBLEMS—CHAPTER 7

Interpret the following abbreviations and symbols without consulting another source.

1. b.i.d.	_____	9. IV	_____
2. p.r.	_____	10. q.i.d.	_____
3. a.c.	_____	11. stat	_____
4. p̄	_____	12. ad.lib.	_____
5. t.i.d.	_____	13. p.c.	_____
6. q.4h	_____	14. IM	_____
7. p.r.n.	_____	15. s̄	_____
8. p.o.	_____		

Give the abbreviations for the following terms without consulting another source.

16. night	_____	23. subcutaneous	_____
17. drop	_____	24. teaspoon	_____
18. milliliter	_____	25. twice daily	_____
19. under the tongue	_____	26. every 3 hours	_____
20. gram	_____	27. after meals	_____
21. 4 times a day	_____	28. before	_____
22. with	_____	29. kilogram	_____

Interpret the following physician's drug orders without consulting another source.

30. Toradol 60 mg IV stat et q.6h p.r.n., pain _____

31. procaine penicillin G 300,000 units IV q.i.d. _____

32. Mylanta 5 mL p.o. 1 h a.c., 1 h p.c., bedtime, et q.2h p.r.n. at noct, gastric upset _____

_____

33. Librium 25 mg p.o. q.6h p.r.n., agitation _____

34. heparin 5,000 units subcut stat _____

35. morphine sulfate 5 mg IV q.4h p.r.n., moderate to severe pain _____

36. digoxin 0.25 mg p.o. daily _____

37. Neo-Synephrine ophthalmic 10% 2 gtt left eye q.30 min × 2 _____

_____

38. Lasix 40 mg IM stat _____

39. Decadron 4 mg IV b.i.d. _____

Refer to the paper-based MAR in Figure 7-5 on page 155 to answer questions 40 through 44.

40. Convert the scheduled times for isosorbide SR to traditional AM/PM times.

_____   _____   _____

41. How many units of heparin will be used to flush the central line at 2200? _____

42. What route is ordered for the Humulin R regular U-100 insulin? _____

43. Interpret the order for Cipro. _____

44. If the administration times for the sliding scale insulin are accurate (30 minutes before meals), at what times will meals be served? (Use traditional AM/PM time.) _____

Refer to the computerized pharmacy MAR in Figure 7-6 on page 156 to answer questions 45 through 49.

45. How often may the patient receive the "as needed" medication, oxycodone? _____

_____

46. What is the ordered dosage for lorazepam? _____

_____

FIGURE 7-5 Paper-based MAR for Chapter 7 Practice Problems (questions 40–44)

PAGE ___1___ of ___1___

MEDICATION ADMINISTRATION RECORD

ORIGINAL ORDER DATE	DATE STARTED/RENEWED	MEDICATION - DOSAGE	ROUTE	SCHEDULE 11-7	7-3	3-11	DATE 11/3/xx 11-7	7-3	3-11	DATE 11/4/xx 11-7	7-3	3-11	DATE 11/5/xx 11-7	7-3	3-11	DATE 11/6/xx 11-7	7-3	3-11
11/3/xx	11/3/xx	heparin lock central line flush (10 units per mL solution) 2 mL b.i.d.	IV		1000	2200												
11/3/xx	11/3/xx	isosorbide SR 40 mg q.8h	PO	2400	0800	1600												
11/3/xx	11/3/xx	Cipro 500 mg q.12h	PO		1000	2200												
11/3/xx	11/3/xx	Humulin N NPH U-100 insulin 15 units q.am	subcut	0700														
11/3/xx	11/3/xx	Humulin R regular U-100 insulin 30 min. ac and bedtime	subcut		0730 1130	1730 2200												
		per sliding scale Blood glucose																
		0-150 3 units 151-250 8 units																
		251-350 13 units 351-400 18 units																
		greater than 400 call Dr.																

PRN MEDICATIONS

11/3/xx	11/3/xx	Tylenol 1,000 mg q.4h p.r.n., headache	PO															

INJECTION SITES

B - RIGHT ARM D - RIGHT ANTERIOR THIGH H - LEFT ABDOMEN L - LEFT BUTTOCKS
C - RIGHT ABDOMEN G - LEFT ARM J - LEFT ANTERIOR THIGH M - RIGHT BUTTOCKS

DATE GIVEN	TIME	INT.	ONE - TIME MEDICATION - DOSAGE	RT.	11-7	7-3	3-11	11-7	7-3	3-11	11-7	7-3	3-11	11-7	7-3	3-11	11-7	7-3	3-11
					SCHEDULE		11-7	DATE			DATE			DATE			DATE		

SIGNATURE OF NURSE ADMINISTERING MEDICATIONS — 11-7 / 7-3 / 3-11

DATE GIVEN | TIME | INT. | MEDICATION-DOSAGE-CONT. | RT.

RECOPIED BY:
CHECKED BY:

Patient, Pat H.
#6-33725-4

ALLERGIES: None Known

47. Interpret the order for ranitidine. _____

48. At what time may the patient receive pain medication again, if needed? _____

49. How many hours are between the scheduled administration times for megestrol? _____

FIGURE 7-6 Computerized pharmacy MAR for Chapter 7 Practice Problems (questions 45–49)

PHARMACY MEDICATION ADMINISTRATION RECORD					_ □ ×

File Edit View Window Help

SMITH, JOHN ID# 667134
SSN = 100-03-6333
DOB = 04/05/1965 (48)
Height = 5' 11", Weight = 175 lb
Location = MED-SURG

Schedule
☑ Continuous   ☑ On-Call
☑ PRN   ☑ One-Time

Start Time: 12/12@0700
Stop Time: 12/12@1700

Allergies: NAFCILLIN, BACTRIM, SULFA/TRIMETHOPRIM, CIPROFLOXACIN HCL

Active Medication	Dosage	Route	Admin Time	Last Action
WITCH HAZEL PAD WITCH HAZEL PADS APPLY TO RECTUM	1 PAD, Q4H PRN	TOPICAL	12/12@0700	GIVEN
OXYCODONE HCL TAB OXYCODONE HCL 5 MG PRN FOR PAIN	5 MG, Q4H PRN	ORAL	12/12@0700	GIVEN
LIDOCAINE OINT LIDOCAINE 5% OINTMENT APPLY TO RECTAL AREA	35 GM TUBE, AS DIRECTED PRN	TOPICAL	12/12@0700	GIVEN
LORAZEPAM INJ LORAZEPAM 2 MG/ML TUBEX FOR ANXIETY	1 MG, Q6H PRN	INTRAVENOUS	12/12@0730	GIVEN
RANITIDINE TAB RANITIDINE 150 MG WITH BREAKFAST AND SUPPER	150 MG, BID	ORAL	12/12@0800	GIVEN
MEGESTROL ACETATE TAB MEGESTROL ACETATE 40 MG	40 MG, BID	ORAL	12/12@0900	GIVEN
FLUCONAZOLE TAB FLUCONAZOLE 100 MG TAB, ORAL	100 MG, DAILY	ORAL	12/12@0900	GIVEN
VANCOMYCIN CAP VANCOMYCIN 250 MG	250 MG, QID	ORAL	12/12@0900	GIVEN
HEMORRHOIDAL HYDROCORTISONE SUPPOSITORY HYDROCORTISONE SUPPOSITORY	1 SUPPOSITORY, Q4H	RECTAL	12/12@0900	GIVEN
HEMORRHOIDAL HYDROCORTISONE SUPPOSITORY HYDROCORTISONE SUPPOSITORY	1 SUPPOSITORY, Q4H	RECTAL	12/12@1300	GIVEN
VANCOMYCIN CAP VANCOMYCIN 250 MG	250 MG, QID	ORAL	12/12@1300	GIVEN
DIGOXIN TAB DIGOXIN 0.125 MG CHECK PULSE RATE	0.125 MG, DAILY AC DINNER	ORAL	12/12@1630	
RANITIDINE TAB RANITIDINE 150 MG WITH BREAKFAST AND SUPPER	150 MG, BID	ORAL	12/12@1700	
MEGESTROL ACETATE TAB MEGESTROL ACETATE 40 MG	40 MG, BID	ORAL	12/12@1700	
VANCOMYCIN CAP VANCOMYCIN 250 MG	250 MG, QID	ORAL	12/12@1700	
HEMORRHOIDAL HYDROCORTISONE SUPPOSITORY HYDROCORTISONE SUPPOSITORY	1 SUPPOSITORY, Q4H	RECTAL	12/12@1700	

Server Time: 12/12/xxxx 15:36

50. Describe the clinical reasoning you would use to prevent this medication error.

Possible Scenario

Suppose a physician wrote an order for **gentamicin 100 mg IV q.8h** for a patient hospitalized with meningitis. The unit secretary transcribed the order as:

gentamicin 100 mg IV q.8h

(12 AM–6 AM–12 PM–6 PM)

The medication nurse checked the order without noticing the discrepancy in the administration times. Suppose the patient received the medication every 6 hours for 3 days before the error was noticed.

Potential Outcome

The patient would have received one extra dose each day, which is equivalent to one third more medication daily than prescribed. Most likely, the physician would be notified of the error, the medication discontinued, and the serum gentamicin levels drawn. The levels would likely be in the toxic range, and the patient's gentamicin levels would be monitored until the levels returned to normal. This patient would be at risk of developing ototoxicity or nephrotoxicity from the overdose of gentamicin.

Prevention

_____

_____

After completing these problems, see pages 649–650 to check your answers.

Be sure to use the online software for additional practice!

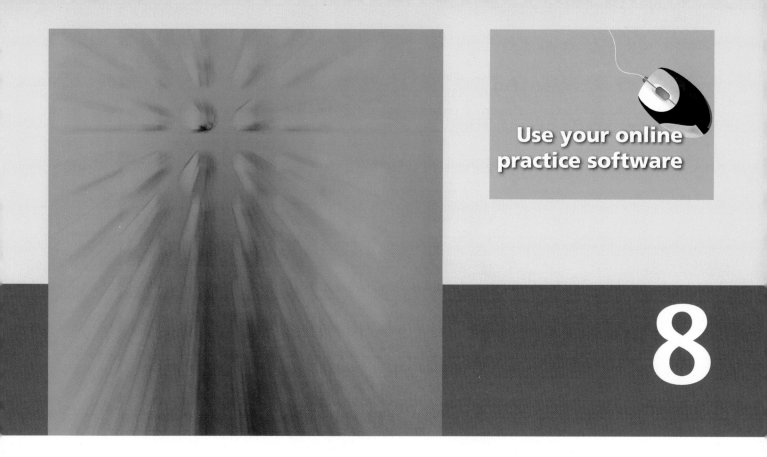

8

Understanding Drug Labels

OBJECTIVES

Upon mastery of Chapter 8, you will be able to read and understand the labels of the medications you have available. To accomplish this, you will also be able to:

- Recognize pertinent information on drug labels including:
    - Drug form
    - Dosage strength
    - Supply dosage or concentration
    - Total volume of drug container
    - Administration route
    - Expiration date
- Differentiate between the brand and generic names of drugs.
- Find the directions for mixing or preparing the supply dosage of drugs, as needed.
- Recognize and follow drug alerts.
- Locate the lot or control number, National Drug Code, barcode symbols, and controlled substance classifications.
- Determine if containers are for single-dose or multidose use.
- Identify combination drugs.
- Describe supply dosage expressed as a ratio or percent.

The drug order prescribes how much of a drug the patient is to receive. The nurse must prepare the order from the drugs on hand. The drug label tells how the available drug is supplied. Examine the various preparations, labels, and dosage strengths of Valium injection, as shown in Figure 8-1.

FIGURE 8-1   Various Valium preparations

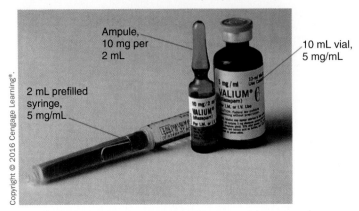

Look at the following common drug labels to learn to recognize pertinent information about the drugs supplied.

BRAND AND GENERIC NAMES

The brand, trade, or proprietary name is the manufacturer's name for a drug. Notice that the brand name is usually the most prominent word on the drug label—set in large type and boldly visible to easily identify and promote the product. It is often followed by the registered sign (®), meaning that both the name and formulation are so designated. The generic, or established, nonproprietary name appears directly under the brand name. Sometimes the generic name is placed inside parentheses. By law, the generic name must be identified on all drug labels.

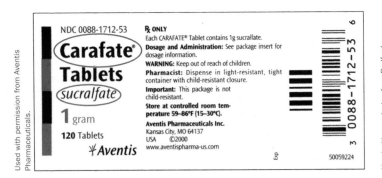

Brand name (Carafate) and generic name (sucralfate)

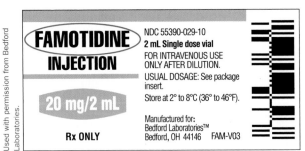

Generic drug (famotidine)

Generic equivalents of many brand-name drugs are ordered as substitutes or allowed by the prescribing practitioner. Because only the generic name appears on these labels, nurses need to carefully cross-check all medications. Failure to do so could cause inaccurate drug identification.

DOSAGE STRENGTH

The dosage strength refers to the dosage *weight* or amount of drug provided in a specific unit of measurement. The dosage strength of Lopid tablets is 600 milligrams (the weight and specific unit of measurement) per tablet. Some drugs, such as penicillin V potassium, have two different but equivalent dosage strengths. Penicillin V potassium has a dosage strength of 250 milligrams (per tablet), or 400,000 units (per tablet). This allows prescribers to order the drug using either unit of measurement.

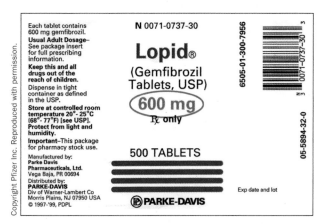

600 milligrams (per tablet)

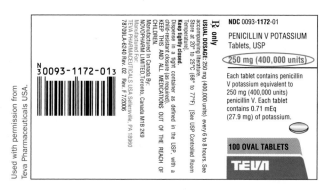

250 milligrams (400,000 units) (per tablet)

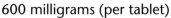

FORM

The form identifies the *structure* and *composition* of the drug. Solid dosage forms for oral use include tablets and capsules. Some powdered or granular medications that are not manufactured in tablet or capsule form can be directly combined with food or beverages and administered. Others must be reconstituted (liquefied) and measured in a precise liquid volume, such as milliliters, drops, or ounces. They may be a crystalloid (clear solution) or a suspension (solid particles in liquid that separate when held in a container).

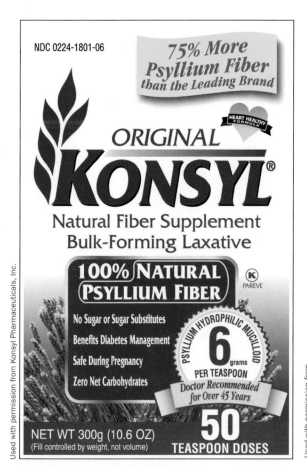

Fiber granular drug added to beverage

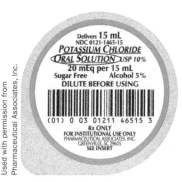

Oral solution

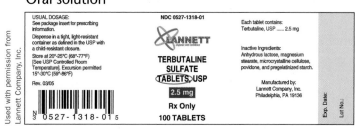

Tablets

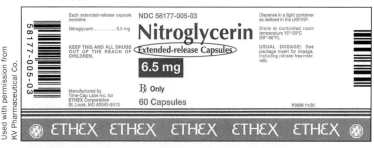

Extended-release capsules

Injectable medications may be supplied in solution or dry powdered form to be reconstituted. Once reconstituted, they are measured in milliliters.

Medications are also supplied in a variety of other forms, such as suppositories, creams, and patches.

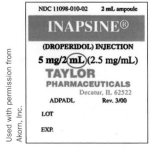

Injectable solution

SUPPLY DOSAGE

The supply dosage refers to both *dosage strength* and *form*. It is read *X amount of medication per some unit of measurement*. For solid-form medications, such as tablets, the supply dosage is *X amount of medication per tablet*. For liquid medications, the supply dosage is the same as the medication's concentration, such as *X amount of medication per milliliter*. Take a minute to read the supply dosage printed on the labels in this section.

Traditionally, it has been common to see the supply dosage expressed in per mL (1 mL) predominantly displayed on the label as with the Nubain label pictured. Occasionally, especially with oral solutions and suspensions, the concentration has been expressed in the usual standard dose, such as 250 mg per 5 mL. However, safety concerns with high-risk medications have led to a new way to express the supply dosage for single-dose and multidose injectable drug products. Compare the Nubain and heparin labels. The heparin supply dosage predominantly displayed is based on the total amount in the container. The amount per mL is printed directly below in smaller text. This strategy is intended to prevent an error from administering too large a dose. Notice that the Nubain label provides the total volume per container, but it is not expressed in supply dosage. The U.S. Pharmacopeial Convention (USP) first issued a requirement in 2009 for labels to state clearly the strength of the entire container of the medication followed by how much of the medication is in 1 milliliter (mL) (U.S. Pharmacopeia, 2013). Until manufacturers comply by revising all medication labels and the supply of older labeled medications is exhausted, extreme caution must be taken when locating the dosage strength.

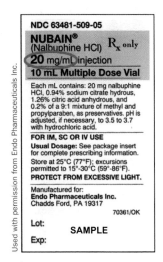

20 milligrams per milliliter

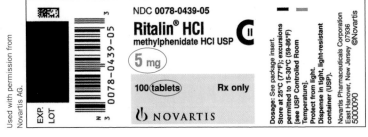

5 milligrams per tablet

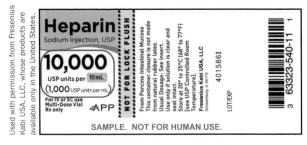

10,000 units per 10 mL (1,000 units per mL)

TOTAL VOLUME

The total volume refers to the *full quantity* contained in a package, bottle, or vial. For tablets and other solid medications, it is the total number of individual items. For liquids, it is the total fluid volume.

All too frequently, dosage strength and total volume are misinterpreted, resulting in medication errors. As of February 1, 2009, a new Food and Drug Administration (FDA) requirement became official that calls for the strength per total volume to be the prominent expression on single- and multidose injectable product labels, followed in close proximity by the strength per mL enclosed in parentheses (Cohen, 2008). Notice the Inapsine (droperidol injection) label on the previous page, which complies with the new rule: 2 mL ampule size, **5 mg/2 mL** (2.5 mg/mL). Clearly providing all of this information lowers the risk of misinterpretation and medication error.

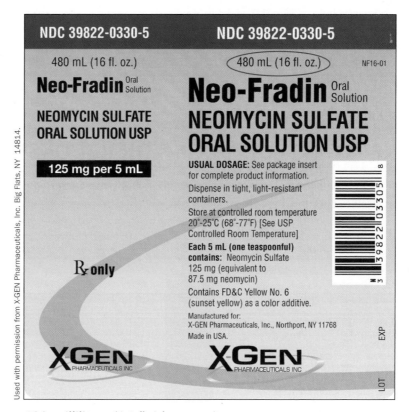

480 milliliters (16 fluid ounces)

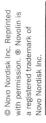 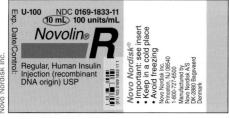

10 milliliters

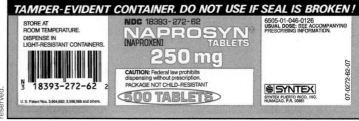

500 tablets

ADMINISTRATION ROUTE

The administration route refers to the *site* (of the body) or the *method of drug delivery* into the patient. Examples of routes of administration include oral, enteral (into the gastrointestinal tract through a tube), sublingual, injection (IV, IM, subcut), otic, optic, topical, rectal, vaginal, and others. Unless specified otherwise, tablets, capsules, and caplets are intended for oral use.

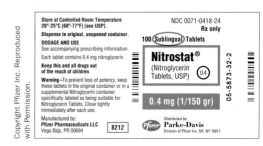

Sublingual

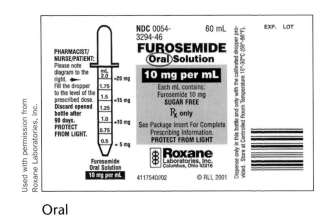

Oral

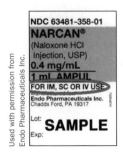

Intramuscular (IM),
subcutaneous (SC),
or intravenous (IV)

DIRECTIONS FOR MIXING OR RECONSTITUTING

Some drugs are dispensed in *powder* form and must be *reconstituted (or mixed) for use.* (Reconstitution is discussed further in Chapters 10 and 12.)

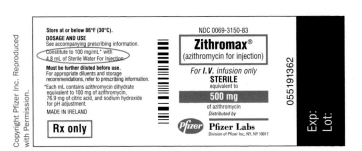

See directions

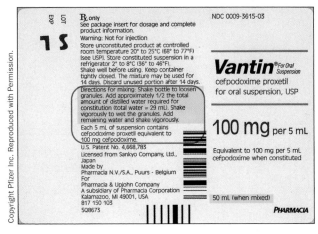

See directions

LABEL ALERTS

Manufacturers may print warnings on the packaging, or special alerts may be added by the pharmacy before dispensing. Look for special storage alerts such as "refrigerate at all times," "keep in a dry place," "replace cap and close tightly before storing," or "protect from light." Reconstituted suspensions may be dispensed already prepared for use, and directions may instruct the health care professional to "shake well before using," as a reminder to remix the components. Read and follow all label instructions carefully.

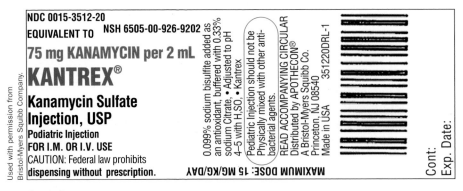

See alert

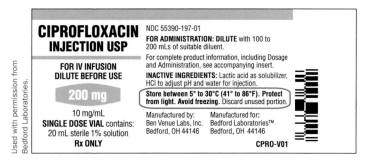

See alert

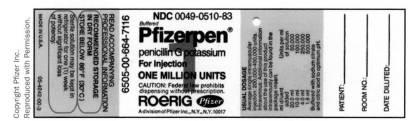

See alerts

NAME OF THE MANUFACTURER

The name of the manufacturer is circled on the following labels.

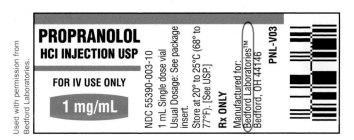

Bedford Laboratories

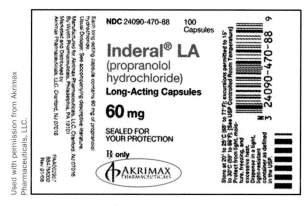

Akrimax Pharmaceuticals, Inc.

EXPIRATION DATE

The medication should be used, discarded, or returned to the pharmacy by the expiration date. Further, note the special expiration instructions given on labels for reconstituted medications. Refer to the discard instructions on the Vantin label on page 164.

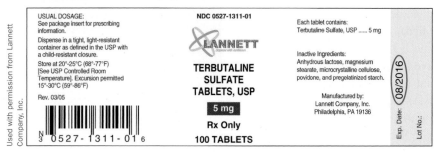

Expiration date: 08/2016

LOT OR CONTROL NUMBERS

Federal law requires all medication packages to be identified with a lot or control number. If a drug is recalled for reasons such as damage or tampering, the lot number quickly identifies the particular group of medication packages to be removed from shelves. This number has been invaluable for vaccine and over-the-counter medication recalls.

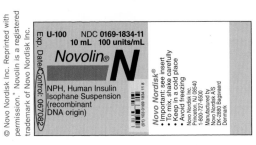

Control number: 067082

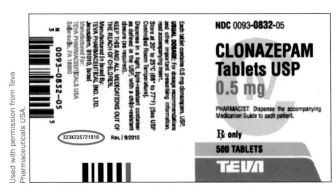

Lot number: 323K235721010

NATIONAL DRUG CODE (NDC)

Federal law requires every prescription medication to have a unique identifying number, much like every U.S. citizen has a unique Social Security number. This number must appear on every manufacturer's label and is printed with the letters "NDC" followed by three discrete groups of numbers.

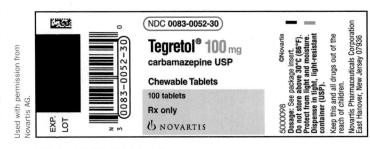

NDC: 0083-0052-30

CONTROLLED SUBSTANCE SCHEDULE

The Controlled Substances Act was passed in May 1971. One of its purposes was to improve the administration and regulation of the production, distribution, and dispensing of controlled substances. Drugs considered controlled substances are classified according to their potential for use and abuse.

Drugs are classified into five numbered levels, or schedules, with the schedules designated by a C (for Controlled) and Roman numerals: Schedule I, II, III, IV, and V. Drugs that have no medical use and highest potential for abuse (such as heroine and LSD) are Schedule I drugs, and those with the lowest potential for abuse are Schedule V drugs.

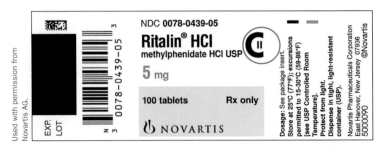

Schedule II

BARCODE SYMBOLS

Barcode symbols are commonly used in retail sales. They also document drug dosing for recordkeeping and stock reordering and can automate medication documentation right at the patient's bedside.

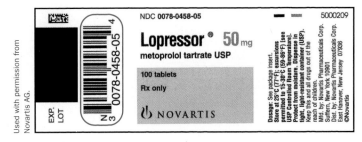

Barcode

UNITED STATES PHARMACOPEIA (USP) AND NATIONAL FORMULARY (NF)

These codes are found on many manufacturer-printed medication labels, and they are placed after the generic drug name. The USP and NF are the two official national lists of approved drugs. Each manufacturer follows special guidelines that determine when to include these initials on a label. Be careful not to mistake these abbreviations for other initials that designate specific characteristics of a drug, such as *SR,* which means *sustained release.*

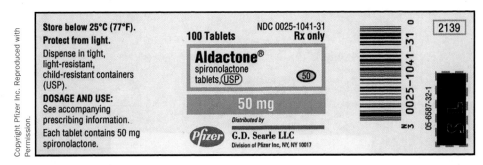

USP

UNIT- OR SINGLE-DOSE LABELS

Most oral medications administered in the hospital setting are available in unit dosage, such as a single capsule or tablet packaged separately in a typical blister pack. The pharmacy provides a 24-hour supply of each drug for the patient. The only major difference in this form of labeling is that the total volume of the container is usually omitted because the volume is 1 tablet or capsule. Likewise, the dosage strength is understood as *per one.* Further, injectable medicines may be packaged in single-dose preparations.

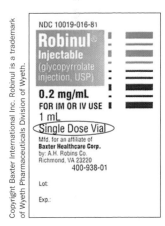

Unit dose
single-use vial

COMBINATION DRUGS

Some medications are a combination of two or more drugs in one form. Read the labels for Percocet and Lortab and notice the different substances that are combined in each tablet. Combination drugs are sometimes prescribed by the number of tablets, capsules, or milliliters to be given rather than by the dosage strength.

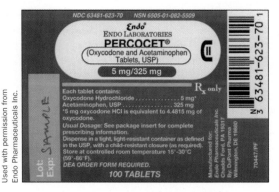

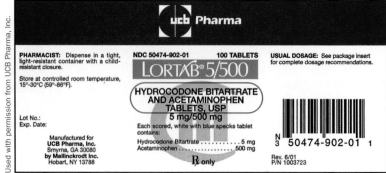

oxycodone and acetaminophen   hydrocodone bitartrate and acetaminophen

SUPPLY DOSAGE EXPRESSED AS A RATIO OR PERCENT

Occasionally, solutions will be ordered and/or manufactured in a supply dosage expressed as a ratio or percent.

RULE

Ratio solutions express the number of grams of the drug per total milliliters of solution.

EXAMPLE ■

Epinephrine 1:1,000 contains 1 g pure drug per 1,000 mL solution:

1 g:1,000 mL = 1,000 mg:1,000 mL = 1 mg:1 mL

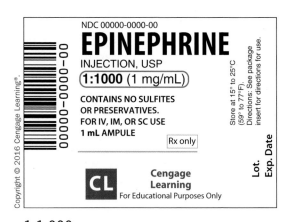

1:1,000

RULE

Percentage (%) solutions express the number of grams of the drug per 100 milliliters of solution.

EXAMPLE ■

Lidocaine 2% contains 2 g pure drug per 100 mL solution:

2 g per 100 mL =

2,000 mg per 100 mL =

20 mg/mL

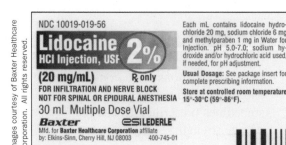

2%

Although these labels look different from many of the other labels, it is important to recognize that the supply dosage can still be determined. Many times the label will have a more commonly identified supply dosage and not just the ratio or percent. Look at the epinephrine and lidocaine labels. On the epinephrine label, the ratio is 1:1,000; the supply dosage can also be identified as 1 mg/mL. On the lidocaine label, the percentage is 2%; the supply dosage can also be identified as 20 mg/mL.

CHECKING LABELS

Practice the Six Rights of safe medication administration: The *right patient* must receive the *right drug* in the *right amount* by the *right route* at the *right time* followed by the *right documentation.* To be absolutely sure the patient receives the right drug, check the label three times.

CAUTION

Before administering a medication to a patient, check the drug label three times:

1. Against the medication order or MAR.

2. Before preparing the medication.

3. After preparing the medication and before administering it.

QUICK REVIEW

Read labels carefully to:

- Identify the drug and the manufacturer.

- Differentiate between brand and generic names, dosage strength, form, supply dosage, total container volume, and administration route.

- Recognize that the drug's supply dosage similarly refers to a drug's weight per unit of measure or concentration.

- Find the directions for reconstitution, as needed.

- Note expiration date and alerts.

- Describe lot or control number, NDC number, and schedule (if controlled substance).

- Identify supply dosage on labels with ratios and percents.

- Be sure that you administer the right drug.

Review Set 20

Use labels A through G to find the information requested in questions 1 through 15. Indicate your answer by letter (A through G).

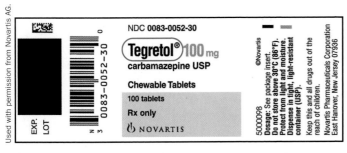

A

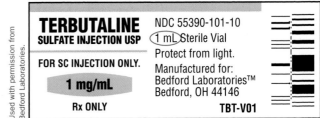

B

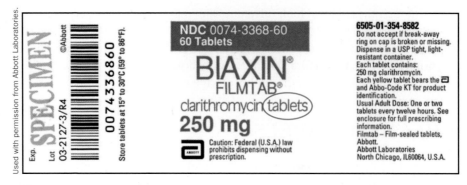

C

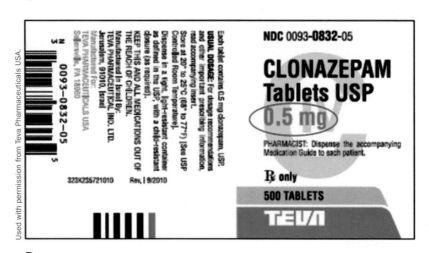

D

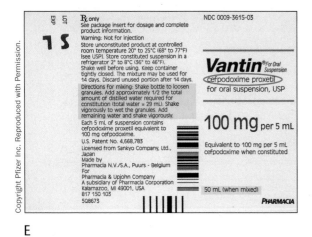

E

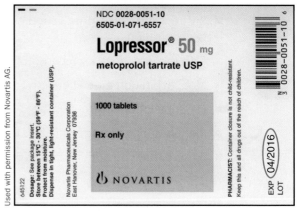

F

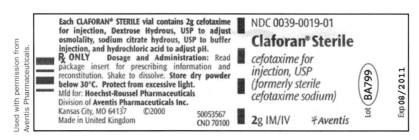

G

1. The total volume of the liquid container is circled. _____

2. The dosage strength is circled. _____

3. The form of the drug is circled. _____

4. The brand name of the drug is circled. _____

5. The generic name of the drug is circled. _____

6. The expiration date is circled. _____

7. The lot number is circled. _____

8. Look at label E and determine how much of the supply drug you will administer to the patient per dose for the order *cefpodoxime 100 mg p.o. q.12h.* _____

9. Look at label A and determine the route of administration. _____

10. Indicate which labels have a visible imprinted barcode symbol. _____

11. Search for and define the meaning and purpose of *Filmtab* on label C. _____

12. Look at label B and determine the supply dosage. _____

13. Look at label F, and determine how much of the supply drug you will administer to the patient per dose for the order *metoprolol 100 mg p.o. daily.* _____

14. Which drug label(s) represent controlled substance(s)? _____

15. Evaluate the potential for abuse of the controlled substance drug(s) identified in question 14.

_____

Refer to the following label to identify the specific drug information described in questions 16 through 21.

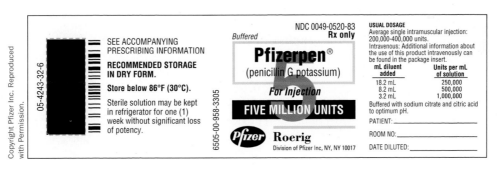

16. Generic name _____

17. Brand name _____

18. Dosage strength _____

19. Route of administration _____

20. National Drug Code _____

21. Manufacturer _____

Refer to the following label to answer questions 22 through 24.

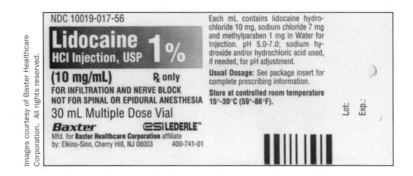

22. The supply dosage of the drug is _____ %.

23. The supply dosage of the drug is _____ g per 100 mL.

24. The supply dosage of the drug is _____ mg per mL.

After completing these problems, see page 650 to check your answers.

CLINICAL REASONING SKILLS

Reading the labels of medications is critical. Make sure that the drug you want is what you have on hand before you prepare it. Let's look at an example of a medication error related to reading the label incorrectly.

ERROR

Not checking the label for correct dosage; not paying attention to safety alert on label

Possible Scenario

A nurse flushed a triple central venous catheter (an IV with three ports). According to hospital policy, the nurse was to flush each port with 10 mL of normal saline followed by 3 mL of heparin flush solution in the concentration of 10 units/mL. The nurse mistakenly picked up a vial of heparin labeled 10,000 units per 10 mL, which is actually 1,000 units in 1 mL. Without rechecking the label, the nurse prepared and administered the heparin flush solution for all three ports. Therefore, the patient received a total of 9,000 units of heparin (1,000 units/mL × 3 mL/port × 3 ports = 9,000 units) instead of a total of 90 units of heparin (10 units/mL × 3 mL/port × 3 ports = 90 units).

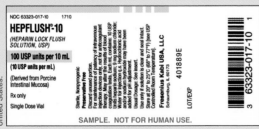

Potential Outcome

The patient in this case received 100 times the ordered dosage and could be at risk for hemorrhage, potentially leading to shock and death. The physician would likely order protamine sulfate to counteract the action of the heparin, but a successful outcome is uncertain based on the critical condition of the patient.

Prevention

There is no substitute for checking the label before administering a medication. The nurse in this case, having drawn three different syringes of medication for the three ports, had three opportunities to catch the error. The similar colors on the two vials may have contributed to the mix-up, but the nurse should also pay attention to the yellow "NOT FOR LOCK FLUSH" alert.

CLINICAL REASONING SKILLS

Many drugs have brand names or generic names that look alike or sound alike. Inattention to detail while preparing medications may lead to administration of the wrong drug, which can have serious consequences. Let's consider the safety risk of two look-alike/sound-alike (LASA) medications.

ERROR

Mixing up two medications with similar names

Possible Scenario

A patient who was receiving hydromorphone, an opioid analgesic for postoperative pain, complained of nausea. The physician had written an order for hydroxyzine 50 mg IM q.3–4h p.r.n., nausea. Instead of retrieving the ordered antiemetic medication, the nurse selected a vial of hydralazine 20 mg/mL, an antihypertensive, from the automated dispensing cabinet. After calculating the dose to be 2.5 mL, the nurse administered the medication by the intramuscular route. Although he still felt nauseous an hour later, the patient tried to amubulate for the first time since surgery with the assistance of the nurse technician but experienced severe dizziness and could not stand at the side of the bed. His blood pressure was taken and noted to have dropped to 92/48 mm/Hg. The nurse called the physician, who ordered vital signs to be taken q.2h and for the patient to remain on bed rest until his blood pressure returned to normal. Eight hours later the patient's blood pressure returned to normal and he was able to get out of bed to a chair. Neither the nurse nor the physician was able to determine the reason for the blood pressure drop.

Potential Outcome

The patient needed an antiemetic medication but received an antihypertensive medication. Besides continuing to suffer from nausea, the patient was inconvenienced and lost needed rest by having vital signs taken more frequently than otherwise would have been required. He was also at risk for a serious injury from a fall due to orthostatic hypotension when attempting to ambulate the first time following surgery.

Prevention

Administering the antihypertensive agent (hydralazine) instead of the antiemetic (hydroxyzine) could lead to a serious adverse drug event. Observe that the first four letters in the drug names are identical. Pharmacies are likely to stock these drugs next to each other on pharmacy shelves or in automated dispensing cabinets. Nurses may also locate these drugs alphabetically on computer screens. Additionally, their similar dosage strengths may not indicate a potential problem to the nurse. The nurse and the physician not recognizing the error is an all too common occurrence. According to the Institute of Medicine (IOM, 2000), most errors and safety issues go undetected and unreported. In order to prevent errors involving the interchange of look-alike/sound-alike drugs, nurses should be aware of, and annually review, the list of such drugs identified by their health care agency.

PRACTICE PROBLEMS—CHAPTER 8

Look at labels A through G and identify the information requested.

Label A:

1. The supply dosage of the drug in milliequivalents is _____.

2. The total volume of the vial is _____.

3. The supply dosage of the drug in milligrams is _____.

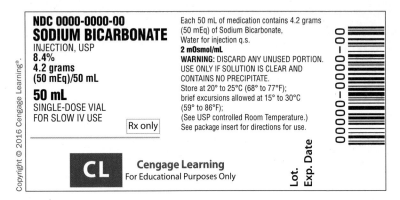

A

Label B:

4. The generic name of the drug is _____.

5. The reconstitution instruction to mix a supply dosage of 100 mg per 5 mL for oral suspension is

_____.

6. The manufacturer of the drug is _____.

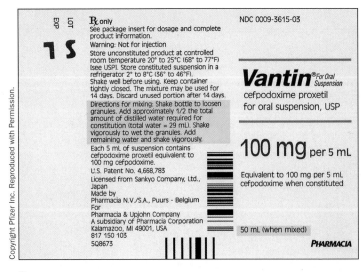

B

Label C:

7. The total volume of the medication container is _____.

8. The supply dosage is _____.

9. How much will you administer to the patient per dose for the order **methotrexate 25 mg IV stat?**

   _____.

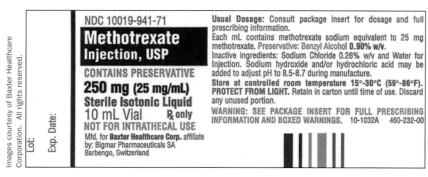

C

Label D:

10. The brand name of the drug is _____.

11. The generic name is _____.

12. The National Drug Code of the drug is _____.

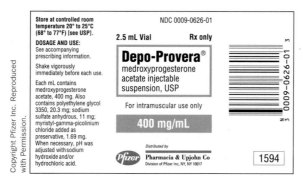

D

Label E:

13. The form of the drug is _____.

14. The total volume of the drug container is _____.

15. The administration route is _____.

E

Label F:

16. The name of the drug manufacturer is _____.

17. The form of the drug is _____.

18. The appropriate temperature for storage of this drug is _____.

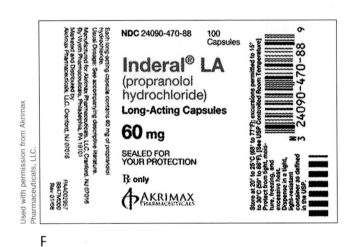

F

Label G:

19. The supply dosage of the drug is _____.

20. The dosage strength of the drug container is _____.

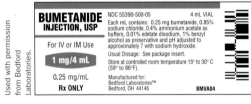

G

Answer questions 21 through 26 referring to labels H and I on the next page.

21. This label represents a unit- or single-dose drug. _____

22. This label represents a combination drug. _____

23. This label represents a drug that may be ordered by the number of tablets or capsules to be administered rather than the dosage strength. _____

24. This label represents a brand name drug. _____

25. What is the administration route for the drug labeled H? _____

26. What is the controlled substance schedule for the drug labeled H? _____

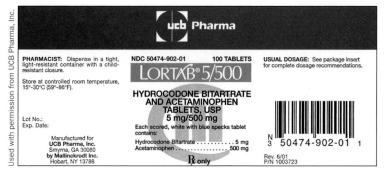

H

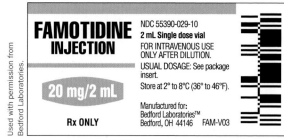

I

Answer questions 27 and 28 referring to label J.

27. Expressed as a percentage, the supply dosage of the drug is _____.

28. The supply dosage is equivalent to _____ g per 100 mL, or _____ mg per mL.

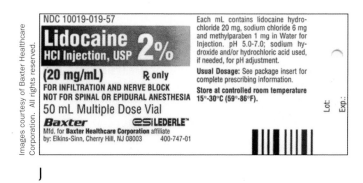

J

29. Describe the clinical reasoning you would use to prevent this medication error.

Possible Scenario

Suppose a physician ordered the antibiotic **Principen .5 g p.o. q.6h**. The writing was not clear on the order, and Prinivil (an antihypertensive medication) 5 mg was sent up by the pharmacy. However, the order was correctly transcribed to the MAR. In preparing the medication, the nurse did not read the MAR or label carefully and administered Prinivil, the wrong medication.

Potential Outcome

A medication error occurred because the wrong medication was given. The patient's infection treatment would be delayed. Furthermore, the erroneous blood pressure drug could have harmful effects.

Prevention

_____

_____

30. Describe the clinical reasoning you would use to prevent this medication error.

Possible Scenario

Suppose a physician wrote the order **Celebrex 100 mg p.o. q.12h** (anti-inflammatory to treat rheumatoid arthritis pain), but the order was difficult to read. The unit secretary and pharmacy interpreted the order as *Celexa* (antidepressant), a medication with a similar spelling. Celexa was written on the MAR.

Potential Outcome

The nurse administered the Celexa for several days, and the patient began complaining of severe knee and hip pain from rheumatoid arthritis. Also, the patient experienced side effects of Celexa, including drowsiness and tremors. A medication error occurred because several health care professionals misinterpreted the order.

Prevention

a) What should have alerted the nurse that something was wrong?

_____

b) What should have been considered to prevent this error?

_____

After completing these problems, see page 650 to check your answers.

Be sure to use the online software for additional practice!

REFERENCES

Cohen, M. R. (2008). ISMP medication error report analysis: Strength misread as total dose [Electronic version]. *Hospital Pharmacy, 43,* 7. Retrieved from http://www.factsandcomparisons.com/assets/hpdatenamed/20080701_July2008_ismp.pdf

Institute of Medicine. (2000). Committee on the Quality of Health Care in America. Kohn, L. T., Corrigan, J. M., and Donaldson, M. S., Editors. To err is human: Building a safer health system. National Academy Press, Washington, DC, page 43.

U.S. Pharmacopeia. (2013). USP-NF injections. U.S. Pharmacopeial Convention. Retrieved from http://www.usp.org/sites/default/files/usp_pdf/EN/USPNF/generalChapterInjections.pdf

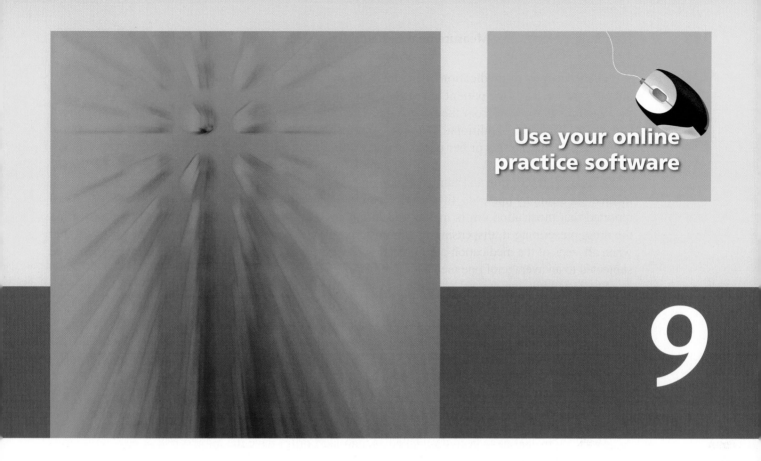

9

Preventing Medication Errors

OBJECTIVES

Upon mastery of Chapter 9, you will be able to identify and prevent the common situations that lead to medication-administration errors. To accomplish this, you will also be able to:

- Describe the consequences and costs of medication errors.
- Cite the incidence of hospital injuries and deaths attributable to medication errors.
- Explore the evidence and rationale for the underreporting of medication errors.
- Name the steps involved in medication administration.
- Identify six common causes of medication errors.
- Identify the role of the nurse in preventing medication errors.
- Describe the role of technology and health care administration in medication error prevention.
- Recognize examples of prescription, transcription, and recording notation errors.
- Correct medical notation errors.
- Describe the requirements of The Joint Commission to prevent medication errors.
- Provide a sound rationale for the critical nature of medication administration and the importance of accurate and safe dosage calculations and medication administration.

Medication administration is one of the primary functions of the nurse and the other health care practitioners in most health care settings. Unfortunately, medication-administration errors are common. Any health care practitioner is potentially at risk for making an error. Several studies addressing the problem indicate that there is no relationship between the incidence of medication errors and the characteristics of the nurses who usually make them (that is, years of practice and education).

The frequency of medication errors made by nurses and the consequences of these errors affect not only the health of the patient but also the overall cost of health care. These medication errors and the reactions that result from them cause increased length of stay, increased cost, patient disability, and death. There are additional indirect consequences as well. These include harm to the nurse involved, in regard to his or her personal and professional status, confidence, and practice (Mayo & Duncan, 2004).

Although prescription and administration mistakes are the most commonly reported, the incidence of medication errors by nurses is difficult to accurately determine. The Institute of Medicine (IOM, 2006) reported that medication errors may occur during any step of the medication process, from procuring the drug, prescribing it, dispensing it, administering it, and monitoring the effects. IOM estimates that when all steps of the medication-administration process are taken into account, hospitalized patients are subjected to an average of one medication error per day.

Studies addressing nurses' perception of medication errors support the existence of underreporting by nurses (Mayo & Duncan, 2004; Stetina, Groves, & Pafford, 2005; Wolf & Serembus, 2004). Other research indicates confusion among nurses about what constitutes a drug error. Failure to administer a medication and administering a medication late are the most underreported errors, because some nurses erroneously perceive that the patients will not be harmed in these situations (Mayo & Duncan, 2004; Stetina et al., 2005).

Statistics indicate that 10% to 18% of all hospital injuries are attributable to medication errors (Mayo & Duncan, 2004). The Institute of Medicine (2006) estimated that at least 400,000 medication errors a year, resulting in $3.5 billion in annual costs, occur in U.S. hospitals and could have been prevented.

Medications that have been designated as high-alert drugs have the highest risk of causing injuries when errors are made. The Joint Commission (1999) identified insulin, opiates and narcotics, injectable potassium chloride, and intravenous anticoagulants as the high-alert medications with the greatest safety risk. A complete list of high-alert medications may be obtained on the Institute for Safe Medication Practices Website, www.ismp.org (see Figure 9-1).

The medication delivery process is complex and involves many individuals and departments. This chapter will focus on the critical role of the nurse in this process and the importance of legible medication orders, correct transcription and interpretation, safe medication administration, and accurate recording.

PRESCRIPTION

The steps involved in safe medication administration begin with the *prescription*, followed by *transcription* and then *administration*. Only those licensed health care providers who have authority by their state to write prescriptions are permitted to do so, such as a medical doctor (MD), an osteopathic doctor (DO), a podiatrist (DPM), a dentist (DDS), a physician's assistant (PA), or an advanced registered nurse practitioner (ARNP).

Although nurses are not the originators of drug prescriptions, they play an important role in preventing errors in the *prescription* step. Refer back to Chapter 7 to review the seven parts of drug orders: patient's name, date and time of the order, name of the drug, amount of the drug (including the unit of measure), route, frequency or specific administration schedule, and the prescriber's name and licensure. It is important to always remember that the practitioner who administers a drug shares the liability for patient injury, even if the medical order was incorrect. The wise nurse always verifies the safety of the drug order by consulting a reputable drug reference, such as the American Hospital Formulary Service *AHFS Drug Information,* published annually by the American Society of Health-System Pharmacists, *Delmar's Nurse's Drug Handbook* published annually by Cengage Learning, and the *Physicians' Desk Reference* published annually by Thomson Reuters. Most hospitals and health care systems have access to electronic drug guides available online, with many accessed directly from the electronic medication administration record (MAR) by clicking on the drug name, such as the Thomson Reuters Micromedex system for point-of-care decision support.

FIGURE 9-1   ISMP's list of high-alert medications

Institute for Safe Medication Practices

ISMP's List of *High-Alert Medications*

High-alert medications are drugs that bear a heightened risk of causing significant patient harm when they are used in error. Although mistakes may or may not be more common with these drugs, the consequences of an error are clearly more devastating to patients. We hope you will use this list to determine which medications require special safeguards to reduce the risk of errors. This may include strategies such as standardizing the ordering, storage, preparation, and administration of these products; improving access to information about these drugs; limiting access to high-alert medications; using auxiliary labels and automated alerts; and employing redundancies such as automated or independent double-checks when necessary. (Note: manual independent double-checks are not always the optimal error-reduction strategy and may not be practical for all of the medications on the list).

Classes/Categories of Medications
adrenergic agonists, IV (e.g., **EPINEPH**rine, phenylephrine, norepinephrine)
adrenergic antagonists, IV (e.g., propranolol, metoprolol, labetalol)
anesthetic agents, general, inhaled and IV (e.g., propofol, ketamine)
antiarrhythmics, IV (e.g., lidocaine, amiodarone)
antithrombotic agents, including: ■ anticoagulants (e.g., warfarin, low-molecular-weight heparin, IV unfractionated heparin) ■ Factor Xa inhibitors (e.g., fondaparinux) ■ direct thrombin inhibitors (e.g., argatroban, bivalirudin, dabigatran etexilate, lepirudin) ■ thrombolytics (e.g., alteplase, reteplase, tenecteplase) ■ glycoprotein IIb/IIIa inhibitors (e.g., eptifibatide)
cardioplegic solutions
chemotherapeutic agents, parenteral and oral
dextrose, hypertonic, 20% or greater
dialysis solutions, peritoneal and hemodialysis
epidural or intrathecal medications
hypoglycemics, oral
inotropic medications, IV (e.g., digoxin, milrinone)
insulin, subcutaneous and IV
liposomal forms of drugs (e.g., liposomal amphotericin B) and conventional counterparts (e.g., amphotericin B desoxycholate)
moderate sedation agents, IV (e.g., dexmedetomidine, midazolam)
moderate sedation agents, oral, for children (e.g., chloral hydrate)
narcotics/opioids ■ IV ■ transdermal ■ oral (including liquid concentrates, immediate and sustained-release formulations)
neuromuscular blocking agents (e.g., succinylcholine, rocuronium, vecuronium)
parenteral nutrition preparations
radiocontrast agents, IV
sterile water for injection, inhalation, and irrigation (excluding pour bottles) in containers of 100 mL or more
sodium chloride for injection, hypertonic, greater than 0.9% concentration

Specific Medications
epoprostenol (Flolan), IV
magnesium sulfate injection
methotrexate, oral, non-oncologic use
opium tincture
oxytocin, IV
nitroprusside sodium for injection
potassium chloride for injection concentrate
potassium phosphates injection
promethazine, IV
vasopressin, IV or intraosseous

Background
Based on error reports submitted to the ISMP National Medication Errors Reporting Program, reports of harmful errors in the literature, and input from practitioners and safety experts, ISMP created and periodically updates a list of potential high-alert medications. During October 2011-February 2012, 772 practitioners responded to an ISMP survey designed to identify which medications were most frequently considered high-alert drugs by individuals and organizations. Further, to assure relevance and completeness, the clinical staff at ISMP, members of our advisory board, and safety experts throughout the US were asked to review the potential list. This list of drugs and drug categories reflects the collective thinking of all who provided input.

© ISMP 2012. Permission is granted to reproduce material with proper attribution for internal use within healthcare organizations. Other reproduction is prohibited without written permission from ISMP. Report actual and potential medication errors to the ISMP National Medication Errors Reporting Program (ISMP MERP) via the website (www.ismp.org) or by calling 1-800-FAIL-SAF(E).

ISMP
INSTITUTE FOR SAFE MEDICATION PRACTICES
www.ismp.org

Verbal Orders

In most health care institutions, the nurse (or other authorized individual, such as a transcriptionist) can receive verbal orders either in person or by phone from licensed physicians or other practitioners who are licensed to prescribe. As the accrediting body for health care organizations and agencies, The Joint Commission (2011) annually publishes Patient Safety Goals. Goal 2 is designed to improve the effectiveness of communication among caregivers. It requires that the authorized individual receiving a verbal or telephone order first **write it down** in the patient's chart or enter it into the computer record; second, **read it back** to the prescriber; and third, **get confirmation** from the prescriber that it is correct. For the nurse to only repeat back the order as heard or repeat it while writing it down is not sufficient to regularly prevent errors, and this is not allowed by The Joint Commission. The order must first be **written** and then it must be **read back** after it is written to ensure that the order is clear to the recipient and in turn **confirmed** by the prescriber giving the order. As with written orders, the nurse must also verify that all seven parts of the verbal order have been included and are accurate. If the nurse has any question or concern about the order, it should be clarified during the conversation. Of course, The Joint Commission advises that in emergency situations, such as a code in the ER, doing a formal read-back would not be feasible and would compromise patient safety. In such cases, a repeat-back is acceptable.

CAUTION

Accepting verbal orders is a major responsibility and a situation that can readily lead to medication errors. Most health care institutions have policies concerning telephone or verbal orders, and the nurse or other authorized staff member should be informed of his or her responsibility in this regard.

TRANSCRIPTION

One of the main causes of medication errors is incorrect *transcription* of the original prescriber's order. Many studies addressing the causes of medication errors identify one of the main sources to be illegible physician handwriting (Stetina et al., 2005). During the transcription process, the transcriber must ensure that the drug order includes all seven parts. If any of the components are absent or illegible, the nurse must obtain or clarify that information prior to signing off and implementing the order.

Further, The Joint Commission and the Institute for Safe Medication Practices have published lists of abbreviations, acronyms, and symbols to avoid in prescriptions and patient records because they have been common sources of errors and can be easily misinterpreted. The Joint Commission first published the Official "Do Not Use" List (Figure 9-2) in 2004 and required that health care organizations publish their own lists of abbreviations not to use. At that time, it also published a list of additional abbreviations, acronyms, and symbols for possible future inclusion in the Official "Do Not Use" List (Figure 9-3). Now they refer health care organizations to the ISMP list of dangerous abbreviations relating to medication use. The ISMP recommends that these abbreviations, symbols, and dose designations be strictly prohibited when communicating medical information (Figure 9-4).

CAUTION

Stay alert to the guidelines and restrictions of The Joint Commission, the ISMP, and your own health care facility regarding abbreviations and medical notation. Acceptable medical communication is subject to abrupt change. Check the websites listed in the references for this chapter to stay up to date.

FIGURE 9-2   The Joint Commission's Official "Do Not Use" List of medical abbreviations, acronyms, and symbols

Official "Do Not Use" List[1]		
Do Not Use	***Potential Problem***	**Use Instead**
U (unit)	Mistaken for "0" (zero), the number "4" (four) or "cc"	Write "unit"
IU (International Unit)	Mistaken for IV (intravenous) or the number 10 (ten)	Write "International Unit"
Q.D., QD, q.d., qd (daily)	Mistaken for each other	Write "daily"
Q.O.D., QOD, q.o.d, qod (every other day)	Period after the Q mistaken for "I" and the "O" mistaken for "I"	Write "every other day"
Trailing zero (X.0 mg)* Lack of leading zero (.X mg)	Decimal point is missed	Write X mg Write 0.X mg
MS	Can mean morphine sulfate or magnesium sulfate	Write "morphine sulfate" Write "magnesium sulfate"
MSO_4 and $MgSO_4$	Confused for one another	

[1] Applies to all orders and all medication-related documentation that is handwritten (including free-text computer entry) or on pre-printed forms.

*Exception: A "trailing zero" may be used only where required to demonstrate the level of precision of the value being reported, such as for laboratory results, imaging studies that report size of lesions, or catheter/tube sizes. It may not be used in medication orders or other medication-related documentation.

FIGURE 9-3   Abbreviations, acronyms, and symbols formerly included in The Joint Commission's list for possible future inclusion in the Official "Do Not Use" List

Problematic Abbreviation/Acronym/Symbol	Potential Error	Preferred Documentation
> (greater than) < (less than)	Misinterpreted as the number "7" (seven) or the letter "L" Confused for one another	Write "greater than" Write "less than"
Abbreviations for drug names	Misinterpreted due to similar abbreviations for multiple drugs	Write drug names in full
Apothecary units	Unfamiliar to many practitioners Confused with metric units	Use metric units
@	Mistaken for the number "2" (two)	Write "at"
cc	Mistaken for U (units) when poorly written	Write "mL" or "ml" or "milliliters" ("mL" is preferred)
μg	Mistaken for mg (milligrams) resulting in one thousand-fold overdose	Write "mcg" or "micrograms"

FIGURE 9-4 ISMP's list of error-prone abbreviations, symbols, and dose designations

Institute for Safe Medication Practices

ISMP's List of *Error-Prone Abbreviations, Symbols*, and *Dose Designations*

The abbreviations, symbols, and dose designations found in this table have been reported to ISMP through the ISMP National Medication Errors Reporting Program (ISMP MERP) as being frequently misinterpreted and involved in harmful medication errors. They should **NEVER** be used when communicating medical information. This includes internal communications, telephone/verbal prescriptions, computer-generated labels, labels for drug storage bins, medication administration records, as well as pharmacy and prescriber computer order entry screens.

Abbreviations	Intended Meaning	Misinterpretation	Correction
μg	Microgram	Mistaken as "mg"	Use "mcg"
AD, AS, AU	Right ear, left ear, each ear	Mistaken as OD, OS, OU (right eye, left eye, each eye)	Use "right ear," "left ear," or "each ear"
OD, OS, OU	Right eye, left eye, each eye	Mistaken as AD, AS, AU (right ear, left ear, each ear)	Use "right eye," "left eye," or "each eye"
BT	Bedtime	Mistaken as "BID" (twice daily)	Use "bedtime"
cc	Cubic centimeters	Mistaken as "u" (units)	Use "mL"
D/C	Discharge or discontinue	Premature discontinuation of medications if D/C (intended to mean "discharge") has been misinterpreted as "discontinued" when followed by a list of discharge medications	Use "discharge" and "discontinue"
IJ	Injection	Mistaken as "IV" or "intrajugular"	Use "injection"
IN	Intranasal	Mistaken as "IM" or "IV"	Use "intranasal" or "NAS"
HS	Half-strength	Mistaken as bedtime	Use "half-strength" or "bedtime"
hs	At bedtime, hours of sleep	Mistaken as half-strength	
IU**	International unit	Mistaken as IV (intravenous) or 10 (ten)	Use "units"
o.d. or OD	Once daily	Mistaken as "right eye" (OD-oculus dexter), leading to oral liquid medications administered in the eye	Use "daily"
OJ	Orange juice	Mistaken as OD or OS (right or left eye); drugs meant to be diluted in orange juice may be given in the eye	Use "orange juice"
Per os	By mouth, orally	The "os" can be mistaken as "left eye" (OS-oculus sinister)	Use "PO," "by mouth," or "orally"
q.d. or QD**	Every day	Mistaken as q.i.d., especially if the period after the "q" or the tail of the "q" is misunderstood as an "i"	Use "daily"
qhs	Nightly at bedtime	Mistaken as "qhr" or every hour	Use "nightly"
qn	Nightly or at bedtime	Mistaken as "qh" (every hour)	Use "nightly" or "at bedtime"
q.o.d. or QOD**	Every other day	Mistaken as "q.d." (daily) or "q.i.d. (four times daily) if the "o" is poorly written	Use "every other day"
q1d	Daily	Mistaken as q.i.d. (four times daily)	Use "daily"
q6PM, etc.	Every evening at 6 PM	Mistaken as every 6 hours	Use "daily at 6 PM" or "6 PM daily"
SC, SQ, sub q	Subcutaneous	SC mistaken as SL (sublingual); SQ mistaken as "5 every;" the "q" in "sub q" has been mistaken as "every" (e.g., a heparin dose ordered "sub q 2 hours before surgery" misunderstood as every 2 hours before surgery)	Use "subcut" or "subcutaneously"
ss	Sliding scale (insulin) or ½ (apothecary)	Mistaken as "55"	Spell out "sliding scale;" use "one-half" or "½"
SSRI	Sliding scale regular insulin	Mistaken as selective-serotonin reuptake inhibitor	Spell out "sliding scale (insulin)"
SSI	Sliding scale insulin	Mistaken as Strong Solution of Iodine (Lugol's)	
i/d	One daily	Mistaken as "tid"	Use "1 daily"
TIW or tiw	3 times a week	Mistaken as "3 times a day" or "twice in a week"	Use "3 times weekly"
U or u**	Unit	Mistaken as the number 0 or 4, causing a 10-fold overdose or greater (e.g., 4U seen as "40" or 4u seen as "44"); mistaken as "cc" so dose given in volume instead of units (e.g., 4u seen as 4cc)	Use "unit"
UD	As directed ("ut dictum")	Mistaken as unit dose (e.g., diltiazem 125 mg IV infusion "UD" misinterpreted as meaning to give the entire infusion as a unit [bolus] dose)	Use "as directed"
Dose Designations and Other Information	**Intended Meaning**	**Misinterpretation**	**Correction**
Trailing zero after decimal point (e.g., 1.0 mg)**	1 mg	Mistaken as 10 mg if the decimal point is not seen	Do not use trailing zeros for doses expressed in whole numbers
"Naked" decimal point (e.g., .5 mg)**	0.5 mg	Mistaken as 5 mg if the decimal point is not seen	Use zero before a decimal point when the dose is less than a whole unit
Abbreviations such as mg. or mL. with a period following the abbreviation	mg mL	The period is unnecessary and could be mistaken as the number 1 if written poorly	Use mg, mL, etc. without a terminal period

FIGURE 9-4   Continued

Institute for Safe Medication Practices

ISMP's List of *Error-Prone Abbreviations, Symbols,* and *Dose Designations* (continued)

Dose Designations and Other Information	Intended Meaning	Misinterpretation	Correction
Drug name and dose run together (especially problematic for drug names that end in "l" such as Inderal40 mg; Tegretol300 mg)	Inderal 40 mg Tegretol 300 mg	Mistaken as Inderal 140 mg Mistaken as Tegretol 1300 mg	Place adequate space between the drug name, dose, and unit of measure
Numerical dose and unit of measure run together (e.g., 10mg, 100mL)	10 mg 100 mL	The "m" is sometimes mistaken as a zero or two zeros, risking a 10- to 100-fold overdose	Place adequate space between the dose and unit of measure
Large doses without properly placed commas (e.g., 100000 units; 1000000 units)	100,000 units 1,000,000 units	100000 has been mistaken as 10,000 or 1,000,000; 1000000 has been mistaken as 100,000	Use commas for dosing units at or above 1,000, or use words such as 100 "thousand" or 1 "million" to improve readability

Drug Name Abbreviations	Intended Meaning	Misinterpretation	Correction
To avoid confusion, do not abbreviate drug names when communicating medical information. Examples of drug name abbreviations involved in medication errors include:			
APAP	acetaminophen	Not recognized as acetaminophen	Use complete drug name
ARA A	vidarabine	Mistaken as cytarabine (ARA C)	Use complete drug name
AZT	zidovudine (Retrovir)	Mistaken as azathioprine or aztreonam	Use complete drug name
CPZ	Compazine (prochlorperazine)	Mistaken as chlorpromazine	Use complete drug name
DPT	Demerol-Phenergan-Thorazine	Mistaken as diphtheria-pertussis-tetanus (vaccine)	Use complete drug name
DTO	Diluted tincture of opium, or deodorized tincture of opium (Paregoric)	Mistaken as tincture of opium	Use complete drug name
HCl	hydrochloric acid or hydrochloride	Mistaken as potassium chloride (The "H" is misinterpreted as "K")	Use complete drug name unless expressed as a salt of a drug
HCT	hydrocortisone	Mistaken as hydrochlorothiazide	Use complete drug name
HCTZ	hydrochlorothiazide	Mistaken as hydrocortisone (seen as HCT250 mg)	Use complete drug name
MgSO4**	magnesium sulfate	Mistaken as morphine sulfate	Use complete drug name
MS, MSO4**	morphine sulfate	Mistaken as magnesium sulfate	Use complete drug name
MTX	methotrexate	Mistaken as mitoxantrone	Use complete drug name
PCA	procainamide	Mistaken as patient controlled analgesia	Use complete drug name
PTU	propylthiouracil	Mistaken as mercaptopurine	Use complete drug name
T3	Tylenol with codeine No. 3	Mistaken as liothyronine	Use complete drug name
TAC	triamcinolone	Mistaken as tetracaine, Adrenalin, cocaine	Use complete drug name
TNK	TNKase	Mistaken as "TPA"	Use complete drug name
ZnSO4	zinc sulfate	Mistaken as morphine sulfate	Use complete drug name

Stemmed Drug Names	Intended Meaning	Misinterpretation	Correction
"Nitro" drip	nitroglycerin infusion	Mistaken as sodium nitroprusside infusion	Use complete drug name
"Norflox"	norfloxacin	Mistaken as Norflex	Use complete drug name
"IV Vanc"	intravenous vancomycin	Mistaken as Invanz	Use complete drug name

Symbols	Intended Meaning	Misinterpretation	Correction
ℨ	Dram	Symbol for dram mistaken as "3"	Use the metric system
ℳ	Minim	Symbol for minim mistaken as "mL"	
x3d	For three days	Mistaken as "3 doses"	Use "for three days"
> and <	Greater than and less than	Mistaken as opposite of intended; mistakenly use incorrect symbol; "< 10" mistaken as "40"	Use "greater than" or "less than"
/ (slash mark)	Separates two doses or indicates "per"	Mistaken as the number 1 (e.g., "25 units/10 units" misread as "25 units and 110" units)	Use "per" rather than a slash mark to separate doses
@	At	Mistaken as "2"	Use "at"
&	And	Mistaken as "2"	Use "and"
+	Plus or and	Mistaken as "4"	Use "and"
°	Hour	Mistaken as a zero (e.g., q2° seen as q 20)	Use "hr," "h," or "hour"
Φ or ⌀	zero, null sign	Mistaken as numerals 4, 6, 8, and 9	Use 0 or zero, or describe intent using whole words

**These abbreviations are included on The Joint Commission's "minimum list" of dangerous abbreviations, acronyms, and symbols that must be included on an organization's "Do Not Use" list, effective January 1, 2004. Visit www.jointcommission.org for more information about this Joint Commission requirement.

INSTITUTE FOR SAFE MEDICATION PRACTICES
www.ismp.org

Many health care institutions are utilizing a computerized physician/prescriber order entry (CPOE) system to help eliminate transcription sources of error. Physicians choose drug orders from a menu screen (Figure 9-5) and then choose the route and dosage strength offered on the following screen (Figure 9-6). These systems can also be implemented with clinical decision support systems (CDSSs). The CDSS may include suggestions or default values for drug dosages, routes, and frequencies. The chance still exists

FIGURE 9-5   A CPOE menu screen allows the user to select a drug

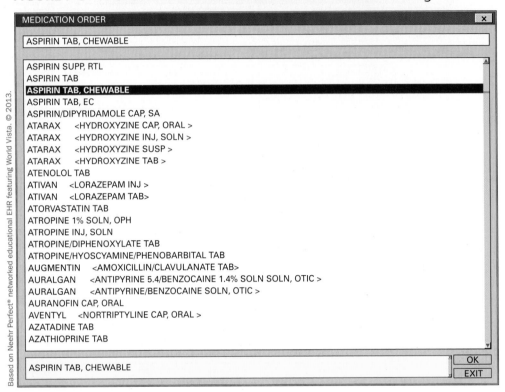

FIGURE 9-6   A CPOE offers options for the dosage, route, and frequency of the drug chosen

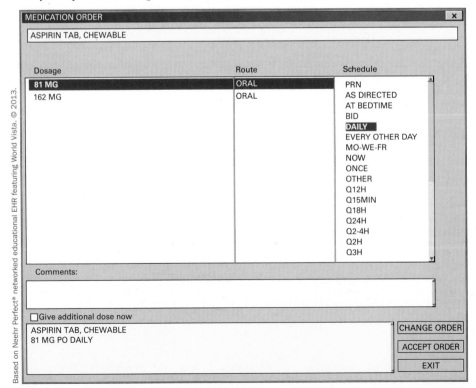

that the order may be entered incorrectly, but the computer system does remove the variable of illegible handwriting and is known to foster a *safety culture*.

SAFE MEDICATION ADMINISTRATION

The Five Rights of medication administration *(right patient, right drug, right amount, right route, and right time)* have been the cornerstones for safe and effective nursing practice in the area of medication administration. A sixth right, *right documentation,* is often added to the list. These Six Rights were introduced in Chapter 7. Thoroughly and consistently following these rights can ensure that nurses administer medications safely.

REMEMBER

Nurses should refer to reputable drug reference resources to validate the safety of the medication as ordered and transcribed. Whoever administers a medication is legally responsible for patient safety. Any medication errors that result also fall under the responsibility of the person who administered the drug, regardless of the primary source of the error.

Right Patient

The administration of a medication to a patient other than the one for whom it was ordered is clearly an error. It is also one that should be easily prevented. Yet the literature shows this to be one of the three most common causes of medication errors. The failure of the nurse to accurately identify a patient is the most common cause for the error. The Joint Commission (2011) has a Patient Safety Goal to improve the accuracy of patient identification when administering medications. The Joint Commission requires that patients be identified with at least two unique person-specific identifiers (neither of which can be the patient's room number), such as name and date of birth or name and patient ID number. Electronic identification technology coding, such as barcoding, that includes two or more person-specific identifiers (not room number) will also comply. Basic nursing education emphasizes the importance of correctly identifying a patient prior to administering a medication, by comparing the two person-specific identifiers with the patient's arm band, medication administration record (MAR), or chart and by asking the patient to state his or her name (as a third identifier). Both steps should be consistently implemented regardless of the nurse's familiarity with the patient or the practice arena.

It is also wise to tell the patient at the time of administration what medication and dosage strength of the drug the nurse is administering. This extra step can often prevent errors, because patients who are familiar with their medications may spot an error or question a drug dosage. This is also an opportunity to engage the patient in medication teaching and learning. However, the nurse should never rely on this practice as the primary means to prevent errors. Instead, this is an extra precaution.

Technological advances in medication administration and documentation have included mechanisms to help prevent errors in this area. Computers installed at the patient's bedside and/or handheld devices that enable the nurse to scan the barcodes on the patient's identification band and on the medications serve as reinforcement to visual checks by the nurse. Few studies have been published in regard to the effectiveness of these systems in preventing errors. However, this additional mechanism to ensure correct patient identification increases efficiency, ensuring that the right patient receives the right drug. The health care industry has invested heavily in technology to help prevent costly medication errors caused by carelessness and distraction.

Right Drug

Nurses can ensure that the right drug criterion is maintained by checking the medication label against the order or MAR at three points during the administration process:

1. On first contact with the drug (removing it from the medication cart, drawer, or shelf)

2. Prior to measuring the drug (pouring, counting, or withdrawing the drug)

3. After preparing the drug, just prior to administration

Distraction in the workplace has been identified as a key reason for error in obtaining the right drug (Pape, Guerra, Muzquiz, & Bryant, 2005). Nurses should take measures to ensure that they are not distracted during this phase of medication administration. Optimally, the physical workplace should provide for the nurse to move to an area without distractions. However, if this is not available, the nurse should be conscious of the need to focus solely on the task at hand and avoid the temptation to multitask while dispensing medications.

In February 2004, the U.S. Food and Drug Administration (FDA) issued a regulation that requires all new pharmaceuticals to be barcoded upon launch into the market (FDA, 2006). Studies by the U.S. Pharmacopeia in 2003 indicated that insulin products have the highest rates of error (Information Technology, 2005). Projections by the FDA indicate that barcoding on prescription drugs will reduce errors in the United States by 500,000 instances over 20 years, with estimated savings of $93 billion in additional health care costs, patient pain, and lost wages (FDA, 2004). This represents a 50% reduction in the medication errors that would otherwise occur without the use of barcoding (FDA, 2004).

Barcodes on drugs are used with a barcode-scanning system and computerized database. At a minimum, the code must contain the drug's National Drug Code. This number uniquely identifies the drug. The process starts as a patient enters the hospital and is given a barcoded patient identification band. The hospital has barcode scanners that are linked to the hospital's electronic medical records system. Before a health care worker administers a medication, he or she scans the patient's barcode, which allows the computer to access the patient's medical records. The health care worker then scans each drug prior to administration. This notifies the computer of each medication to be administered. The information is compared to the patient's database to ensure a match. If there is a problem, the health care worker receives an error message and investigates the problem.

Nurses are responsible for being knowledgeable about the actions, indications, and contraindications of the medications they administer. The constant changes that are occurring in health care delivery and the steady influx of new medications being released into the market have challenged the individual nurse's ability to meet this responsibility. A valid and current drug-reference system should be available in every practice setting. The nurse should not hesitate to seek information about any medication that is unfamiliar. The prescribing clinician should be contacted for clarification or confirmation for any medication order that appears inappropriate or incorrect.

Automated dispensing cabinets (ADCs) (Figure 9-7) have been utilized in many health care settings since the 1980s and are now used in the majority of hospitals. There are many safety measures in place with the use of this technology, but the possibility still exists that the patient may receive the wrong medication. It is important that the correct medication be stocked by the pharmacy in the correct location within the ADC to avoid mistakes in drug selection (ISMP, 2008a). In a survey conducted by the ISMP (2008b), nurses reported that at least half of the ADCs were not located in areas free from distractions. Nurses also reported that they always or frequently wait in line to access the ADC, and one third of the respondents indicated that they often remove multiple patients' medications at a time. This identified "workaround" is known to lead to drug administration errors. Recognizing that few resources exist to guide health care organizations in the safest use of this technology, the ISMP has developed and posted guidelines that include 12 interdisciplinary core processes for safe use of automated dispensing cabinets.

CAUTION

When medications are distributed with automated dispensing cabinets, follow the ISMP *Core Processes* for safe ADC use (ISMP, 2008a).

1. Provide ideal environmental conditions for the use of ADCs.

2. Ensure ADC system security.

3. Use pharmacy-profiled ADCs.

4. Identify and include information that should appear on the ADC screen.

5. Select and maintain proper ADC inventory.

6. Select appropriate ADC configuration (e.g., lidded compartments are preferred to matrix drawers).

7. Define and implement safe ADC restocking processes.

8. Develop procedures to ensure the accurate withdrawal of medications from the ADC.

9. Establish strict criteria for ADC system overrides.

10. Standardize processes for transporting medications from the ADC to the patient's bedside.

11. Eliminate the process for returning medications directly to their original ADC location.

12. Provide staff education and competency validation.

FIGURE 9-7 The Pyxis MedStation® is an example of an automated dispensing cabinet (ADC) system

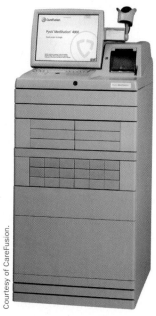

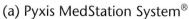

(a) Pyxis MedStation System®

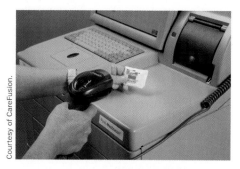

(b) Pyxis Barcode Scanner®

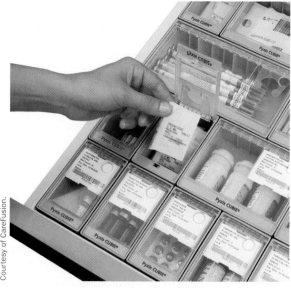

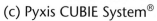

(c) Pyxis CUBIE System®

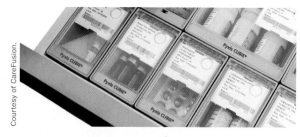

(d) Pyxis CUBIE System®

In addition, nurses who practice in a setting utilizing this technology should continue to implement the three checks described at the beginning of this section to avoid administering the wrong drug: during retrieval, preparation, and administration. Review the information about reading drug labels in Chapter 8 to ensure that all of the important information is confirmed.

A common preventable medication error is interchanging look-alike/sound-alike (LASA) medication pairs—prescribing and administering one for the other. The Joint Commission (2011) Patient Safety Goal 3 addresses this issue and posts online an extensive list of LASA medications that pose the greatest risk for medication errors, including drugs such as ephedrine and epinephrine, hydromorphone injection and morphine injection, hydroxyzine and hydralazine, OxyContin (controlled release) and oxycodone (immediate release). Hospitals are independently required to list at least 10 look-alike/sound-alike drug pairs commonly prescribed and administered in their institution for their caregivers to monitor. A survey conducted by the Institute for Safe Medication Practices (ISMP, 2009a) indicated that compliance with The Joint Commission National Patient Safety Goal 3 for LASA drugs has been high, with rates of at least 95% for hospitals. Yet 27% of staff nurses responding were still uncertain whether their organization maintained a list of LASA drug name pairs. To reduce the risk of errors, all clinical staff, but especially nurses administering medications, must know the hospital's list of LASA drugs and its importance to patient safety.

The ISMP and the Food and Drug Administration (FDA) also suggest the use of "Tall Man" lettering to differentiate drugs with look-alike names (ISMP, 2010b). Using this method, the drug name is highlighted by various means such as uppercase letters, colors, bolding, and italics to call attention to the dissimilarities between look-alike drug names; the FDA-approved Tall Man list is shown in Figure 9-8. Tall Man lettering is being used in many hospitals on computerized physician/prescriber order entry (CPOE) screens, automated dispensing cabinet (ADC) screens, computer-generated medication administration records (MARs), computer-generated pharmacy labels, preprinted standard orders, and medication shelf labels.

The Joint Commission (2011) National Patient Safety Goal 8 addresses the practice of reconciling the right medications across the continuum of care, beginning with admission and following the patient through transfers within the health care facility (such as from a hospital intensive care unit to a medical floor) and back home or to a long-term care facility. A complete list of current medications the patient is taking at home (including dosage, route, and frequency) is created and documented upon admission, ideally before prescribing any new medications. The medications ordered for the patient while under care are compared to this list and discrepancies are reconciled and documented. Likewise, when the patient is transferred to another unit within the hospital or to another facility, or discharged to home, the up-to-date, reconciled medication list is communicated and documented. Strict adherence to these standards will prevent many medication errors of transcription, omission, duplication, and drug interactions.

Right Amount

Illegible prescriber's handwriting, transcription error, miscalculation of the amount, or misreading of the label can result in errors involving the administration of an incorrect dose of a medication. The need for each nurse to carefully read and clarify drug orders and recheck drug labels has been previously discussed. Transcription errors involving dosage can be avoided if nurses consult drug references to confirm the dosage of medications when they are in doubt. The Joint Commission's Official "Do Not Use" List (Figure 9-2) will also help eliminate dosage problems for those medications ordered daily, ordered every other day, or measured in units.

Two nurses must check some potent high-alert drugs, such as insulin or heparin, which are common sources of errors. Drug labels with product strength statements written as "mg per mL" are often misunderstood by health care practitioners as total drug content even when the total amount of the container is printed elsewhere on the label. Such errors with high-alert medications such as heparin could result in improper dosing with serious outcomes, including death (U.S. Pharmacopeial Convention, 2012). For this reason, the U.S. Pharmacopeial Convention (USP) recently announced a change in labeling requirements for both heparin sodium injection USP and heparin lock flush solution USP, which became

FIGURE 9-8   FDA-approved list of generic drug names with Tall Man letters from the FDA and ISMP lists

ISMP Institute for Safe Medication Practices

FDA and ISMP Lists of
Look-Alike Drug Names with Recommended Tall Man Letters

FDA-Approved List of Generic Drug Names with Tall Man Letters	
Drug Name with Tall Man Letters	**Confused with**
aceta**ZOLAMIDE**	aceto**HEXAMIDE**
aceto**HEXAMIDE**	aceta**ZOLAMIDE**
bu**PROP**ion	bus**PIR**one
bus**PIR**one	bu**PROP**ion
chlorpro**MAZINE**	chlorpro**PAMIDE**
chlorpro**PAMIDE**	chlorpro**MAZINE**
clomi**PHENE**	clomi**PRAMINE**
clomi**PRAMINE**	clomi**PHENE**
cyclo**SERINE**	cyclo**SPORINE**
cyclo**SPORINE**	cyclo**SERINE**
DAUNOrubicin	**DOXO**rubicin
dimenhy**DRINATE**	diphenhydr**AMINE**
diphenhydr**AMINE**	dimenhy**DRINATE**
DOBUTamine	**DOP**amine
DOPamine	**DOBUT**amine
DOXOrubicin	**DAUNO**rubicin
glipi**ZIDE**	gly**BURIDE**
gly**BURIDE**	glipi**ZIDE**
hydr**ALAZINE**	hydr**OXY**zine
hydr**OXY**zine	hydr**ALAZINE**
medroxy**PROGESTER**one	methyl**PREDNIS**olone - methyl**TESTOSTER**one
methyl**PREDNIS**olone	medroxy**PROGESTER**one - methyl**TESTOSTER**one
methyl**TESTOSTER**one	medroxy**PROGESTER**one - methyl**PREDNIS**olone
ni**CAR**dipine	**NIFE**dipine
NIFEdipine	ni**CAR**dipine
predniso**LONE**	predni**SONE**
predni**SONE**	predniso**LONE**
sulf**ADIAZINE**	sulfi**SOXAZOLE**
sulfi**SOXAZOLE**	sulf**ADIAZINE**
TOLAZamide	**TOLBUT**amide
TOLBUTamide	**TOLAZ**amide
vin**BLAS**tine	vin**CRIS**tine
vin**CRIS**tine	vin**BLAS**tine

effective on May 1, 2013 (ISMP, 2013). This requirement follows the 2009 FDA recommendation that first advocated that labels clearly state the strength of the entire container of the medication followed by how much of the medication is in 1 mL (Cohen, 2008). Heparin labels must now print the strength per total volume as the primary expression of strength followed in close proximity by strength per milliliter (U.S. Pharmacopeia, 2013). Compare the old and new versions of the heparin labels (Figure 9-9). Vials labeled with either the old or new version would contain the same concentration and total volume of medication, but with the revised label it is more obvious that using the entire container may provide an excessive amount of heparin.

FIGURE 9-9   **(a)** Old version heparin label; **(b)** New version heparin label

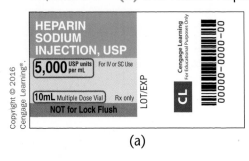
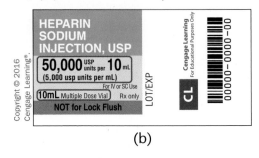

(a)   (b)

CAUTION

Heparin is a high-alert medication. Read heparin labels very carefully. Health care agencies are transitioning from old to new regulations for label content and design. Both labels may be available until current supplies are depleted. To avoid serious medication errors, always identify the concentration of the supply as well as the total volume in the container.

While medication errors are known to be the most common type of medical error in general, the risk of harm from dosage errors is a significant risk in the pediatric population. Increased caution must be taken when administering medication to children because of the greater frequency of weight-based dosage calculations, fractional dosage, and the need for decimal points in calculations (The Joint Commission, 2008b).

Ensuring that the patient receives the right amount when administering parenteral fluids is equally important. Electronic infusion pumps have enabled nurses to have greater control over the rate of infusion of intravenous solutions and medications, thereby reducing medication errors. The newest innovation with infusion pumps is the Smart Pump, which is equipped with computer software that includes a library of medications and dosage guidelines (ISMP, 2009b). Other infusion pumps, such as the patient-controlled analgesia (PCA) pump and the insulin pump, have enabled patients to be active participants in their own care (FDA, 2010a). Although infusion pump technology has increased administration safety, one cannot rely fully on these devices. Because electronic infusion pumps are primarily used for patients who require a precise delivery of fluids or critical medications, errors can result in serious consequences to the patient. The Food and Drug Administration (FDA) is concerned with the number of adverse events associated with the use of infusion pumps. Some of these events are attributed to user error, while others have been associated with pump malfunction. The FDA Infusion Pump Improvement Initiative (2010b) addresses infusion pump safety problems. Along with establishing additional safety requirements for infusion pump manufacturers, the FDA is increasing user awareness with a new infusion pump website (http://www.fda.gov/MedicalDevices/ProductsandMedicalProcedures/GeneralHospitalDevicesandSupplies/InfusionPumps/default.htm). It is the responsibility of the nurse to be trained on the proper use of infusion pumps and to be watchful for potential problems associated with emerging technologies.

Teaching effective dosage calculation methods is the main purpose of this text. The need for each nurse to estimate the correct dosage prior to calculating the exact amount is stressed throughout the book.

The inclusion of this commonsense approach to calculating dosages is crucial in preventing errors in dosage calculation. Calculating, preparing, and administering the wrong dose of a drug are preventable medication errors. Full attention to accurate dosage calculations will ensure that you avoid such liabilities.

Right Route

Errors involving the route of medication administration can occur for several reasons. One of the most common problems has already been addressed: that of illegible prescriber's handwriting. Another common error relates to the nurse's knowledge of medications and their dosage forms. Nurses are usually familiar with medications commonly ordered and administered in their area of practice, but the nurse should consult a drug information source to confirm that the correct route is ordered for an unfamiliar medication, particularly in regard to injectable forms of medications.

Nurses should also be alert to the need to change or clarify administration forms or routes for the patient receiving medication through a feeding tube, such as a nasogastric or surgically inserted gastric tube. Medication errors related to this route of administration may occur due to administering multiple medications that are incompatible, preparing the medications improperly, or using improper administration techniques (ISMP, 2010d). Sometimes the patient may not be allowed any oral intake (NPO status) or may have a nasogastric tube but the medications are ordered for oral administration. Prescribers may order time-released or enteric-coated medications to be administered via a feeding tube but not realize that medications must be crushed or dissolved to be administered. The Institute for Safe Medication Practices (2010e) provides a comprehensive drug list of oral dosage forms that should not be crushed, including the rationale for the restriction. Such situations require the nurse to contact the prescriber for a change in the medication form or route or to seek clarification for the drug to be administered safely and correctly. Enteral infusion pumps are often used to administer liquid nutrients and medications by the gastrointestinal route. These pumps may be used with patients who also have intravenous infusion pumps or other pumps in place. Serious adverse events as a result of misconnections of tubing have been reported due to a mix-up with electronic infusion devices as well as tubing regulated by manual devices (The Joint Commission, 2006). To ensure that the patient receives the ordered medication by the right route, it is recommended that the tube or catheter from the patient be traced to the point of origin before connecting any new device or infusion. Additionally, a "line reconciliation" should be conducted to recheck connections and trace all patient tubes and catheters to their sources upon a patient's arrival at a new setting as part of the handoff process (The Joint Commission, 2006). It is the nurse's responsibility to be alert to potential errors of all kinds that may interfere with patient safety and rights.

Right Time

Medication orders should include the frequency with which a drug is to be administered or the specific administration schedule. Computerized hospital drug administration systems automatically indicate these times on the medication administration record. The nurse is responsible for checking these records to be sure they are accurate. For example, a physician writes an order for an antibiotic to be given q.i.d., or 4 times a day. The computer system might transcribe these times to 9:00 AM, 1:00 PM, 5:00 PM, and 9:00 PM. The nurse should recognize that an antibiotic should be administered at regular intervals around the clock so that the 4 doses would be 6 hours apart. The right time for the order should have been q.6h or *every 6 hours.* The nurse should contact the physician to clarify the order.

The Joint Commission has recognized the problem of misinterpretation of time and frequency in medication orders. It has taken steps to prevent common errors in regard to the time a drug is to be administered, by prohibiting the use of some abbreviations related to dosing frequency (Figure 9-2). For example, the notation to give a drug q.d. has frequently been transcribed as q.i.d., with the period being mistaken for an *i,* resulting in a daily medication being administered four times a day instead of once daily.

Right Documentation

The last step in medication administration is correct documentation. The policy in most institutions directs nurses to administer a medication prior to documentation. Numerous studies indicate that fatigue and lack of time are factors that contribute to medication errors. Nurses who prioritize their time may find that they give medications correctly but fail to document that they have done so. This omission can result in unintentional overmedication of the patient when the follow-on nurse responds as though the drug was not given. Many of the new ADCs document drug administration at the time the drug is removed from the machine. This ensures that administration is documented, but an error occurs if the patient does not take the medication. In that situation, the nurse must follow the institution's policy for clarifying or deleting the initial documentation. Often, this is a time-consuming process, but if omitted, it can result in undermedication of the patient.

THE NURSE'S CRITICAL ROLE IN MEDICATION ERROR PREVENTION

As the largest segment of the health care workforce, nurses are essential to reducing medication errors and improving patient outcomes. In the Institute of Medicine (2006) landmark report, *Preventing Medication Errors,* the most effective way to reduce errors was identified as a partnership between patients and their health care providers. Communication between nurses and patients should be open, with nurses not only talking to patients, but listening to them as well. To this end, The Joint Commission (2002) launched a Speak Up™ campaign to urge patients to take a larger role in preventing errors by becoming more active participants in their care. When administering medications, nurses should be prepared for and encourage patients' questions. By way of brochures, buttons, and posters displayed in health care facilities, patients are instructed to use six strategies to avoid medication mistakes at the hospital or clinic (Figure 9-10).

Additionally, the number of medication errors may be reduced by making greater use of information technologies when prescribing and administering medications. Nurses cannot be expected to keep up with all the relevant information on all the medications they administer. Using point-of-care reference information provided with the electronic medical record or by automated dispensing units, the Internet, or downloaded content on personal digital assistants (PDAs) will enhance the nurse's ability to apply critical reasoning when making judgments related to medication administration. Yet, while technological interventions such as smart infusion pumps, patient-controlled analgesia, computerized physician/provider order entry (CPOE), automated dispensing cabinets (ADCs), automated medication dispensing machines (AMDMs), electronic medical records (EMRs), and barcoding identification have contributed to improved patient care, there is considerable data on incidences of adverse events while using these tools (The Joint Commission, 2008a). As health technologies are increasingly adopted by health care organizations, nurses must be mindful of the safety risks and preventable adverse events that these new innovations may bring about. Still, some nurses will be involved in medication errors and they must be aware of the appropriate response. Whenever a medication error is identified, the nurse must follow the health organization's procedure for reporting. This enables organizations to track errors and implement improvement processes aimed at preventing repeat errors. Organizations have also been encouraged to have specific plans in place in order to guide health providers in the appropriate manner to disclose harmful errors to patients and family members (ISMP, 2006). Many organizations have participated in the Medication Errors Reporting Program (MERP), a confidential national voluntary reporting program. The ISMP publishes *Medication Safety Alerts* that provide vital information about medication and device errors and adverse drug reactions (ISMP, 2010a). Nurses may also receive a monthly safety newsletter, *ISMP Medication Safety Alert! Nurse Advise-ERR,* specifically designed to meet the needs of frontline nurses who are actively involved with medication administration (ISMP, 2010c). Another source for error-prevention advice, provided on the Website of The Joint Commission (2008b), is the *Sentinel Event Alert,* which includes reduction strategies for sentinel events that occur with significant frequency.

FIGURE 9-10   The Joint Commission Speak Up™ Program—Tips for patients to reduce medication errors

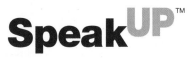

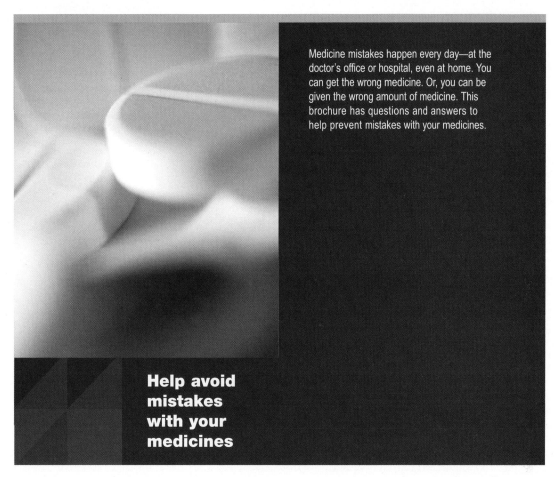

Medicine mistakes happen every day—at the doctor's office or hospital, even at home. You can get the wrong medicine. Or, you can be given the wrong amount of medicine. This brochure has questions and answers to help prevent mistakes with your medicines.

Help avoid mistakes with your medicines

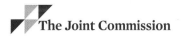
The Joint Commission

My Medicine List

Medication* (include amount you take and how often or what time of day)

vitamins————————————————————————

————————————————————————————

herbs, diet supplements, natural remedies——————————

————————————————————————————

alcohol, recreational drugs————————————————

————————————————————————————

FIGURE 9-10   Continued

Who is responsible for your medicines?

A lot of people—including you!

- Doctors check all of your medicines to make sure they are OK to take together. They will also check your vitamins, herbs, diet supplements or natural remedies.

- Pharmacists will check your new medicines to see if there are other medicines, foods or drinks you should not take with your new medicines. This helps to avoid a bad reaction.

- Nurses and other caregivers may prepare medicines or give them to you.

- You need to give your doctors, pharmacists and other caregivers a list of your medicines. This list should have your

  prescription medicines
  over-the-counter medicines (for example, aspirin)
  vitamins
  herbs
  diet supplements
  natural remedies
  amount of alcohol you drink each day or week
  recreational drugs

This brochure has a wallet card for your list of medicines.

What should you know about your medicines?

- Make sure you can read the handwriting on the prescription. If you can't read it, the pharmacist may not be able to read it either. You can ask to have the prescription printed.

- Read the label. Make sure it has your name on it and the right medicine name.

- Make sure that you understand all of the instructions for your medicines.

- If you have doubts about a medicine, ask your doctor, pharmacist or caregiver about it.

What if you forget the instructions for taking a medicine or are not sure about taking it?

Call your doctor or pharmacist. Don't be afraid to ask questions about any of your medicines.

What can you do at the hospital or clinic to help avoid mistakes with your medicines?

- Make sure your doctors, nurses and other caregivers check your wristband and ask your name before giving you medicine. Some patients get a medicine that was supposed to go to another patient.

- Don't be afraid to tell a caregiver if you think you are about to get the wrong medicine.

- Know what time you should get a medicine. If you don't get it then, speak up.

- Tell your caregiver if you don't feel well after taking a medicine. Ask for help immediately if you think you are having a side effect or reaction.

- You may be given IV (intravenous) fluids. Read the bag to find out what is in it. Ask the caregiver how long it should take for the liquid to run out. Tell the caregiver if it's dripping too fast or too slow.

- Get a list of your medicines—including your new ones. Read the list carefully. Make sure it lists everything you are taking. If you're not well enough to do this, ask a friend or relative to help.

Questions to ask your doctor or pharmacist

- How will this new medicine help you?

- Are there other names for this medicine? For example, does it have a brand or generic name?

- Is there any written information about the medicine?

- Can you take this medicine with your allergy? Remind your doctor about your allergies and reactions you have had to medicines.

- Is it safe to take this medicine with your other medicines? Is it safe to take it with your vitamins, herbs and supplements?

- Are there any side effects of the medicine? For example, upset stomach. Who can you call if you have side effects or a bad reaction? Can they be reached 24 hours a day, seven days a week?

- Are there specific instructions for your medicines? For example, are there any foods or drinks you should avoid while taking it?

- Can you stop taking the medicine as soon as you feel better? Or do you need to take it until it's gone?

- Do you need to swallow or chew the medicine? Can you cut or crush it if you need to?

- Is it safe to drink alcohol with the medicine?

www.jointcommission.org

The goal of the Speak Up™ program is to help patients become more informed and involved in their health care.

My Medicine List

Name ————————————————

Blood Type ————————————————

Allergies ————————————————

Emergency Contact ————————————————

List all of your
prescription medicines
over-the-counter medicines (for example, aspirin)
vitamins
herbs
diet supplements
natural remedies
amount of alcohol you drink each day or week
recreational drugs

It's important to include this information in case of an emergency.
Carry this card with you. Share it with your pharmacist, doctor and other caregivers.

Medication* (include amount you take and how often or what time of day)

prescription ————————————————

————————————————

————————————————

over-the-counter (for example, aspirin) ————————————————

————————————————

————————————————

————————————————

    Throughout this text there are **Clinical Reasoning Skills** that require critical thinking. They are designed to alert you to common medication errors and to practice how to prevent them. Combating errors requires diligent adherence to safety standards prescribed by organizations such as The Joint Commission, the Institute of Medicine, the Institute for Safe Medication Practices, and your health care agency. Stay alert by practicing the *Six Rights of safe medication administration,* regularly reading prevention publications, and spotting and reporting medication errors.

SUMMARY

In conclusion, medication administration is a critical nursing skill that can lead to costly errors, morbidity, and death if not carried out correctly. It is the nurse's responsibility to ensure that the right patient receives the right drug, in the right amount, by the right route, at the right time, and with the right documentation. The nurse who administers a medication is legally liable for medication errors whether the primary cause was an unsafe order, an incorrect transcription, a wrong drug, an inaccurate dosage calculation, an improper preparation, or an administration error.

Review Set 21

1. What are the Six Rights of safe medication administration?

   _____

2. Using The Joint Commission's Official "Do Not Use" List, correct the notations in the following medication order: NPH insulin 20.0 U SC qd

   _____

3. Safe medication administration requires that you check the drug against the order three times:

   1) when you first make contact with the drug (such as removing it from the medication drawer),

   2) when you measure it, and 3) _____.

4. Give two examples of acceptable patient identification according to The Joint Commission, using two unique person-specific identifiers.

   _____.

5. True or False? The nurse who administers a drug based on an incorrect or unsafe medication order shares legal liability for patient injury that results from that drug. _____.

6. According to the Institute of Medicine landmark report, *Preventing Medication Errors,* what strategy is the most effective way to reduce errors?

   a. partnership between the patient and health care providers

   b. double-checking insulin dosage

   c. checking medications three times

   d. safe use of prescribing, dispensing, and recording technologies

   e. strict adherence to the ISMP's List of Error-Prone Abbreviations, Symbols, and Dose Designations

7. Identify one common "workaround" known to lead to drug administration errors during the use of an automated dispensing cabinet (ADC). _____.

8. Where are the two barcodes located that are scanned during medication administration? _____

   _____.

9. Name four drugs or drug categories that have the highest risk of causing injuries when errors are made. How are these drugs designated? _____

   _____.

10. To ensure the accuracy of the order, what nursing actions should you implement following the receipt of a verbal or telephone order from a licensed prescribing practitioner?

   _____

After completing these problems, see page 650 to check your answers.

CLINICAL REASONING SKILLS

It is important for the nurse to check the label on each medication administered, regardless of the medication dispensing mechanism.

ERROR

Failing to check the medication label

Possible Scenario

Suppose a physician orders a diuretic for an adult with congestive heart failure: Lasix 40 mg p.o. b.i.d. The Lasix is supplied in 20 mg tablets. The nurse plans to administer 2 tablets and use an automated medication dispensing machine. The nurse chooses the correct medication from the computer screen. The medication drawer, which should contain the medication, opens. The nurse removes 2 tablets without reading the label, goes to the patient's room, and administers the medication. The medication the nurse removed was Lanoxin 0.25 mg tablets (a cardiac glycoside). The pharmacy technician incorrectly stocked the medication drawer.

Potential Outcome

Although the patient has an order for Lanoxin 0.25 mg p.o. daily, he had already received his dose for the day. At this point, he has received three times the correct amount. He becomes nauseated, and when the nurse checks his pulse, it is 40 beats per minute. The nurse notifies the doctor of the change in the patient's condition. As the one who administered the incorrect medication, the nurse clearly shares responsibility for the medication error.

Prevention

The nurse should read the label on each medication and compare it to the order or MAR three times before administering the drug. If the nurse had checked the label as the drug was removed from the medication drawer, the error could have been prevented. And the nurse had two more opportunities to prevent this error: prior to calculating the dose (the amount should have been 40 mg, not 0.25 mg) and prior to administering the medication.

CLINICAL REASONING SKILLS

The nurse should ensure that the medication ordered can be administered by the right route.

ERROR

Opening a time-released capsule and administering it through a nasogastric tube

Possible Scenario

Suppose a patient is hospitalized to treat a stroke. The physician's orders state to continue all of the patient's home medications. One of the medications is oral theophylline 100 mg, to be administered daily as a 24-hour extended-release capsule (Theo-24) for the treatment of asthma. The patient is unable to swallow as a result of the stroke, and all of his medications must be given through his nasogastric tube. The nurse opens the capsule and dissolves the contents in water and administers it via the nasogastric tube. The patient begins complaining of palpitations, and his pulse increases to 180 beats per minute. The nurse evaluates the changes in the patient's condition and realizes the error.

Potential Outcome

The physician would be notified of the error, and a peak level of theophylline would be ordered. If the patient had a history of cardiac problems, the sympathetic stimulation caused by the theophylline could result in anginal pain or an acute myocardial infarction. The patient would be treated symptomatically until his theophylline blood levels returned to therapeutic range.

Prevention

The nurse should have recognized that a time-released medication could not safely be administered through a nasogastric tube. The physician should have been contacted to obtain orders for a different dosage form of the medication.

PRACTICE PROBLEMS—CHAPTER 9

1. Which of the following statements is/are true?

   a) Statistics show that 5% of all hospital injuries are attributable to medication errors.

   b) According to the Institute of Medicine, most medication errors occur during the administration step of the medication process.

   c) A nurse with more experience and education is less likely to make medication errors.

   d) The medication delivery process involves many individuals and departments.

   e) c and d

2. True or False? Studies indicate that nurses' education and years of practice are closely correlated to the incidence of medication errors. _____

3. True or False? Ten percent (10%) to 18% of patient injuries are attributable to preventable medication errors. _____

4. True or False? Administering a drug late is a frequently underreported medication error. _____

5. True or False? Illegible prescriber's handwriting is a major contributor to transcription errors. _____

6. Fill in the blanks of the following statement. "The right _____ must receive the right _____ in the right _____ by the right _____ at the right _____, followed by the right _____."

7. What are the three steps of medication administration?

   _____

8. The nurse can ensure that the patient receives the right drug by checking the drug label three times. When should the nurse perform these label checks?

   _____

9. Which of the following medical notations is (are) written in the recommended format?

   0.75 mg   *.2 cm*   *q.d.* _____

10. Describe a nursing action to prevent medication errors when receiving verbal drug orders.

   _____

11. Cite four of the direct and/or indirect costs of medication errors.

   _____

12. Describe the strategy or strategies you would implement to prevent this potential medication error.

Possible Scenario

Suppose the physician writes the following order: Dilacor XR 240 mg p.o. q.d.

The order is transcribed as *Dilacor XR 240 mg p.o. q.i.d.,* and the medication is scheduled for administration at 0600, 1200, 1800, and 2400 on the medication administration record.

The nurse reviews the order prior to obtaining the medication for administration. The nurse notices the XR following the name of the medication and recognizes that the letters usually indicate a sustained-release form of medication. The nurse consults the current *AHFS Drug Information* resource and finds that the drug is a sustained-release formula and is only to be given once daily. The nurse reviews the original orders and notes that there was a transcription error. The medication administration record is corrected, and the patient receives the correct amount of medication at the correct time.

Potential Outcome

Had the nurse administered the medication at each of the times indicated on the medication administration record, the patient would have received four times the intended dosage. The drug's therapeutic effect is a decrease in the cardiac output and decrease in blood pressure. However, the toxic effects caused by overdosing could have resulted in congestive heart failure. The patient's life would have been jeopardized.

Prevention

_____

_____

After completing these problems, see pages 650–651 to check your answers.

🖱 Be sure to use the online software for additional practice!

REFERENCES

Cohen, M. R. (2008). ISMP medication error report analysis: Strength misread as total dose [Electronic version]. *Hospital Pharmacy, 43,* 7. Retrieved from http://www.factsandcomparisons.com/assets/hpdatenamed/20080701_July2008_ismp.pdf

Information Technology: Drug company announces individual bar coding on all insulin vials [Electronic version]. *Medical Letter on the CDC & FDA,* March 13, 2005.

Institute for Safe Medication Practices. (2006). Medication safety alert. Harmful errors: How will your facility respond? Retrieved from http://www.ismp.org/Newsletters/acutecare/articles/20061005.asp

Institute for Safe Medication Practices. (2008a). Guidance on the interdisciplinary safe use of automated dispensing cabinets. Retrieved from http://www.ismp.org/Tools/guidelines/ADC_Guidelines_Final.pdf

Institute for Safe Medication Practices. (2008b). Medication safety alert. ADC survey shows some improvements, but unnecessary risks still exist. Retrieved from http://www.ismp.org/Newsletters/acutecare/articles/20080117.asp

Institute for Safe Medication Practices. (2009a). Medication safety alert. Survey on LASA drug name pairs. Retrieved from http://www.ismp.org/Newsletters/acutecare/articles/ 20090521.asp

Institute for Safe Medication Practices. (2009b). Proceedings from the ISMP summit on the use of smart infusion pumps: Guidelines for safe implementation and use. Retrieved from http://www.ismp.org/tools/guidelines/smartpumps/printerVersion.pdf

Institute for Safe Medication Practices. (2010a). Medication safety alerts. Retrieved from http://www.ismp.org/Newsletters/acutecare/default.asp

Institute for Safe Medication Practices. (2010b). Medication safety alert. ISMP updates its list of drug name pairs with TALL Man Letters. Retrieved from http://www.ismp.org/Newsletters/acutecare/articles/20101118.asp

Institute for Safe Medication Practices. (2010c). Medication safety alert. Nurse Advise-ERR. Retrieved from http://www.ismp.org/Newsletters/nursing/default.asp

Institute for Safe Medication Practices. (2010d). Medication safety alert. Preventing errors when administering drugs via an enteral feeding tube. Retrieved from http://www.ismp.org/ Newsletters/acutecare/ articles/20100506.asp

Institute for Safe Medication Practices. (2010e). J. F. Mitchell, PharmD. ISMP Tool, Oral forms that should not be crushed. Retrieved from http://www.ismp.org/Tools/DoNotCrush.pdf

Institute for Safe Medication Practices. (2013). National alert network. Important change with heparin labels. Retrieved from http://www.ismp.org/NAN/files/NAN-20130610.pdf

Institute of Medicine. (2006). Report Brief—Preventing medication errors. Retrieved from http://www .iom.edu/~/media/Files/Report%20Files/2006/Preventing-Medication-Errors-Quality-Chasm-Series/ medicationerrorsnew.pdf

The Joint Commission. (1999). Sentinel event alert, Issue 11. High-alert medications and patient safety. Retrieved from http://www.jointcommission.org/assets/1/18/SEA_11.pdf

The Joint Commission. (2002). Facts about Speak Up™ initiatives. Retrieved from http://www .jointcommission.org/assets/1/18/Facts_Speak_Up.pdf

The Joint Commission. (2006). Sentinel event alert, Issue 36. Tubing misconnections—A persistent and potentially deadly occurrence. Retrieved from http://www.jointcommission.org/assets/1/18/ SEA_36.PDF

The Joint Commission. (2008a). Sentinel event alert, Issue 42. Safely implementing health information and converging technologies. Retrieved from http://www.jointcommission.org/assets/1/18/SEA_42.PDF

The Joint Commission. (2008b). Sentinel event alert, Issue 39. Preventing pediatric medication errors. Retrieved from http://www.jointcommission.org/assets/1/18/SEA_39.PDF

The Joint Commission. (2011). National patient safety goals. Retrieved from http://www.jointcommission .org/standards_information/npsgs.aspx

Mayo, A. M., & Duncan, D. (2004). Nurse perceptions of medication errors: What we need to know for patient safety [Electronic version]. *Journal of Nursing Quality Care, 19,* 3.

Pape, T. M., Guerra, D. M., Muzquiz, M., & Bryant, J. B. (2005). Innovative approaches to reducing nurses' distractions during medication administration. *Journal of Continuing Nursing Education, 36,* 3.

Stetina, P., Groves, M., & Pafford, L. (2005). Managing medication errors—A qualitative study. *Medsurg Nursing, 14,* 3.

U.S. Food and Drug Administration (FDA). (2004). HHS announces new requirements for bar codes on drugs and blood to reduce risks of medication errors. Retrieved from http://www.fda.gov/NewsEvents/ Newsroom/PressAnnouncements/2004/ucm108250.htm

U.S. Food and Drug Administration (FDA). (2006). Guidance for industry: Bar code label requirements. Retrieved from http://www.fda.gov/OHRMS/DOCKETS/98fr/05d-0202-gdl0002.pdf

U.S. Food and Drug Administration (FDA). (2010a). Infusion pumps. Retrieved from http://www .fda.gov/MedicalDevices/ProductsandMedicalProcedures/GeneralHospitalDevicesandSupplies/ InfusionPumps/default.htm

U.S. Food and Drug Administration (FDA). (2010b). Infusion pump improvement initiative. Retrieved from http://www.fda.gov/downloads/MedicalDevices/ProductsandMedicalProcedures/ GeneralHospitalDevicesandSupplies/InfusionPumps/UCM206189.pdf

U.S. Pharmacopeia. (2013). USP-NF injections. U.S. Pharmacopeial Convention. Retrieved from http:// www.usp.org/sites/default/files/usp_pdf/EN/USPNF/generalChapterInjections.pdf

U.S. Pharmacopeial Convention. (2012). USP announces change in labeling requirement for total strength of heparin to help minimize medication errors. Retrieved from http://us.vocuspr.com/Newsroom/ ViewAttachment.aspx?SiteName=uspharm&Entity=PRAsset&AttachmentType=F&EntityID=10 9618&AttachmentID=d49328ac-0f15-496b-b7b9-32cc4ac47773

Wolf, Z. R., & Serembus, J. F. (2004). Medication errors: Ending the blame game. *Nursing Management, 35,* 8.

SECTION 2 SELF-EVALUATION

Directions

1. Round decimals to two places. Round temperatures to one decimal place.

2. Reduce fractions to lowest terms.

Chapter 3—Systems of Measurement

Express the following amounts in proper medical notation.

1. six-tenths gram   _____

2. four teaspoons   _____

3. two hundred fifty thousand units   _____

4. one-half milliliter   _____

5. one-half fluid ounce   _____

Interpret the following notations.

6. 4 gtt   _____

7. 0.25 mg   _____

8. 125 mcg   _____

9. 2 T   _____

10. 0.25 L   _____

Chapters 4 and 5—Conversions

Convert each of the following to the equivalent units indicated.

11. 350 mcg   =   _____ mg   =   _____ g

12. 1.2 g   =   _____ mg   =   _____ mcg

13. 4 T   =   _____ t   =   _____ mL

14. 5 fl oz   =   _____ mL   =   _____ L

15. 56 oz   =   _____ lb   =   _____ kg

16. 56.2 mm   =   _____ cm   =   _____ in

17. 198 lb   =   _____ kg   =   _____ g

18. 11.59 kg   =   _____ g   =   _____ lb

19. A patient is told to take $\frac{1}{2}$ t of a medication. What is the equivalent dose amount in milliliters?
_____ mL

20. A patient is being treated for an infection with two 250 mg tablets of cephalexin four times daily for 10 days. How many grams will he receive in the total dose amount over 10 days? _____ g

21. A full-term infant that weighs less than 2,500 g at birth is considered small for gestational age (SGA). Would a full-term infant with a birth weight of 6 lb 4 oz be SGA? _____

22. Your patient drinks the following for breakfast: 3 fl oz orange juice, 8 fl oz coffee with 1 fl oz cream, and 4 fl oz water. Your patient's total fluid intake is _____ mL.

Convert the following times as indicated. Designate AM or PM where needed.

Traditional Time	International Time
23. 11:35 PM	_____
24. _____	1844
25. 8:03 AM	_____

Convert the following temperatures as indicated.

26. 38°C _____ °F

27. _____ °C 101.5°F

28. 37.2°C _____ °F

Chapter 6—Equipment Used in Dosage Measurement

Draw an arrow to demonstrate the correct measurement of the doses given.

29. 1.5 mL

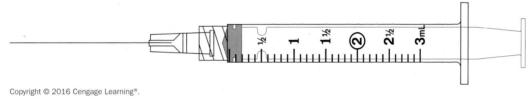

30. 0.33 mL

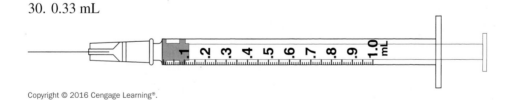

31. 44 units U-100 insulin

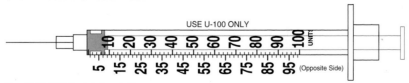

32. 37 units U-100 insulin

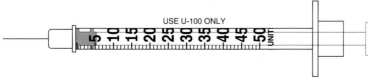

33. $1\frac{1}{2}$ t

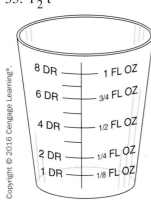 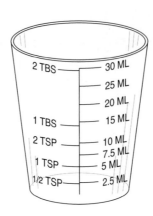

Chapters 7 and 8—Interpreting Drug Orders and Understanding Drug Labels

Use label A to identify the information requested for questions 34 through 36.

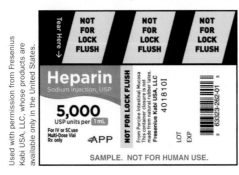

A

34. The generic name is _____.

35. The route of administration intended for this tablet is _____.

36. Interpret this order: **nitroglycerin 400 mcg SL stat.** _____

_____

Use label B to identify the information requested for questions 37 through 39.

37. The supply dosage is _____.

38. The National Drug Code is _____.

39. Interpret: **heparin 3,750 units subcut q.8h.** _____

_____

Use label C to identify the information requested for questions 40 and 41.

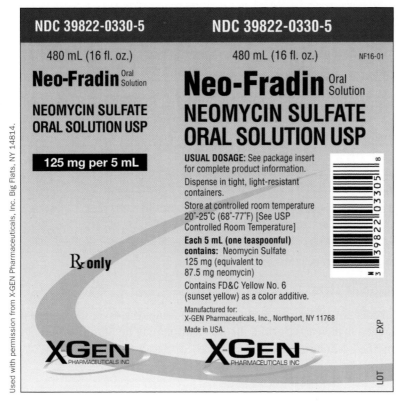

C

40. The generic name is _____.

41. The supply dosage is _____.

Chapter 9—Preventing Medication Errors

42. Using abbreviations from both The Joint Commission and Institute for Safe Medication Practices (ISMP) sources, correct the medical notation of the following order.

    Heparin 5000 U SC qd _____

43. Complete the following statement that defines the Six Rights of safe medication administration.

    "The right patient must receive the right . . . _____

    _____."

Section 2 Board Examination Practice

To obtain licensure, you will be required to pass a board examination. The following problems represent the various types of items on the NCLEX-RN® (National Council Licensure Examination for Registered Nurses) and NCLEX-PN® (National Council Licensure Examination for Practical Nurses) exams. Whether you will be taking one of these board examinations or one from another licensure board, alternate test items such as these are good practice. For additional practice, go to the online practice software that accompanies this text to respond to more interactive test items, including those using the calculator tool.

44. NCLEX *Fill-in-the-Blank* Item

A medication order is written for 0.25 mg of medication. The supplied dosage is expressed in mcg. What would be an equivalent ordered dosage expressed in the supplied unit of measure?

Answer: _____

45. NCLEX *Multiple-Choice One-Response* Item

A hospital nursing unit is preparing signs for the medication room, to alert the staff to look-alike/sound-alike (LASA) drugs that have been associated with medication errors. Which of the following would be an example of the recommended use of Tall Man letters? (Place a check mark beside the correct answer.)

Answer:

    a.   CHLORPROmazine – CHLORPROpamide   _____

    b.   **PREDNISONE – PREDNISOLONE**   _____

    c.   DOBUTamine – DOPamine   _____

    d.   VINBLASTINE – VINCRISTINE   _____

46. NCLEX *Fill-in-the-Blank* Item

If a patient who has an order for **hydromorphone (Dilaudid) 2 mg IV q.4h p.r.n., *severe pain*** received the medication at 5:00 PM, when is the earliest time the medication may be administered again if requested? Write your answer using the 24-hour clock.

Answer: _____

47. NCLEX *Exhibit* Item

Look at the syringe pictured. What is the amount of medication contained in the syringe? (Place a check mark beside the correct answer.)

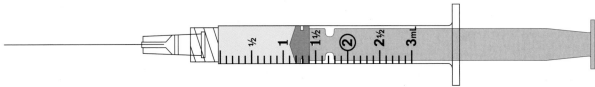

Answer:

    a.   0.12 mL   _____

    b. $1\frac{1}{2}$ mL   _____

    c.   1.2 mL   _____

    d.   1.4 mL   _____

48. NCLEX *Drag-and-Drop / Ordered-Response* Item

Copy the parts of a medication order from the box onto the list in the proper sequence.

Answer:

| 650 mg |
| acetaminophen (Tylenol) |
| fever greater than 101°F |
| p.o. |
| p.r.n. |
| q.4h |

_____

_____

_____

_____

_____

_____

49. NCLEX *Multiple-Response* Item

A medication is ordered to be administered q.i.d. Which of the following possible administration times would be appropriate? (Place a check mark beside all that apply.)

a. 0400, 0800, 1200, 1600, 2000, 2400 _____

b. 0730, 1330, 1830, 2230 _____

c. 2:00 AM, 6:00 AM, 10:00 AM, 2:00 PM, 6:00 PM, 10:00 PM _____

d. 0800, 1200, 2000, 2400 _____

e. 7:00 AM, 12:00 PM, 5:00 PM, 10:00 PM _____

50. NCLEX *Hot Box* Item

Place an X on the circled section of the label that identifies the supply dosage of the medication.

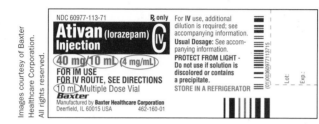

After completing these problems, see pages 651–653 to check your answers. Give yourself 2 points for each correct answer.

Perfect score = 100   My score = _____

Minimum mastery score = 86 (43 correct)

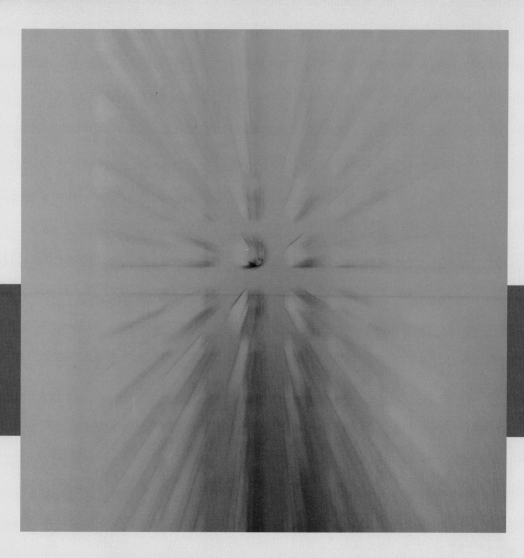

Drug Dosage Calculations

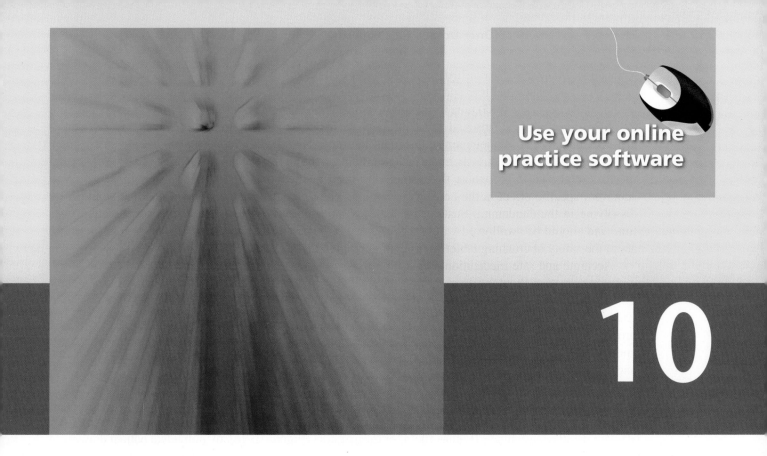

10

Oral Dosage of Drugs

OBJECTIVES

Upon mastery of Chapter 10, you will be able to apply clinical reasoning skills to prepare safe and accurate oral dosages of drugs. To accomplish this, you will also be able to:

- Gather current information about the drug.
- Retrieve the right drug in the correct supply dosage strength.
- Convert all units of measurement to the same system and same size units.
- Estimate the reasonable amount of the drug to be administered.
- Use ratio-proportion to calculate drug dosage.
- Calculate the dose amount (number) of tablets or capsules required to administer oral prescribed dosages.
- Calculate the volume of liquid per dose when the prescribed dosage is in solution form.
- Measure oral dose amounts.

Medications for oral administration are supplied in a variety of forms, such as tablets, capsules, and liquids. They are usually ordered to be administered by mouth, or *p.o.,* which is an abbreviation for the Latin phrase *per os.* To reduce errors in dosage calculations, safety organizations have recommended that all medications supplied to hospital patient care areas be provided in unit-dose packaging, preferably in the original package from the manufacturer (Cohen, 2007). This is not always possible, because hospital pharmacies are frequently supplied with large bulk containers of tablets, capsules, and drugs for injection. Whenever possible, hospital pharmacists should repackage medication into unit doses for distribution to inpatient areas.

When a liquid form of a drug is unavailable, children and many elderly patients may need to have a tablet crushed or a capsule opened and mixed with a small amount of food or fluid to enable them to swallow the medication. Many of these crushed medications and oral liquids also may be ordered to be given enterally or into the gastrointestinal tract via a specially placed tube. Such tubes and their associated enteral routes include the *nasogastric* (NG) tube from nares to stomach, the *nasojejunal* (NJ) tube from nares to jejunum, the *gastrostomy tube* (GT) inserted directly through the abdomen into the stomach, the *jejunum tube* (J-tube) that goes directly into the jejunum of the small intestines, and the *percutaneous endoscopic gastrostomy* (PEG) tube that is placed directly into a patient's stomach through the abdominal wall.

It is important to recognize that some solid-form medications are intended to be given whole to achieve a specific effect in the body. For example, enteric-coated medications protect the stomach by dissolving in the duodenum. Sustained-release capsules allow for gradual release of medication over time and should be swallowed whole. Consult a drug reference or the pharmacist if you are in doubt about the safety of crushing tablets or opening capsules.

Accurate and safe medication preparation requires that the nurse understand the medication order, gather information about the drug, retrieve the right drug in the correct supply dosage strength, accurately calculate the dose amount, and select the proper equipment for accurate measurement of the dose. An error can be made at any point in this process. To help you to avoid costly errors, the examples and problems in Section 3 will lead you through the process of critically thinking about the medication and supply dosage before performing dosage calculations, because all are related. A knowledgeable and safety-minded nurse is the best defense against calculation errors.

To foster clinical reasoning skills, extra clinical information will be provided in this and the next chapters to detail how the dosage calculation skill is an integral step in the safe preparation and administration of medication. Simple illustrations will be used in examples to simulate medications supplied either by floor stock in medication cabinets (Figure 10-1a) or refrigerators (Figure 10-1c), by individual patient drawers in a unit-dose cart (Figure 10-2a), or by drawers in an automated dispensing cabinet (Figures 10-3a, b).

FIGURE 10-1 (**a**) Stock medication cabinet; (**b**) Sample stock drug labels; (**c**) Stock medication refrigerator; (**d**) Sample refrigerated drug label

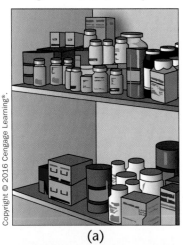

(a)

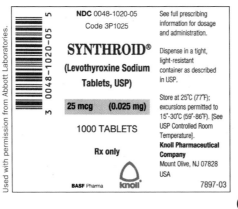

(b)

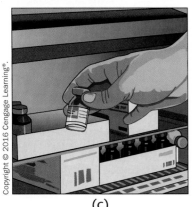

(c)

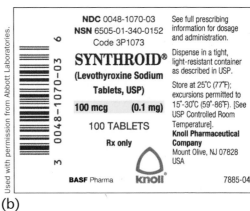

(d)

FIGURE 10-2 **(a)** Unit-dose medication cart with individual patient drawers stocked with 24-hour supply of ordered medication for each patient; **(b)** Example of rectangular box with sample unit-dose drug labels used in text to illustrate one unit-dose drawer stocked with 24-hour supply for one patient that includes four cefadroxil, two labetatol, and three ibuprofen

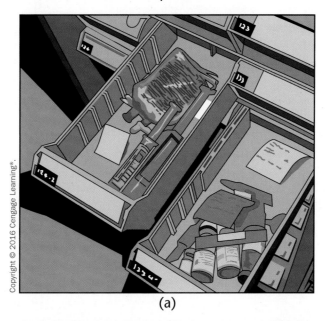

(a)

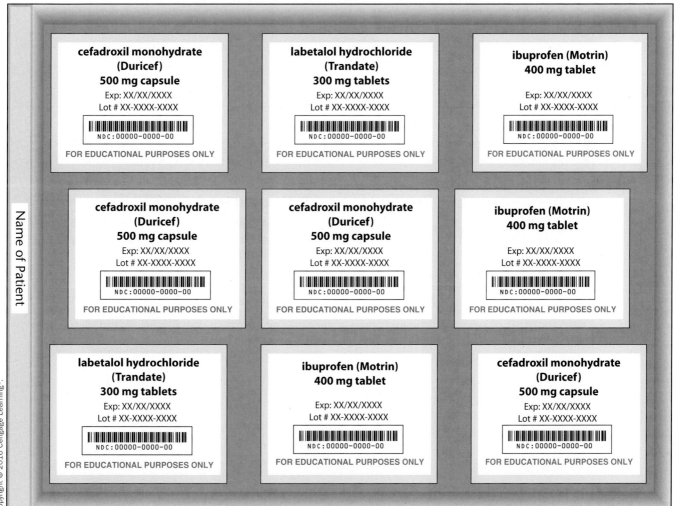

(b)

FIGURE 10-3   **(a)** Automated dispensing cabinet (ADC) matrix drawer; **(b)** Automated dispensing cabinet (ADC) individual cubbies; **(c)** Example of image that will be used in text to illustrate a matrix drawer, stocked with supply of sample unit-dose drug labels depicting look-alike/sound-alike (LASA) drugs; **(d)** Example of image that will be used in text to illustrate a cubby, stocked with supply of sample unit-dose drug labels

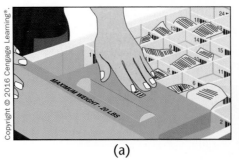

(a)

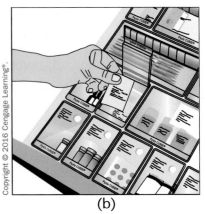

(b)

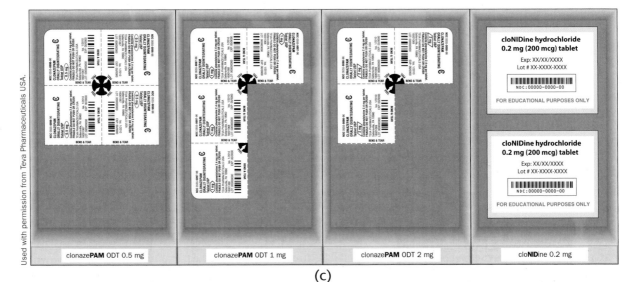

| clonaze**PAM** ODT 0.5 mg | clonaze**PAM** ODT 1 mg | clonaze**PAM** ODT 2 mg | clo**NID**ine 0.2 mg |

(c)

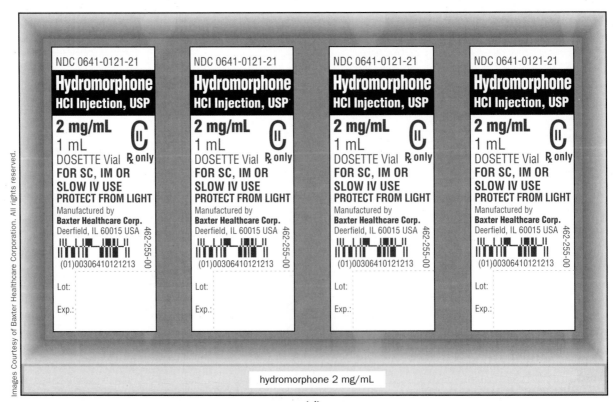

hydromorphone 2 mg/mL

(d)

Drawers in an automated dispensing cabinet (ADC) may be configured many different ways. Two common configurations are the matrix drawer (Figure 10-3a), containing multiple open compartments for different medications and a drawer with individual closed compartments or cubbies (Figure 10-3b). When retrieving medications from a matrix drawer, care must be taken to be sure the drug is removed from the correct compartment. Read the label cautiously before removing the package from the ADC, especially with look-alike/sound-alike drugs (recall Chapter 9). When medication is stored in a closed cubby, the lid for only the requested medication will open.

CAUTION

Carefully read all medication labels to be sure the ADC is stocked with the right medication and is not malfunctioning.

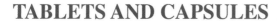

TABLETS AND CAPSULES

Complicated calculations are rarely necessary when preparing tablets or capsules for administration. Usually, the amount required for the ordered dose is one or two pills. Medications with a limited recommended dosage range are often only manufactured in one dosage strength per tablet or capsule. Medications with a wide range of recommended dosages are supplied in capsules or tablets with a variety of strengths, or in scored tablets or caplets that are specially prepared for accurate splitting into half or quarter tablets (Figure 10-4a and b). Only tablets that have scored lines should be split. Research (Verrue et al., 2011) has shown that splitting tablets that are not scored may result in uneven parts and in inaccurate dosage (Figure 10-4c). For high-risk medications, even small deviations in dosage could have serious consequences. It is safer to give whole tablets, but when pill splitting is necessary, use of a pill-splitting device (Figure 10-4d) will result in a more even, but not an exact, split (Verrue et al., 2011). Capsules, geltabs, unscored tablets, and enteric-coated or sustained-release preparations should never be split.

FIGURE 10-4 **(a)** Caplet scored in halves; **(b)** Tablet scored in quarters; **(c)** Uneven split of unscored caplet and tablet; **(d)** Pill-splitting device

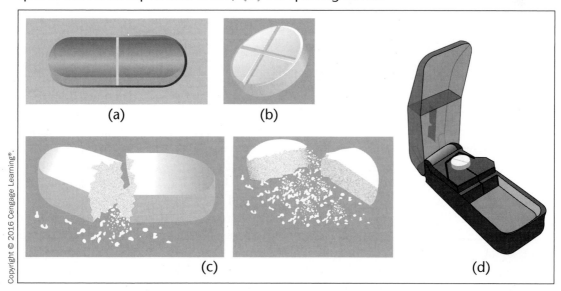

CAUTION

It is safest and most accurate to give the fewest number of whole, undivided tablets possible. Do not split tablets unless they are scored. Do not split capsules, geltabs, enteric-coated, or sustained-release pills.

EXAMPLE 1 ■

The doctor's order reads: sucralfate 1 g p.o. q.i.d. a.c. and at bedtime

As a safety-minded nurse, you gather information about the medication and your patient before determining the amount to give. You consult your drug reference and find that sucralfate, an antiulcer agent, is supplied in 1 g tablets and 500 mg per 5 mL oral suspension. The recommended adult dosage is 1 g q.i.d. 1 hour before meals and at bedtime or 2 g b.i.d. upon waking and at bedtime. The recommended children's dosage is 500 mg q.i.d. 1 hour before meals and at bedtime. Administration guidelines state that tablets should be administered on an empty stomach 1 hour before meals and at bedtime. Guidelines also state that tablets should not be crushed, broken, or chewed. Before selecting the form of the drug to use, the nurse will need to assess whether the patient is able to swallow medication. For this example, we will assume that the patient is an adult who is able to swallow tablets without difficulty.

FIGURE 10-5   (a) Label for stock bottle of sucralfate (Carafate) 1 g tablets; (b) Example of hospital pharmacy-repackaged sucralfate in unit-dose package

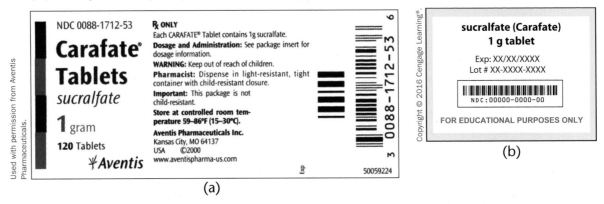

The label pictured in Figure 10-5a is from a stock bottle containing 120 tablets of sucralfate (Carafate) in 1 g tablets. It should be obvious to the nurse that, for the ordered dosage, no calculation is necessary and 1 tablet should be administered to the patient at the scheduled time. While this task seems simple, caution must be taken to ensure the right medication in the right amount is given. In a study reported by the Institute of Medicine (IOM, 2006) of the adverse drug events in U.S. hospitals attributed to administration errors, 10% resulted from faulty drug-identity checking and 10% from faulty dose verification.

There are several options for supplying this medication to the patient unit. Less commonly, the nurse might locate and select the correct stock-supply bottle with the pictured label among many stock medication bottles in a medication supply cabinet. The nurse would remove exactly one tablet from the bottle and return the bottle to the supply cabinet in the correct spot before proceeding to the patient's room. More commonly, the one tablet would be supplied individually in a unit-dose package supplied directly from the manufacturer or in a unit-dose package prepared by the hospital pharmacist, with the drug name and dosage typed on the label as shown in Figure 10-5b. If the hospital uses the unit-dose supply system, the medication will be retrieved from individually labeled patient drawers stocked by the pharmacy daily. It is becoming more common for nurses to find ordered medications in labeled cubicles or cubbies in automated dispensing cabinets (ADCs). While unit-dose distribution systems have been credited with a decrease in medication errors, mistakes still do happen (Cohen, 2007). To avoid errors, the nurse must take the time to select the correct drug in the correct amount from the correct patient unit-dose drawer (such as in Figure 10-2a) or the correctly labeled ADC compartment (such as in Figure 10-3b). The nurse must verify that the medication found in the compartment was stocked correctly by the pharmacy. As you can see, even with the simplest calculation, errors may be made if the nurse omits any steps of the medication administration process.

Let's consider another order that requires identification of the correct dosage strength.

EXAMPLE 2 ▪

The doctor's order reads: clarithromycin 500 mg p.o. q.12h

Clarithromycin, an anti-infective indicated for a variety of infections, is supplied in 250 mg and 500 mg tablets, 500 mg extended-release tablets, and 125 mg per 5 mL and 250 mg per 5 mL oral suspension. Before proceeding with the dosage calculation, the nurse will need to determine which of the available supplied dosage forms are most appropriate for the patient. For this example, we will again assume that the patient is an adult who is able to swallow tablets without difficulty. Depending on the indication, the usual adult dosage is 250 to 500 mg q.12h or 1,000 mg once daily as XL (extended-release) tablets. The nurse should determine that an oral suspension is not necessary and that the extended-release tablet is not the form ordered. The nurse may now proceed to calculate one dose from the available oral tablets pictured, either from a floor stock cabinet (Figure 10-6a) or from an ADC located in the medication room stocked with hospital pharmacy-repackaged unit dosages (Figure 10-6b).

FIGURE 10-6   (a) Label for stock bottles of clarithromycin (Biaxin Filmtab) 250 mg and 500 mg tablets; (b) Hospital pharmacy-repackaged clarithromycin in unit dosages of 250 mg and 500 mg tablets

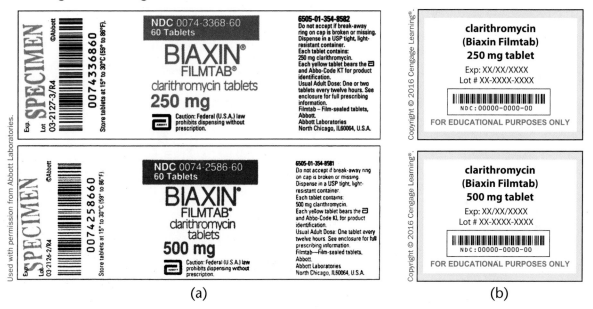

(a)   (b)

Whether the hospital uses the floor-stock distribution system or a unit-dose supply, the calculation is simple. In both instances, two dosage choices are supplied: 250 mg and 500 mg tablets. It should be obvious to the nurse that, for the ordered dosage, the best choice is to select one 500 mg tablet and administer it at the scheduled time.

Now let's consider an order that requires a little more clinical reasoning.

EXAMPLE 3 ▪

The doctor's order reads: clonazepam 1.5 mg p.o. t.i.d.

Clonazepam is an anticonvulsant given to adults and children for seizures or panic disorder. There are many options for administration. It is supplied in 0.5 mg, 1 mg, and 2 mg tablets and also in 0.125 mg, 0.25 mg, 0.5 mg, 1 mg, and 2 mg orally disintegrating tablets. The usual adult dosage range is 0.5 mg 3 times a day, which may be increased gradually based on the patient's response, up to a maximum daily dosage of 20 mg if necessary. The usual dosage for children is based on weight, so the dosage varies greatly depending on the age and size of the child. As you can see, the wide range of dosage strengths is needed for this type of medication. An orally disintegrating tablet (ODT) is a solid form that is designed to be placed directly on the tongue, dissolve within 60 seconds, and then be swallowed with saliva. ODTs differ from sublingual tablets, because they are meant to be absorbed in the gastrointestinal tract and are therefore considered to be administered by the oral route. ODTs do not necessarily result in a faster therapeutic onset, but may be the preferred form for patients with difficulty in swallowing traditional solid oral-dose forms, such as pediatric and geriatric patients. It would be unusual for a specific nursing unit to stock all of the possible dose forms of this medication in the stock cabinet or the ADC. Let's consider the following potential supply in the ADC.

Figure 10-7 illustrates ADC cubbies with prepackaged unit-dose packets of the orally disintegrating tablet (ODT) form of clonazepam: (a) 0.5 mg, (b) 1 mg, (c) 2 mg, and (d) hospital pharmacy-repackaged clonidine hydrochloride 0.2 mg tablets.

ADC cubicle drawers may be customized in various configurations to meet the needs of specific nursing units. Figure 10-7 illustrates one row that would be located in a larger drawer with many different medications in individual cubbies. ADCs will often contain a combination of medications in original unit-dose packages from the manufacturer (Figure 10-7a, 10-7b, 10-7c), as well as medications the pharmacy has repackaged in unit doses (Figure 10-7d).

FIGURE 10-7   Clonazepam and clonidine unit-dose packages

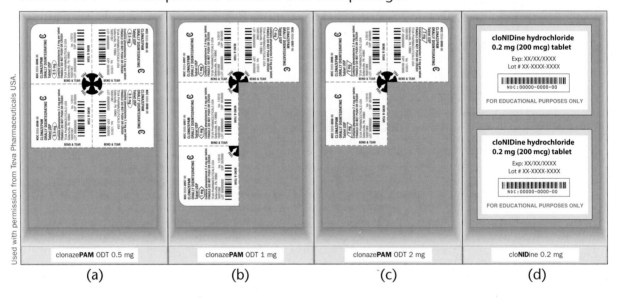

Used with permission from Teva Pharmaceuticals USA.

clonazePAM ODT 0.5 mg	clonazePAM ODT 1 mg	clonazePAM ODT 2 mg	cloNIDine 0.2 mg
(a)	(b)	(c)	(d)

The pictured drawer shows medications ordered alphabetically and by dosage strength. Did you notice something unusual in the typing of the drug names on the compartment labels? Clonazepam and clonidine, located in adjacent cubbies, are on the list of look-alike/sound-alike (LASA) drugs. To reduce the risk of mistaken drug identity, the labels have been printed with Tall Man letters. The ADC supplies only the oral disintegrating tablet (ODT) form of clonazepam. The traditional solid oral-dose form of this drug is a scored tablet and may be split into halves. Because ODTs dissolve rapidly, handling should be kept to a minimum. These tablets are not scored, which will limit the administration options.

We will be administering the medication to an adult patient. Recall that the order is for clonazepam 1.5 mg. None of the tablets is supplied in that dosage. The tablets are not scored, so the nurse can only use a combination of whole tablets to calculate the correct dose amount. The only possible option is to administer one 1 mg tablet with one 0.5 mg tablet for a total dosage of 1.5 mg. It is important to stop and THINK about all the implications for safe medication administration.

THREE-STEP APPROACH TO DOSAGE CALCULATIONS

As the previous examples demonstrate, most of the calculations for tablets and capsules will be simple. At times, the calculations will be more complex if the dosage ordered is in a different unit than the supplied dosage or when the computations involve decimals. Additionally, medications in liquids and solutions will require more exact measurements and calculations.

The following simple Three-Step Approach has been proven to reduce anxiety about calculations and ensure that your results are accurate. Take notice that you will be asked to think or estimate before you attempt to calculate the dosage. Learn and memorize this simple Three-Step Approach, and use it for every dosage calculation every time.

REMEMBER

Three-Step Approach to Dosage Calculations

Step 1	**Convert**	Ensure that all measurements are in the same system of measurement and the same-size unit of measurement. If not, convert before proceeding.
Step 2	**Think**	Estimate what is a *reasonable amount* of the drug to administer.
Step 3	**Calculate**	Set up a proportion to calculate the drug dosage. The ratio for the drug you have on hand is equivalent to the ratio for the desired drug.

$$\frac{\text{Dosage on hand}}{\text{Amount on hand}} = \frac{\text{Dosage desired}}{\text{X Amount desired}}$$

Let's carefully examine each of the three steps as essential and consecutive rules of accurate dosage calculation.

RULE

| Step 1 | **Convert** | Be sure that all measurements are in the same system and all units are in the same size, converting when necessary. |

Many medications are both ordered and supplied in the same system of measurement and in the same-size unit of measurement. This makes dosage calculation easy, because no conversion is necessary. When this is not the case, then you must convert to the same system or the same units. Let's look at two examples where conversion may be a necessary first step in dosage calculation.

EXAMPLE 1 ■

The physician's order reads: clarithromycin 0.5 g p.o. q.12h

Recall from the previous example that clarithromycin (Biaxin) is supplied in 250 mg and 500 mg tablets (Figure 10-6), but the order is written in the unit grams. This is an example of a medication order written and supplied in the same system (metric) but in different-size units (g and mg). That's not a problem. A drug order written in grams but supplied in milligrams will just have to be converted to the same-size unit. We will now perform the first step of the Three-Step Approach: convert.

MATH TIP

In most cases, it is more practical to convert to the smaller unit (such as g to mg). This usually eliminates the decimal or fraction, keeping the calculation in whole numbers.

To continue with Example 1, you should convert 0.5 gram to milligrams. Notice that milligrams are smaller units and converting eliminates the decimal fraction. Use ratio-proportion to convert. Recall that a proportion is a relationship comparing two ratios. Keep the *known* information on the left side of the proportion and the *unknown* on the right. Refer back to Chapter 4 about using ratio-proportion to convert between systems of measurement, as needed.

Equivalent: 1 g = 1,000 mg

$$\frac{1\ g}{1{,}000\ mg} \diagdown\hspace{-1.1em}\diagup \frac{0.5\ g}{X\ mg}$$ Cross-multiply

$X = 1{,}000 \times 0.5$ 0.500. Move the decimal 3 places to the right to multiply by 1,000. Add zeros to complete the operation.

$X = 500\ mg$ Label the units to match the unknown X.

Now you can see that the order and one of the supply choices you have on hand are in the same amount: 500 mg.

Order: clarithromycin 500 mg p.o. q.12h

Supply: clarithromycin 500 mg tablet

There is no need to proceed to steps 2 and 3. The nurse should select one 500 mg tablet of clarithromycin and administer it at the scheduled time.

EXAMPLE 2 ▪

Let's now consider another situation for an order of clonazepam.

The physician's order reads: clonazepam 500 mcg p.o. t.i.d.

In a previous example, we learned that the traditional solid oral-dosage form of clonazepam is supplied in 0.5 mg, 1 mg, and 2 mg scored tablets. For this example, the pharmacy stocked the ADC with repackaged unit-dose packets in the dosages pictured in Figure 10-8.

The Three-Step Approach should be used to calculate this dose. We will again begin with the first step: convert.

The supplied dosages of clonazepam are measured in 1 mg and 2 mg, but the order is expressed in mcg. Before proceeding with calculations, the units of measure must match. Converting the larger unit (mg) of the supplied dosage to the smaller unit (mcg) in the order will avoid the use of decimals.

The known equivalent converts this one.

Equivalent: 1 mg = 1,000 mcg

What is the mcg equivalent of 2 mg?

$$\frac{1\ mg}{1{,}000\ mcg} \diagdown\hspace{-1.1em}\diagup \frac{2\ mg}{X\ mcg}$$ Cross-multiply

$X = 2{,}000\ mcg$ Label the units to match the unknown X.

2 mg = 2,000 mcg

Now the order looks like this:

Order: clonazepam 500 mcg p.o. t.i.d.

Supply: clonazepam 1,000 mcg per tablet or clonazepam 2,000 mcg per tablet

FIGURE 10-8 ADC with various dosages of hospital pharmacy-repackaged clonazepam and clonidine hydrochloride in a matrix drawer

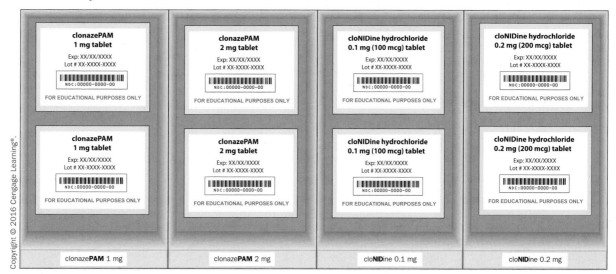

RULE

Step 2   **Think**   Carefully consider what is the reasonable amount of the drug that should be administered.

Now that the two supplied dosages are expressed in the same unit as the order, the nurse will need to decide which supplied dosage to use. Step 2 asks you to logically conclude what amount should be given. Before you go on to Step 3, you may be able to picture in your mind a reasonable amount of medication to be administered, as was demonstrated in the previous example. You know that 500 mcg is half of 1,000 mcg and is one fourth of 2,000 mcg. The tablets are only scored in half, so it is not possible to use the 2,000 mcg tablet. You should calculate the dose using the 1,000 mcg tablet and expect that the answer will be less than one tablet or exactly one half. *Basically, Step 2 asks you to stop and think before you go any further.*

RULE

Step 3   **Calculate**   Ratio for the dosage you have on hand equals the ratio for the desired dosage.

Always double-check your estimated amount from Step 2 with the ratio-proportion method. When setting up the first ratio to calculate a drug dosage, use the supply dosage or the drug concentration information available on the drug label. This is the drug you *have on hand*. Set up the second ratio using the drug order or the *dosage desired* and the amount or volume you will give the patient. This is the unknown or X. Keep the *known* information on the left side of the proportion and the *unknown* on the right.

REMEMBER

$$\frac{\text{Dosage on hand}}{\text{Amount on hand}} = \frac{\text{Dosage desired}}{\text{X Amount desired}}$$

MATH TIP
When solving dosage problems for drugs supplied in tablets or capsules, the amount on hand is always 1, because the supply dosage is per 1 tablet or capsule.

Now you are ready to complete the example with Step 3: calculate.

Order: *clonazepam 500 mcg p.o. t.i.d.*

Supply: clonazepam 1 mg per tablet converted to 1,000 mcg per tablet

Dosage on hand = 1,000 mcg

Amount on hand = 1 tablet

Dosage desired   = 500 mcg

Amount desired = X tablet(s)

$$\frac{\text{Dosage on hand}}{\text{Amount on hand}} = \frac{\text{Dosage desired}}{\text{X Amount desired}}$$

$$\frac{1,000 \text{ mcg}}{1 \text{ tablet}} \diagdown\!\!\!\!\diagup \frac{500 \text{ mcg}}{\text{X tablet(s)}}$$ Cross-multiply

$$1,000\text{X} = 500$$

$$\frac{1,000\text{X}}{1,000} = \frac{500}{1,000}$$ Simplify: Divide both sides of the equation by the number before the unknown X.

$$\text{X} = 0.5$$ 0.500. Move the decimal 3 places to the left to divide by 1,000. Use a leading zero for emphasis in your final answer.

$$\text{X} = \tfrac{1}{2} \text{ tablet}$$ Label the units to match the unknown X.

Give $\frac{1}{2}$ of the clonazepam 1 mg tablet orally three times daily. The calculations verify your estimate from Step 2.

Remember that proportions compare like things. Therefore, you must first convert all units to the same system and to the same size. As pointed out in Chapter 4, the ratio must follow the same sequence. The proportion is set up so that like units are across from each other. The numerators of each represent the weight of the dosage, and denominators represent the amount. It is important to keep like units in order, such as mg as the numerators (on top) and tablets as the denominator (on bottom). And, it is important to keep the known on the left side of the proportion and the unknown (X) on the right. Labeling units also helps you to recognize if you have set up the equation in the proper sequence.

Let's examine three more examples of oral dosages supplied in capsules and tablets, to reinforce the three basic steps. With practice you will be ready to solve dosage calculations such as these on your own.

EXAMPLE 3 ▪

Order: *levothyroxine sodium 0.05 mg p.o. daily*

Synthroid (levothyroxine), a thyroid hormone replacement, is supplied in 25 mcg, 50 mcg, 75 mcg, 88 mcg, 100 mcg, 112 mcg, 125 mcg, 137 mcg, 150 mcg, 175 mcg, 200 mcg, and 300 mcg tablets. All Synthroid tablets are round, color coded, and scored. Levothyroxine is also given by injection. The usual dosage for adults is 50 to 125 mcg daily but may be reduced to 12.5 to 75 mcg per day for geriatric patients. It is also given to children. It would be highly unlikely that a patient unit would stock all of these supply dosages. For this example, the medication will be acquired from a stock medication cabinet. Two stock bottles of Synthroid are located side by side on the shelf in 25 mcg and 100 mcg dosage strengths (Figure 10-9). Do you know which bottle you would choose?

FIGURE 10-9 Synthroid (levothryroxine sodium) stock medication bottles containing: **(a)** 25 mcg and; **(b)** 100 mcg scored tablets

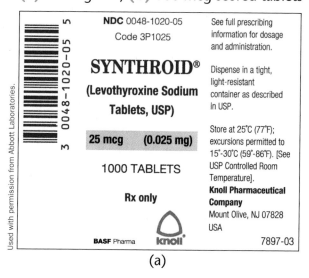

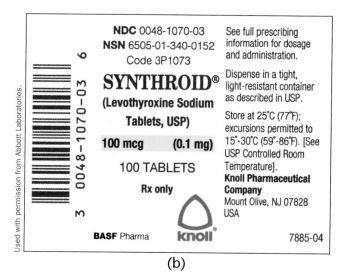

(a)   (b)

| Step 1 | **Convert** | At first look, you might think a conversion is necessary. The order is written as 0.05 mg, but the available supply dosages are 25 mcg and 100 mcg. But on these labels the dosage is provided in both mcg and mg (mg in parentheses). You have two choices. You may calculate this example using the supply dosage in mg, with no conversion needed. The computation will include decimals, and extra care must be taken to avoid a mistake. You may also convert the ordered dosage from 0.05 mg to an equivalent in mcg, which will eliminate the decimal; then you will use the supply dosage in mcg. Let's work this example by first converting. |

Convert to the same-size units. Remember the math tip: Convert larger unit (mg) to smaller unit (mcg) and you will eliminate the decimal fraction.

Approximate equivalent: 1 mg = 1,000 mcg

$$\frac{1 \text{ mg}}{1,000 \text{ mcg}} \diagdown \frac{0.05 \text{ mg}}{X \text{ mcg}}$$ Cross-multiply

$X = 1,000 \times 0.05$ 0.050. Move the decimal 3 places to the right. Add zero to complete the operation.

$X = 50$ mcg   Label the units to match the unknown X.

Order: **levothyroxine sodium 0.05 mg = 50 mcg**

Supply: Synthroid (levothyroxine sodium) 25 mcg tablets

| Step 2 | **Think** | As soon as you convert the ordered dosage of Synthroid 0.05 mg to Synthroid 50 mcg, you suspect that the 25 mcg supply would be the best to use and that you want to give more than 1 tablet for each dose. In fact, you want to give twice the supply dosage, which is the same as 2 tablets. |

Avoid getting confused by the way the original problem is presented. Be sure that you recognize which is the dosage ordered or desired and which is the supply dosage per the amount on hand. A common error is to misread the information and mix up the ratios in Step 3. This demonstrates the importance of thinking (Step 2) before you calculate.

Step 3 **Calculate** $\dfrac{\text{Dosage on hand}}{\text{Amount on hand}} = \dfrac{\text{Dosage desired}}{\text{X Amount desired}}$

$$\frac{25 \text{ mcg}}{1 \text{ tablet}} \diagdown\kern-1.6em\diagup \frac{50 \text{ mcg}}{\text{X tablets}}$$ Cross-multiply

$$25X = 50$$

$$\frac{25X}{25} = \frac{50}{25}$$ Simplify: Divide both sides of the equation by the number before the unknown X.

$$X = 2 \text{ tablets}$$ Label the units to match the unknown X.

Give 2 tablets of Synthroid orally daily.

EXAMPLE 4 ■

Order: **nitroglycerin 0.6 mg SL stat, repeat in 5 minutes if no relief of angina**

Nitroglycerin, an antianginal, is used for the treatment of acute and long-term management of angina pectoris, characterized by episodic severe chest pain. Nitroglycerin is supplied in many different dosage forms and may be administered by a variety of routes (Figure 10-10). Sublingual tablets are available in 0.3 mg, 0.4 mg, and 0.6 mg dosages and extended-release capsules in 2.5 mg, 6.5 mg, and 9 mg dosages. Compare the dosage strengths between the sublingual tablets and oral capsules. Nitroglycerin is rapidly absorbed when given sublingually but undergoes significant metabolism when given orally, leading to decreased bioavailability, thereby requiring a higher dosage to be effective.

In this example, the nurse will provide the medication to an adult patient in an emergency department. In this hospital, the medications are located in a stock medication cabinet in a central medication room.

FIGURE 10-10 Nitroglycerin (Nitrostat) stock medication bottles containing: **(a)** 0.3 mg sublingual tablets; **(b)** 6.5 mg extended-release capsules; **(c)** 0.4 mg sublingual tablets, and; **(d)** 9 mg extended-release capsules

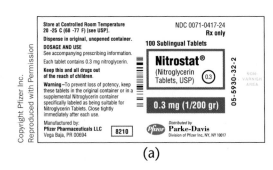

(a)

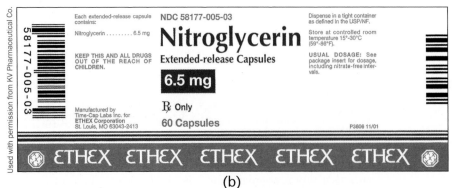

(b)

Continues

FIGURE 10-10   *Continued*

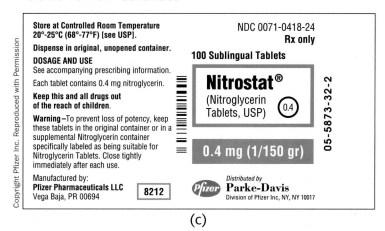

(c)

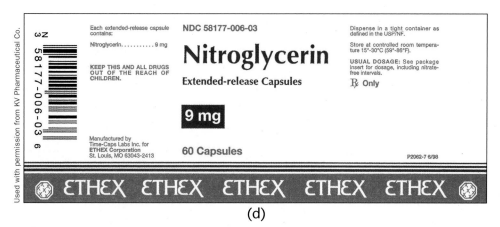

(d)

Step 1   **Convert**   Consider the dosage strength on the Nitrostat labels: 0.3 mg (1/200 gr) and 0.4 mg (1/150 gr). The order is written using the metric unit milligram. Why would the pharmaceutical company also include the dose in the apothecary unit grain (gr)? Although The Joint Commission recommends discontinuing the use of the apothecary system, this medication is an example of a drug that has traditionally been prescribed and is still labeled using apothecary notation. In this example, the order is written in milligrams and the supplied dosage strengths are all provided in the same unit of measure, so no conversion is needed. Be careful to find the metric dosage strength, and avoid being distracted by the apothecary dosage found on the labels.

Step 2   **Think**   There are four possible supply dosages to use. You might first glance at the supply bottle with 6.5 mg capsules, but after carefully reading the label, you would realize that it is not the correct medication. It is more than ten times the dosage ordered and is in the extended-release capsule form, which cannot be given by the sublingual route. Additionally, neither of the extended-release capsules would be appropriate for a stat medication order to treat an acute condition. That leaves two possible choices. Mathematically, either 0.3 mg or 0.4 mg could be used to calculate a 0.6 mg dosage. Recall the recommendation to use whole tablets whenever possible and only divide tablets that are scored. The 0.4 mg tablet is not scored. That leaves only one choice in this situation: the 0.3 mg SL tablet. You anticipate that you will need to give more than 1 tablet, or exactly 2.

Step 3   **Calculate**   Order: nitroglycerin 0.6 mg SL stat

Supply: nitroglycerin 0.3 mg sublingual tablets

$$\frac{\text{Dosage on hand}}{\text{Amount on hand}} = \frac{\text{Dosage desired}}{\text{X Amount desired}}$$

$$\frac{0.3 \text{ mg}}{1 \text{ tablet}} \diagdown\diagup \frac{0.6 \text{ mg}}{\text{X tablet(s)}}$$ Cross-multiply

$$0.3X = 0.6$$

$$\frac{0.3X}{0.3} = \frac{0.6}{0.3}$$ Simplify: Divide both sides of the equation by the number before the unknown X.

$$X = 2 \text{ tablets}$$ Label the units to match the unknown X.

Give 2 tablets Nitrostat sublingually immediately for angina. Repeat in 5 minutes if no relief.

EXAMPLE 5 ■

Order: Lasix 10 mg p.o. b.i.d.

Lasix (furosemide), a loop diuretic, is supplied for oral use in 20 mg, 40 mg, and 80 mg tablets or 10 mg/mL and 8 mg/mL oral solutions. It also may be given by injection. It is ordered for both adults and children with medical conditions that require a reduction in excess fluid. Depending on the indication, the usual adult oral dosage ranges from 20 mg to 80 mg total per day, given in one or two doses. The usual dosage for children is based on weight. In this example, the nurse will provide the medication in tablet form to an adult patient. Medications are distributed in this hospital by ADCs located in the unit medication rooms. Notice that LASA (look-alike/sound-alike) drugs are supplied in adjacent cubbies (Figure 10-11).

FIGURE 10-11   Illustrated ADC matrix drawer with hospital pharmacy-repackaged: **(a)** fluoxetine (Prozac) 10 mg capsules; **(b)** furosemide (Lasix) 20 mg tablets; **(c)** furosemide (Lasix) 40 mg tablets, and; **(d)** furosemide (Lasix) 80 mg tablets

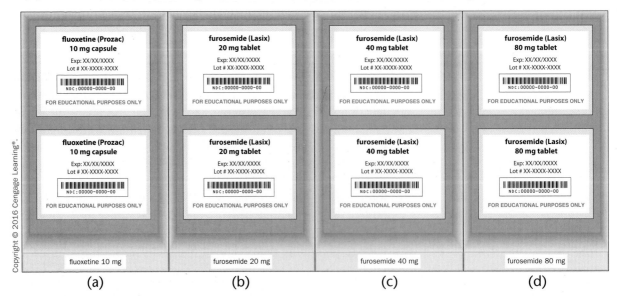

Step 1   **Convert**   No conversion is necessary. The units are in the same system (metric) and the same size (mg).

Step 2   **Think**   There are three possible supply dosages to use. You might first glance at the compartment a with the fluoxetine 10 mg capsules, but after carefully reading, you would realize that it is not the correct medication, and instead you choose the furosemide 20 mg tablet from compartment (b). You anticipate that you will need to give less than one tablet, or exactly one half.

Step 3   **Calculate**   Order: Lasix 10 mg p.o. b.i.d.

Supply: furosemide (Lasix) 20 mg per tablet

$$\frac{\text{Dosage on hand}}{\text{Amount on hand}} = \frac{\text{Dosage desired}}{\text{X Amount desired}}$$

$$\frac{20 \text{ mg}}{1 \text{ tablet}} \diagdown\diagup \frac{10 \text{ mg}}{\text{X tablet(s)}}$$ Cross-multiply

$$20\text{X} = 10$$

$$\frac{20\text{X}}{20} = \frac{10}{20}$$ Simplify: Divide both sides of the equation by the number before the unknown X.

$$\text{X} = \tfrac{1}{2} \text{ tablet}$$ Label the units to match the unknown X.

Give $\tfrac{1}{2}$ tablet Lasix orally twice a day.

The calculations verify your estimate from Step 2. But in this case, when you go to administer the medication, you will find that the 20 mg tablet is not scored. When you look closely at the three furosemide tablets, you will find that each tablet is a different size and shape. The 20 mg tablets are white, oval, and not scored. The 40 mg tablets are white, round, and are scored in half. The 80 mg tablets are white, round, have faceted edges, and are not scored. You will not be able to split the 20 mg tablet, and the other two choices will not work for this order either. The first thing you might question is the accuracy of your calculations. However, you double-check and find that the calculations are correct. The second thing you might question is the original order. Furosemide 10 mg given twice a day will provide a total of 20 mg, which is within the usual dosage range but on the low end. Is there an alternative supply that would work for this order? You realize that furosemide is supplied in 10 mg/mL oral solution, which would provide the correct dosage. Because this form is not supplied in the ADC, it is probably not frequently administered to adult patients on this unit. You should verify the order with the prescriber, and once the order is confirmed in this dosage, ask that the hospital pharmacy deliver the oral solution for this patient.

The previous examples illustrated five different scenarios that you may encounter when calculating and preparing oral medications for administration. Now you are ready to apply all three steps of this logical approach to dosage calculations. The same three steps will be used to solve both oral and parenteral dosage calculation problems. It is most important that you develop the ability to reason for the answer or estimate before you calculate the amount to give. Health care professionals can unknowingly make errors if they rely solely on a calculation method rather than first asking themselves what the answer should be. As a nurse or allied health professional, you are expected to be able to reason sensibly, solve problems, and justify your judgments rationally. With these same skills, you gained admission to your educational program and to your profession. While you sharpen your math skills, your ability to think and estimate are your best resources for avoiding errors. Use ratio-proportion as a calculation tool to validate the dose amount you anticipate should be given, rather than the reverse. If your reasoning is sound, you will find that the dosages you compute make sense and are accurate. For example, you would question any calculation that directs you to administer 5 tablets of any medication.

CAUTION

The maximum number of tablets or capsules for a single dose is usually 3. Stop, think, and recheck your calculation if a single dose requires more. Question all orders that exceed that amount.

QUICK REVIEW
Simple Three-Step Approach to Dosage Calculations

Step 1. **Convert** If necessary, convert to units of the same system and the same size.

Step 2 **Think** Estimate a reasonable amount to give.

Step 3 **Calculate** The ratio for the dosage you have on hand equals the ratio for the dosage desired.

$$\frac{\text{Dosage on hand}}{\text{Amount on hand}} = \frac{\text{Dosage desired}}{\text{X Amount desired}}$$

- For most dosage calculation problems, convert to the smaller-size unit. Example: g → mg

- Consider the reasonableness of the calculated amount to give. Example: you would question giving more than 3 tablets or capsules per dose for oral administration.

- Carefully select the correct drug to match the order and dose amount.

- Only scored tablets may be divided in halves or quarters.

Review Set 22

For questions 1 through 8, calculate the correct number of tablets or capsules to be administered per dose. Tablets are scored in half.

1. Order: *chlorpropamide 0.1 g p.o. daily*

   Supply: chlorpropamide 100 mg tablets, scored in halves

   Give: _____ tablet(s)

2. Order: *bethanechol 15 mg p.o. t.i.d.*

   Supply: bethanechol 10 mg tablets, scored in halves

   Give: _____ tablet(s)

3. Order: *hydrochlorothiazide 12.5 mg p.o. t.i.d.*

   Supply: hydrochlorothiazide 25 mg tablets, scored in halves

   Give: _____ tablet(s)

4. Order: *digoxin 0.125 mg p.o. daily*

   Supply: digoxin 0.25 mg tablets, scored in halves

   Give: _____ tablet(s)

5. Order: *ibuprofen 600 mg p.o. b.i.d.*

   Supply: ibuprofen 200 mg unscored tablets

   Give: _____ tablet(s)

6. Order: levofloxacin 0.5 g p.o. daily

   Supply: levofloxacin 500 mg unscored tablets

   Give: _____ tablet(s)

7. Order: levothyroxine 0.1 mg p.o. daily

   Supply: levothyroxine 50 mcg tablets, scored in halves

   Give: _____ tablet(s)

8. Order: clorazepate 7.5 mg p.o. q.i.d.

   Supply: clorazepate 3.75 mg capsules

   Give: _____ capsule(s)

Calculate 1 dose for each of the medication orders for questions 9 through 16. The labels lettered A through I are the drugs you have available, supplied in stock medication bottles in a locked cabinet in a central medication room. Indicate the letter corresponding to the label you select.

9. Order: carbamazepine 0.2 g p.o. t.i.d.

   Select: _____

   Give: _____

10. Order: potassium chloride 20 mEq p.o. daily

    Select: _____

    Give: _____

11. Order: digoxin 375 mcg p.o. daily

    Select: _____

    Give: _____

12. Order: sulfasalazine 1 g p.o. b.i.d.

    Select: _____

    Give: _____

13. Order: levothyroxine sodium 0.2 mg p.o. daily

    Select: _____

    Give: _____

14. Order: digoxin 0.5 mg p.o. daily

    Select: _____

    Give: _____

15. Order: gabapentin 0.1 g p.o. t.i.d.

    Select: _____

    Give: _____

16. Order: gemfibrozil 0.6 g p.o. daily

    Select: _____

    Give: _____

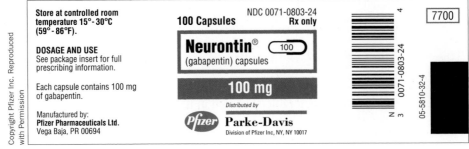

Store at controlled room temperature 15°- 30°C (59°- 86°F).

DOSAGE AND USE
See package insert for full prescribing information.

Each capsule contains 100 mg of gabapentin.

Manufactured by:
Pfizer Pharmaceuticals Ltd.
Vega Baja, PR 00694

NDC 0071-0803-24
100 Capsules   **Rx only**

Neurontin® (100)
(gabapentin) capsules

100 mg

Distributed by
Pfizer **Parke-Davis**
Division of Pfizer Inc, NY, NY 10017

7700

0071-0803-24
05-5810-32-4

A

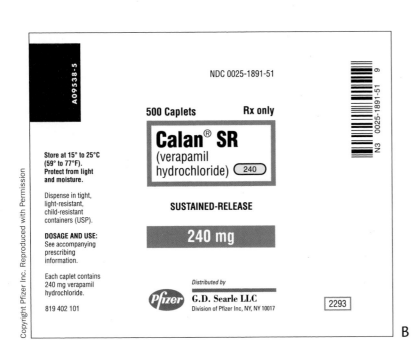

A09538-5

NDC 0025-1891-51

500 Caplets   **Rx only**

Calan® SR
(verapamil hydrochloride) (240)

SUSTAINED-RELEASE

240 mg

Store at 15° to 25°C (59° to 77°F).
Protect from light and moisture.

Dispense in tight, light-resistant, child-resistant containers (USP).

DOSAGE AND USE:
See accompanying prescribing information.

Each caplet contains 240 mg verapamil hydrochloride.

819 402 101

Distributed by
Pfizer **G.D. Searle LLC**
Division of Pfizer Inc, NY, NY 10017

2293

N3 0025-1891-51 9

B

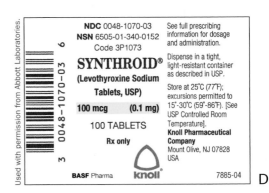

NDC 0048-1070-03
NSN 6505-01-340-0152
Code 3P1073

SYNTHROID®

(Levothyroxine Sodium Tablets, USP)

100 mcg   **(0.1 mg)**

100 TABLETS

Rx only

See full prescribing information for dosage and administration.

Dispense in a tight, light-resistant container as described in USP.

Store at 25°C (77°F); excursions permitted to 15°-30°C (59°-86°F). [See USP Controlled Room Temperature].
Knoll Pharmaceutical Company
Mount Olive, NJ 07828 USA

BASF Pharma   **knoll®**

0048-1070-03 6

7885-04

D

Each tablet contains 600 mg gemfibrozil.
Usual Adult Dosage–
See package insert for full prescribing information.
Keep this and all drugs out of the reach of children.
Dispense in tight container as defined in the USP.
**Store at controlled room temperature 20°- 25°C (68°- 77°F) [see USP].
Protect from light and humidity.**
Important–This package for pharmacy stock use.

Manufactured by:
Parke Davis Pharmaceuticals, Ltd.
Vega Baja, PR 00694
Distributed by:
PARKE-DAVIS
Div of Warner-Lambert Co
Morris Plains, NJ 07950 USA
© 1997-'99, PDPL

N 0071-0737-30

Lopid®

(Gemfibrozil Tablets, USP)

600 mg
℞ only

500 TABLETS

Ⓟ **PARKE-DAVIS**

6505-01-300-7956

N3 0071-0737-30 3

05-5894-32-0

Exp date and lot

C

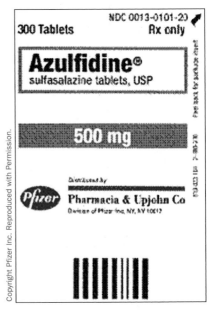

300 Tablets   NDC 0013-0101-20 **Rx only**

Azulfidine®
sulfasalazine tablets, USP

500 mg

Distributed by
Pfizer **Pharmacia & Upjohn Co**
Division of Pfizer Inc, NY, NY 10017

E

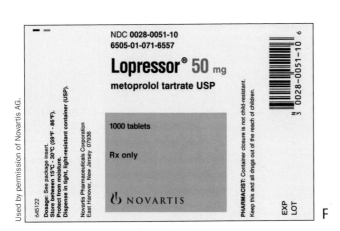

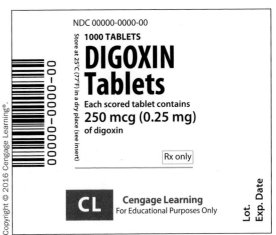

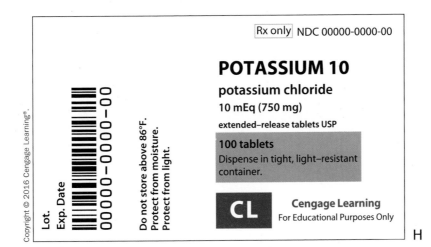

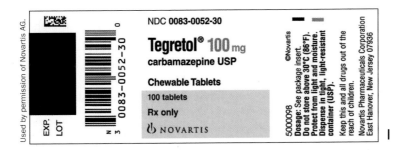

Questions 17 through 30 depict medication administration simulation exercises. The medications are stocked for each individual patient in unit-dose carts by the pharmacy once every 24 hours (review Figure 10-2a, b). Prepare the medications for each patient, using the Three-Step Approach. Refer to a nursing drug guide, such as the annual *2013 Delmar Nurse's Drug Handbook*, to answer specific questions about the medication prior to administering.

Patient #1 (questions 17 through 19) is scheduled to receive the following medications at 0800. The patient's stocked unit-dose drawer with pharmacy-repackaged medications is pictured below. The full supply of medications needed for 24 hours should be in the ADC; therefore, multiple packets of the same medication are included in random order as stocked.

Patient #1

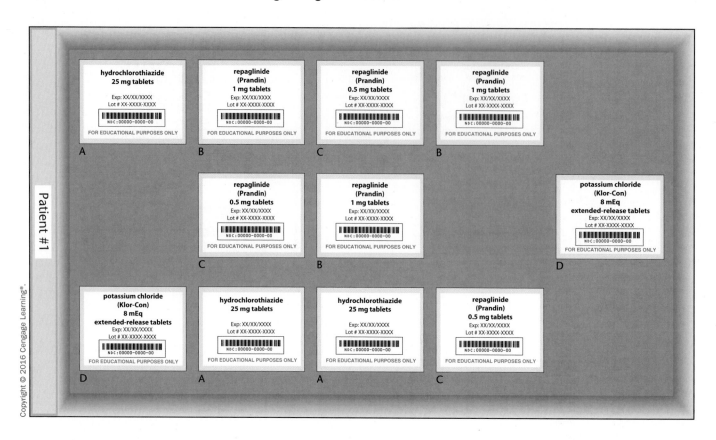

17. Order: repaglinide 1.5 mg t.i.d. with meals

    a. Look up repaglinide in your drug guide. For what condition(s) is repaglinide indicated? _____
        _____

    b. What supply dosages (dosage strengths) and forms may be available from the pharmaceutical
        manufacturer? _____

    c. What is the usual recommended adult dosage range? _____

    d. Identify the letter of the supplied dosage strength you will use to calculate 1 dose. _____

    e. Give: _____ tablet(s)

18. Order: hydrochlorothiazide 12.5 mg p.o. t.i.d

    a. For what condition(s) is hydrochlorothiazide indicated? _____

    b. What supply dosages (dosage strengths) and forms may be available from the pharmaceutical
        manufacturer? _____

    c. What is the usual recommended adult dosage range? _____

    d. Identify the letter of the supplied dosage strength you will use to calculate 1 dose. _____

    e. Give: _____ tablet(s)

19. Order: Klor-Con 16 mEq p.o. daily

    a. For what condition(s) is Klor-Con indicated? _____

    b. What supply dosages (dosage strengths) and forms may be available from the pharmaceutical
        manufacturer? _____

   c. What is the usual recommended adult dosage range? _____

   d. Identify the letter of the supplied dosage strength you will use to calculate 1 dose. _____

   e. Give: _____ tablet(s)

Patient #2 (questions 20 through 22) is scheduled to receive the following routine medications at 2100. The patient's unit-dose drawer is stocked with pharmacy-repackaged medications as pictured below. As in the previous scenario, multiple packets of the same medication are stocked in the drawer in random order. As you can see, there are four cefadroxil monohydrate capsules (E), two labetalol hydrochloride tablets (F), and three ibuprofen tablets (G) for p.r.n. use.

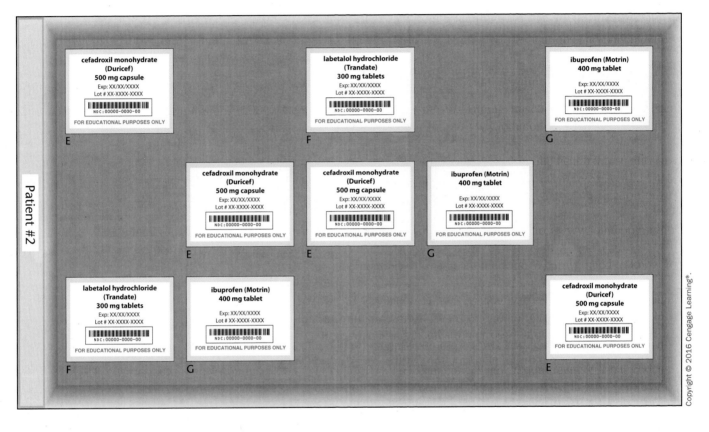

20. Order: **Trandate 150 mg p.o. b.i.d**

   a. For what condition(s) is Trandate indicated? _____

   b. What supply dosages (dosage strengths) and forms may be available from the pharmaceutical manufacturer? _____

   c. What is the usual recommended adult dosage range? _____

   d. Identify the letter of the supplied dosage strength you will use to calculate 1 dose. _____

   e. Give: _____ tablet(s)

21. Order: **ibuprofen 800 mg p.o. t.i.d.**

   a. For what condition(s) is ibuprofen indicated? _____

   b. What supply dosages (dosage strengths) and forms may be available from the pharmaceutical manufacturer? _____

   c. What is the usual recommended adult dosage range? _____

   d. Identify the letter of the supplied dosage strength you will use to calculate 1 dose. _____

   e. Give: _____ tablet(s)

22. Order: *cefadroxil monohydrate 1 g p.o. b.i.d.*

    a. For what condition(s) is cefadroxil indicated? _____

    b. What supply dosages (dosage strengths) and forms may be available from the pharmaceutical manufacturer? _____

    c. What is the usual recommended adult dosage range? _____

    d. Identify the letter of the supplied dosage strength you will use to calculate 1 dose. _____

    e. Give: _____ capsule(s)

Patient #3 (questions 23 through 30) complains of pain rated 8 on a 1-to-10 scale at 1800. Controlled substances are located in a double-locked medication supply cabinet with stock bottles of medications located on shelves as pictured below.

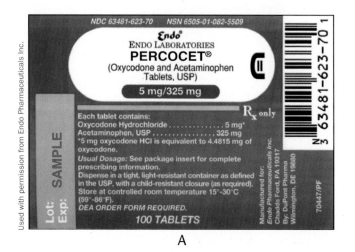

A

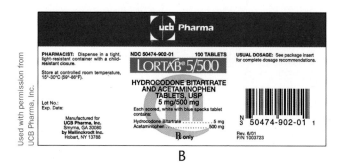

B

23. Order: *oxycodone 5 mg/acetaminophen 325 mg 1 to 2 tablets p.o. q.6h p.r.n., moderate to moderately severe pain*

    a. For what condition(s) is oxycodone indicated? _____

    b. For what condition(s) is acetaminophen indicated? _____

    c. What dosage variations of oxycodone with acetaminophen can be supplied in tablet or capsule form? _____

24. What is the usual recommended adult dosage range? _____

25. Identify the drugs that are different in the two supplied combination medications. Refer to Figure 9-8: *FDA and ISMP Lists of Look-Alike Drug Names with Recommended Tall Man Letters* (on page 191). Write the drug names, using Tall Man letters. _____

    _____

26. Identify the letter of the supplied dosage strength you will use to calculate 1 dose. _____

27. To administer the p.r.n., medication at the right time, what is the latest time the patient should have received the previous dose? _____

28. Give: _____ tablet(s)

29. What is the maximum recommended daily dosage of acetaminophen? _____

30. If this patient receives the maximum ordered dosage in 24 hours, will the maximum recommended daily dosage be exceeded? _____

After completing these problems, see pages 653–655 to check your answers.

ORAL LIQUIDS

Oral liquids are supplied in solution form and contain a specific amount of drug in a given amount of solution or suspension, as stated on the label. In solving dosage problems when the drug is supplied in solid form, you calculated the number of tablets or capsules that contained the prescribed dosage. The supply container label indicates the amount of medication per 1 tablet or 1 capsule. For medications supplied in liquid form, you must calculate the volume of the liquid that contains the prescribed dosage of the drug. The supply dosage noted on the label may indicate the amount of drug per 1 milliliter (Figure 10-12) or per multiple milliliters of solution, such as 125 mg per 5 mL (Figure 10-13a) or 20 mEq per 15 mL (Figure 10-14c).

The Three-Step Approach can be used to solve liquid oral dosage calculations in the same way that solid-form oral dosages are calculated. Let's apply the three steps to dosage calculations in a few examples.

EXAMPLE 1 ■

Order: *oxycodone 15 mg p.o. q.3h p.r.n., moderate to severe pain*

Oxycodone is an opioid analgesic Schedule II controlled substance used to treat moderate to severe pain. It may be used in adults and children. The usual adult oral dosage is 5 to 10 mg q.3 to 4h as needed, but a larger dosage may be required for chronic pain relief. The patient in this example is an adult with terminal cancer, being cared for in his home by hospice. The patient has difficulty swallowing pills, and the hospice nurse has decided that an oral solution would be indicated at this time. Oral solution is available in 5 mg per 5 mL in a 500 mL bottle and in a concentrated oral solution in 20 mg/mL in a 30 mL bottle with a dropper. A stock bottle of oxycodone hydrochloride oral concentrate solution has been dispensed (Figure 10-12).

FIGURE 10-12   Stock bottle of oxycodone hydrochloride oral concentrate solution 20 mg/mL

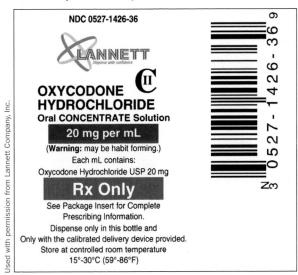

Step 1	Convert	The order is in the metric unit milligrams. The supply is 20 mg/mL. The ordered unit is the same as the supplied unit. No conversion is needed.
Step 2	Think	The ordered dosage is 15 mg every 3 hours, but the usual dosage is 5 to 10 mg every 3 to 4 hours. This ordered dosage is higher than the usual dosage, but this patient has a chronic condition. Larger dosages may be required for chronic conditions. The ordered dosage of 15 mg is $1\frac{1}{2}$ times more than the high end of the usual dosage. This seems reasonable for a patient with terminal cancer pain. The supply is 20 mg/mL, so you expect the 15 mg dosage to be slightly less than 1 mL.

Step 3   **Calculate** $\dfrac{\text{Dosage on hand}}{\text{Amount on hand}} = \dfrac{\text{Dosage desired}}{\text{X Amount desired}}$

$$\dfrac{20\ \text{mg}}{1\ \text{mL}} \diagbox \dfrac{15\ \text{mg}}{\text{X mL}}$$ Cross-multiply

$$20\text{X} = 15$$

$$\dfrac{20\text{X}}{20} = \dfrac{15}{20}$$ Simplify: Divide both sides
of the equation by the number
before the unknown X.

$$\text{X} = 0.75\ \text{mL}$$ Label the units to match the
unknown X.

The patient should be given 0.75 mL of the oxycodone hydrochloride oral concentrate solution, using the dropper provided with the bottle. This confirms your estimate.

EXAMPLE 2 ■

Order: *cefaclor 100 mg p.o. q.8h for 7 days*

Cefaclor is a second-generation cephalosporin, a broad-spectrum anti-infective used to treat a variety of infections. It is used in adults and children and administered only by the oral routes. It is supplied in 250 mg and 500 mg capsules; 125 mg, 187 mg, 250 mg, and 375 mg chewable tablets; 375 mg and 500 mg extended-release tablets; and 125 mg per 5 mL, 187 mg per 5 mL, 250 mg per 5 mL, and 375 mg per 5 mL strawberry-flavored oral suspension. Your patient for this example is an 18-month-old child weighing 10 kg who is evaluated in an urgent care clinic and being treated for a respiratory infection. The usual child dosage is 6.7 to 13.4 mg/kg every 8 hours. In Chapter 13, you will learn how to calculate and verify dosages based on weight, but for this example, you may assume that the ordered dosage is appropriate. Medications are dispensed as a courtesy in this urgent care clinic. Four dosage strengths of cefaclor are available in stock (Figure 10-13).

Step 1   **Convert**   The order is in the metric unit milligrams. All supplied dosages are also in millgrams. No conversion is needed.

FIGURE 10-13   Cefaclor oral suspension: (a) 125 mg per 5 mL; (b) 187 mg per 5 mL; (c) 250 mg per 5 mL, and; (d) 375 mg per 5 mL

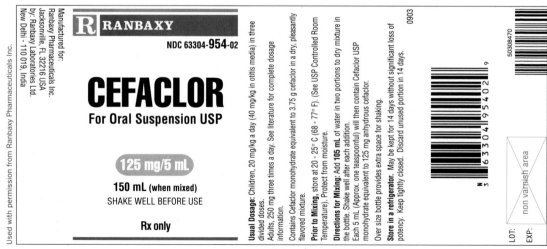

(a)

Continues

FIGURE 10-13 *Continued*

Manufactured for:
Ranbaxy Pharmaceuticals Inc.
Jacksonville, FL 32216 USA
by: Ranbaxy Laboratories Ltd.
New Delhi - 110 019, India

R RANBAXY

NDC 63304-**955**-04

CEFACLOR
For Oral Suspension USP

187 mg/5 mL

100 mL (when mixed)
SHAKE WELL BEFORE USE

Rx only

Usual Dosage: Children, 20 mg/kg a day (40 mg/kg in otitis media) in three divided doses.
Adults, 250 mg three times a day. See literature for complete dosage information.

Contains Cefaclor monohydrate equivalent to 3.74 g cefaclor in a dry, pleasantly flavored mixture.

Prior to Mixing, store at 20 - 25° C (68 - 77° F). (See USP Controlled Room Temperature). Protect from moisture.

Directions for Mixing: Add **70 mL** of water in two portions to dry mixture in the bottle. Shake well after each addition.
Each 5 mL (Approx. one teaspoonful) will then contain Cefaclor USP monohydrate equivalent to 187 mg anhydrous cefaclor.

Over size bottle provides extra space for shaking.

Store in a refrigerator. May be kept for 14 days without significant loss of potency. Keep tightly closed. Discard unused portion in 14 days.

0903

50308490

LOT:
EXP:

non varnish area

(b)

Manufactured for:
Ranbaxy Pharmaceuticals Inc.
Jacksonville, FL 32216 USA
by: Ranbaxy Laboratories Ltd.
New Delhi - 110 019, India

R RANBAXY

NDC 63304-**956**-02

CEFACLOR
For Oral Suspension USP

250 mg/5 mL

150 mL (when mixed)
SHAKE WELL BEFORE USE

Rx only

Usual Dosage: Children, 20 mg/kg a day (40 mg/kg in otitis media) in three divided doses.
Adults, 250 mg three times a day. See literature for complete dosage information.

Contains Cefaclor monohydrate equivalent to 7.5 g cefaclor in a dry, pleasantly flavored mixture.

Prior to Mixing, store at 20 - 25° C (68 - 77° F). (See USP Controlled Room Temperature). Protect from moisture.

Directions for Mixing: Add **105 mL** of water in two portions to dry mixture in the bottle. Shake well after each addition.
Each 5 mL (Approx. one teaspoonful) will then contain Cefaclor USP monohydrate equivalent to 250 mg anhydrous cefaclor.

Over size bottle provides extra space for shaking.

Store in a refrigerator. May be kept for 14 days without significant loss of potency. Keep tightly closed. Discard unused portion in 14 days.

0903

50308510

LOT:
EXP:

non varnish area

(c)

Manufactured for:
Ranbaxy Pharmaceuticals Inc.
Jacksonville, FL 32216 USA
by: Ranbaxy Laboratories Ltd.
New Delhi - 110 019, India

R RANBAXY

NDC 63304-**957**-04

CEFACLOR
For Oral Suspension USP

375 mg/5 mL

100 mL (when mixed)
SHAKE WELL BEFORE USE

Rx only

Usual Dosage: Children, 20 mg/kg a day (40 mg/kg in otitis media) in three divided doses.
Adults, 250 mg three times a day. See literature for complete dosage information.

Contains Cefaclor monohydrate equivalent to 7.5 g cefaclor in a dry, pleasantly flavored mixture.

Prior to Mixing, store at 20 - 25° C (68 - 77° F). (See USP Controlled Room Temperature). Protect from moisture.

Directions for Mixing: Add **70 mL** of water in two portions to dry mixture in the bottle. Shake well after each addition.
Each 5 mL (Approx. one teaspoonful) will then contain Cefaclor USP monohydrate equivalent to 375 mg anhydrous cefaclor.

Over size bottle provides extra space for shaking.

Store in a refrigerator. May be kept for 14 days without significant loss of potency. Keep tightly closed. Discard unused portion in 14 days.

0903

50308540

LOT:
EXP:

non varnish area

(d)

Step 2   **Think**   Which supplied dosage will you select? All four choices could be used. The supplied dosages of 125 mg per 5 mL and 250 mg per 5 mL seem to be the easiest to calculate; but will both provide a total volume for the full 7 days of therapy? Let's check.

100 mg given 3 times per day = 300 mg

300 mg per day given for 7 days = 2,100 mg total

Both bottles contain 150 mL when mixed.

Cefaclor 125 mg per 5 mL: $\dfrac{125\ mg}{5\ mL} \bowtie \dfrac{X\ mg}{150\ mL}$ Cross-multiply

$$5X = 18{,}750$$

$$\frac{5X}{5} = \frac{18{,}750}{5}$$ Simplify: Divide both sides of the equation by the number before the unknown X.

$$X = 3{,}750\ mg$$ Label the units to match the unknown X.

Cefaclor 250 mg per 5 mL: $\dfrac{250\ mg}{5\ mL} \bowtie \dfrac{X\ mg}{150\ mL}$ Cross-multiply

$$5X = 37{,}500$$

$$\frac{5X}{5} = \frac{37{,}500}{5}$$ Simplify: Divide both sides of the equation by the number before the unknown X.

$$X = 7{,}500\ mg$$ Label the units to match the unknown X.

Both bottles will supply enough medication for the 7-day total dosage of 2,100 mg. Let's consider both dosage strengths in our calculations.

If the dosage strength with a concentration of 125 mg per 5 mL is used, then it would be expected that slightly less than 5 mL would be required to provide 100 mg. If the 250 mg per 5 mL concentration is selected, then less than $\frac{1}{2}$ of the 5 mL would be needed, or slightly less than 2.5 mL.

Step 3   **Calculate**   Order: *cefaclor 100 mg p.o. q.8h*

Supply: cefaclor 125 mg per 5 mL

$$\frac{\text{Dosage on hand}}{\text{Amount on hand}} = \frac{\text{Dosage desired}}{\text{X Amount desired}}$$

$$\frac{125\ mg}{5\ mL} \bowtie \frac{100\ mg}{X\ mL}$$ Cross-multiply

$$125X = 100 \times 5$$

$$125X = 500$$

$$\frac{125X}{125} = \frac{500}{125}$$ Simplify: Divide both sides of the equation by the number before the unknown X.

$$X = 4\ mL$$ Label the units to match the unknown X.

Give 4 mL of the cefaclor (concentration 125 mg per 5 mL) orally four times daily.

Order: *cefaclor 100 mg p.o. q.8h*

Supply: cefaclor 250 mg per 5 mL

$$\frac{\text{Dosage on hand}}{\text{Amount on hand}} = \frac{\text{Dosage desired}}{\text{X Amount desired}}$$

$$\frac{250 \text{ mg}}{5 \text{ mL}} \diagdown\diagup \frac{100 \text{ mg}}{\text{X mL}}$$ Cross-multiply

$$250X = 100 \times 5$$

$$250X = 500$$

$$\frac{250X}{250} = \frac{500}{250}$$ Simplify: Divide both sides of the equation by the number before the unknown X.

$$X = 2 \text{ mL}$$ Label the units to match the unknown X.

Give 2 mL of the cefaclor (concentration 250 mg per 5 mL) orally four times daily.

Both calculations confirm your estimates. You may choose to administer either one, depending on the equipment you select to use.

Notice that in both supplied dosage strengths in Example 2, the supply quantity is the same (5 mL), but the dosage strength (weight) of the medication is different (125 mg per 5 mL versus 250 mg per 5 mL). This results in the calculated dose volume (amount to give) being different (4 mL versus 2 mL). This difference is the result of each liquid's concentration. *Cefaclor 125 mg per 5 mL* is half as concentrated as *cefaclor 250 mg per 5 mL.* In other words, there is half as much drug in 5 mL of the *125 mg per 5 mL* supply as there is in 5 mL of the *250 mg per 5 mL* supply. Likewise, *cefaclor 250 mg per 5 mL* is twice as concentrated as *cefaclor 125 mg per 5 mL.* The more concentrated solution allows you to give the patient less volume per dose for the same dosage. This is significant when administering medication to infants and small children when a smaller quantity is needed. Think about this carefully until it is clear.

CAUTION

Think before you calculate. It is important to estimate before you apply any formula. In this way, if you make an error in math or if you set up the problem incorrectly, your thinking will alert you to try again.

EXAMPLE 3 ■

Order: *potassium chloride 30 mEq p.o. b.i.d. for 2 doses*

Potassium is an electrolyte essential for many physiologic responses such as transmission of nerve impulses and contraction of cardiac, skeletal, and smooth muscle. Potassium supplements are administered either by the oral or intravenous route to treat or prevent potassium depletion, which may be a side effect of some medications. For the prevention of hypokalemia during diuretic therapy, the recommended adult dosage is 20 to 40 mEq in 1 to 2 divided doses, but a single dose should not exceed 20 mEq. For the treatment of hypokalemia, the recommended dosage is 40 to 100 mEq/day in divided doses. The oral form of potassium chloride is supplied in 8 mEq, 10 mEq, and 20 mEq extended-release tablets; 8 mEq, 10 mEq, and 20 mEq extended-release capsules; 20 mEq per 15 mL and 40 mEq per 15 mL oral solution; 20 mEq and 25 mEq powder packets for oral solution; and 20 mEq packets for oral suspension. As you can see, there are a number of options for the ordered dosage.

The patient for this example is an adult patient admitted to the hospital for scheduled surgery the next day. The patient has been taking diuretics and potassium supplements for a number of years. Compare the recommended dosage to the ordered dosage. What might you be able to conclude about the indication for this order? The ordered dosage falls within the dosage range for the treatment of hypokalemia, not the prevention of hypokalemia. This is likely a higher dosage than the patient usually takes at home, and the preoperative lab work may have revealed a low serum potassium level. The nurse should check the most recent lab results before proceeding with this order and be prepared to explain the increased dosage to the patient. Medications are distributed in this hospital by ADCs located in the unit medication rooms (Figure 10-14).

FIGURE 10-14 Illustrated ADC matrix drawer with hospital pharmacy-repackaged potassium chloride extended-release tablets: **(a)** 8 mEq; **(b)** 20 mEq, and; **(c)** prepackaged unit-dose cups of 20 mEq oral solution

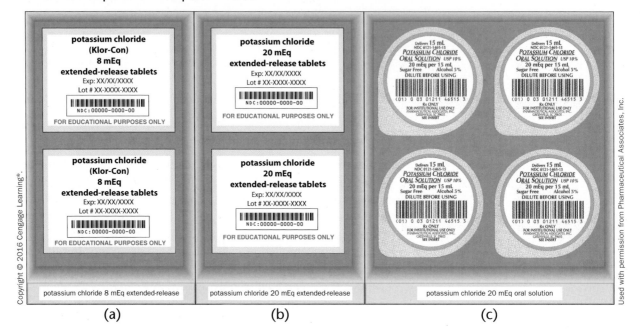

(a)   (b)   (c)

Step 1	**Convert**	The order is in a miscellaneous unit of measure, mEq (milliequivalents). Recall from Chapter 3 that there is no standard equivalent between mEq and other systems of measurement. Conversion should never be necessary, and the supplied medication used must also be measured in mEq. All three supplied dosages are measured in mEq. No conversion is needed.
Step 2	**Think**	The order is for 30 mEq of potassium chloride, but none of the supplied dosages will provide the exact amount. Using the 8 mEq or 20 mEq tablets would require whole and partial tablets to equal the ordered amount. Remember: In order to split tablets, they must be scored. Do you think the extended-release tablets are scored? Probably not. Extended-release tablets should be administered whole without crushing or chewing, so using either of these tablets is not recommended. The only option for this problem is the 20 mEq per 15 mL oral solution. You will need more than one 15 mL unit-dose cup, but less than the 30 mL contained in 2 cups. Remove two unit-dose cups from the ADC.
Step 3	**Calculate**	$\dfrac{\text{Dosage on hand}}{\text{Amount on hand}} = \dfrac{\text{Dosage desired}}{\text{X Amount desired}}$

$$\frac{20\ \text{mEq}}{15\ \text{mL}} \diagdown\!\!\!\diagup \frac{30\ \text{mEq}}{\text{X mL}} \qquad\qquad \text{Cross-multiply}$$

$$20\text{X} = 30 \times 15$$

$$20\text{X} = 450$$

$$\frac{20X}{20} = \frac{450}{20}$$
Simplify: Divide both sides of the equation by the number before the unknown X.

$$X = 22.5 \text{ mL}$$
Label the units to match the unknown X.

The patient should be given 22.5 mL of the potassium chloride oral solution. This confirms your estimate. But now how will you administer it? Can you measure 22.5 mL in a calibrated medication cup? Check the image below (Figure 10-15).

FIGURE 10-15   Calibrated medication cup showing measurements in mL and cc (recall that cc is an obsolete, prohibited unit for dosage measurement)

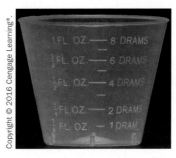
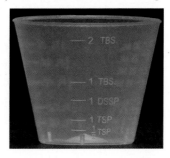
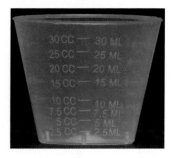

As you can see, 22.5 mL is not a calibration on a standard medication cup. You will have to think of a more precise way to measure this dose.

You could deliver one of the unit-dose cups, then measure the extra you would need. If you use one full 15 mL unit-dose cup, how much more will you need from the second unit-dose cup?

22.5 mL − 15 mL = 7.5 mL

Can you measure this amount in a calibrated medication cup? Yes; 7.5 mL is a calibration on the medication cup. Give the patient one full unit-dose cup and measure an additional 7.5 mL from the second unit-dose cup in the calibrated medication cup. It is recommended that potassium in powdered or liquid form be further diluted in 3 to 8 fl oz of water or juice. You should consult your patient before diluting, to clarify personal preference of water or juice and the amount of fluid the patient can tolerate. If the patient is unable to finish the entire mixture, the patient will not receive the correct dosage and you will not be able to accurately document the dosage that was administered.

EXAMPLE 4 ■

Order: *potassium chloride 40 mEq p.o. daily*

The doctor orders potassium chloride for another patient on diuretic therapy in need of potassium supplement. You have potassium chloride available as shown in the ADC, Figure 10-14c. How many fluid ounces of potassium chloride will you administer?

Step 1	**Convert**	The order is in a miscellaneous unit of measure, mEq (milliequivalents). Recall from Chapter 3 that there is no standard equivalent between mEq and other systems of measurement. Conversion should never be necessary, and the supplied medication used must also be measured in mEq. The supplied dosage is measured in mEq. No conversion is needed.
Step 2	**Think**	The order is for 40 mEq of potassium chloride, and two doses of the 20 mEq oral solution will provide exactly that amount; therefore, you would assume that you are going to be using twice the given dosage.

Step 3   **Calculate** $\dfrac{\text{Dosage on hand}}{\text{Amount on hand}} = \dfrac{\text{Dosage desired}}{\text{X Amount desired}}$

$$\dfrac{20 \text{ mEq}}{15 \text{ mL}} \diagdown\diagup \dfrac{40 \text{ mEq}}{\text{X mL}}$$ Cross-multiply

$$20X = 40 \times 15$$

$$20X = 600$$

$$\dfrac{20X}{20} = \dfrac{600}{20}$$ Simplify: Divide both sides of the equation by the number before the unknown X.

$$X = 30 \text{ mL}$$ Label the units to match the unknown X.

The order calls for 30 mL of potassium chloride to be administered to the patient. However, the question was to calculate how many fluid *ounces* of potassium chloride was ordered to be administered. Therefore, we must convert the 30 mL (metric measure) of potassium chloride into fluid ounces (household measure). You learned in Chapter 3 that the approximate equivalent is 30 mL = 1 fl oz. Because 30 mL is approximately 1 fl oz, you would administer 1 fl oz of potassium chloride to the patient.

For more practice, let's go back to Example 3 and calculate how many fluid ounces that dose would be equivalent to. The dose is 22.5 mL.

Convert   Approximate equivalent: 1 fl oz = 30 mL

$$\dfrac{1 \text{ fl oz}}{30 \text{ mL}} \diagdown\diagup \dfrac{\text{X fl oz}}{22.5 \text{ mL}}$$ Cross-multiply

$$30X = 22.5$$

$$\dfrac{30X}{30} = \dfrac{22.5}{30}$$ Simplify: Divide both sides of the equation by the number before the unknown X.

$$X = 0.75 \quad \text{or} \quad \tfrac{3}{4} \text{ fl oz}$$ Label the units to match the unknown X.

QUICK REVIEW

Look again at Steps 1 through 3 as a valuable dosage calculation checklist.

Step 1   **Convert**   Be sure that all measurements are in the same system and all units are the same size.

Step 2   **Think**   Carefully estimate the reasonable amount of the drug that you should administer.

Step 3   **Calculate** $\dfrac{\text{Dosage on hand}}{\text{Amount on hand}} = \dfrac{\text{Dosage desired}}{\text{X Amount desired}}$

Review Set 23

For questions 1 through 15, calculate 1 dose of the drugs ordered.

1. Order: **morphine sulfate (Roxanol) oral solution 30 mg p.o. q.4h p.r.n., pain**

   Supply: Roxanol Oral Solution 20 mg per 5 mL

   Give: _____ mL

2. Order: *penicillin V potassium 1 g p.o. 1 h preop dental surgery*

   Supply: penicillin V potassium oral suspension 250 mg (400,000 units) per 5 mL

   Give: _____ mL

3. Order: *amoxicillin 100 mg p.o. q.i.d.*

   Supply: 80 mL bottle of amoxicillin (Amoxil) oral pediatric suspension 200 mg per 5 mL

   Give: _____ mL

4. Order: *Tylenol 0.325 g p.o. q.4h p.r.n., pain*

   Supply: acetaminophen (Tylenol) oral solution 325 mg per 5 mL

   Give: _____ t

5. Order: *promethazine HCl 25 mg p.o. at bedtime pre-op*

   Supply: promethazine HCl oral solution 6.25 mg/t

   Give: _____ mL

6. Order: *dicloxacillin 125 mg p.o. q.6h*

   Supply: dicloxacillin suspension 62.5 mg per 5 mL

   Give: _____ t

7. Order: *Pediazole 300 mg p.o. q.6h*

   Supply: erthromycin and sulfisoxazole (Pediazole) oral suspension 200 mg per 5 mL

   Give: _____ mL

8. Order: *cefaclor suspension 225 mg p.o. b.i.d.*

   Supply: cefaclor oral suspension 375 mg per 5 mL

   Give: _____ mL

9. Order: *Septra suspension 400 mg p.o. b.i.d.*

   Supply: trimethoprim and sulfamethoxazole (Septra) oral suspension 200 mg per 5 mL

   Give: _____ mL

10. Order: *Elixophyllin 0.24 g p.o. stat*

    Supply: theophylline (Elixophyllin) elixir 80 mg per 5 mL

    Give: _____ mL

11. Order: *Trilisate liquid 750 mg p.o. t.i.d.*

    Supply: choline magnesium salicylate (Trilisate) liquid 500 mg per 5 mL

    Give: _____ mL

12. Order: *digoxin elixir 0.25 mg p.o. daily*

    Supply: digoxin elixir 50 mcg/mL

    Give: _____ mL

13. Order: *Zyvox 0.6 g p.o. q.12h*

    Supply: linezolid (Zyvox) oral suspension 100 mg per 5 mL

    Give: _____ fl oz

14. Order: *cephalexin 375 mg p.o. t.i.d.*

    Supply: cephalexin oral suspension 250 mg per 5 mL

    Give: _____ t

15. Order: *oxacillin sodium 0.25 g p.o. q.8h*

    Supply: oxacillin sodium oral suspension 125 mg per 2.5 mL

    Give: _____ t

For questions 16 through 21, the medications are usually stocked for each individual patient in unit-dose carts by the pharmacy once every 24 hours. But these medications require refrigeration; therefore, the pharmacy has supplied stock bottles labeled on the back of the bottle with individual patient names and hospital identification, and stored in the medication refrigerator as pictured below. Prepare the medications for each patient, using the Three-Step Approach. Refer to a nursing drug guide, such as the annual *2013 Delmar Nurse's Drug Handbook,* to answer specific questions about the medication prior to administering.

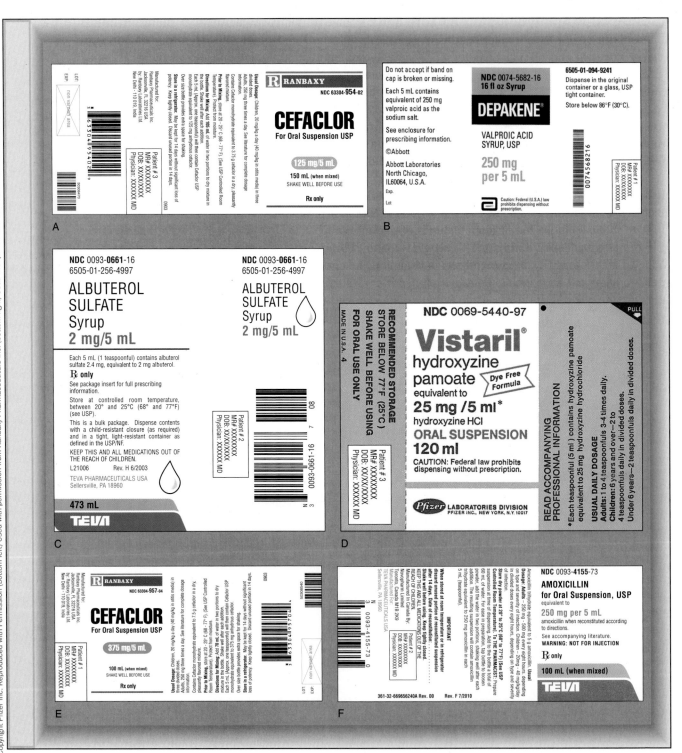

Patient #1 (questions 16 and 17) is scheduled to receive the following medications at 0800.

16. Order: *cefaclor 300 mg p.o. q.8h*

    a. For what condition(s) is cefaclor indicated? _____

    b. What oral dosage strengths of cefaclor are manufactured? _____

    _____

    c. Is using a tablet or capsule a possible option for this ordered dosage? _____

    d. What is the usual recommended adult dosage range? _____

    e. Identify the letter of the supplied dosage(s) you will retrieve from the stocked medication refrigerator to calculate 1 dose. _____

    f. Give: _____ mL

    Mark correct amount on the oral syringe:

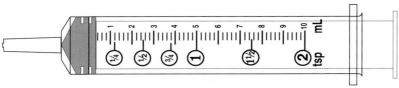

Copyright © 2016 Cengage Learning®.

17. Order: *valproic acid 150 mg p.o. b.i.d.*

    a. For what condition(s) is valproic acid indicated? _____

    b. What oral dosage strengths of valproic acid are manufactured?

    _____

    c. Is using a tablet or capsule a possible option for this ordered dosage? _____

    d. What is the usual recommended adult dosage range? _____

    e. Identify the letter of the supplied dosage(s) you will retrieve from the stocked medication refrigerator to calculate 1 dose. _____

    f. Give: _____ mL

    Mark correct amount on the oral syringe:

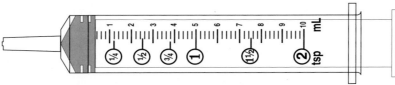

Copyright © 2016 Cengage Learning®.

Patient #2 (questions 18 and 19) is scheduled to receive the following medications at 2100.

18. Order: **amoxicillin 500 mg p.o. q.12h**

    a. For what condition(s) is amoxicillin indicated? _____

    b. What oral dosage strengths of amoxicillin are manufactured?

        _____

    c. Is using a tablet or capsule a possible option for this ordered dosage? _____

    d. What is the usual recommended adult dosage range? _____

    e. Identify the letter of the supplied dosage strength(s) you will retrieve from the stocked medication refrigerator to calculate 1 dose. _____

    f. Give: _____ mL

Mark correct amount on the oral syringe:

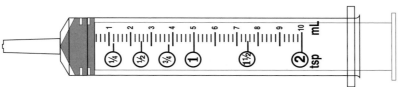

19. Order: **albuterol sulfate 5 mg p.o. t.i.d.**

    a. For what condition(s) is albuterol sulfate indicated? _____

    b. What oral dosage strengths of albuterol are manufactured?

        _____

    c. Is using a tablet or capsule a possible option for this ordered dosage? _____

    d. What is the usual recommended adult dosage range? _____

    e. Identify the letter of the supplied dosage strength(s) you will retrieve from the stocked medication refrigerator to calculate 1 dose. _____

    f. Give: _____ mL

Mark correct amount on the oral syringe:

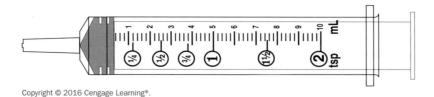

Patient #3 (questions 20 and 21) is scheduled to receive the following medications at 1400.

20. Order: *hydroxyzine 15 mg p.o. on call radiology*

   a. For what condition(s) is hydroxyzine indicated? _____

   b. What oral dosage strengths of hydroxyzine are manufactured?

   _____

   c. Is using a tablet or capsule a possible option for this ordered dosage? _____

   d. What is the usual recommended adult dosage range? _____

   e. Do you think this patient is more likely an adult or a child? _____

   Why? _____

   f. Identify the letter of the supplied dosage strength(s) you will retrieve from the stocked medication refrigerator to calculate 1 dose. _____

   g. Give: _____ mL

Mark correct amount on the oral syringe:

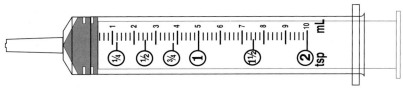

Copyright © 2016 Cengage Learning®.

21. Order: *cefaclor 100 mg p.o. q.8h*

   a. For what condition is cefaclor indicated? *Recall from question #16.* _____

   b. What oral dosage strengths of cefaclor are manufactured? *Recall from question #16.* _____

   c. Is using a tablet or capsule a possible option for this ordered dosage? _____

   d. What is the usual recommended adult dosage range? *Recall from question #16.* _____

   e. Do you think this patient is more likely an adult or a child? _____

   f. Identify the letter of the supplied dosage(s) you will retrieve from the stocked medication refrigerator to calculate 1 dose. _____

   g. Give: _____ mL

Mark correct amount on the oral syringe:

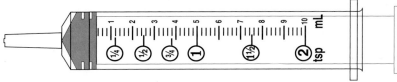

Copyright © 2016 Cengage Learning®.

Questions 22 through 30 will give you additional practice using the Three-Step Approach to prepare dosages for oral solutions. Medications are prepared and labeled by the pharmacy in individually filled unit-dose syringes and supplied to each patient's labeled drawer in the unit-dosage cart. Use your drug guide to look up the medication orders and supplied dosages as you did in questions 16 through 21. Then calculate and confirm the measurement of each dosage.

22. Order: **metoclopramide 10 mg p.o. 30 min a.c. and at bedtime**

    Pharmacy-supplied dose:

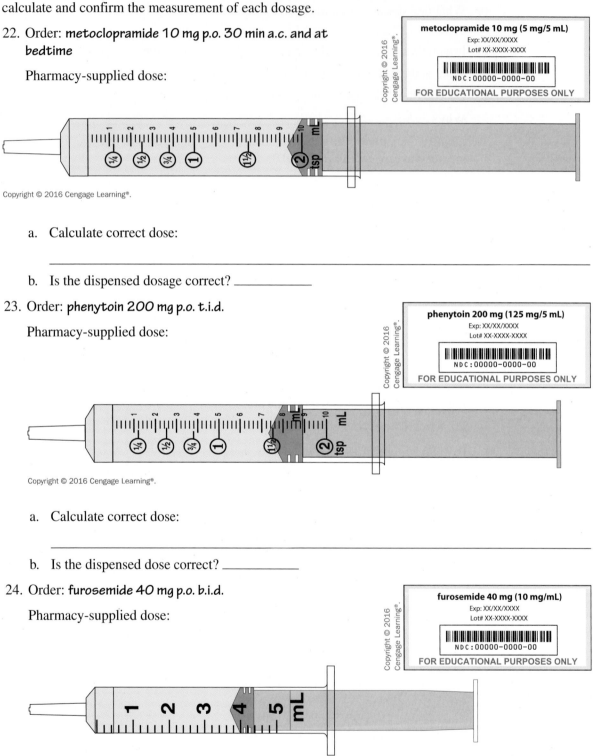

    a. Calculate correct dose:

    _____

    b. Is the dispensed dosage correct? _____

23. Order: **phenytoin 200 mg p.o. t.i.d.**

    Pharmacy-supplied dose:

    a. Calculate correct dose:

    _____

    b. Is the dispensed dose correct? _____

24. Order: **furosemide 40 mg p.o. b.i.d.**

    Pharmacy-supplied dose:

    a. Calculate correct dose:

    _____

    b. Is the dispensed dose correct? _____

25. Order: **furosemide 60 mg p.o. daily**

    Pharmacy-supplied dose:

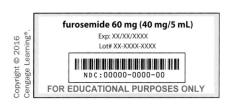

furosemide 60 mg (40 mg/5 mL)
Exp: XX/XX/XXXX
Lot# XX-XXXX-XXXX
N D C : 00000-0000-00
FOR EDUCATIONAL PURPOSES ONLY

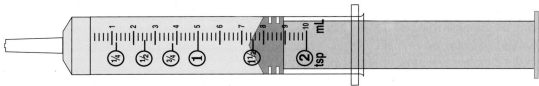

   a. Calculate correct dose:

   _____

   b. Is the dispensed dose correct? _____

26. Order: **ranitidine 75 mg p.o. b.i.d.**

    Pharmacy-supplied dose:

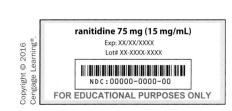

ranitidine 75 mg (15 mg/mL)
Exp: XX/XX/XXXX
Lot# XX-XXXX-XXXX
N D C : 00000-0000-00
FOR EDUCATIONAL PURPOSES ONLY

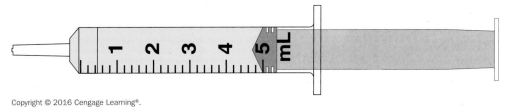

   a. Calculate correct dose:

   _____

   b. Is the dispensed dose correct? _____

27. Order: **promethazine 12.5 mg p.o. a.c. and at bedtime**

    Pharmacy-supplied dose:

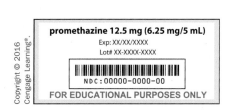

promethazine 12.5 mg (6.25 mg/5 mL)
Exp: XX/XX/XXXX
Lot# XX-XXXX-XXXX
N D C : 00000-0000-00
FOR EDUCATIONAL PURPOSES ONLY

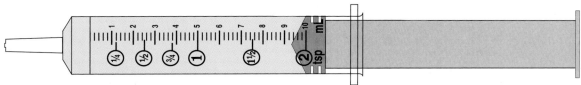

   a. Calculate correct dose:

   _____

   b. Is the dispensed dose correct? _____

28. Order: *digoxin 250 mcg p.o. daily*

    Pharmacy-supplied dose:

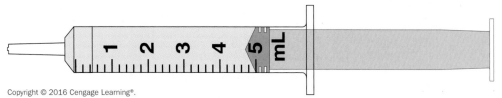

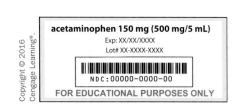

    a. Calculate correct dose:

    _____

    b. Is the dispensed dose correct? _____

29. Order: *acetaminophen 150 mg p.o. q.4h fever greater
    than 102°F*

    Pharmacy-supplied dose:

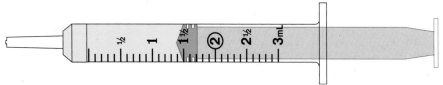

    a. Calculate correct dose:

    _____

    b. Is the dispensed dose correct? _____

30. Order: *acetaminophen 80 mg p.o. q.6h times four doses
    today*

    Pharmacy-supplied dose:

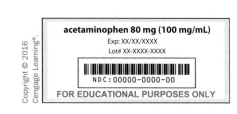

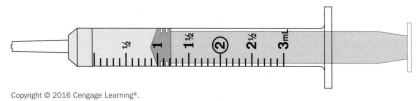

    a. Calculate correct dosage: _____

    b. Is the dispensed dose correct? _____

After completing these problems, see pages 655–659 to check your answers.

SUMMARY

Let's examine where you are in mastering the skill of dosage calculations. You have learned to convert equivalent units within systems of measurements and from one system to another. You have also applied this conversion skill to the calculation of oral dosages—both solid and liquid forms. By now, you know that solving dosage problems requires that all units of measurement first be expressed in the same system and in the same size.

Next, you learned to think through the dosage ordered and dosage supplied, to retrieve the right drug, and to estimate the amount to be given. *To minimize medication errors, it is essential that you consider the reasonableness of the amount before applying a calculation method or formula.*

Finally, you have learned to set up and solve a drug dosage proportion of two equivalent ratios with one unknown, X. This method is so simple and easy to recall that it will stick with you throughout your career:

$$\frac{\text{Dosage on hand}}{\text{Amount on hand}} = \frac{\text{Dosage desired}}{\text{X Amount desired}}$$

Review the Clinical Reasoning Skills and work the Practice Problems for Chapter 10. If you are having difficulty, get help from an instructor before proceeding to Chapter 11. Continue to concentrate on accuracy. Keep in mind that one error can become a serious mistake when you are calculating the dosages of medicines. Medication administration is a legal responsibility. Remember: When you give a medication, you are legally responsible for your actions.

CLINICAL REASONING SKILLS

Inaccuracy in dosage calculation is often attributed to errors in calculating the dosage. Many medication errors can be avoided by first asking the question, "What is the reasonable amount to give?"

ERROR

Incorrect calculation and not assessing the reasonableness of the calculation before administering the medication

Possible Scenario

The physician ordered phenobarbital 60 mg p.o. b.i.d. for a patient with seizures. The pharmacy supplied *phenobarbital 30 mg per tablet*. The nurse did not use Step 2 to think about the reasonable dosage and calculated the dosage this way:

$$\frac{\text{Dosage on hand}}{\text{Amount on hand}} = \frac{\text{Dosage desired}}{\text{X Amount desired}}$$

$$\frac{30 \text{ mg}}{1 \text{ tablet}} \diagdown\!\!\!\!\diagup \frac{60 \text{ mg}}{\text{X tablets}}$$

$$30X = 60$$

$$\frac{30X}{30} = \frac{60}{30}$$

$$X = 20 \text{ tablets} \qquad \textbf{(Answer is incorrect! But what if the nurse did not realize this?)}$$

Suppose the nurse then gave the patient 20 tablets of the 30 mg per tablet of phenobarbital. The patient would have received 600 mg of phenobarbital, or 10 times the correct dosage. This is a serious error.

Potential Outcome

The patient would likely develop signs of phenobarbital toxicity, such as nystagmus (rapid eye movement), ataxia (lack of coordination), central nervous system depression, respiratory depression, hypothermia, and hypotension. When the error was caught and the physician notified, the patient would likely be given doses of charcoal to hasten the elimination of the drug. Depending on the severity of the symptoms, the patient would likely be moved to the intensive care unit for monitoring of respiratory and neurological status.

Prevention

This medication error could have been prevented if the nurse had used the three-step method and estimated for the reasonable dosage of the drug to give. The order is for 60 mg of phenobarbital, and the available drug has 30 mg per tablet, so the nurse should give 2 tablets. The incorrect calculation that indicated such a large number of tablets to give per dose should have alerted the nurse to a possible error.

Ratio-proportion $\frac{\text{Dosage on hand}}{\text{Amount on hand}} = \frac{\text{Dosage desired}}{\text{X Amount desired}}$ should be used to verify thinking about the *reasonable* dosage. Further, the nurse should double-check the math to find the error.

$$\frac{\text{Dosage on hand}}{\text{Amount on hand}} \diagdown\diagup \frac{\text{Dosage desired}}{\text{X Amount desired}}$$

$$\frac{30 \text{ mg}}{1 \text{ tablet}} = \frac{60 \text{ mg}}{\text{X tablets}}$$

$$30X = 60$$

$$\frac{30X}{30} = \frac{60}{30}$$

$$X = 2 \text{ tablets} \qquad \textbf{CORRECT (Not 20 tablets)}$$

CLINICAL REASONING SKILLS

Oral suspensions used for medications prescribed for children frequently are supplied in various dosage strengths per teaspoon or 5 mL. This allows for dosage adjustments according to the weight of the child. Nurses should exercise caution when identifying the dosage strength ordered and administered.

ERROR

Not recognizing that oral suspensions frequently are supplied in different concentrations and documenting the wrong dosage strength in the medical record

Possible Scenario

After being treated for a few days for a respiratory infection, a child's condition worsens and his parents take him to an urgent care clinic. While taking an admission history, the nurse learned that the child had been taking 1 teaspoon of amoxicillin three times a day. Unfamiliar with the various concentrations of this suspension drug, the nurse wrote in the medical record that the child had been receiving 250 mg of amoxicillin with each dose. In fact, amoxicillin is supplied in three dosage strengths: 200 mg per 5 mL, 250 mg per 5 mL, and 400 mg per 5 mL. The child was actually taking 1 teaspoon of the 400 mg per 5 mL concentration. The nurse documented an incorrect medication history.

Potential Outcome

The health care provider who examines the child would need an accurate medical history to evaluate the prescribed treatment and determine the best course of action for the child's current condition. The incorrect dosage documented by the nurse was almost half the dosage the child was receiving. Based on this erroneous information, the provider might come to the wrong conclusion that the child was not provided a therapeutic dosage to treat the infection.

Prevention

The nurse should have questioned the parents further to determine what concentration of amoxicillin was prescribed. If they were unsure of the dosage, then the nurse should document this in the record. When the amount of a medication is provided by the number of tablets, capsules, milliliters, or ounces, always verify the dosage strength. Many oral medications are supplied in more than one strength or concentration. Do not make assumptions; refer to a reputable drug reference to verify the available dosage strengths.

| **CLINICAL REASONING SKILLS** | Medication errors can be caused by setting up problems incorrectly. Let's look at an example to identify the nurse's error. |

ERROR

Incorrectly using the ratio-proportion method of dosage calculation

Possible Scenario

Suppose the physician ordered Keflex 80 mg p.o. q.i.d. for a child with an upper respiratory infection, and the Keflex is supplied in an oral suspension with 250 mg per 5 mL. The nurse decided to calculate the dosage using the ratio-proportion method and set up the problem this way:

$$\frac{80 \text{ mg}}{5 \text{ mL}} \diagdown \frac{250 \text{ mg}}{X \text{ mL}}$$

$$80X = 1,250$$

$$\frac{80X}{80} = \frac{1,250}{80}$$

$$X = 15.6 \text{ mL} \qquad \textbf{INCORRECT}$$

The nurse gave the child 15 mL of Keflex for 2 doses. The next day, as the nurse prepared the medication in the medication room, another nurse observed the nurse pouring 15 mL into a medicine cup and asked about the dosage. At that point, the nurse preparing the medication realized the error.

Potential Outcome

The child could develop complications from the overdosage of Keflex, such as renal impairment and liver damage. When the physician was notified of the error, the physician would likely order the medication discontinued and the child's blood urea nitrogen (BUN) and liver enzymes monitored. An incident report would be filed and the family would be notified of the error.

Prevention

This type of calculation error occurred because the nurse set up the ratio-proportion problem incorrectly. The dosage on hand and amount on hand were not both set up on the left (or same) side of the proportion. The problem should have been calculated this way:

$$\frac{250 \text{ mg}}{5 \text{ mL}} \diagdown \frac{80 \text{ mg}}{X \text{ mL}}$$

$$250X = 400$$

$$\frac{250X}{250} = \frac{400}{250}$$

$$X = 1.6 \text{ mL} \qquad \textbf{CORRECT}$$

In addition, had the nurse used **Step 2: Think** of the Three-Step Approach, the nurse would have estimated that the dose required was less than 5 mL, not more. You should **think first, and then calculate.** In calculating ratio-proportion problems, remember to keep the weight of the medication and the amount of the *known* together on the left side of the proportion, and the weight and the amount of the *unknown* together on the right side. In this scenario, the patient would have received almost 10 times the amount of medication ordered by the physician each time the nurse committed the error. You can use ratio-proportion to determine how many mg of Keflex the child received in the scenario.

$$\frac{250 \text{ mg}}{5 \text{ mL}} \diagdown \frac{X \text{ mg}}{15 \text{ mL}}$$

$$5X = 3,750$$

$$X = 750 \text{ mg, not } 80 \text{ mg as ordered}$$

Obviously, the nurse did not think through for the reasonable amount and either miscalculated the dosage three times or did not bother to calculate the dosage again, preventing identification of the error.

PRACTICE PROBLEMS—CHAPTER 10

For questions 1 through 30, calculate 1 dose of the following drug orders.

1. Order: **tolbutamide 250 mg p.o. b.i.d.**

   Supply: tolbutamide 0.5 g scored tablets

   Give: _____ tablet(s)

2. Order: **codeine 30 mg p.o. q.4h p.r.n., pain**

   Supply: codeine 15 mg scored tablets

   Give: _____ tablet(s)

3. Order: **levothyroxine 75 mcg p.o. daily**

   Supply: levothyroxine 150 mcg scored tablets

   Give: _____ tablet(s)

4. Order: **phenobarbital 10 mg p.o. t.i.d.**

   Supply: phenobarbital elixir 20 mg per 5 mL

   Give: _____ mL

5. Order: **cephalexin 500 mg p.o. q.i.d.**

   Supply: cephalexin 250 mg per 5 mL

   Give: _____ mL

6. Order: **propranolol 20 mg p.o. q.i.d.**

   Supply: propranolol 10 mg unscored tablets

   Give: _____ tablet(s)

7. Order: **amoxicillin 400 mg p.o. q.6h**

   Supply: amoxicillin 250 mg per 5 mL

   Give: _____ mL

8. Order: **chlorpropamide 150 mg p.o. b.i.d.**

   Supply: chlorpropamide 100 mg scored tablets

   Give: _____ tablet(s)

9. Order: **acetaminophen 1 g p.o. q.6h p.r.n., pain**

   Supply: acetaminophen 325 mg and 500 mg unscored tablets

   Select: _____ mg tablets

   Give: _____ tablet(s)

10. Order: **codeine 15 mg p.o. daily**

    Supply: codeine 30 mg scored tablets

    Give: _____ tablet(s)

11. Order: **propranolol 30 mg p.o. q.i.d.**

    Supply: propranolol 20 mg scored tablets

    Give: _____ tablet(s)

12. Order: **levothyroxine 300 mcg p.o. daily**

    Supply: levothyroxine 0.3 mg scored tablets

    Give: _____ tablet(s)

13. Order: **furosemide 60 mg p.o. daily**

    Supply: furosemide 40 mg scored tablets

    Give: _____ tablet(s)

14. Order: **Tylenol c̄ codeine 15 mg p.o. daily**

    Supply: Tylenol with 7.5 mg codeine unscored tablets

    Give: _____ tablet(s)

15. Order: **penicillin V potassium 0.5 g p.o. q.6h**

    Supply: penicillin V potassium 250 mg scored tablets

    Give: _____ tablet(s)

16. Order: **enalapril 7.5 mg p.o. daily**

    Supply: enalapril 5 mg scored and 10 mg scored tablets

    Select: _____ mg tablets

    Give: _____ tablet(s)

17. Order: **penicillin V potassium 375 mg p.o. q.i.d.**

    Supply: penicillin V potassium 250 mg per 5 mL

    Give: _____ mL

18. Order: **neomycin 1 g p.o. q.6h**

    Supply: neomycin 500 mg unscored tablets

    Give: _____ tablet(s)

19. Order: **triazolam 0.25 mg p.o. bedtime**

    Supply: triazolam 0.125 mg unscored tablets

    Give: _____ tablet(s)

20. Order: **Roxanol 30 mg p.o. q.4h p.r.n., pain**

    Supply: morphine sulfate (Roxanol) oral solution 20 mg/mL

    Give: _____ mL

21. Order: **dexamethasone 750 mcg p.o. b.i.d.**

    Supply: dexamethasone 0.75 mg scored tablets and 1.5 mg scored tablets

    Select: _____ mg tablets

    Give: _____ tablet(s)

22. Order: **Edecrin 12.5 mg p.o. b.i.d.**

    Supply: ethcynic acid (Edecrin) 25 mg scored tablets

    Give: _____ tablet(s)

23. Order: **bethanechol 50 mg p.o. t.i.d.**

    Supply: bethanechol 25 mg scored tablets

    Give: _____ tablet(s)

24. Order: **erythromycin stearate 0.5 g p.o. q.12h**

    Supply: erythromycin stearate 250 mg unscored tablets

    Give: _____ tablet(s)

25. Order: **glyburide 2.5 mg p.o. daily**

    Supply: glyburide 1.25 mg scored tablets

    Give: _____ tablet(s)

26. Order: **clorazepate 7.5 mg p.o. q.AM**

    Supply: clorazepate 3.75 mg scored tablets

    Give: _____ tablets

27. Order: **phenobarbital 45 mg p.o. daily**

    Supply: phenobarbital 15 mg scored, 30 mg scored, and 60 mg scored tablets

    Select: _____ mg tablets

    Give: _____ tablet(s)

28. Order: **acetaminophen 240 mg p.o. q.4h p.r.n., pain or temperature greater than 102°F**

    Supply: acetaminophen drops 80 mg per 0.8 mL

    Give: _____ mL

29. Order: **acetaminophen 80 mg p.o. q.4h p.r.n., pain or temperature greater than 102°F**

    Supply: acetaminophen liquid 160 mg/t

    Give: _____ mL

30. Order: **warfarin 7.5 mg p.o. daily**

    Supply: warfarin 2.5 mg scored tablets

    Give: _____ tablet(s)

See the two handwritten and two electronic medication administration records (MARs) and accompanying labels A through R provided on pages 260–263 for stock supply on the following pages for questions 31 through 49. Calculate 1 dose of each of the drugs prescribed. Indicate the letter corresponding to the label that you select.

PAGE ____ of ____

	ORIGINAL ORDER DATE	DATE STARTED/RENEWED	MEDICATION - DOSAGE	ROUTE	SCHEDULE			DATE 1/5/xx			DATE			DATE			DATE		
					11-7	7-3	3-11	11-7	7-3	3-11	11-7	7-3	3-11	11-7	7-3	3-11	11-7	7-3	3-11
31.	1/5/xx	1/5	Tegretol 200 mg b.i.d.	PO		0900	2100		0900GP	2100 MS										
32.	1/5/xx	1/5	nitroglycerin extended-release 6.5 mg b.i.d.	PO		0900	2100		0900GP	2100 MS										
33.	1/5/xx	1/5	sucralfate 1,000 mg b.i.d.	PO		0900	2100		0900GP	2100 MS										
34.	1/5/xx	1/5	Feldene 20 mg daily	PO		0900			0900GP											

MEDICATION ADMINISTRATION RECORD

PRN MEDICATIONS

INJECTION SITES

					B - RIGHT ARM	D - RIGHT ANTERIOR THIGH	H - LEFT ABDOMEN	L - LEFT BUTTOCKS
					C - RIGHT ABDOMEN	G - LEFT ARM	J - LEFT ANTERIOR THIGH	M - RIGHT BUTTOCKS

DATE GIVEN	TIME	INT.	ONE - TIME MEDICATION - DOSAGE	RT.	11-7	7-3	3-11	11-7	7-3	3-11	11-7	7-3	3-11	11-7	7-3	3-11	11-7	7-3	3-11
					SCHEDULE			DATE 1/5/xx			DATE			DATE			DATE		

SIGNATURE OF NURSE ADMINISTERING MEDICATIONS

11-7		
7-3	GP G. Pickar, R.N.	
3-11	MS M. Smith, R.N.	

DATE GIVEN	TIME	INT.	MEDICATION-DOSAGE-CONT.	RT.
			RECOPIED BY:	
			CHECKED BY:	

Patient, Mary Q.

ID # 786522391

ALLERGIES: NKA

31. Select: _____ Give: _____

32. Select: _____ Give: _____

33. Select: _____ Give: _____

34. Select: _____ Give: _____

PAGE _____ of _____

	ORIGINAL ORDER DATE	DATE STARTED / RENEWED	MEDICATION - DOSAGE	ROUTE	SCHEDULE 11-7	SCHEDULE 7-3	SCHEDULE 3-11	DATE 11-7	1/5/xx 7-3	3-11	DATE 11-7	7-3	3-11	DATE 11-7	7-3	3-11	DATE 11-7	7-3	3-11
									MEDICATION ADMINISTRATION RECORD										
35.	1/5/xx	1/5	Synthroid 0.2 mg daily	PO		0900			GP 0900										
36.	1/5/xx	1/5	terbutaline 5 mg q.6h 3x per day	PO		0700 1300	1900	1	0700 GP 1300 GP	GP 1900									
37.	1/5/xx	1/5	metronidazole 1 g b.i.d.	PO		0900	2100		GP 0900	2100 MS									
38.	1/5/xx	1/5	clonazepam 500 mcg b.i.d.	PO		0900	2100		GP 0900	2100 MS									
39.	1/5/xx	1/5	Aldactone 0.1 g daily	PO		0900			GP 0900										

PRN MEDICATIONS

INJECTION SITES

B - RIGHT ARM   D - RIGHT ANTERIOR THIGH   H - LEFT ABDOMEN   L - LEFT BUTTOCKS
C - RIGHT ABDOMEN   G - LEFT ARM   J - LEFT ANTERIOR THIGH   M - RIGHT BUTTOCKS

DATE GIVEN	TIME	INT.	ONE - TIME MEDICATION - DOSAGE	RT.	11-7	7-3	3-11	11-7	7-3	3-11	11-7	7-3	3-11	11-7	7-3	3-11	11-7	7-3	3-11
					SCHEDULE			DATE 1/5/xx			DATE			DATE			DATE		

SIGNATURE OF NURSE ADMINISTERING MEDICATIONS

11-7		
7-3	GP G. Pickar, R.N.	
3-11	MS M. Smith, R.N.	

DATE GIVEN	TIME	INT.	MEDICATION-DOSAGE-CONT.		RT.
			RECOPIED BY:		
			CHECKED BY:		

Patient, John Q.

ID # 233418763

ALLERGIES: NKA

35. Select: _____   Give: _____

36. Select: _____   Give: _____

37. Select: _____   Give: _____

38. Select: _____   Give: _____

39. Select: _____   Give: _____

File   View   Reports   Due List   Tools   Help

| Missing Dose | Medication Log | Medication Admin History | Allergies | CPRS Med Order | Flag |

DOE, JANE Q (FEMALE) ID# 678522
SSN = 100-03-6420
DOB = 05/05/1950 (64)
Height = 5'2'', ' Weight = 129 LB
Location = MED-SURG

Start Time: 12/16@0700   Stop Time: 12/16@2100

Schedule Types:
☑ Continuous   ☑ On-Call
☑ PRN   ☑ One-Time

ALLERGIES: No known allergies   ADRs: NO ADRS ON FILE

Ver	Active Medication	Dosage	Route	Admin Time	Last Action

XXX	GEMFIBROZIL TAB
	  GEMFIBROZIL 600 MG
	  BID AC
		0.6 G, BID AC	ORAL	12/16@0730	GIVEN

XXX	LEVOTHYROXINE TAB LEVOTHYROXINE 100 MCG	200 MCG, DAILY	ORAL	12/16@0900	GIVEN
XXX	POTASSIUM CHLORIDE ORAL SOLUTION POTASSIUM CHLORIDE 20 MEQ PER 15 ML	40 MEQ, BID	ORAL	12/16@0900	GIVEN
XXX	METOPROLOL TAB METOPROLOL 50 MG	100 MG, BID	ORAL	12/16@0900	GIVEN

XXX	GEMFIBROZIL TAB
	  GEMFIBROZIL 600 MG
	  BID AC
		0.6 G, BID AC	ORAL	12/16@1630	

XXX	POTASSIUM CHLORIDE ORAL SOL POTASSIUM CHLORIDE 20 MEQ PER 15 ML	40 MEQ, BID	ORAL	12/16@1700	
XXX	METOPROLOL TAB METOPROLOL 50 MG	100 MG, BID	ORAL	12/16@1700	
XXX	DIGOXIN TAB DIGOXIN 250 MCG	0.5 MG, DAILY	ORAL	12/16@1700	
XXX	OXYCODONE/ACETAMINOPHEN TAB OXYCODONE/ACETAMINOPHEN 5 MG/325 MG	5 MG, Q4H, PRN HEADACHE	ORAL		

| Cover Sheet | ○ Unit Dose | ○ IVP/IVPB | ○ IV |

Scanner Status: **Ready**   Enable Scanner

Server Time: 12/16/XXXX 11:03

40. Digoxin at 5:00 PM   Select: _____   Give: _____

41. Potassium Chloride at 5:00 PM   Select: _____   Give: _____

42. Gemfibrozil before dinner   Select: _____   Give: _____

43. Levothyroxine at 9:00 AM   Select: _____   Give: _____

44. Metoprolol at 5:00 PM   Select: _____   Give: _____

45. Oxycodone/Acetaminophen   Select: _____   Give: _____
    at 3:00 PM

File   View   Reports   Due List   Tools   Help

| Missing Dose | Medication Log | Medication Admin History | Allergies | CPRS Med Order | Flag |

SNEEHR, SARA (FEMALE) ID# 467834
SSN = 100-03-6421
DOB = 09/16/1955 (59)
Height = 5'10", Weight = 175 LB
Location = MED-SURG

Start Time: 12/16@0900   Stop Time: 12/16@2100

Schedule Types:
☑ Continuous   ☑ On-Call
☑ PRN   ☑ One-Time

ALLERGIES: No known allergies   ADRs: NO ADRS ON FILE

Ver	Active Medication	Dosage	Route	Admin Time	Last Action
XXX	FUROSEMIDE TAB FUROSEMIDE 20 MG	20 MG, BID	ORAL	12/16@0900	GIVEN
XXX	PROPRANOLOL CAP PROPRANOLOL 60 MG	60 MG, BID	ORAL	12/16@0900	GIVEN
XXX	POTASSIUM CHLORIDE TAB POTASSIUM CHLORIDE 10 MEQ	20 MEQ, DAILY	ORAL	12/16@0900	GIVEN
XXX	FUROSEMIDE TAB FUROSEMIDE 20 MG	20 MG, BID	ORAL	12/16@1700	
XXX	PROPRANOLOL CAP PROPRANOLOL 60 MG	60 MG, BID	ORAL	12/16@1700	
XXX	RANITIDINE TAB RANITIDINE 150 MG	300 MG, BEDTIME	ORAL	12/16@2100	

| Cover Sheet | ○ Unit Dose | ○ IVP/IVPB | ○ IV |

Scanner Status: **NOT Ready**   Enable Scanner

Server Time: 12/16/XXXX 11:00

46. Ranitidine at bedtime   Select: _____   Give: _____

47. Propranolol at 5:00 PM   Select: _____   Give: _____

48. Furosemide at 5:00 PM   Select: _____   Give: _____

49. Potassium Chloride at 9:00 AM Select: _____   Give: _____

Each extended-release capsule contains:

Nitroglycerin . . . . 6.5 mg

KEEP THIS AND ALL DRUGS OUT OF THE REACH OF CHILDREN.

Manufactured by Time-Cap Labs Inc. for ETHEX Corporation St. Louis, MO 63043-2413

NDC 58177-005-03

Nitroglycerin

Extended-release Capsules

6.5 mg

℞ Only

60 Capsules

Dispense in a tight container as defined in the USP/NF.

Store at controlled room temperature 15°-30°C (59°-86°F).

USUAL DOSAGE: See package insert for dosage, including nitrate-free intervals.

P3806 11/01

ETHEX   ETHEX   ETHEX   ETHEX   ETHEX

A

Store below 86°F (30°C)

Dispense in tight, light-resistant containers (USP).

DOSAGE AND USE
See accompanying prescribing information. One capsule per day.

Each capsule contains 20 mg piroxicam.

IMPORTANT: This closure is not child-resistant.

CAUTION: Federal law prohibits dispensing without prescription.

NDC 0069-3230-66

100 Capsules

Feldene®
(piroxicam)   20

20 mg

Pfizer **Pfizer Labs**
Division of Pfizer Inc, NY, NY 10017

6505-01-137-4628   2

05-4300-00-5
MADE IN USA

1292

B

NDC 0088-1712-53

Carafate®
Tablets
sucralfate

1 gram

120 Tablets

❦ *Aventis*

℞ ONLY

Each CARAFATE® Tablet contains 1g sucralfate.

Dosage and Administration: See package insert for dosage information.

WARNING: Keep out of reach of children.

Pharmacist: Dispense in light-resistant, tight container with child-resistant closure.

Important: This package is not child-resistant.

Store at controlled room temperature 59–86°F (15–30°C).

Aventis Pharmaceuticals Inc.
Kansas City, MO 64137
USA   ©2000
www.aventispharma-us.com

0088-1712-53   6

Exp   50059224

C

NDC 0083-0052-30

Tegretol® 100 mg

carbamazepine USP

Chewable Tablets

100 tablets

Rx only

ↄ NOVARTIS

0083-0052-30   0

EXP.
LOT

©Novartis

5000098
Dosage: See package insert. Do not store above 30°C (86°F). Protect from light and moisture. Dispense in tight, light-resistant container (USP).

Keep this and all drugs out of the reach of children.

Novartis Pharmaceuticals Corporation
East Hanover, New Jersey 07936

D

Delivers **15 mL**
NDC 0121-1465-15
POTASSIUM CHLORIDE
ORAL SOLUTION USP 10%
20 mEq per 15 mL
Sugar Free   Alcohol 5%
DILUTE BEFORE USING

(01) 0 03 01211 46515 3

Rx ONLY
FOR INSTITUTIONAL USE ONLY
PHARMACEUTICAL ASSOCIATES, INC.
GREENVILLE, SC 29605
SEE INSERT

E

Store below 25°C (77°F).

Protect from light.

Dispense in tight, light-resistant, child-resistant containers (USP).

DOSAGE AND USE:
See accompanying prescribing information.

Each tablet contains 500 mg metronidazole.

NDC 0025-1821-50

50 Tablets   **Rx only**

Flagyl®
metronidazole
tablets USP   500

500 mg

Pfizer **G.D. Searle LLC**
Division of Pfizer Inc, NY, NY 10017
Distributed by

2281

0025-1821-50   9

05-6605-32-0

LOT
EXP

F

USUAL DOSAGE:
See package insert for prescribing information.

Dispense in a tight, light-resistant container as defined in the USP with a child-resistant closure.

Store at 20°-25°C (68°-77°F) [See USP Controlled Room Temperature]. Excursion permitted 15°-30°C (59°-86°F)

Rev. 03/05

NDC 0527-1318-01

LANNETT
Dispense with confidence

**TERBUTALINE
SULFATE
TABLETS, USP**

2.5 mg

Rx Only

100 TABLETS

Each tablet contains:
Terbutaline, USP ...... 2.5 mg

Inactive Ingredients:
Anhydrous lactose, magnesium stearate, microcrystalline cellulose, povidone, and pregelatinized starch.

Manufactured by:
Lannett Company, Inc.
Philadelphia, PA 19136

Exp. Date:

Lot No.:

N 3 0527-1318-01 5

G

Instructions to the Patient
Use immediately upon opening individual tablet blister.
Fragile: Do not push tablets through blister packaging.

1. Note: Check for the correct dosage strength.
2. Bend and tear perforation to separate blister.

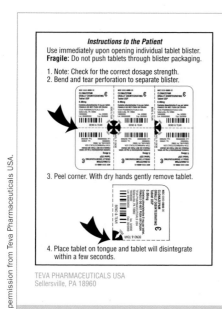

3. Peel corner. With dry hands gently remove tablet.

4. Place tablet on tongue and tablet will disintegrate within a few seconds.

TEVA PHARMACEUTICALS USA
Sellersville, PA 18960

NDC 0555-0096-96

**CLONAZEPAM
ORALLY DISINTEGRATING
Tablets USP**
0.5 mg

Each tablet contains 0.5 mg clonazepam, USP.

Phenylketonurics: Contains phenylalanine 2.4 mg per tablet.

Pharmacist: Dispense the enclosed Medication Guide to each patient. Dispense one "Instruction to the Patient Sheet" with each prescription.

Rx only

60 TABLETS (10 blister cards of 6 tablets each)

TEVA

H

NDC 0048-1070-03
NSN 6505-01-340-0152
Code 3P1073

SYNTHROID®
(Levothyroxine Sodium Tablets, USP)

100 mcg   (0.1 mg)

100 TABLETS

Rx only

BASF Pharma

knoll

See full prescribing information for dosage and administration.

Dispense in a tight, light-resistant container as described in USP.

Store at 25°C (77°F); excursions permitted to 15°-30°C (59°-86°F). [See USP Controlled Room Temperature].

Knoll Pharmaceutical Company
Mount Olive, NJ 07828 USA

7885-04

3 0048-1070-03 6

I

NDC 0039-0067-50

Lasix® 20mg

furosemide

500 Tablets ✦**Aventis**

Rx ONLY
Each LASIX® Tablet contains 20mg furosemide. **Dosage and Administration:** See package insert for dosage information. **WARNING:** Keep out of reach of children. Do not use if bottle closure seal is broken. **Pharmacist:** Dispense in well-closed, light-resistant container with child-resistant closure. **Store at room temperature.**
Hoechst-Roussel Pharmaceuticals
Division of Aventis Pharmaceuticals Inc.
Kansas City, MO 64137 USA   ©2000
www.aventispharma-us.com

3 0039-0067-50 9

50058803 50058803 50058803

J

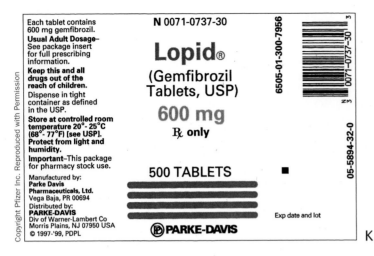

Each tablet contains 600 mg gemfibrozil.

Usual Adult Dosage– See package insert for full prescribing information.

Keep this and all drugs out of the reach of children.

Dispense in tight container as defined in the USP.

Store at controlled room temperature 20°- 25°C (68°- 77°F) [see USP]. Protect from light and humidity.

Important–This package for pharmacy stock use.

Manufactured by: Parke Davis Pharmaceuticals, Ltd. Vega Baja, PR 00694

Distributed by: **PARKE-DAVIS** Div of Warner-Lambert Co Morris Plains, NJ 07950 USA © 1997-'99, PDPL

N 0071-0737-30

Lopid®

(Gemfibrozil Tablets, USP)

600 mg

℞ only

500 TABLETS

Ⓟ **PARKE-DAVIS**

6505-01-300-7956

0071-0737-30

05-5894-32-0

Exp date and lot

K

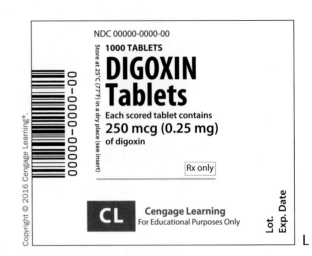

NDC 00000-0000-00

1000 TABLETS

Store at 25°C (77°F) in a dry place (see insert)

DIGOXIN
Tablets

Each scored tablet contains

250 mcg (0.25 mg)

of digoxin

Rx only

00000-0000-00

CL **Cengage Learning** For Educational Purposes Only

Lot. Exp. Date

L

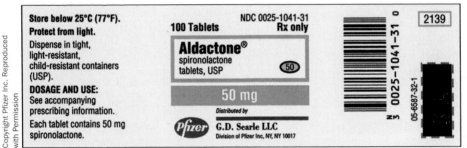

Store below 25°C (77°F).

Protect from light.

Dispense in tight, light-resistant, child-resistant containers (USP).

DOSAGE AND USE: See accompanying prescribing information.

Each tablet contains 50 mg spironolactone.

100 Tablets

NDC 0025-1041-31

Rx only

Aldactone® spironolactone tablets, USP

50

50 mg

Distributed by

Pfizer **G.D. Searle LLC** Division of Pfizer Inc, NY, NY 10017

2139

0025-1041-31

05-6587-32-1

M

NDC 0028-0051-10
6505-01-071-6557

Lopressor® **50** mg

metoprolol tartrate USP

1000 tablets

Rx only

Ⓤ **NOVARTIS**

645122

Dosage: See package insert. **Store between 15°C - 30°C (59°F - 86°F). Protect from moisture. Dispense in tight, light-resistant container (USP).**

Novartis Pharmaceuticals Corporation East Hanover, New Jersey 07936

PHARMACIST: Container closure is not child-resistant. Keep this and all drugs out of the reach of children.

0028-0051-10

EXP
LOT

N

NDC 63481-623-70   NSN 6505-01-082-5509

Endo® ENDO LABORATORIES **PERCOCET®** (Oxycodone and Acetaminophen Tablets, USP)

5 mg/325 mg

℞ only

C II

Each tablet contains:
Oxycodone Hydrochloride . . . . 5 mg*
Acetaminophen, USP . . . . 325 mg
*5 mg oxycodone HCl is equivalent to 4.4815 mg of oxycodone.

Usual Dosage: See package insert for complete prescribing information.
Dispense in a tight, light-resistant container as defined in the USP, with a child-resistant closure (as required). Store at controlled room temperature 15°-30°C (59°-86°F).
DEA ORDER FORM REQUIRED.

100 TABLETS

SAMPLE

Lot:
Exp:

Manufactured for: Endo Pharmaceuticals Inc. Chadds Ford, PA 19317 By: DuPont Pharma Wilmington, DE 19880

70447/PF

63481-623-70

O

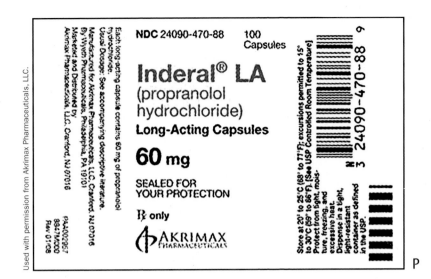

P

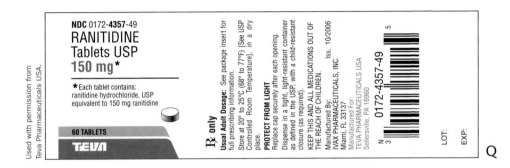

Q

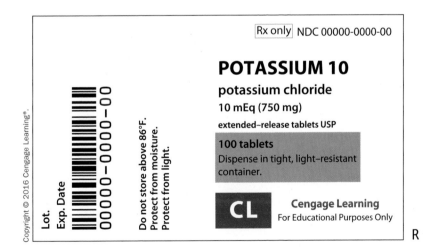

R

50. Describe the strategy to prevent this medication error.

Possible Scenario

Suppose the physician ordered *penicillin V potassium 5 mL (250 mg) p.o. q.i.d.* for a patient with an upper respiratory tract infection. The pharmacy supplied penicillin V potassium 125 mg per 5 mL. In a rush to administer the medication on time, the nurse read the order as *penicillin V potassium 5 mL,* checked the label for penicillin V potassium, and poured that amount and administered the drug. In a hurry, the nurse failed to recognize that 5 mL of the supply dosage of 125 mg per 5 mL did not provide the ordered dosage of 250 mg and underdosed the patient.

Potential Outcome

The patient received one half of the ordered dosage of antibiotic needed to treat the respiratory infection. If this error was not caught, the patient's infection would not be halted. This would add to the patient's illness time and might lead to a more severe infection. Additional tests might be required to determine why the patient was not responding to the medication.

Prevention

_____

_____

After completing these problems, see pages 660–661 to check your answers.

Be sure to use the online software for additional practice!

REFERENCES

Cohen, M. R. (2007). *Medication errors*, 2nd ed., American Pharmacists Association, Washington, D.C. p. 257.

Institute of Medicine. (2006). Report Brief—Preventing medication errors. Retrieved from http://www.iom.edu/~/media/Files/Report%20Files/2006/Preventing-Medication-Errors-Quality-Chasm-Series/medicationerrorsnew.pdf

Verrue, C., Mehuys, E., Boussery, K., Remon, J., & Petrovic, M. (2011). Tablet-splitting: A common yet not so innocent practice. *Journal of Advanced Nursing, 67*(1), 26–32. doi: 10.1111/j.1365-2648.2010.05477.x

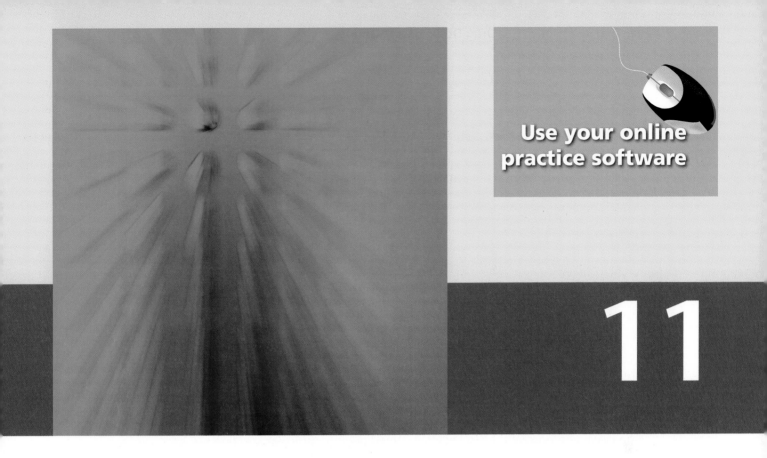

11

Parenteral Dosage of Drugs

OBJECTIVES

Upon mastery of Chapter 11, you will be able to apply clinical reasoning skills to prepare safe and accurate parenteral dosages of drugs. To accomplish this, you will also be able to:

- Gather current information about the drug.
- Retrieve the right drug in the correct supply dosage strength.
- Apply the Three-Step Approach to dosage calculation: convert, think, and calculate using ratio-proportion.
- Verify drug and dosage with a second nurse for high-alert medications and for wasting of controlled substances.
- Measure correct dose amounts.
- Collaborate with patients and families regarding their medications, including safe administration at home.

The term *parenteral* is used to designate routes of administration other than gastrointestinal, such as the injection routes of intramuscular (IM), subcutaneous (subcut), intradermal (ID), and intravenous (IV). In this chapter, IM, subcut, and IV injections will be emphasized. Intravenous flow-rate calculations are discussed in Chapters 15 through 17.

Intramuscular indicates an injection given into a muscle, such as promethazine given IM for nausea and vomiting. *Subcutaneous* means an injection given into the subcutaneous tissue, such as an insulin injection given subcut for the management of diabetes. *Intravenous* refers to an injection given directly into a vein, either by direct injection (IV push) or diluted in a larger volume of intravenous fluid and administered as part of an intravenous infusion. When a patient has an IV site or IV infusing, the IV injection route is frequently used to administer parenteral drugs rather than the IM route. *Intradermal* (ID) means an injection given under the skin, such as an allergy test or tuberculin skin test.

INJECTABLE SOLUTIONS

Most parenteral medications are supplied in liquid or solution form and packaged in dosage vials, ampules, or prefilled syringes (Figure 11-1). Injectable drugs are measured in syringes.

FIGURE 11-1   Parenteral solutions

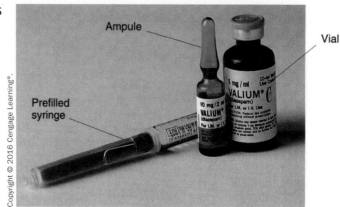

RULE

The maximum dose volume to be administered per intramuscular injection site for:

1. An average 150 lb adult = 3 mL (maximum for deltoid site is 1 mL)

2. Children ages 6 to 12 years = 2 mL

3. Children birth to age 5 years = 1 mL

For example, if you must give an adult patient 4 mL of a drug, divide the dose into two injections of 2 mL each. The condition of the patient must be considered when applying this rule. Adults or children who have decreased muscle or subcutaneous mass or poor circulation may not be able to tolerate the maximum dose volumes.

Administering medications by the intravenous (IV) route requires a number of skills. The first skill is calculating and measuring the ordered dosage. Some drugs may then be injected directly into the infusion port located on the side of the IV tubing. For safety, other drugs may need to be diluted further so that a less concentrated solution enters the vein. The nurse must also infuse the medications at the safe recommended rate. Some medications may be given rapidly (as quickly as one minute), others as a slow push over a matter of minutes, while many others will be injected into a small IV piggyback bag to infuse at an even slower rate. In this chapter you will learn the first skill: calculating and measuring the ordered dosage. In Chapters 15 and 17, you will learn more skills for diluting and managing the flow rate of intravenous medications and solutions.

To solve parenteral dosage problems, apply the same Three-Step Approach used for the calculation of oral dosages.

REMEMBER

Step 1	**Convert**	Ensure that all units of measurement are in the same system and all units are the same size.
Step 2	**Think**	Estimate the logical amount.
Step 3	**Calculate**	$\dfrac{\text{Dosage on hand}}{\text{Amount on hand}} = \dfrac{\text{Dosage desired}}{\text{X Amount desired}}$

Use the following rules to help you decide which size syringe to select to administer parenteral dosages.

RULE

As you calculate parenteral dosages:

1. Round the amount to be administered (X) to tenths if the amount is greater than 1 mL, and measure it in a 3 mL syringe.

2. Round amounts of less than 1 mL to hundredths, and measure all amounts less than 0.5 mL in a 1 mL syringe.

3. Amounts of 0.5 to 1 mL, calculated in tenths, can be accurately measured in either a 1 mL or 3 mL syringe.

Let's look at some examples of rounding volumes and of appropriate syringe selections for the dosages to be measured and review how to read the calibrations. Refer to Chapter 6, *Equipment Used in Dosage Measurement,* regarding how to measure medication in a syringe. To review, the top black ring of the plunger should align with the desired calibration, not the raised midsection and not the bottom ring. Look carefully at the illustrations that follow.

EXAMPLE 1 ■

Measure 0.33 mL in a 1 mL syringe. The exact amount is measured with this syringe. No rounding needed.

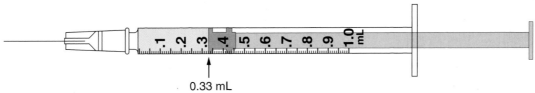

0.33 mL

EXAMPLE 2 ■

Round 1.33 mL to 1.3 mL, and measure in a 3 mL syringe. The syringe is calibrated in tenths, so rounding is necessary to measure the desired amount.

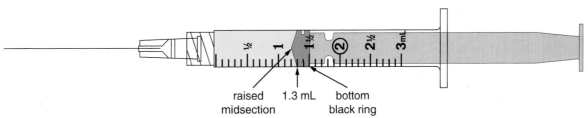

raised   1.3 mL   bottom
midsection   black ring

EXAMPLE 3 ■

Measure 0.6 mL in either a 1 mL or a 3 mL syringe. (Notice that the amount is measured in tenths and is greater than 0.5 mL, so the 3 mL syringe would be acceptable.)

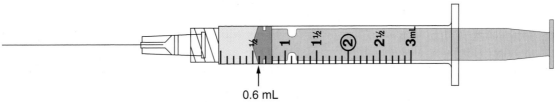

0.6 mL

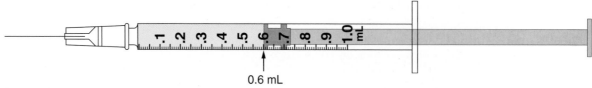

EXAMPLE 4 ■

Measure 0.65 mL in a 1 mL syringe. (Notice that the amount is measured in hundredths and is less than 1 mL.) The volume would need to be rounded if a 3 mL syringe was used. However, the 1 mL syringe would provide a more precise dose.

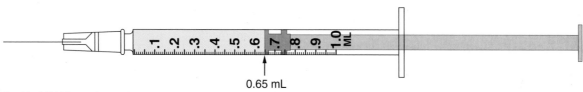

An amber color has been added to selected syringe drawings throughout the text *to simulate a specific amount of medication,* as indicated in the example or problem. Because the color used may not correspond to the actual color of the medications named, **it must not be used as a reference for identifying medications.**

Let's look at some examples of parenteral dosage calculations, utilizing all aspects of accurate dosage calculation and safe preparation of medications, including:

- collecting data about the drug
- selecting supplied dosage
- calculating the amount to give using the Three-Step Approach
- measuring the dose with appropriate equipment for medication administration

EXAMPLE 1 ■

Order: Dilaudid 3 mg IM q.6h p.r.n., severe pain

Dilaudid is the brand name for the opioid analgesic hydromorphone HCl. It is indicated for moderate to severe pain. It is supplied in liquid, tablets, suppositories, and a solution for injection. The solution for intramuscular, subcutaneous, or intravenous injection is available in 1 mg/mL, 2 mg/mL, 4 mg/mL, and highly concentrated as 10 mg/mL. The recommended adult dosage to be administered by the intramuscular (IM) route is 1 to 2 mg q.4 to 6h up to 3 to 4 mg for severe pain as needed.

For this example, you will administer the medication to a hospitalized adult who is experiencing surgical pain. You will retrieve the drug from the unit automated dispensing cabinet (ADC). Hydromorphone is categorized as a Schedule II controlled substance; therefore, inventory is verified each time the medication is used. Most ADCs will only open the specific individual cubby containing the controlled substance. If the whole amount is not needed, the remainder must be wasted (meaning the rest is discarded) according to policy and witnessed by another nurse. The ADC cubby drawer that opens contains vials of hydromorphone, as illustrated in Figure 11-2.

FIGURE 11-2　ADC cubby with prepackaged vials of hydromorphone HCl 2 mg/mL

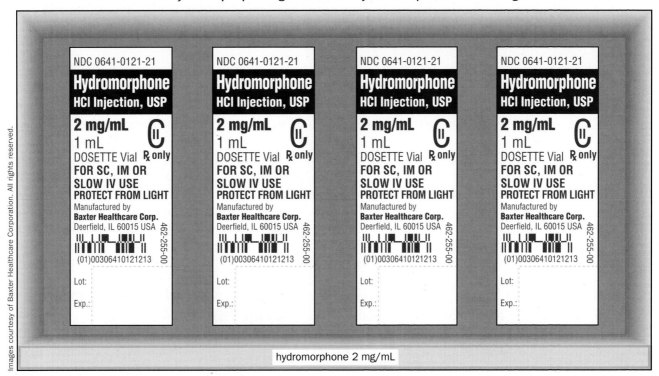

Let's complete the dosage calculation using the Three-Step Approach.

Step 1　**Convert**　For the ordered dose of 3 mg, no conversion is necessary. The units are in the same system (metric) and the same size (mg).

Step 2　**Think**　The supply is 2 mg/mL. Each single-dose vial contains a total of 1 mL. Two vials will be needed to administer the 3 mg dose. Because 3 mg is $1\frac{1}{2}$ times as much as 2 mg, the volume for this dose should be $1\frac{1}{2}$ times 1 mL, or exactly 1.5 mL.

Step 3　**Calculate**　$\dfrac{\text{Dosage on hand}}{\text{Amount on hand}} = \dfrac{\text{Dosage desired}}{\text{X Amount desired}}$

$\dfrac{2\text{ mg}}{1\text{ mL}} \diagdown\!\!\!\!\diagup \dfrac{3\text{ mg}}{\text{X mL}}$　　Cross-multiply

$2\text{X} = 3$

$\dfrac{2\text{X}}{2} = \dfrac{3}{2}$　　Simplify: Divide both sides of the equation by the number before the unknown X.

$\text{X} = 1.5\text{ mL}$　　Label the units to match the unknown X.

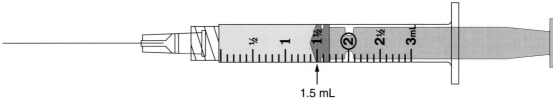

1.5 mL

Measure 1 mL of hydromorphone from the first vial and an additional 0.5 mL from the second vial for a total of 1.5 mL. The remaining 0.5 mL cannot be saved for a later dose and must be wasted and witnessed by another nurse. If the syringe is prepackaged with a needle attached, check to be sure that the correct needle is used according to the patient's size.

EXAMPLE 2 ■

Order: *famotidine 20 mg IV q.12h*

Famotidine is an H_2 receptor-blocking drug used to treat gastric ulcers. Low doses of the oral forms are available over the counter (a common brand being Pepcid) for the relief and prevention of heartburn. Solution for injection is available by prescription in 10 mg/mL concentration. Injections of famotidine are only given by the intravenous (IV) route, not intramuscular (IM) or subcutaneous (subcut) routes. The recommended adult dosage is 20 mg IV q.12h.

For this example, the adult patient is hospitalized for gastric ulcer disease. This hospital unit supplies a 24-hour supply for each patient in labeled unit-dose drawers or in the unit medication refrigerator. Famotidine should be stored at 2° to 8°C (36° to 46°F). You retrieve one vial containing the following label (Figure 11-3) from the unit medication refrigerator.

FIGURE 11-3 Famotidine multidose vial in unit medication refrigerator

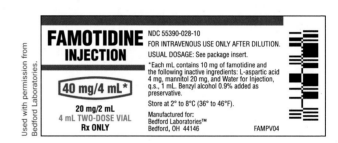

Complete the dosage calculation.

Step 1 **Convert** For the ordered dose of 20 mg, no conversion is necessary. The units are in the same system (metric) and the same size (mg).

Step 2 **Think** Let's look at this label. The drug reference described the supplied dosage concentration as 10 mg/mL, yet this label lists two other concentrations: 40 mg per 4 mL and 20 mg per 2 mL. Can you see that all of these concentrations are equal? Let's view them as equivalent fractions to see this more clearly.

$$\frac{10 \text{ mg}}{1 \text{ mL}} = \frac{20 \text{ mg}}{2 \text{ mL}} = \frac{40 \text{ mg}}{4 \text{ mL}}$$

Sometimes manufacturers label medications with the concentrations including the most commonly used dosages. You can see that the amount needed for the ordered dosage is 2 mL. This seems easy, but errors can be made if the label is read too quickly and the nurse assumes that the large 40 mg in red type is per 1 mL. This is a common oversight and in this case could lead to administering 4 times the ordered dosage.

Step 3 **Calculate**

$$\frac{\text{Dosage on hand}}{\text{Amount on hand}} = \frac{\text{Dosage desired}}{\text{X Amount desired}}$$

$$\frac{20 \text{ mg}}{2 \text{ mL}} \diagup\hspace{-1.2em}\diagdown \frac{20 \text{ mg}}{\text{X mL}}$$ Cross-multiply

$$20\text{X} = 40$$

$$\frac{20\text{X}}{20} = \frac{40}{20}$$ Simplify: Divide both sides of the equation by the number before the unknown X.

$$\text{X} = 2 \text{ mL}$$ Label the units to match the unknown X.

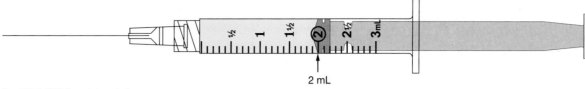

2 mL

Measure 2 mL in a 3 mL syringe, being careful to remove only the amount needed for 1 dose. This vial has been supplied for the 2 doses given in a 24-hour period. The vial should be labeled with the date and time it was opened, initialed by the nurse, and returned to the unit medication refrigerator. Notice the instructions on the label: "FOR INTRAVENOUS USE ONLY AFTER DILUTION." The solution is too concentrated to give directly into the IV tubing. It will need to be further diluted in a syringe or IV piggyback bag. In Chapter 15, you will learn more about calculations used to manage IV medications and infusions.

EXAMPLE 3 ■

Order: *digoxin 0.375 mg IV daily*

Digoxin is a cardiac glycoside used to treat congestive heart failure and cardiac arrhythmias. It is supplied in tablets, injectable solution, and pediatric elixir. Recommended dosages vary depending on indication, route, and urgency of treatment. The maintenance dosage for patients who have been on a stabilized dosage is 0.125 to 0.5 mg per day given orally (p.o.) or by intravenous (IV) injection. Digoxin is not administered by the intramuscular (IM) or subcutaneous (subcut) routes.

For this example, the adult patient has been admitted to the hospital for surgery. The patient has been taking an oral maintenance dose of digoxin for 2 years, but will need to be given the usual dose by IV while NPO following surgery. You will retrieve the medication from the unit automated dispensing cabinet (ADC). The ADC drawer that opens contains cubbies located side by side, as illustrated in Figure 11-4.

FIGURE 11-4   Illustrated ADC matrix drawer with prepackaged vials: **(a)** box containing digoxin 500 mcg per 2 mL single-dose vials; **(b)** dexamethasone 4 mg/mL single-dose vials; **(c)** dexamethasone 10 mg/mL single-dose vials

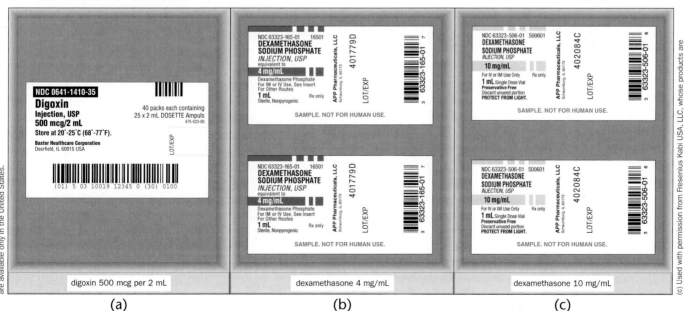

Complete the dosage calculation.

Step 1   **Convert**   Select one vial from the box of single-dose vials of digoxin in the first compartment. For the ordered dose of 0.375 mg, a conversion is necessary. The units are in the same system (metric), but the ordered size units are mg and the supply is labeled as mcg. Remember that converting the larger unit (mg) to the smaller unit (mcg) will eliminate the decimal fraction. Convert the ordered units.

Equivalent: 1 mg = 1,000 mcg

$$\frac{1\ mg}{1,000\ mcg} \diagdown \frac{0.375\ mg}{X\ mcg}$$ Cross-multiply

X = 1,000 × 0.375   0.375. Move the decimal 3 places to the right to multiply by 1,000.

X = 375 mcg   Label the units to match the unknown X.

Order equivalent: **digoxin 375 mcg IV daily**

Supply: digoxin 500 mcg per 2 mL

Step 2   **Think**   375 mcg is less than 500 mcg.

The amount to give will be less than 2 mL but more than 1 mL.

Step 3   **Calculate** $$\frac{Dosage\ on\ hand}{Amount\ on\ hand} = \frac{Dosage\ desired}{X\ Amount\ desired}$$

$$\frac{500\ mcg}{2\ mL} \diagdown \frac{375\ mcg}{X\ mL}$$ Cross-multiply

500X = 750

$$\frac{500X}{500} = \frac{750}{500}$$ Simplify: Divide both sides of the equation by the number before the unknown X.

X = 1.5 mL   Label the units to match the unknown X.

Measure 1.5 mL in a 3 mL syringe to administer as directed through an injection port on the IV tubing.

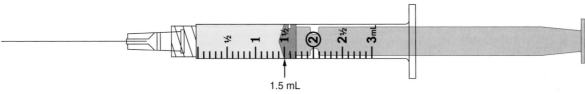

1.5 mL

EXAMPLE 4 ■

Order: **Robinul 100 mcg IM stat**

Glycopyrrolate (Robinul) is an anticholinergic given as a one-time dose to inhibit salivation and excessive respiratory secretions prior to surgery or as adjunctive management of peptic ulcer disease. It is available in tablets and in solution for injection in 0.2 mg/mL concentration. The recommended adult dosage for control of secretions during surgery is 4.4 mcg/kg IM 30 to 60 min preop.

For this example, you will prepare a one-time dosage for a patient scheduled for surgery. This medication is not part of the usual inventory in the ADC, so the pharmacy has delivered a single dose of the medication (Figure 11-5) to the hospital unit, labeled with the specific patient's name. You will learn to calculate medication based on body weight in Chapter 13.

Complete the dosage calculation.

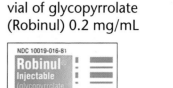
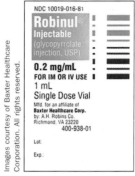

FIGURE 11-5 Single-dose vial of glycopyrrolate (Robinul) 0.2 mg/mL

| Step 1 | **Convert** | For the ordered dose of 100 mcg, a conversion is necessary. The units are in the same system (metric), but the ordered size units are mcg and the supply is labeled as mg. Remember that converting the larger unit (mg) to the smaller unit (mcg) will eliminate the decimal fraction. Convert the supply units. |

Equivalent: 1 mg = 1,000 mcg

$$\frac{1 \text{ mg}}{1,000 \text{ mcg}} \diagdown \diagup \frac{0.2 \text{ mg}}{X \text{ mcg}}$$ Cross-multiply

$$X = 1,000 \times 0.2$$ 0.200. Move the decimal 3 places to the right. Add zeros to complete the operation.

$$X = 200 \text{ mcg}$$ Label the units to match the unknown X.

Order: **Robinul 100 mcg IM stat**

Supply equivalent: Robinul 200 mcg/mL

| Step 2 | **Think** | 100 mcg is less than 200 mcg, or exactly half. The amount needed will be half of 1 mL, or 0.5 mL. |

| Step 3 | **Calculate** | $\dfrac{\text{Dosage on hand}}{\text{Amount on hand}} = \dfrac{\text{Dosage desired}}{X \text{ Amount desired}}$ |

$$\frac{200 \text{ mcg}}{1 \text{ mL}} \diagdown \diagup \frac{100 \text{ mcg}}{X \text{ mL}}$$ Cross-multiply

$$200X = 100$$

$$\frac{200X}{200} = \frac{100}{200}$$ Simplify: Divide both sides of the equation by the number before the unknown X.

$$X = 0.5 \text{ mL}$$ Label the units to match the unknown X.

The dose volume is less than the maximum for an adult intramuscular (IM) injection. Measure 0.5 mL in a 3 mL or 1 mL syringe for injection in one muscle site. If the syringe is prepackaged with a needle attached, check to be sure that the correct needle is used according to the patient's size.

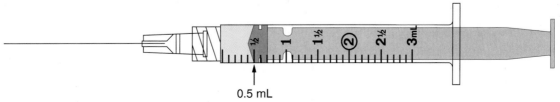

0.5 mL

EXAMPLE 5 ■

Order: **diphenhydramine 25 mg IM q.6h p.r.n., itching**

Diphenhydramine is an antihistamine used to treat allergic reactions, motion sickness, insomnia, and symptoms of Parkinson's disease. The oral forms are available over the counter under many brand names, the most recognizable being Benadryl. The solution for injection is available by prescription in 50 mg/mL concentration. The recommended adult dosage to be given by the intramuscular (IM) or intravenous (IV) route is 10 to 50 mg, up to 100 mg if needed, and not to exceed 400 mg per day.

For this example, the adult patient is complaining of itching. After checking to be sure that it has been at least 6 hours since the previous dose, you retrieve the medication from the unit automated dispensing cabinet (ADC). The ADC drawer that opens contains cubbies located side by side, as illustrated in Figure 11-6. Take care to read the labels closely. Both drugs are labeled with generic names that begin with "di" and include "HCl." Additionally, the dosage strength of the concentration is 50 mg for both. The use of "Tall Man" letters to spell out diphenhydrAMINE alerts you that this medication is on the list of look-alike/sound-alike drugs. Select one single-dose vial of diphenhydrAMINE HCl 50 mg/mL from the supply box and read the label on the vial to check for the "right drug" again.

FIGURE 11-6 Illustrated ADC matrix drawer with prepackaged vials: **(a)** diltiazem HCl 50 mg per 10 mL in individual single-dose vials; **(b)** box containing diphenhydramine HCl 50 mg/mL single-dose vials

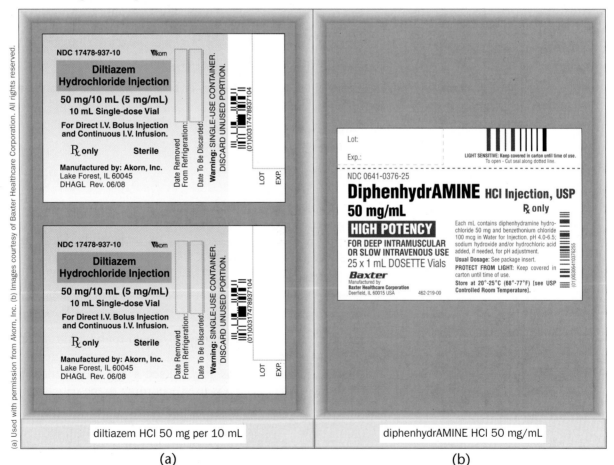

Let's complete the dosage calculation using the Three-Step Approach.

Step 1	**Convert**	For the ordered dose of 25 mg, no conversion is necessary. The units are in the same system (metric) and the same size (mg).
Step 2	**Think**	25 mg is half of 50 mg. You will need half of 1 mL, or exactly 0.5 mL.

Step 3 **Calculate** $\dfrac{\text{Dosage on hand}}{\text{Amount on hand}} = \dfrac{\text{Dosage desired}}{\text{X Amount desired}}$

$$\dfrac{50\ \text{mg}}{1\ \text{mL}} \diagdown \dfrac{25\ \text{mg}}{\text{X mL}}$$ Cross-multiply

$$50\text{X} = 25$$

$$\dfrac{50\text{X}}{50} = \dfrac{25}{50}$$ Simplify: Divide both sides of the equation by the number before the unknown X.

$$\text{X} = 0.5\ \text{mL}$$ Label the units to match the unknown X.

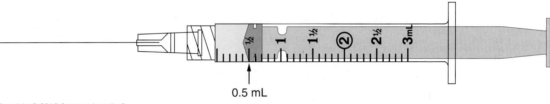

0.5 mL

Measure 0.5 mL of diphenhydrAMINE in a 3 mL syringe or 1 mL syringe for injection in one muscle site. If the syringe is prepackaged with a needle attached, check to be sure that the correct needle is used according to the patient's size.

EXAMPLE 6 ■

Order: **ketorolac 25 mg IM q.6h p.r.n., severe pain**

Ketorolac tromethamine is a nonsteroidal, anti-inflammatory drug used for severe acute pain in adults, usually postoperatively. It is supplied in tablets, ophthalmic solution, and solution for injection. The recommended adult dosage for the intramuscular (IM) or intravenous (IV) route is 15 mg to 30 mg q.6h, not to exceed 120 mg daily. It is not classified as a controlled substance, as are the opioid analgesics also used for severe pain. If the whole amount is not needed, the remainder may be discarded according to policy, without a witness.

For this example, the adult patient is recovering in the hospital one day after surgery. The patient complains of pain, rating the severity as a 9 on a scale of 0 to 10. After checking to be sure that it has been at least 6 hours since the previous dose, the medication will be retrieved from the unit automated dispensing cabinet (ADC). The ADC drawer that opens contains cubbies located side by side, as illustrated in Figure 11-7.

Let's complete the first two steps of the dosage calculation before deciding which supply to remove from the ADC.

Step 1 **Convert** For the ordered dose of 25 mg, no conversion is necessary. The units of the order and all supplied dosages are in the same system (metric) and the same size (mg).

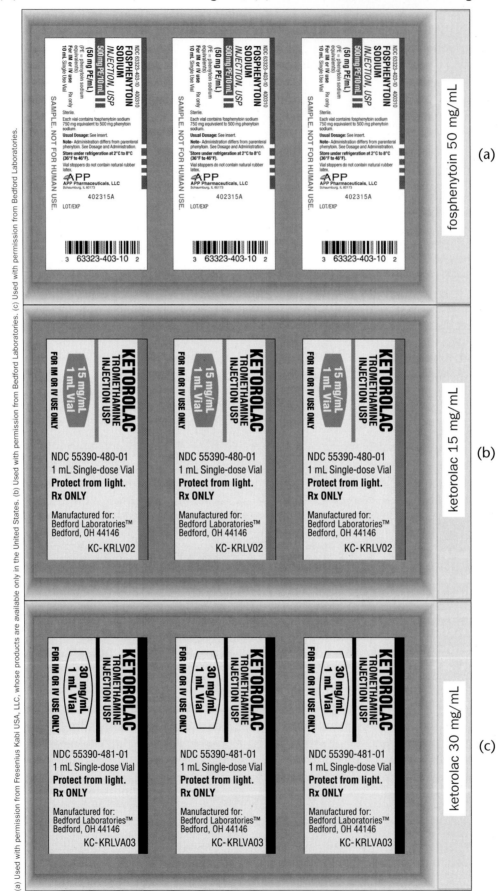

Step 2 **Think** There are two possible supply dosages to use. In order to administer the 25 mg dose using the 15 mg/mL concentration, more than 1 mL but less than 2 mL will be needed, supplied in two 1 mL vials. Using the 30 mg/mL concentration, slightly less than 1 mL and only one 1 mL vial would be needed. Although either supply would provide a dose volume less than the maximum for an adult intramuscular (IM) injection, it would be more practical to select one 30 mg/mL vial.

Step 3 **Calculate**

$$\frac{\text{Dosage on hand}}{\text{Amount on hand}} = \frac{\text{Dosage desired}}{\text{X Amount desired}}$$

$$\frac{30 \text{ mg}}{1 \text{ mL}} \times \frac{25 \text{ mg}}{\text{X mL}}$$ Cross-multiply

$$30X = 25$$

$$\frac{30X}{30} = \frac{25}{30}$$ Simplify: Divide both sides of the equation by the number before the unknown X.

$$X = 0.833 \text{ mL} = 0.83 \text{ mL}$$ Label the units to match the unknown X.

(Rounded to hundredths to measure in 1 mL syringe. Verifies estimate.)

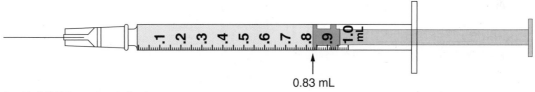

0.83 mL

Measure 0.83 mL of ketorolac tromethamine 30 mg/mL in a 1 mL syringe. If the syringe is prepackaged with a needle attached, check to be sure that the correct needle is used according to the patient's size. Discard remaining solution as per hospital policy.

REMEMBER

Dosages measured in hundredths (such as 0.83 mL) and all amounts less than 0.5 mL should be prepared in a 1 mL syringe that is calibrated in hundredths. However, if the route is intramuscular (IM), you may need to change needles to achieve a more appropriate length.

EXAMPLE 7 ■

Order: Ativan 4 mg IV stat

Lorazepam, the generic name for Ativan, is an antianxiety drug. It may also be given before surgery as a sedative and to treat continuous seizures called *status epilepticus*. It is available in tablets, oral solution, and solution for injection. The recommended adult dosage for a preanesthetic intramuscular (IM) injection is 0.05 mg/kg up to a maximum of 4 mg/kg. The standard dosage for status epilepticus is 4 mg intravenously (IV) injected at 2 mg per minute, which may be repeated as needed in 10 to 15 minutes.

For this example, you will administer the medication to a hospitalized adult who is experiencing status epilepticus and receiving this medication as a one-time stat dose. You will retrieve the drug from the unit automated dispensing cabinet (ADC) matrix drawer, but most ADCs will be programed to only open a specific individual cubby containing the controlled substance. Lorazepam (Ativan) is categorized as a Schedule IV controlled substance. Inventory is verified each time the medication is used. If the whole amount is not needed, the remainder must be wasted according to policy and witnessed by a second nurse. The ADC screen provides an option of using two different supplies of lorazepam (Ativan), as pictured in Figure 11-8.

FIGURE 11-8   Illustrated ADC matrix drawer with prepackaged vials of lorazepam (Ativan): **(a)** 2 mg/mL individual multidose vials; **(b)** box containing 4 mg/mL single-dose vials

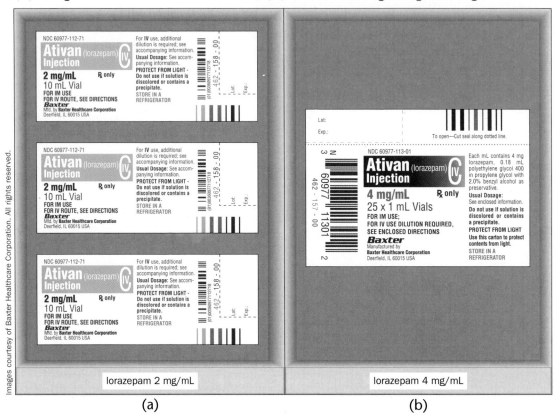

Complete the first two steps of the dosage calculation before removing the supply from the ADC.

Step 1	**Convert**	For the ordered dose of 4 mg, no conversion is necessary. The units of the order and all supplied dosages are in the same system (metric) and the same size (mg).
Step 2	**Think**	There are two possible supply dosages to use. The 2 mg/mL concentration, in compartment a, is supplied in a 10 mL vial. That means that the total dosage available in the vial equals 20 mg.

$$\frac{2 \text{ mg}}{\text{mL}} \diagup\!\!\!\diagdown \frac{\text{X mg}}{10 \text{ mL}}$$

$$\text{X} = 20 \text{ mg (per 10 mL vial)}$$

After administering the 4 mg dose, the 16 mg remaining would need to be wasted and witnessed. The 4 mg/mL concentration is supplied in 1 mL single-dose vials. The full dose would be used, so none would need to be wasted. This supply is the best choice. You anticipate that you will need to give 1 mL of the single-dose vial. Remove one vial from the supply box and read the label again to double-check.

Step 3 **Calculate** $\dfrac{\text{Dosage on hand}}{\text{Amount on hand}} = \dfrac{\text{Dosage desired}}{\text{X Amount desired}}$

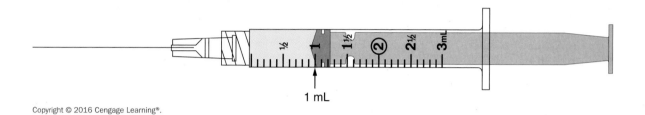

$\dfrac{4 \text{ mg}}{1 \text{ mL}} \diagdown \dfrac{4 \text{ mg}}{\text{X mL}}$ Cross-multiply

$4X = 4$

$\dfrac{4X}{4} = \dfrac{4}{4}$ Simplify: Divide both sides of the equation by the number before the unknown X.

$X = 1 \text{ mL}$ Label the units to match the unknown X.

1 mL

You will probably want to figure this calculation in your head. It is obvious that you want to give 1 mL. But make a habit of writing down the desired dosage, the supplied dosage, and the supplied quantity. Slowing yourself down just a little and seeing the numbers written down may prevent an error caused by reading the labels too quickly. The important decision in this example is selecting the correct supply strength.

The desired amount for this dose is measured using a 3 mL syringe and will be injected slowly through an injection port on the IV tubing. Techniques used to manage the rate of infusions for medications given by direct IV, or "slow IV push," will be addressed in Chapter 15.

QUICK REVIEW

- To solve parenteral dosage problems, apply the Three-Step Approach to dosage calculations:

Step 1 **Convert**

Step 2 **Think**

Step 3 **Calculate** $\dfrac{\text{Dosage on hand}}{\text{Amount on hand}} = \dfrac{\text{Dosage desired}}{\text{X Amount desired}}$

- Prepare a maximum of 3 mL per IM injection site for an average-size adult, 1 mL per site for adult deltoid site, 2 mL for children ages 6 through 12, and 0.5 to 1 mL for children under age 6.

- Calculate dose volumes and prepare injectable fractional doses in a syringe using these guidelines:

  - Standard doses more than 1 mL: Round to tenths and measure in a 3 mL syringe. The 3 mL syringe is calibrated to 0.1 mL increments. Example: 1.53 mL is rounded to 1.5 mL and drawn up in a 3 mL syringe.

  - Small (less than 0.5 mL) doses: Round to hundredths and measure in a 1 mL syringe. Critical care and children's doses less than 1 mL calculated in hundredths should also be measured in a 1 mL syringe. The 1 mL syringe is calibrated in 0.01 mL increments. Example: 0.257 mL is rounded to 0.26 mL and drawn up in a 1 mL syringe.

  - Amounts of 0.5 to 1 mL calculated in tenths can be accurately measured in either a 1 mL or 3 mL syringe.

Review Set 24

For questions 1 through 6, let's focus only on the mathematical aspects of dosage calculation to reinforce the Three-Step Approach and the dosage calculation formula. These problems will present different medication orders for drugs we have already worked with in the examples in this chapter. Use the labels provided for the supplied dosage, and draw an arrow on the syringe for the correct dose amount.

1. Order: Dilaudid 1.5 mg IM q.6h p.r.n., severe pain

   Give: _____ mL

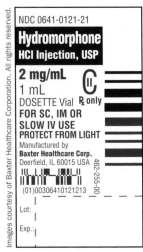

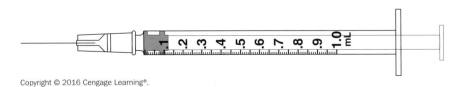

2. Order: digoxin 0.25 mg IV daily

   Give: _____ mL

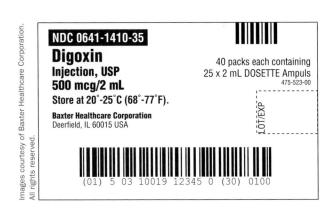

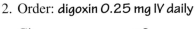

3. Order: ketorolac 25 mg IM q.6h p.r.n., severe pain

   Give: _____ mL

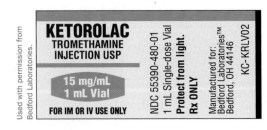

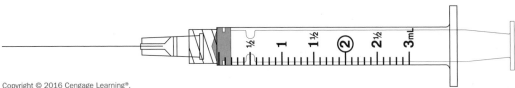

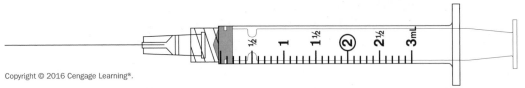

4. Order: Robinul 125 mcg IM stat

Give: _____ mL

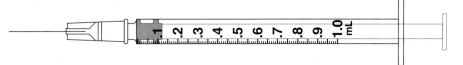

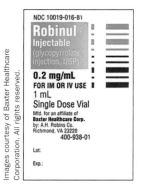

5. Order: diphenhydramine 10 mg IM q.6h p.r.n., itching

Give: _____ mL

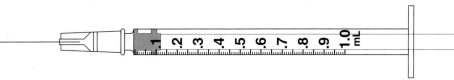

6. Order: Ativan 3.4 mg IM × 1 dose pre-op

Give: _____ mL

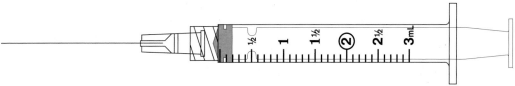

For questions 7 through 12, the medications are stocked by the pharmacy in unit-dose carts once every 24 hours at 1900 for each individual patient. For these medication-preparation simulations, utilize all aspects of safe dosage preparation and calculation of medications, including collecting data about the drug, selecting the supplied dosage, computing the dose, and measuring with equipment for medication administration. Refer to a nursing drug guide, such as the *Delmar Nurse's Drug Handbook,* to answer specific questions about the medication prior to administering.

Questions 7 through 9: The nurse is preparing to give Patient #1 the following routine and p.r.n. medications at 0800. The patient's unit-dose drawer is stocked with individual medication vials labeled as pictured below.

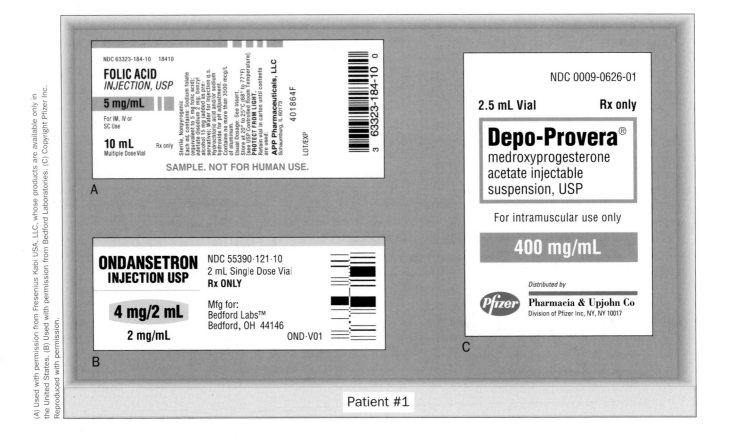

Patient #1

7. Order: **folic acid 1,000 mcg IM daily for 10 days**

   a. For what condition(s) is folic acid indicated? _____

   b. What dosage strengths of folic acid may be supplied in solution for injection? _____
   _____

   c. By what parenteral routes may folic acid be administered? _____

   d. What is the usual recommended adult dosage range? _____

   e. Identify the letter of the label showing the supplied dosage strength that you will use to calculate one dose. _____

   f. Give: _____ mL

g. Mark the correct amount on the syringe:

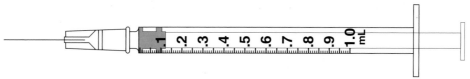

8. Order: *medroxyprogesterone acetate 1 g IM stat*

    a. For what condition(s) is medroxyprogesterone acetate indicated? _____

    b. What dosage strengths of medroxyprogesterone acetate may be supplied in solution for injection? _____

    c. By what parenteral routes may medroxyprogesterone acetate be administered? _____

    d. What is the usual recommended adult dosage range? _____

    e. Identify the letter of the label showing the supplied dosage strength that you will use to calculate one dose. _____

    f. Give: _____ mL

    g. Mark the correct amount on the syringe:

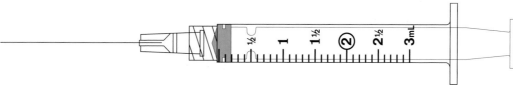

9. Order: *ondansetron 3 mg slow IV push × 1 dose stat*

    a. For what condition(s) is ondansetron indicated? _____

    b. What dosage strengths of ondansetron may be supplied in solution for injection? _____

    _____

    c. By what parenteral routes may ondansetron be administered? _____

    d. What is the usual recommended adult dosage range? _____

    e. Identify the letter of the label showing the supplied dosage strength that you will use to calculate one dose. _____

    f. Give: _____ mL (Administer as directed through an injection port on the IV tubing.)

    g. Mark correct amount on the syringe:

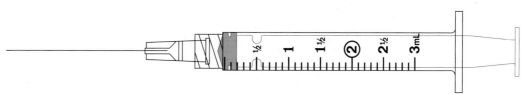

Questions 10 through 12: The nurse is preparing to give Patient #2 the following routine and p.r.n. medications at 2100. The patient's unit-dose drawer is stocked with individual medication vials labeled as pictured below.

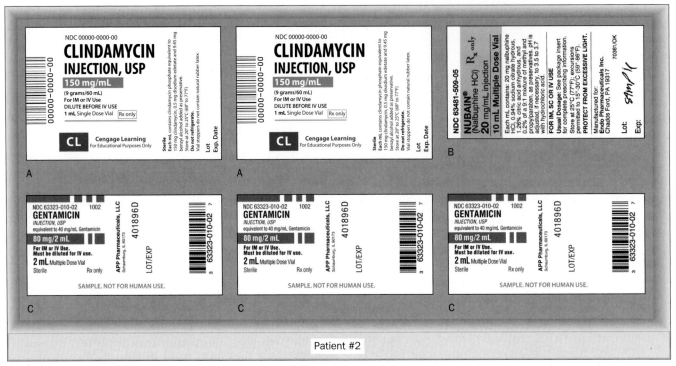

Patient #2

10. Order: *gentamicin 70 mg IV PB q.8h*

    a. For what condition(s) is gentamicin indicated? _____

    b. What dosage strengths of gentamicin may be supplied in solution for injection? _____

    _____

    c. By what parenteral routes may gentamicin be administered? _____

    d. What is the usual recommended adult dosage range? _____

    e. Identify the letter of the label showing the supplied dosage strength that you will use to calculate one dose. _____

    f. Give: _____ mL (Inject into recommended-size piggyback bag.)

    g. Mark correct amount on the syringe:

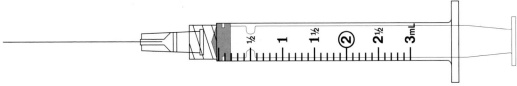

11. Order: *clindamycin 0.6 g IV PB q.12h*

    a. For what condition(s) is clindamycin indicated? _____

    b. What dosage strengths of clindamycin may be supplied in solution for injection? _____

    _____

    c. By what parenteral routes may clindamycin be administered? _____

    d. What is the usual recommended adult dosage range? _____

    e. Identify the letter of the label showing the supplied dosage strength that you will use to calculate one dose. _____

    f. Give: _____ mL (Inject into recommended-size piggyback bag.)

    g. Mark correct amount on the syringe:

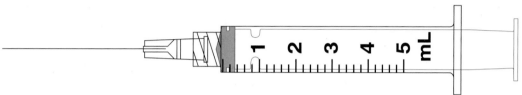

12. Order: *nalbuphine HCl 5 mg subcut q.4h p.r.n., pain*

    a. For what condition(s) is nalbuphine indicated? _____

    b. What dosage strengths of nalbuphine may be supplied in solution for injection? _____

    _____

    c. By what parenteral routes may nalbuphine be administered? _____

    d. What is the usual recommended adult dosage range? _____

    e. Identify the letter of the label showing the supplied dosage strength that you will use to calculate one dose. _____

    f. Give: _____ mL

    g. Mark correct amount on the syringe:

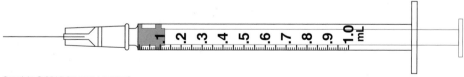

For questions 13 through 20, the medications will be retrieved from an automated dispensing cabinet (ADC) matrix drawer, as illustrated, to administer a variety of different orders. Utilize all aspects of safe dosage calculation of medication, including collecting data about the drug, selecting the supply dosage, computing the dose, and measuring with equipment for medication administration. Refer to a nursing drug guide, such as the *Delmar Nurse's Drug Handbook,* to answer specific questions about the medication prior to administering.

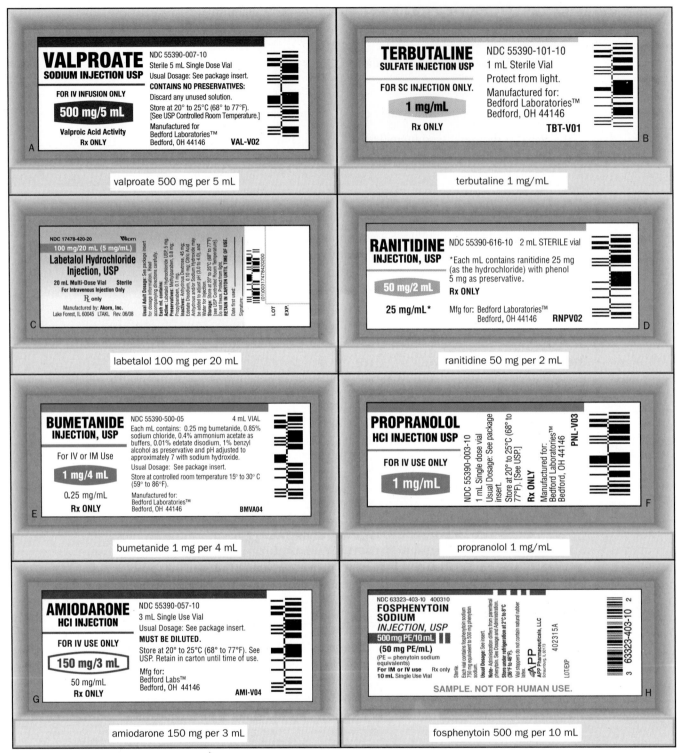

VALPROATE SODIUM INJECTION USP	NDC 55390-007-10 Sterile 5 mL Single Dose Vial Usual Dosage: See package insert. **CONTAINS NO PRESERVATIVES:** Discard any unused solution. Store at 20° to 25°C (68° to 77°F). [See USP Controlled Room Temperature.] Manufactured for Bedford Laboratories™ Bedford, OH 44146
FOR IV INFUSION ONLY **500 mg/5 mL** Valproic Acid Activity **Rx ONLY** A	VAL-V02

valproate 500 mg per 5 mL

TERBUTALINE SULFATE INJECTION USP	NDC 55390-101-10 1 mL Sterile Vial Protect from light. Manufactured for: Bedford Laboratories™ Bedford, OH 44146
FOR SC INJECTION ONLY. **1 mg/mL** **Rx ONLY**	TBT-V01 B

terbutaline 1 mg/mL

NDC 17478-420-20 Akorn **100 mg/20 mL (5 mg/mL)** **Labetalol Hydrochloride Injection, USP** 20 mL Multi-Dose Vial Sterile For Intravenous Injection Only Rx only Manufactured by: Akorn, Inc. Lake Forest, IL 60045 LTAKL Rev. 06/08	

labetalol 100 mg per 20 mL

RANITIDINE INJECTION, USP	NDC 55390-616-10 2 mL STERILE vial *Each mL contains ranitidine 25 mg (as the hydrochloride) with phenol 5 mg as preservative.
50 mg/2 mL **Rx ONLY** 25 mg/mL*	Mfg for: Bedford Laboratories™ Bedford, OH 44146 RNPV02 D

ranitidine 50 mg per 2 mL

BUMETANIDE INJECTION, USP	NDC 55390-500-05 4 mL VIAL Each mL contains: 0.25 mg bumetanide, 0.85% sodium chloride, 0.4% ammonium acetate as buffers, 0.01% edetate disodium, 1% benzyl alcohol as preservative and pH adjusted to approximately 7 with sodium hydroxide.
For IV or IM Use **1 mg/4 mL** 0.25 mg/mL **Rx ONLY** E	Usual Dosage: See package insert. Store at controlled room temperature 15° to 30° C (59° to 86°F). Manufactured for: Bedford Laboratories™ Bedford, OH 44146 BMVA04

bumetanide 1 mg per 4 mL

PROPRANOLOL HCl INJECTION USP	NDC 55390-003-10 1 mL Single dose vial Usual Dosage: See package insert. Store at 20° to 25°C (68° to 77°F). [See USP.] Rx ONLY Manufactured for: Bedford Laboratories™ Bedford, OH 44146 PNL-V03
FOR IV USE ONLY **1 mg/mL**	F

propranolol 1 mg/mL

AMIODARONE HCl INJECTION	NDC 55390-057-10 3 mL Single Use Vial Usual Dosage: See package insert. **MUST BE DILUTED.** Store at 20° to 25°C (68° to 77°F). See USP. Retain in carton until time of use.
FOR IV USE ONLY **150 mg/3 mL** 50 mg/mL **Rx ONLY** G	Mfg for: Bedford Labs™ Bedford, OH 44146 AMI-V04

amiodarone 150 mg per 3 mL

NDC 63323-403-10 400310 **FOSPHENYTOIN SODIUM** INJECTION, USP **500 mg PE/10 mL** **(50 mg PE/mL)** (PE = phenytoin sodium equivalents) **For IM or IV use** Rx only 10 mL Single Use Vial	Each vial contains fosphenytoin sodium 750 mg equivalent to 500 mg phenytoin sodium. See Dosage and Administration. Note—Administration differs from parenteral phenytoin. See Dosage and Administration. Store under refrigeration at 2°C to 8°C (36°F to 46°F). Vial stoppers do not contain natural rubber latex. APP APP Pharmaceuticals, LLC 402315A LOT/EXP 3 63323-403-10 2
SAMPLE. NOT FOR HUMAN USE.	H

fosphenytoin 500 mg per 10 mL

(A, B, D, E, F, G) Used with permission from Bedford Laboratories. (C) Used with permission from Akorn, Inc. (H) Used with permission from Fresenius Kabi USA, LLC, whose products are available only in the United States.

13. Order: **terbutaline 250 mcg subcut stat and repeat q.15 to 30 min if no significant improvement**

    a. For what condition(s) is terbutaline indicated? _____

    b. What dosage strengths of terbutaline may be supplied in solution for injection? _____

_____

   c. By what parenteral routes may terbutaline be administered? _____

   d. What is the usual recommended adult dosage range? _____

   e. Identify the letter of the label showing the supplied dosage strength that you will use to calculate one dose. _____

   f. Give: _____ mL

   g. Mark correct amount on the syringe:

14. Order: **bumetanide 500 mcg slow IV push stat**

   a. For what condition(s) is bumetanide indicated? _____

   b. What dosage strengths of bumetanide may be supplied in solution for injection? _____

     _____

   c. By what parenteral routes may bumetanide be administered? _____

   d. What is the usual recommended adult dosage range? _____

   e. Identify the letter of the label showing the supplied dosage strength that you will use to calculate one dose. _____

   f. Give: _____ mL (Administer as directed through an injection port on the IV tubing.)

   g. Mark correct amount on the syringe:

15. Order: **ranitidine 35 mg IV q.6h**

   a. For what condition(s) is ranitidine indicated? _____

   b. What dosage strengths of ranitidine may be supplied in solution for injection? _____

     _____

   c. By what parenteral routes may ranitidine be administered? _____

   d. What is the usual recommended adult dosage range? _____

   e. Identify the letter of the label showing the supplied dosage strength that you will use to calculate one dose. _____

   f. Give: _____ mL (Dilute further, as directed, in a large syringe or IV piggyback bag.)

   g. Mark correct amount on the syringe:

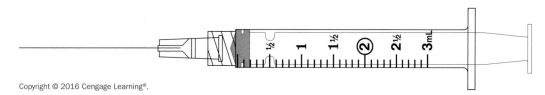

16. Order: *valproate sodium 420 mg IV PB q.12h*

    a. For what condition(s) is valproate indicated? _____

    b. What dosage strengths of valproate may be supplied in solution for injection? _____

        _____

    c. By what parenteral routes may valproate be administered? _____

    d. What is the usual recommended adult dosage range? _____

    e. Identify the letter of the label showing the supplied dosage strength that you will use to
        calculate one dose. _____

    f. Give: _____ mL (Inject into the recommended-size IV piggyback bag.)

    g. Mark correct amount on the syringe:

17. Order: *propranolol 2 mg IV slow push stat*

    a. For what condition(s) is propranolol indicated? _____

    b. What dosage strengths of propranolol may be supplied in solution for injection? _____

        _____

    c. By what parenteral routes may propranolol be administered? _____

    d. What is the usual recommended adult dosage range? _____

    e. Identify the letter of the label showing the supplied dosage strength that you will use to
        calculate one dose. _____

    f. Give: _____ mL (Administer as directed through an injection port on the IV tubing.)

    g. Mark correct amount on the syringe:

18. Order: *amiodarone 360 mg IV PB (over 6 h at 1 mg/min)*

    a. For what condition(s) is amiodarone indicated? _____

    b. What dosage strengths of amiodarone may be supplied in solution for injection? _____

        _____

    c. By what parenteral routes may amiodarone be administered? _____

    d. What is the usual recommended adult dosage range? _____

    e. Identify the letter of the label showing the supplied dosage strength that you will use to
        calculate one dose. _____

    f. Give: _____ mL (Inject into a recommended-size IV piggyback bag.)

g. Mark correct amount on the syringe:

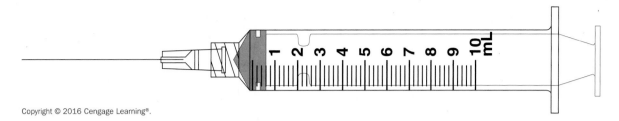

19. Order: **fosphenytoin 280 mg IV daily until tolerating PO fluids**

   a. For what condition(s) is fosphenytoin indicated? _____

   b. What dosage strengths of fosphenytoin may be supplied in solution for injection? _____

   _____

   c. By what parenteral routes may fosphenytoin be administered? _____

   d. What is the usual recommended adult dosage range? _____

   e. Identify the letter of the label showing the supplied dosage strength that you will use to calculate one dose. _____

   f. Give: _____ mL (Dilute further, as directed, in a large syringe or IV piggyback bag.)

   g. Mark correct amount on the syringe:

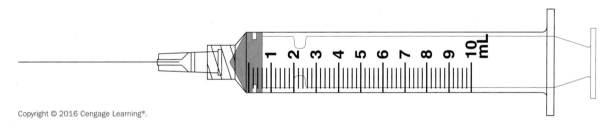

20. Order: **labetalol 18 mg IV bolus stat**

   a. For what condition(s) is labetalol indicated? _____

   b. What dosage strengths of labetalol may be supplied in solution for injection? _____

   _____

   c. By what parenteral routes may labetalol be administered? _____

   d. What is the usual recommended adult dosage range? _____

   e. Identify the letter of the label showing the supplied dosage strength that you will use to calculate one dose ._____

   f. Give: _____ mL

   g. Mark correct amount on the syringe:

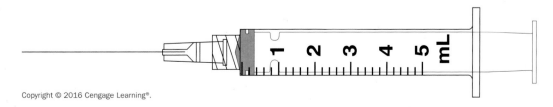

After completing these problems, see pages 661–667 to check your answers.

HIGH-ALERT PARENTERAL MEDICATIONS

The Institute for Safe Medication Practices (ISMP) defines high-alert medications as "drugs that bear a heightened risk of causing significant patient harm when they are used in error" (ISMP, 2011). The ISMP has published a list of classes/categories of high-alert medications and specific medications that require special safeguards to reduce the risk of errors leading to devastating consequences. Heparin (antithrombotic agent) and insulin (antidiabetic agent) have been identified as two of the high-alert medications with the greatest safety risk. In addition to dosage calculation errors, fatal dosing errors have been associated with confusing various concentrations of the drug, reading drug labels incorrectly, and making mistakes in filling automated dispensing cabinets (ADCs). Other fatal errors have occurred when insulin and heparin have been mixed up. Heparin and insulin are both measured in units, administered by the subcutaneous or intravenous route, and supplied in multidose vials that may look similar. Additionally, both of these drugs are used on a daily basis on nursing units and may be placed near each other on a counter or medication cart. Many hospitals require double verification before administration of high-alert drugs. The double-check should include the chart order, the product selected, the calculated dose, and the dose drawn up.

FIGURE 11-9 Sample high-alert medications: **(a)** heparin lock flush 100 units/mL; **(b)** regular human insulin 100 units/mL

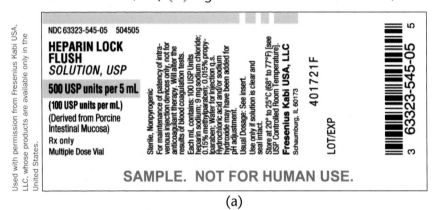

(a)

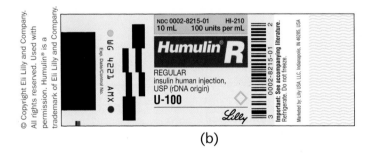

(b)

Consider the two sample insulin and heparin labels pictured in Figure 11-9. Imagine that they are sitting side by side on a counter in the medication room. As the nurse prepares to flush an intravenous access port with the standard 1 mL of heparin flush, the insulin vial is picked up by mistake. There is no second nurse available in the medication room to do an independent check, so the nurse measures 1 mL from the insulin vial and brings only the syringe to another nurse at the nurses' station to check. Soon after the 100 units of insulin are injected into the IV, the patient starts to show signs of severe hypoglycemia, a life-threatening condition. The shortcut the nurse took to verify the dose is considered a "work-around." The risk of medication errors increases when nurses "work around" standard policies and procedures because the planned method is time consuming or inconvenient.

In this chapter, we will practice calculating and drawing up heparin and insulin to be administered subcutaneously (subcut), along with some basic intravenous (IV) heparin calculations. You will learn more-advanced skills for complex orders and the intravenous (IV) administration of these and other high-risk drugs in Chapter 17.

Heparin

Anticoagulants are used to prevent the formation or extension of blood clots, a condition known as thrombosis. Contrary to a common misconception, anticoagulants do not dissolve clots. Hemorrhage is a potential life-threatening adverse reaction. Subcutaneous heparin may be administered as a prophylaxis for thromboembolism prior to and following surgery. IV locks, which are venous access ports without continuous IV fluid infusing, will be injected periodically with very low doses of heparin to maintain patency by preventing clots from forming at the insertion site. Treatment for thrombosis is initially started with intravenous heparin or heparin-like drugs for rapid results. Heparin therapy frequently consists of a combination of intermittent IV boluses (large doses to achieve a rapid, therapeutic effect) and continuous IV infusions. In this section, you will practice calculation for subcutaneous injections and IV boluses. You will learn to calculate doses to manage continuous IV heparin infusions according to protocols in Chapter 17.

CAUTION

Heparin is a high-alert medication. Read heparin labels very carefully. Health care agencies are transitioning from old to new regulations for label content and design in response to a recent announcement by the US Pharmacopeial Convention (USP). Heparin labels must now print the strength per total volume as the primary expression of strength followed in close proximity by strength per milliliter (ISMP, 2013a). Both labels may be available until current supplies are depleted. To avoid serious medication errors always identify the concentration of the supply as well as the total volume in the container.

In the following four examples, the supply dosages will be retrieved from the ADC matrix drawer illustrated in Figure 11-10.

EXAMPLE 1 ■

Order: **heparin 5,000 units subcut 2 h prior to surgery**

For this example, the patient is at risk for thromboembolism and the patient is scheduled for routine surgery. Heparin solution for injection is supplied in 10 units/mL, 100 units/mL, 1,000 units/mL, 5,000 units/mL, 7,500 units/mL, 10,000 units/mL, 20,000 units/mL, and 40,000 units/mL—each in single-dose and multidose vials. The usual recommended adult dosage for prophylaxis of thromboembolism is 5,000 units 2 h preop, then q.8 to 12 h. You will retrieve the heparin supply dosage from the ADC (Figure 11-10).

Complete the dosage calculation using the Three-Step Approach.

Step 1	**Convert**	No conversion is ever necessary for heparin. The order and the supplied dosages are always in the same unit of measurement—units.
Step 2	**Think**	There is a supply dosage, as represented in Figure 11-10(b), that is identical to the ordered dose: 5,000 units/mL. The total volume in the vial is also 1 mL. Using this vial will leave no remaining solution to store. Another option is the 10,000 units/mL supply in a 10 mL multidose vial, Figure 11-10(d). Selecting this vial would require calculating a dose and discarding the remaining medication or storing the vial until after surgery. The 5,000 units/mL 1 mL vial is the better choice.
Step 3	**Calculate**	No calculation is needed. It is obvious that 1 mL will be needed. The order is for 5,000 units and 5,000 units per mL is available; therefore you will give 1 mL from that vial.

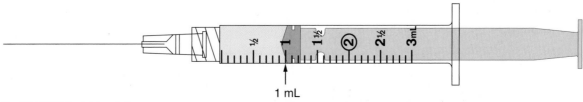

1 mL

FIGURE 11-10   Illustrated ADC matrix drawer with vials of heparin in various concentrations: **(a)** Heparin lock flush 100 units/10 mL (10 units/mL) single-dose vial; **(b)** Heparin 5,000 units/1 mL; **(c)** Heparin 10,000 units/10 mL (1,000 units/mL) multidose vial; **(d)** Heparin 50,000 units/5 mL (10,000 units/mL) multidose vial

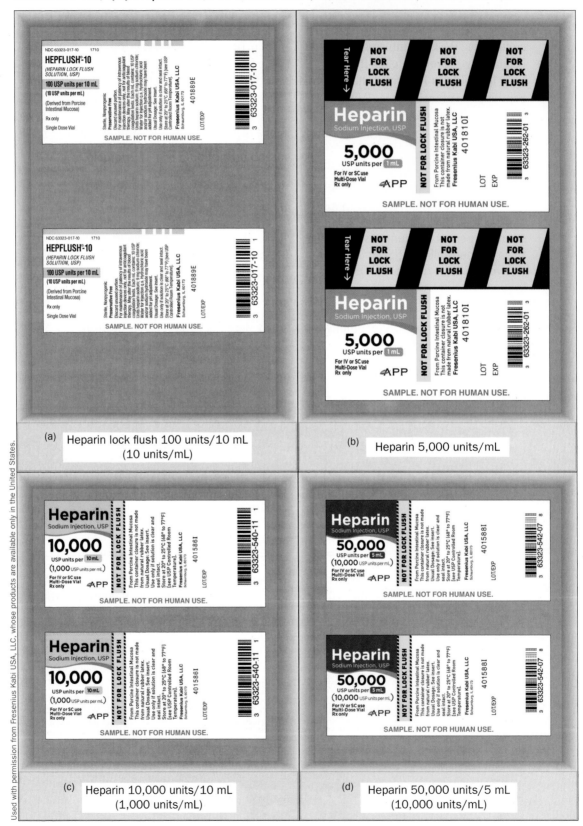

Double check the label and measure 1 mL of heparin from the 5,000 units/mL supply. Provide the order, vial, and syringe to another nurse for independent verification and documentation. If the syringe is prepackaged with a needle attached, check to be sure the correct needle is used for a subcutaneous injection site. Heparin is usually administered in the abdomen.

EXAMPLE 2 ■

Order: **Flush PICC line with 3 mL heparin-lock flush 10 units/mL q.12h**

For this example, the patient will need an IV access port for an extended period of time. A peripherally inserted central line (PICC) is a longer IV catheter that may require flushing with a low concentration of heparin solution to remain patent. Heparin solution for flushing IV locks is supplied in 10 units/mL and 100 units/mL. The usual recommended dosage for a lock is an injection of 10 to 100 units/mL heparin solution in sufficient quantity to fill the entire IV catheter to the tip. Hospital policy usually specifies the required dosage strength and amount for PICC lines for each facility, generally ranging from 3 to 6 mL.

Complete the dosage calculation using the Three-Step Approach.

Step 1	**Convert**	No conversion is ever necessary for heparin. The order and the supplied dosages are always in the same unit of measurement—units.
Step 2	**Think**	There is one supply dosage as represented in Figure 11-10(a) that is appropriate for this heparin flush: 10 units/mL. The other supply dosages (1,000 units/mL, 5,000 units/mL, and 10,000 units/mL) far exceed the recommended concentration. The total volume in the vial shown in Figure 11-10(a) is 10 mL. Remove the vial of 10 units/mL strength, and check to be certain the vial removed is in the strength or the concentration desired.
Step 3	**Calculate**	No calculation is needed. The order specifies the concentration and the volume in mL.

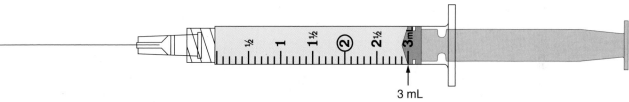

3 mL

Measure 3 mL of heparin from the supplied vial of 10 units/mL. Provide the order, the vial, and the syringe to another nurse for independent verification and documentation.

EXAMPLE 3 ■

Order: **heparin 8,000 units IV bolus ASAP prior to initiation of continuous heparin infusion**

There are various options for the treatment of thrombosis with heparin, including subcutaneous injections ranging from q.8 to 12 h, intermittent direct IV doses, and continuous IV infusions. Some hospitals have approved protocols for heparin therapy, which you will learn about in Chapter 17. The recommended dosage is often based on the patient's weight and is adjusted by conducting periodic blood tests. The patient in this example will be receiving a bolus loading dose of heparin by direct IV, followed by a continuous IV heparin infusion.

Complete the dosage calculation using the Three-Step Approach.

Step 1	**Convert**	No conversion is ever necessary for heparin. The order and the supplied dosages are always in the same unit of measurement—units.
Step 2	**Think**	There are 3 possible supply dosage strengths represented in Figure 11-10 that could be used. The 5,000 units/mL, Figure 11-10(b), supply dosage

may be used, but because the total volume in the vial is only 1 mL, 2 vials would be needed. Both the 10 mL vial of 1,000 units/mL, Figure 11-10(c), and the 10 mL vial of 10,000 units/mL, Figure 11-10(d), would supply the full ordered dosage. Compare these two concentrations. The amount needed from the 10,000 units/mL vial would be a very small and highly concentrated amount. Even small variations when measuring in a syringe would be significant. By contrast, the amount needed from the 1,000 units/mL vial would be a larger and more diluted amount. Variations when measuring this concentration would be much less significant. Heparin protocols often specify the use of this concentration for IV boluses. Because 8,000 units is 8 times larger than 1,000 units, you will need 8 times 1 mL, or exactly 8 mL. Unlike subcutaneous and intramuscular injections, larger volumes may be administered safely by the intravenous route. The 1,000 units/mL 10 mL vial is the better choice. Select one vial and check the label to be certain it is the desired concentration.

Step 3   **Calculate** $\dfrac{\text{Dosage on hand}}{\text{Amount on hand}} = \dfrac{\text{Dosage desired}}{\text{X Amount desired}}$

$$\dfrac{1,000 \text{ units}}{1 \text{ mL}} \diagdown \dfrac{8,000 \text{ units}}{\text{X mL}} \qquad \text{Cross-multiply}$$

$$1,000\text{X} = 8,000$$

$$\dfrac{1,000\text{X}}{1,000} = \dfrac{8,000}{1,000} \qquad$$ Simplify: Divide both sides of the equation by the number before the unknown X.

$$\text{X} = 8 \text{ mL} \qquad$$ Label the units to match the unknown X.

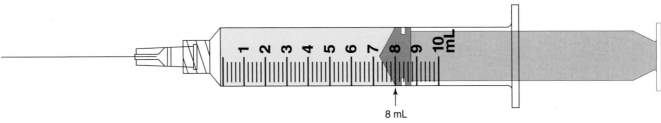

8 mL

Measure 8 mL of heparin in a 10 mL syringe from the 1,000 units/mL supply. Provide the order, vial, and syringe to another nurse for independent verification and documentation.

EXAMPLE 4 ▪

Order: D$_5$W 500 mL c̄ heparin 25,000 units IV at 1,000 units/h

The patient in Example 3 received the bolus, which will now be followed by a continuous infusion. Frequently, IV solutions with heparin additive come premixed or prepared by the hospital pharmacy. But there may be situations when a nurse will need to mix the IV solution for continuous infusion.

Complete the dosage calculation using the Three-Step Approach.

Step 1   **Convert**   No conversion is ever necessary for heparin. The order and the supplied dosages are always in the same unit of measurement—units.

Step 2   **Think**   The 10,000 units/mL supply dosage is the only vial depicted in Figure 11-10(d) that will provide 25,000 units. There is a total of 50,000 units in the 5 mL vial. This order for 25,000 units is half of the total volume in the vial, or 2.5 mL. Select one 10,000 units/mL vial, and check the label to be certain it is the desired concentration.

Step 3 **Calculate** $\dfrac{\text{Dosage on hand}}{\text{Amount on hand}} = \dfrac{\text{Dosage desired}}{\text{X Amount desired}}$

$$\frac{10{,}000 \text{ units}}{1 \text{ mL}} \underset{\times}{\times} \frac{25{,}000 \text{ units}}{\text{X mL}}$$ Cross-multiply

$$10{,}000\text{X} = 25{,}000$$

$$\frac{10{,}000\text{X}}{10{,}000} = \frac{25{,}000}{10{,}000}$$ Simplify: Divide both sides of the equation by the number before the unknown X.

$$\text{X} = 2.5 \text{ mL}$$ Label the units to match the unknown X.

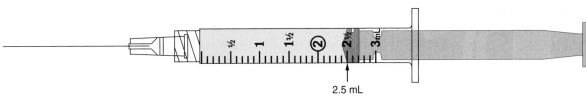

2.5 mL

Measure 2.5 mL of heparin from the 10,000 units/mL supply in a 3 mL syringe. Provide the order, vial, and syringe to another nurse for independent verification and documentation. Add the heparin solution to the 500 mL IV PB bag of 5% dextrose in water (D_5W) through the injection port. Label with the patient's name, drug name and concentration, dosage and amount added, date and time prepared, and your signature. You will learn about managing the rate of continuous IV infusions in Chapters 15 and 17.

Insulin

Insulin, a hormone made in the pancreas, is necessary for the metabolism of glucose, proteins, and fats. Patients who are deficient in insulin (insulin-dependent diabetics) are required to take insulin by injection daily. Insulin is a ready-to-use solution that is measured in units. The common supply dosage of insulin is 100 units per mL, which is abbreviated on the label as U-100. Insulin is also available as 500 units per mL (U-500). This supply dosage is used in special circumstances for diabetic patients with marked insulin resistance (such as daily requirements of more than 200 units).

MATH TIP
Think: U-100 = 100 units per mL
Think: U-500 = 500 units per mL

CAUTION
Accuracy in insulin preparation and administration is critical. Inaccuracy is potentially life threatening. It is essential for nurses to understand the information on the insulin label, to correctly interpret the insulin order, and to select the correct syringe to accurately measure insulin for administration. It is critical to understand that U-500 insulin (500 units/mL) is five times as concentrated as U-100 insulin (100 units/mL). **Extreme caution must be exercised in the administration of U-500 insulin, because inadvertent overdose may result in irreversible insulin shock and death.**

Insulin Labels

Figure 11-11 identifies the essential components of insulin labels. The insulin label includes important information. For example, the *brand* and *generic names,* the *supply dosage* or *concentration,* and the *storage* instructions are details routinely found on most parenteral drug labels. Chapter 8 explained these and other typical drug-label components. Compare the U-100 and U-500 insulin labels to find important identifiers and differences.

FIGURE 11-11   **(a)** U-100 insulin label; **(b)** U-500 insulin label

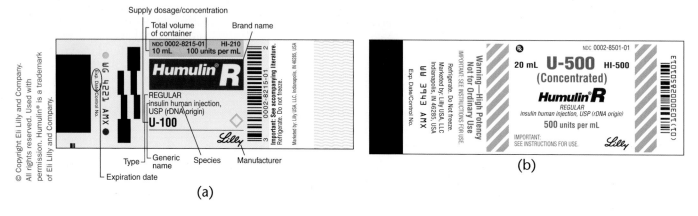

(a)

(b)

Insulin Action Times

Insulin is categorized by action times, as described by McCulloch (2008).

- Rapid-acting (analog)—5 to 15 min, peak in 45 to 75 min, 2–4 h duration: *lispro, aspart, and glulisine*
- Short-acting—30 min, peak in 2 to 4 h, 5–8 h duration: *regular*
- Intermediate-acting—2 h, peak in 6 to 10 h, 18–28 h duration: *NPH*
- Long-acting (analog)—2 h, no peak, 6–24 h duration: *detemir and glargine*

Regular and NPH insulin are the two types that have traditionally been used most frequently, and they are often mixed. Regular human insulin is synthesized in the laboratory to be structurally identical to human insulin. NPH human insulin is a suspension of human insulin mixed with protamine and zinc to create an intermediate-acting insulin with a slower onset of action and a longer duration than that of regular human insulin. Notice the uppercase, bold letters on these two insulin types: R for regular insulin (Figure 11-11a) and N for NPH insulin (Figure 11-12g). These letters are important visual identifiers when selecting the insulin type. Further, note the different concentrations of regular insulin: regular U-100 (100 units/mL) and regular U-500 (500 units/mL)(Figure 11-11).

An insulin analog is the newest type of insulin that has been chemically modified to either act faster or slower than the type of insulin naturally made by the body. Lispro, aspart, and glulisine are rapid-acting analogs. Detemir and glargine are long-acting analogs. According to the American Diabetes Association, most people with Type I diabetes should use insulin analogs to reduce hypoglycemia risk (American Diabetes Association, 2013).

FIGURE 11-12 Labels for insulin types grouped by action times

Rapid acting (labels a–c)

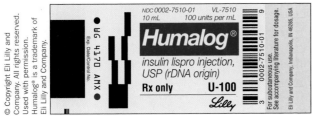

(a)

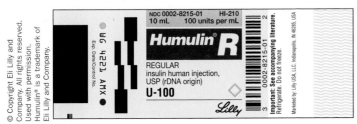

(b)

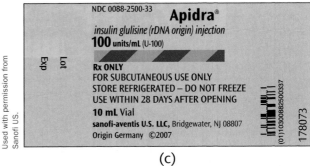

(c)

Short acting (labels d–f)

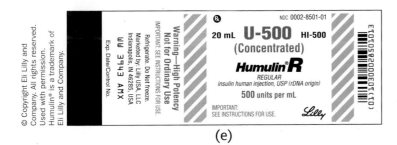

(d)

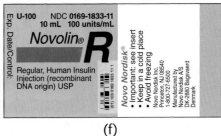

(f)

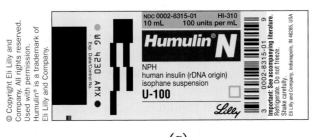

(e)

Intermediate acting (labels g and h)

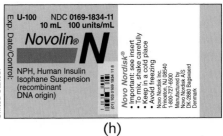

(g)

(h)

Continues

FIGURE 11-12 *Continued*

Long acting (labels i and j)

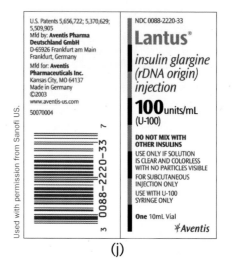

(i)

(j)

Premixed, Combination Insulin

Premixed insulin preparations contain two types of insulin—rapid or short acting with intermediate acting—in the same insulin vial or pen. This is a convenience for patients who are in a treatment plan using a standard ratio of these insulins, reducing the number of injections required. Several premixed insulin combinations are commercially available. Figure 11-13 (a–c) depicts three of these preparations.

FIGURE 11-13 Premixed, combination insulins

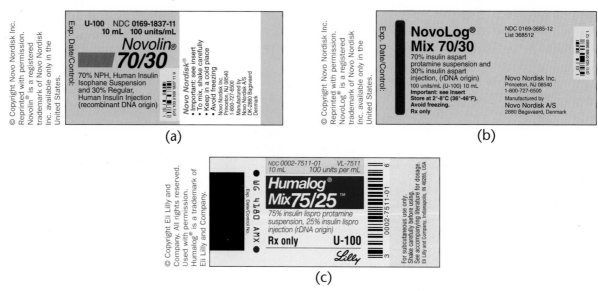

(a)

(b)

(c)

It is important to carefully read the labels to understand what types of insulin are included in each combination. Notice that Novolin 70/30 (Figure 11-13a) includes 70% NPH U-100 insulin, an intermediate-acting agent, and 30% regular U-100 insulin, a short-acting agent, in each unit. Therefore, if the physician orders 10 units of 70/30 U-100 insulin, the patient would receive 7 units of NPH insulin (70%, or 0.7×10 units = 7 units) and 3 units of regular insulin (30%, or 0.3×10 units = 3 units) in the 70/30 concentration. If the physician orders 20 units of 70/30 insulin, the patient would receive 14 units ($0.7 \times 20 = 14$) of NPH and 6 units ($0.3 \times 20 = 6$) of regular insulin.

The Humalog Mix 75/25 U-100 insulin concentration is 75% of insulin lispro protamine suspension, an intermediate-acting agent, and 25% of insulin lispro solution, a rapid-acting agent. Therefore, if the physician orders 24 units of Humalog 75/25 U-100 insulin, the patient would receive 18 units of insulin lispro protamine suspension (75%, or 0.75 × 24 units = 18 units) and 6 units of insulin lispro solution (25%, or 0.25 × 24 units = 6 units).

It is easy to mistake one 70/30 preparation for another. For example, check out the differences between the labels for Novolin 70/30 (Figure 11-13a) and NovoLog 70/30 (Figure 11-13b). The Novolin is a combination of NPH and regular U-100 insulins, but the NovoLog is a combination of aspart protamine and aspart. These all have different action times, and selecting the wrong combination could be a serious and life-threatening error.

CAUTION

Insulin repeatedly is at or near the top of the list of high-alert medications that can lead to errors and patient harm (Cohen, 2007; Grissinger, 2010; Hahn, 2007; ISMP, 2011; Onufer, 2002). Avoid a potentially life-threatening medication error. Carefully read the label, and compare it to the drug order to ensure that you select the correct action time, strength, and type of insulin.

Interpreting the Insulin Order

Insulin orders must be written clearly and contain specific information to ensure correct administration and prevent errors. An insulin order should contain:

1. The *brand and generic names* and the *action time.* Patients are instructed to stay with the same manufacturer's brand-name insulin. Slight variations between brands can affect an individual's response. Verify with the patient, both the usual brand name used and the actual insulin supplied before administration. Look for one of the four insulin action times: rapid acting (e.g., lispro), short acting (e.g., regular), intermediate acting (e.g., NPH), or long acting (e.g., detemir).

2. The *supply dosage (concentration)* and *number of units* to be given—for example, U-100 regular insulin 40 units.

3. The *route* of administration and *time* or *frequency.* All insulin may be administered subcutaneously (subcut), and regular U-100 insulin may additionally be administered intravenously (IV).

EXAMPLES ■

Humulin R regular U-100 insulin 14 units subcut stat

Novolin N NPH U-100 insulin 24 units subcut $\frac{1}{2}$ hour $\bar{a}$ breakfast

Insulin Administration

The primary route of insulin administration is by subcutaneous injection. Regular U-100 insulin can also be administered intravenously. The schedule and frequency for insulin administration vary based on the needs of the individual patient. The insulin pump is one method for insulin administration (Figure 11-14). Insulin pumps deliver rapid- or short-acting insulin 24 hours a day through a catheter placed under the skin. Pumps can be programmed to deliver a basal rate and/or bolus doses. Basal insulin is delivered continuously over 24 hours to keep blood glucose levels within a target range between meals and overnight. The basal rate can be programmed to deliver different rates at different times of the day and night. Bolus doses can be delivered at mealtimes to provide control for additional food intake.

FIGURE 11-14   Insulin pumps

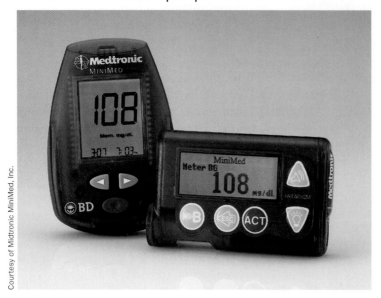

Courtesy of Midtronic MiniMed, Inc.

Measuring Insulin in an Insulin Syringe

The insulin syringe and the measurement of insulin were introduced in Chapter 6. This critical skill warrants your attention again. Once you understand (a) how insulin is packaged, (b) about different concentrations (i.e., U-100 or U-500), and (c) how to use the insulin syringe, you will find insulin dosage simple.

RULE

- Measure U-100 insulin in a U-100 insulin syringe only. Do not use a 3 mL or 1 mL syringe to measure U-100 insulin.

- Use U-100 insulin syringes to measure U-100 insulin only. Do not measure other drugs supplied in units in a U-100 insulin syringe.

- Measure U-500 insulin in a 1 mL syringe. Take extra precautions, when measuring and administering U-500 insulin, to note that the concentration is 500 units/mL. Correct dosage requires a calculation.

- Two nurses must check insulin dosage *before* administration to the patient.

Measuring U-100 insulin with the insulin syringe is simple. The insulin syringe makes it possible to obtain a correct dosage without mathematical calculation. Let's look at three different U-100 insulin syringes. They are the *standard* (100 unit) capacity and the *Lo-Dose* (50 unit and 30 unit) capacity.

Standard U-100 Insulin Syringe

Recall from Chapter 6 that the standard U-100 insulin syringe (Figure 11-15) is a dual-scale syringe with 100 units/mL capacity. It is calibrated on one side in even-numbered 2-unit increments (2, 4, 6, . . .), with every 10 units labeled (10, 20, 30, . . .). It is calibrated on the opposite side in odd-numbered 2-unit increments (1, 3, 5, . . .), with every 10 units labeled (5, 15, 25, . . .). It is not necessary to use the dosage calculation formula to measure the volume for preparing U-100 insulin. The insulin syringe is specially designed to measure a dose of insulin in units. The important skill is correctly reading the syringe calibrations.

FIGURE 11-15   Standard U-100 insulin syringe

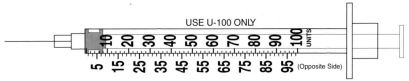

Copyright © 2016 Cengage Learning®.

EXAMPLE ▪

Order: **Lantus U-100 insulin 73 units subcut daily at 0900**

Lantus insulin (Figure 11-16) is a brand name for the long-acting insulin glargine, with duration of up to 24 hours. For this example, the patient is an adult with insulin-dependent diabetes, admitted to the hospital for a medical problem unrelated to diabetes. Prior to the morning dose of insulin, the point-of-care blood glucose measurement supported the need for insulin therapy. On this nursing unit, the pharmacy supplies a multidose vial of Lantus to the patient's unit-dose drawer. Apply the Three-Step Approach to measure and prepare the order.

FIGURE 11-16   U-100 insulin glargine (Lantus), 10 mL multidose vial in unit-dose drawer

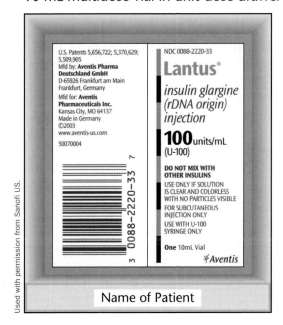

Step 1	**Convert**	No conversion needed. Order and supply for insulin will always be in units.
Step 2	**Think**	Because there are 100 units in each mL, one dose of 73 units will be less than 1 mL, so there should be at least 10 doses available in one 10 mL multidose vial. If this vial has been used before, the date and time it was opened should be checked for expiration according to hospital policy. Turning the syringe to view the odd-numbered side and counting by 2 units for each calibration line, the correct amount should be found between 65 and 75 units.
Step 3	**Calculate**	Although no dosage calculation is necessary, counting by 2s can be confusing, especially for odd numbers. 75 units − 73 units = 2 units. One calibration line on the standard 100-unit U-100 syringe equals 2 units. Starting at 75 units on the odd-unit scale, count 1 calibration line down from the 75-unit mark toward the 65-unit mark. The filled syringe verifies estimate.

Again, what seems like a simple measurement requires careful attention to the details of the syringe: find the correct side of the syringe to view the measurement, and recognize the value of each calibration. After drawing up insulin, provide the order, vial, and syringe to another nurse for independent verification and documentation.

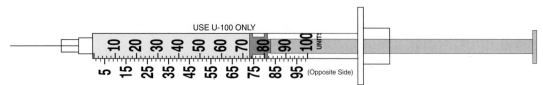

CAUTION

Look carefully at the increments on the standard U-100 insulin syringe with the dual scale. The volume from one mark to the next (on either side) is 2 units. You are probably comfortable counting by twos for even numbers; however, pay closer attention when counting by twos with odd numbers.

Lo-Dose U-100 Insulin Syringes

Recall from Chapter 6 that the 50-unit Lo-Dose U-100 insulin syringe (Figure 11-17a) is a single-scale syringe with 50 units per 0.5 mL capacity. It is calibrated in 1-unit increments with every 5 units labeled (5, 10, 15, . . .) up to 50 units. The 30-unit Lo-Dose U-100 insulin syringe (Figure 11-17b) is a single-scale syringe with 30 units per 0.3 mL capacity. It is also calibrated in 1-unit increments with every 5 units labeled (5, 10, 15, . . .) up to 30 units. The enlarged 50-unit and 30-unit calibration of these syringes provides more space between increment lines, making it easier to read and use for measuring low dosages of insulin, resulting in a more accurate dose.

It is not necessary to use the dosage calculation formula to measure the volume of U-100 insulin. The U-100 insulin syringe is specially designed to measure a dose of insulin in units.

FIGURE 11-17 **(a)** 50-unit U-100 insulin syringe; **(b)** 30-unit U-100 insulin syringe

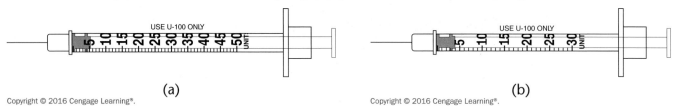

(a)

(b)

EXAMPLE 1 ■

Order: *NovoLog 70/30 U-100 insulin 32 units subcut daily at 0700*

NovoLog insulin is a brand name for the premixed combination insulin with 70% of the intermediate-acting insulin aspart protamine suspension and 30% of the rapid-acting insulin aspart with a duration of 18 to 24 hours. For this example, the patient is an adult with insulin-dependent diabetes, admitted to the hospital for a medical problem unrelated to diabetes. Prior to the morning dose of insulin, the point-of-care blood glucose measurement supported the need for insulin therapy. On this nursing unit, the pharmacy supplies a multidose vial of NovoLog (Figure 11-18) to the patient's unit-dose drawer.

FIGURE 11-18 U-100 NovoLog Mix 70/30, 10 mL multidose vial in unit-dose drawer

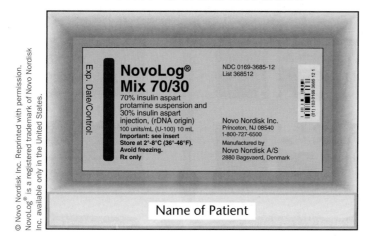

Exp. Date/Control:

NovoLog®
Mix 70/30
70% insulin aspart
protamine suspension and
30% insulin aspart
injection, (rDNA origin)
100 units/mL (U-100) 10 mL
Important: see insert
Store at 2°-8°C (36°-46°F).
Avoid freezing.
Rx only

NDC 0169-3685-12
List 368512

Novo Nordisk Inc.
Princeton, NJ 08540
1-800-727-6500
Manufactured by
Novo Nordisk A/S
2880 Bagsvaerd, Denmark

(01) 103 0169 3685 12 1

Name of Patient

Apply the Three-Step Approach.

Step 1	**Convert**	No conversion needed. Order and supply for insulin will always be in units.
Step 2	**Think**	The ordered dose is greater than 30 units but less than 50 units. Choose the 50-unit syringe. Because the syringe measures 50 units in each 0.5 mL, one dose of 32 units will be less than 0.5 mL, so there should be at least 20 doses available in one 10 mL multidose vial. If this vial has been used before, the date and time it was opened should be checked for expiration according to hospital policy. Each calibration line on the 50-unit Lo-Dose U-100 syringe is equal to 1 unit of insulin. After counting by 1 unit for each calibration line, the correct amount should be found between 30 and 35 units.
Step 3	**Calculate**	No calculation is necessary. Draw up NovoLog 70/30 to the 32 unit line, as shown on the filled syringe. After drawing up insulin, provide the order, vial, and syringe to another nurse for independent verification and documentation.

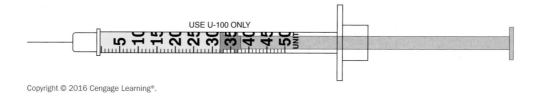

USE U-100 ONLY

5 10 15 20 25 30 35 40 45 50 UNIT

Copyright © 2016 Cengage Learning®.

EXAMPLE 2 ∎

Order: **Humalog U-100 insulin 12 units subcut stat**

Humalog insulin is a brand name for the rapid-acting insulin lispro, with an onset of action within 15 minutes. For this example, the patient is an adult admitted through the emergency department, with a diagnosis of pneumonia. The point-of-care blood glucose measurement indicated a higher-than-normal level. In the emergency department, the pharmacy supplies rapid- and short-acting multidose vials of insulin in the automated dispensing cabinet (ADC). The ADC drawer that opens contains cubbies located side by side, as illustrated in Figure 11-19.

FIGURE 11-19   Illustrated ADC matrix drawer with 10 mL multidose vials: **(a)** Humalog U-100; **(b)** Humulin R U-100; **(c)** Humulin R U-500

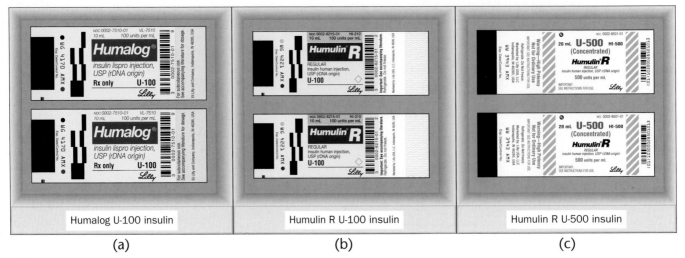

Humalog U-100 insulin	Humulin R U-100 insulin	Humulin R U-500 insulin
(a)	(b)	(c)

Apply the Three-Step Approach.

Step 1	**Convert**	No conversion needed. Order and supply for insulin will always be in units.
Step 2	**Think**	All three insulin vials look similar. They are all manufactured by Lilly and begin with the same three letters: "Hum." Compare the labels closely. From the left, the first supply dosage is the rapid-acting insulin lispro (Figure 11-19a), the second is the short-acting regular insulin (Figure 11-19b), and the third is also a regular insulin but in the very concentrated form of 500 units per mL (Figure 11-19c). Choose a vial of the Humalog insulin from the first compartment. The ordered dosage is small and less than 30 units. If available, use the 30-unit Lo-Dose insulin syringe. Each interval on the 30-unit Lo-Dose U-100 insulin syringe is equal to 1 unit of insulin. After counting by 1 unit for each calibration line, the correct amount should be found between 10 and 15 units.
Step 3	**Calculate**	No calculation is necessary. Draw up Humalog U-100 insulin to the 12-unit line. The filled syringe depicts this amount. After drawing up insulin, provide the order, vial, and syringe to another nurse for independent verification and documentation.

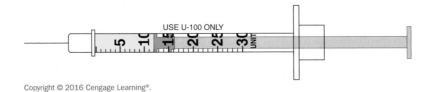

Combination Insulin Dosage

The patient may have two types of insulin—a rapid- or short-acting agent combined with an intermediate-acting agent—prescribed to be administered at the same time. When possible, a premixed U-100 insulin preparation is prescribed (Figure 11-13). However, if the preparation desired is not available, then the nurse must combine the U-100 insulins. To avoid injecting the patient twice, it is common practice to draw up both insulins into the same syringe.

Rapid- or short-acting insulins are injectable solutions; therefore, they do not need to be mixed and should be clear in appearance. Intermediate-acting insulins are suspensions that need to be gently rolled to be mixed before using, and therefore are cloudy in appearance. Long-acting insulins are clear but are never combined with other insulins. The clear insulin solution is always drawn up before the cloudy insulin suspension.

RULE

Draw up clear insulin first, and then draw up cloudy insulin. Rapid-acting and short-acting (regular, lispro, aspart) insulins are clear. Intermediate-acting (NPH) insulin is cloudy.

THINK: *first clear, then cloudy.*

THINK: *first rapid-acting or short-acting insulin, then intermediate-acting insulin.*

EXAMPLE 1 ■

Order: NovoLog U-100 insulin 12 units with Novolin N NPH U-100 40 units subcut ā breakfast

The patient in this example requires an injection of both Novolin N, the intermediate-acting insulin isophane suspension, and NovoLog, the brand name of the rapid-acting insulin aspart. Recall that the patient in Example 1 on page 302 received 32 units from one vial of NovoLog 70/30 U-100 insulin, which provided a specific 70/30 ratio of the rapid- and intermediate-acting forms of insulin aspart. Compare the labels closely in Figure 11-20. The premixed combination insulin can't be used in this situation, because the patient's needs require a ratio of approximately 23% rapid-acting and approximately 77% intermediate-acting insulin which is unavailable in a premixed form. Therefore, doses for each individual insulin have been ordered.

FIGURE 11-20 **(a)** 10 mL multidose vials of Novolin N and NovoLog U-100 insulin provided in patient's drawer; **(b)** U-100 NovoLog Mix 70/30 for comparison

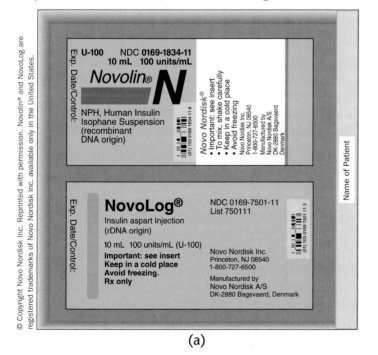

(a)

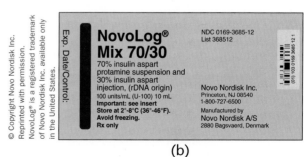

(b)

| Step 1 | **Convert** | No conversion needed. Order and supply for insulin will always be in units. |
| Step 2 | **Think** | To accurately draw up both insulins into the same syringe, you will need to know the total units of both insulins: 12 + 40 = 52 units. Withdraw 12 units of the NovoLog U-100 insulin (clear), and then withdraw 40 units of the |

Novolin N U-100 insulin (cloudy) up to the 52-unit mark. In this case, the smallest-capacity syringe you can use is the standard U-100 insulin syringe. The even-numbered side should be used, and, counting by 2 units for each calibration line, the correct amount for the NovoLog 12 units should be found between 10 and 14 units. The total amount in the syringe after drawing up the Novolin N will be 52 units and, again using the even-numbered side, should be found between 50 and 54 units.

Step 3   **Calculate**   10 units + 2 units = 12 units. One calibration line equals 2 units. Starting at 10 units, count 1 calibration line toward 12 units on the even-numbered side. 50 units + 2 units = 52 units on the even-numbered side. Starting at 50 units, count 1 calibration line toward 52 units on the even-numbered side. The filled syringe demonstrates the measurement. Notice that the NPH insulin is drawn up last and is closest to the needle in the diagram. In reality, the drugs mix right away. Provide the order, vials, and syringe to another nurse for independent verification after drawing up each insulin.

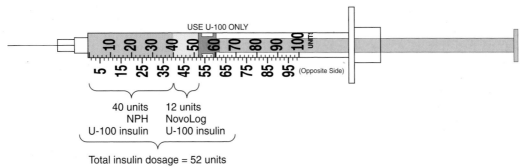

USE U-100 ONLY

40 units
NPH
U-100 insulin

12 units
NovoLog
U-100 insulin

Total insulin dosage = 52 units

There are two very important precautions to take when drawing two different forms of insulin into one syringe. One precaution is to draw an accurate amount of both insulins. If too much of the first insulin is drawn into the syringe, this may be corrected by expelling the extra amount prior to drawing the second insulin. But when the second insulin is drawn up, the insulins mix immediately. Therefore, if the syringe is overfilled with the second insulin, the extra amount cannot be expelled without also expelling some of the first insulin. The remaining insulin would not be the right dosage. Also, another nurse must complete an independent verification after each insulin is drawn up.

A second precaution is to prevent any of the first insulin from entering the vial when inserting the needle to draw up the second insulin. Consider that the rapid- or short-acting (clear) insulins are used when a fast therapeutic response is necessary. By drawing these insulins up first with a sterile, unused syringe, there is no chance of introducing the slower-acting intermediate (cloudy) insulin into the multidose vial. Care is also taken to prevent the opposite from happening when the needle is inserted into the second insulin vial. The pressure that exists inside the closed vial should be taken into consideration. If the pressure inside the vial is less than outside the vial, more pull must be used on the plunger to withdraw the solution. This leads to the formation of small bubbles that may interfere with the measurement of an accurate dose. Injecting an amount of air equal to the dose desired creates an increase in internal pressure, causing the insulin to leave the vial and enter the syringe with little or no pull. This technique should be used prior to withdrawing both insulins, but the additional advantage with the second insulin is that the chance that any of the insulin already in the syringe will be pulled into the vial is decreased. For this to be possible, air equal to the amount of insulin must be injected into both vials prior to withdrawing the first insulin. But do not inject extra air, because this will build up unnecessary pressure in the multidose vials.

CAUTION

When withdrawing two insulins into the same syringe:

▪ Take extra care to accurately withdraw both amounts, especially with the second draw.

▪ Inject air into both insulin vials equal to the amount of insulin required to increase pressure in the vials to make it easier to withdraw accurate doses.

The second example gives step-by-step directions for this procedure. Look closely at Figures 11-21 and 11-22, which demonstrate the procedure, as you study Example 2.

FIGURE 11-21   Procedure for drawing up combination insulin dosage: 10 units Novolin R regular U-100 insulin with 30 units Novolin N NPH U-100 insulin

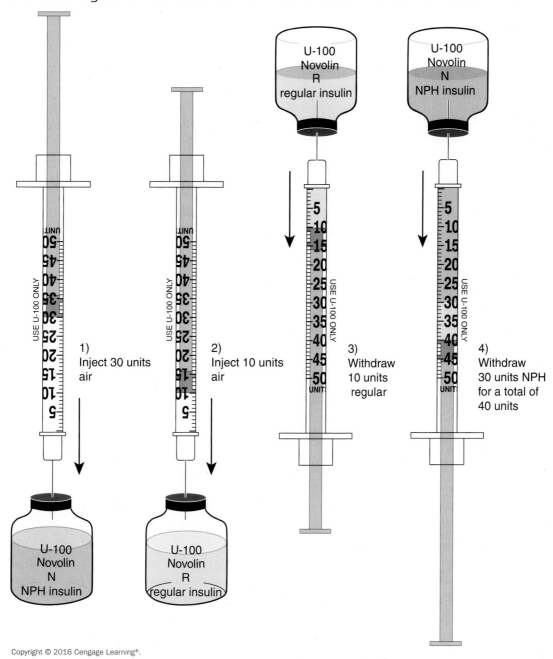

1) Inject 30 units air

2) Inject 10 units air

3) Withdraw 10 units regular

4) Withdraw 30 units NPH for a total of 40 units

FIGURE 11-22 Combination insulin dosage

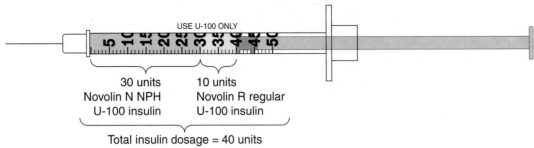

30 units
Novolin N NPH
U-100 insulin

10 units
Novolin R regular
U-100 insulin

Total insulin dosage = 40 units

EXAMPLE 2 ■

The physician orders Novolin R regular U-100 insulin 10 units with Novolin N NPH U-100 insulin 30 units subcut $\frac{1}{2}$ hour ā dinner.

1. Draw back and inject 30 units of air into the NPH insulin vial (cloudy liquid). Remove needle.

2. Draw back and inject 10 units of air into the regular insulin vial (clear liquid), leaving the needle in the vial.

3. Turn the vial of regular U-100 insulin upside down, and draw out the insulin to the 10-unit mark on the U-100 syringe, making sure all air bubbles are removed. Provide the order, vial, and syringe to another nurse for independent verification.

4. Roll the vial of the NPH U-100 insulin in your hands to mix; do not shake it. Insert the needle into the NPH insulin vial, turn the vial upside down, and slowly draw back to the 40-unit mark, being careful not to exceed the 40-unit calibration. Provide the order, vial, and syringe to another nurse for independent verification. In Figure 11-22, 10 units of regular U-100 + 30 units of NPH U-100 = 40 units of insulin total.

CAUTION

If you withdraw too much of the second insulin (NPH), you must discard the entire medication and start over.

CAUTION

Long-acting types of insulin should not be combined or diluted with any other insulin preparations. Combining long-acting insulin with other insulin solutions may interfere with blood sugar control, which could be serious and life threatening.

Insulin Coverage—The "Sliding Scale"

A special insulin order is sometimes needed to "cover" a patient's increasing blood glucose (sugar) level that is not yet regulated. Because a short onset of action is needed, a rapid-acting insulin (such as lispro) or a short-acting insulin (such as regular) will be used. The physician will specify the amount of insulin in units, which "slide" up or down based on a specific blood glucose level range. Sliding scales are individualized for each patient. Here's an example with a sliding-scale order.

EXAMPLE ▪

Order: Humalog U-100 insulin subcut a.c. at bedtime per sliding scale

Humalog is a brand name of insulin lispro, a rapid-acting agent with an onset within 5 to 15 minutes. For this example, the patient is an adult who had major abdominal surgery and is slowly returning to a regular diet. Yesterday, the pharmacy technician delivered a multidose 10 mL vial of Humalog (Figure 11-23), and the remaining amount is stored in the patient's unit-dose drawer. Until he fully recovers, blood glucose levels will be monitored before each meal (a.c.) and at bedtime. The dose of insulin the nurse will administer will be based on a sliding scale (Figure 11-24). The point-of-care glucose measurement before the evening meal was 290 mg/dL.

FIGURE 11-23 Humalog U-100 insulin 10 mL multidose vial in unit-dose drawer

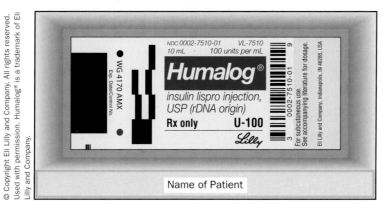

FIGURE 11-24 Sample insulin sliding-scale orders

INSULIN SLIDING SCALE

Insulin Dose	Glucose Reading (mg/dL)
No coverage	Glucose less than 160
2 units	160 to 220
4 units	221 to 280
6 units	281 to 340
8 units	341 to 400
Hold insulin; call MD stat.	401+

Copyright © 2016 Cengage Learning®.

Apply the Three-Step Approach.

Step 1 **Convert** No conversion needed. Order and supply for insulin will always be in units.

Step 2 **Think** There is a glucose range of 281 to 340; 290 is greater than 281 but less than 340, so the insulin coverage for this range should be used. The amount of the coverage, 6 units, is a very small amount; therefore, a Lo-Dose syringe would be the best choice to deliver the most accurate amount. Choose the 30-unit Lo-Dose syringe if available; otherwise, the 50-unit Lo-Dose syringe could be used. The 6-unit increment should fall between 5 and 10 units.

Step 3 **Calculate** No calculation is necessary, but accurate measurement is essential. Starting at 5 units, count 1 calibration line toward 10 units. The filled syringe demonstrates this amount. Yes, this seems obvious. But remember that this is a high-alert medication and simple insulin measurement errors with potentially fatal consequences are all too common. Avoid distractions and take your time when measuring insulin and other high-alert medications. After drawing up insulin, provide the order, point-of-care glucose measurement, vial, and syringe to another nurse for independent verification and documentation.

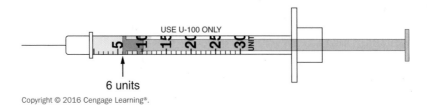

USE U-100 ONLY

6 units

CAUTION

Choose the smallest-capacity U-100 insulin syringe available for accurate U-100 insulin measurement. Use standard and Lo-Dose U-100 syringes to measure U-100 insulin only. Although the Lo-Dose U-100 insulin syringes only measure a maximum of 30 or 50 units, they are still intended for the measurement of U-100 insulin only.

Be cautious when measuring. Remember: The Lo-Dose U-100 syringes are calibrated in 1-unit increments; the standard U-100 insulin syringe is calibrated in 2-unit increments on the even and odd scales.

Prefilled U-100 Insulin Pens

A variety of insulin pen injectors is currently available for patient use (Figure 11-25a). The reusable U-100 pen is equipped with a disposable cartridge filled with 3 mL of either a single U-100 insulin or a premixed combination of U-100 insulins for a total of 300 units of insulin per cartridge (Figure 11-25b).

FIGURE 11-25   **(a)** Sample reusable U-100 insulin pen; **(b)** Sample U-100 insulin pen cartridge label

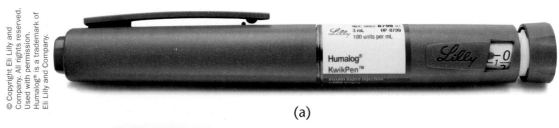

(a)

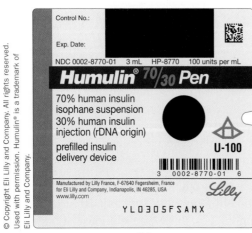

(b)

The availability of pen injectors has afforded patients an easy and accurate method for self-administering insulin. There are several advantages over using vials: (1) each pen is individually labeled with the patient's name, (2) the insulin in the pen cartridge is in a form ready for administration, and (3) less nursing time is required to prepare and administer the insulin. However, the Institute for Safe Medication Practices cautions that insulin pens used in the hospital setting can lead to cross contamination and must not be used between patients. They cited evidence of 700 patients in a New York hospital at risk for human immunodeficiency virus (HIV), hepatitis B, and hepatitis C from cross-contamination with insulin pens (ISMP, 2013b).

The ordered dosage is measured by turning the dose dial until the correct number of units is displayed in the dose window (Figure 11-26). Some of the newer pens are available with a digital display of dose information that can be easily misread if the pen is held upside down. For instance, a dose of 51 units looks like 15 units when the pen is held incorrectly, as shown in Figure 11-27.

The insulin pen cartridge is marked to estimate the amount used or remaining for additional doses but is not intended to measure individual doses. In order to administer a correct dose, after adding a new cartridge and before each additional dose, the pen must be primed by releasing a small amount of insulin.

FIGURE 11-26 Parts of an insulin pen with cartridge

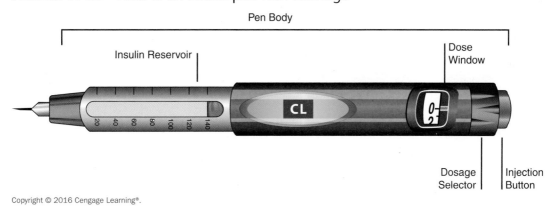

FIGURE 11-27 Digital insulin pen: (a) held correctly, displaying 51 units; (b) held upside down, which makes it appear to display 15 units instead of 51 units

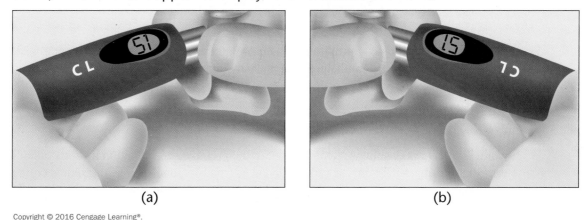

(a)   (b)

EXAMPLE 1 ■

Order: **Humalog U-100 insulin 12 units subcut a.c. breakfast**

Humalog U-100 insulin is a brand name for the rapid-acting insulin lispro, with an onset of action within 15 minutes. For this example, the patient is an adult with insulin-dependent diabetes, admitted to the hospital for a medical problem unrelated to diabetes. At home the patient uses an insulin injector pen, which was ordered for hospital use. Prior to the morning dose of insulin, the point-of-care blood glucose measurement supported the need for insulin therapy. The cartridge attached to the syringe has been used for previous doses, and the amount remaining is pictured below.

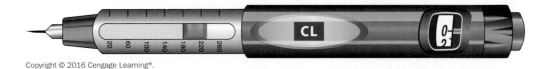

Apply the Three-Step Approach.

Step 1	**Convert**	No conversion needed. Order and supply for insulin will always be in units.
Step 2	**Think**	Current supply remaining in cartridge is approximately 180 units. After administration of the 12-unit insulin dose, the remaining amount should be between the 180- and 140-unit marks.
Step 3	**Calculate**	180 units – 12 units = 168 units (verifies estimated amount remaining)

Dial the ordered amount until the dosage window reaches the correct number of units. After dialing the insulin amount, provide the order and insulin pen to another nurse for independent verification and documentation.

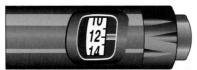

The amount remaining in the cartridge after administration of the insulin dose is pictured below.

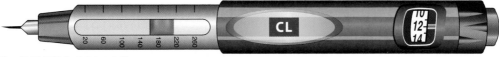

The remaining volume approximates the calculated amount; the amount injected is correct, and the pen functioned properly. Store the pen with the cartridge attached for later use.

EXAMPLE 2 ■

Order: **Novolin 70/30 U-100 insulin 36 units subcut at 1600**

Novolin 70/30 U-100 insulin is a brand name for the premixed combination insulin containing 70% of the intermediate-acting NPH human insulin isophane suspension and 30% of the short-acting regular human insulin. The combined action has a duration of 16 to 24 hours. For this example, the patient is again an adult with insulin-dependent diabetes, admitted to the hospital for a medical problem unrelated to diabetes. The pharmacy supplies insulin pens to the nursing units for patient use. Prior to the afternoon dose of insulin, the point-of-care blood glucose measurement supported the need for insulin therapy. The cartridge attached to the syringe has been used for previous doses, and the amount remaining is pictured below.

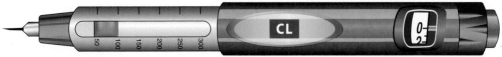

Apply the Three-Step Approach.

Step 1	**Convert**	No conversion needed. Order and supply for insulin will always be in units.
Step 2	**Think**	Current supply remaining in cartridge is slightly less than 50 units. There should be enough to administer the 36-unit dose. The pen should not allow the dial to be turned farther than the amount left in the cartridge. After administration of the 36-unit insulin dose, the remaining amount should be slightly above the zero mark, with a volume less than 1 dose.
Step 3	**Calculate**	45 units (approximate remaining volume) − 36 units = 9 units (verifies estimated amount remaining)

Dial the ordered amount until the dosage window reaches the correct number of units. After dialing the insulin amount, provide the order and insulin pen to another nurse for independent verification and documentation.

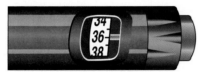

Copyright © 2016 Cengage Learning®.

The amount remaining in the cartridge after administration of the insulin dose is pictured below.

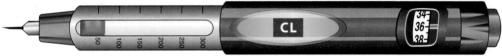

Copyright © 2016 Cengage Learning®.

The remaining volume approximates the calculated amount; the amount injected is correct, and the pen functioned properly. There is an insufficient amount for another dose, so discard the cartridge and needle safely. Store the pen for later use for this patient.

U-500 Insulin

Since its introduction to the market in 1997, the use of a concentrated form of insulin, U-500 insulin, has been on the rise. This may be due to the higher incidence of obesity in American society, the increased use of insulin pumps, and trends to maintain tighter glucose control in hospitalized patients. While the manufacture of a syringe to measure U-500 insulin has been recommended by safety experts, no special safety device is available as yet. The standard 1 mL syringe is used to measure U-500 insulin doses in the hospital. To be safe, physicians should prescribe the exact dosage and dose amount with the order. If you are unsure of the order, be sure to ask for clarification. Do not guess! U-500 insulin is concentrated and is five times as potent as U-100 insulin. **Dosage errors can be life threatening.** Always double-check calculations and preparation with two nurses.

EXAMPLE 1 ■

Order: **Humulin R regular U-500 insulin 140 units (0.28 mL) subcut stat**

Humulin R regular U-500 insulin differs in concentration from U-100 insulin, but both are short-acting insulins that have an effect within 30 minutes. For this example, your patient is a 56-year-old, 360-pound female who has been insulin dependent for most of her life. She has become increasingly resistant to insulin and now requires larger doses of insulin to meet her metabolic needs. She was admitted to the hospital due to uncontrolled hyperglycemia on U-100 insulin. This is the first time she has had U-500 insulin ordered. A supply of rapid-acting and short-acting insulins is stored in the automated dispensing cabinet (ADC) cubbies, as pictured in Figure 11-28. Apply the Three-Step Approach to this clinical situation.

FIGURE 11-28 Illustrated ADC matrix drawer with 10 mL multidose vials: (a) Humalog U-100; (b) Humulin R U-100; (c) Humulin R U-500

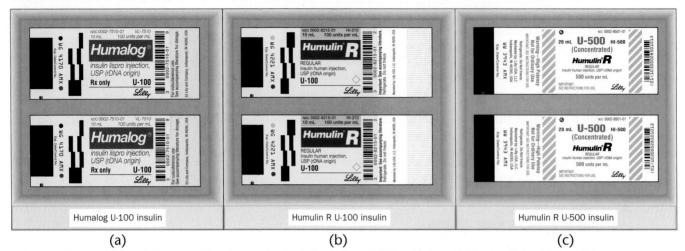

(a)	(b)	(c)
Humalog U-100 insulin	Humulin R U-100 insulin	Humulin R U-500 insulin

Step 1	**Convert**	No conversion needed. Order and supply for insulin will always be in units.
Step 2	**Think**	The prescriber has ordered U-500 insulin both in the dosage (units) and the volume (mL). This is a safe practice, but the nurse must verify that the ordered volume is correct before administration. You correctly choose the insulin in compartment (c). Remember that U-500 insulin is five times more concentrated than U-100 insulin. Consider first that U-100 insulin is very simple to calculate in mL because there are 100 units per 1 mL; therefore, 140 units of U-100 insulin would be more than 1 mL but less than 2 mL—actually, 1.4 mL. So 140 units of U-500 insulin would require $\frac{1}{5}$ of that amount, or approximately 0.3 mL. Because U-500 insulin is concentrated for 500 units/mL, 140 units of U-500 insulin is $\frac{140}{500}$, or less than $\frac{1}{2}$ of 1 mL—approximately 0.3 mL. Because a U-500 insulin syringe has not yet been manufactured, you will measure the U-500 insulin in a 1 mL syringe for an exact measurement.
Step 3	**Calculate**	Use ratio-proportion to determine the exact volume required.

$$\frac{500 \text{ units}}{1 \text{ mL}} \times \frac{140 \text{ units}}{X \text{ mL}} \qquad \text{Cross-multiply}$$

$$500X = 140$$

$$\frac{500X}{500} = \frac{140}{500} \qquad \text{Simplify: Divide both sides of the equation by the number before the unknown X.}$$

$$X = 0.28 \text{ mL} \qquad \text{Label the units to match the unknown X.}$$

Use a standard 1 mL syringe to draw up the dose of U-500 insulin. Prior to administration, provide the order, vial, and syringe to another nurse for independent verification.

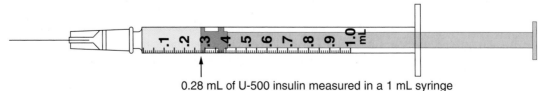

0.28 mL of U-500 insulin measured in a 1 mL syringe

EXAMPLE 2 ■

You need to provide discharge teaching for self-administration of U-500 insulin for your patient in the last example, who is going home. She was accustomed to using U-100 insulin and the standard U-100 syringe prior to admission to the hospital, having used them most of her adult life. Because there is currently no U-500 insulin syringe available on the market, patients requiring U-500 doses at home must be taught to self-administer with traditional U-100 insulin syringes designed for U-100 insulin, *even though many U-100 insulin syringes are still marked "USE U-100 ONLY" on the barrel*. The patient is very knowledgeable about daily glucose testing and adaptation of insulin dosage. Before considering discharge teaching for your patient, let's examine the standard 1 mL syringe and U-100 syringe side by side (Figure 11-29). As you can see, knowing that a U-100 insulin syringe has a direct relationship to the 1 mL syringe will be applicable to using the U-100 syringe for measuring U-500 insulin. Compare the syringes in Figure 11-29 to see how the U-100 and U-500 insulin syringe measurements compare to the measurements on a standard 1 mL syringe. Because U-500 insulin is five times more concentrated than U-100 insulin, the measurements on the U-100 syringe are equivalent to five times more U-500 insulin than U-100 insulin. This may be difficult for patients to comprehend and will necessitate extensive patient teaching and return demonstration prior to discharge. For patient safety, it is also wise to create a chart, such as the one shown in Figure 11-30, with various U-500 dosages and the comparable units as measured in a U-100 syringe.

FIGURE 11-29 Comparison of 1 mL and U-100 syringes: **(a)** Standard U-100 insulin syringe; **(b)** 1 mL syringe marked for U-100 insulin; **(c)** 1 mL syringe marked for U-500 insulin; **(d)** Standard U-100 syringe marked for U-500 insulin

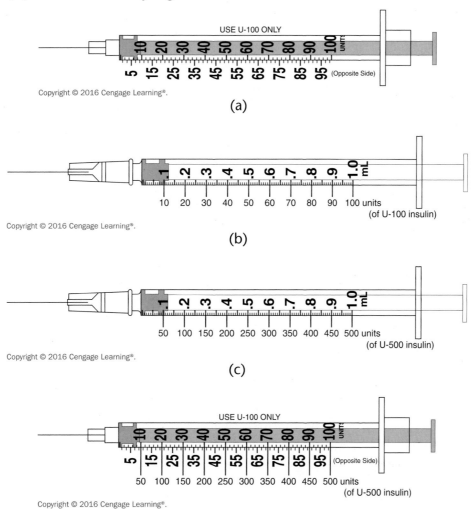

Step 1	**Convert**	No conversion needed. Order and supply for insulin will always be in units.
Step 2	**Think**	The patient needs to draw up U-500 insulin in a U-100 syringe. The U-500 insulin is five times more concentrated than U-100 insulin; therefore, the equivalent volume in a U-100 syringe will be $\frac{1}{5}$ the volume that the U-100 insulin would measure. 140 units $\times \frac{1}{5} = 28$ units

Step 3   **Calculate**

$$\frac{140 \text{ units}}{500 \text{ units}} \underset{\diagdown}{\overset{\diagup}{\diagup}} \frac{X \text{ units}}{100 \text{ units}}$$

$$500X = 14,000$$

$$\frac{500X}{500} = \frac{14,000}{500}$$

$$X = 28 \text{ unit mark on U-100 syringe} = 140 \text{ units of U-500}$$

The calculation verifies your estimate. Instruct the patient to draw up 140 units of U-500 insulin at the 28-unit mark on the U-100 insulin syringe.

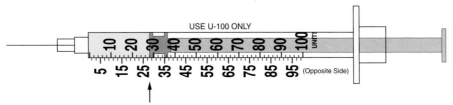

28-unit mark on the U-100 insulin syringe = 140 units (U-500)

Although your patient has been using the standard U-100 syringe, this is an opportune time to explain how this amount could also be measured in the Lo-Dose 50-unit and 30-unit syringes.

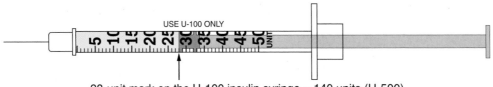

28-unit mark on the U-100 insulin syringe = 140 units (U-500)

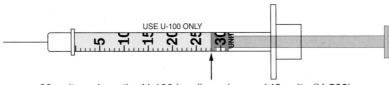

28-unit mark on the U-100 insulin syringe = 140 units (U-500)

Use the following rule to calculate U-500 insulin doses to measure in a U-100 insulin syringe or in a 1 mL syringe. Figure 11-30 provides a conversion table that is useful for patient teaching.

RULE

- Divide prescribed U-500 insulin dose (actual units) by 5 = Volume (unit) markings on a U-100 insulin syringe.

- Divide prescribed U-500 insulin dose (actual units) by 500 = Volume (mL) markings on a 1 mL syringe.

FIGURE 11-30 Conversion for U-500 insulin dose when measuring in a U-100 insulin syringe or a 1 mL syringe

U-500 Insulin (dose in units)	U-100 Insulin Syringe (volume in units)	1 mL Syringe (volume in mL)
25	5	0.05
50	10	0.1
75	15	0.15
100	20	0.2
125	25	0.25
150	30	0.3
175	35	0.35
200	40	0.4
225	45	0.45
250	50	0.5
275	55	0.55
300	60	0.6
325	65	0.65
350	70	0.7
375	75	0.75
400	80	0.8
425	85	0.85
450	90	0.9
475	95	0.95
500	100	1
Dose (U-500 units)	Calculation: Divide dose (U-500 units) by 5	Calculation: Divide dose (U-500 units) by 500

Avoiding Insulin Dosage Errors

Insulin dosage errors are costly and, unfortunately, too common. They can be avoided by following two important rules.

RULE

1. Insulin dosages must be checked by two nurses. To be considered an independent verification, the check by the second nurse must occur away from the first nurse, with no prior knowledge of the first nurse's calculations.

2. When combination dosages are prepared, two nurses must verify each step of the process.

QUICK REVIEW

- Carefully read the physician's order, and match the supply dosage for type, brand, and concentration of insulin.

- Always measure U-100 insulin in a U-100 insulin syringe.

- An insulin syringe is used *only* to measure U-100 insulin. Insulin syringes must not be used to measure other medications measured in units or U-500 insulin preparations, except by patients who self-medicate with U-500 insulin in the home setting.

- Use the smallest-capacity U-100 insulin syringe possible to most accurately measure U-100 insulin doses.

- When drawing up combination insulin doses, think *clear first, then cloudy.*

- Do not mix long-acting insulin with any other insulin or solution.

- Avoid insulin dosage errors. Obtain independent verification by a second nurse.

- There are 100 units per mL for U-100 insulin.

- There are 500 units per mL for U-500 insulin.

- In the hospital, measure U-500 insulin in a 1 mL syringe after careful dosage calculation.

- Be prepared to teach a patient how to measure U-500 insulin with a U-100 insulin syringe at home.

Review Set 25

Questions 1 through 4: For each of the following heparin labels, match the letter(s) of the concentration of the supply dosage with the most appropriate use. Select all that apply.

1. Flush IV locks to maintain patency _____

2. IV bolus to treat thrombosis _____

3. Prepare IV PB bag for continuous infusion to treat thrombosis _____

4. Subcutaneous injection to prevent thrombosis _____

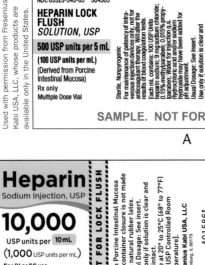

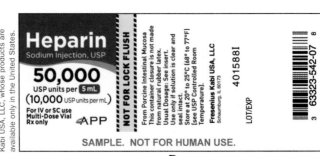

For questions 5 through 10, look at the insulin label and identify:

- Brand name
- Generic name
- Action time (rapid acting, short acting, intermediate acting, or long acting)
- Concentration in units per mL
- Syringe you would select to measure a prescribed dosage

5. Brand name   _____

   Generic name   _____

   Action time   _____

   Concentration   _____

   Syringe   _____

6. Brand name   _____

   Generic name   _____

   Action time   _____

   Concentration   _____

   Syringe   _____

7. Brand name   _____

   Generic name   _____

   Action time   _____

   Concentration   _____

   Syringe   _____

8. Brand name   _____

   Generic name   _____

   Action time   _____

   Concentration   _____

   Syringe   _____

9. Brand name   _____

   Generic name   _____

   Action time   _____

   Concentration   _____

   Syringe   _____

Label 5 (Humulin R):

NDC 0002-8215-01   HI-210
10 mL   100 units per mL

Humulin® R

REGULAR
insulin human injection,
USP (rDNA origin)
U-100

Lilly

Important: See accompanying literature.
Refrigerate. Do not freeze.
Marketed by: Lilly USA, LLC, Indianapolis, IN 46285, USA

Label 6 (Novolin N):

U-100   NDC 0169-1834-11
10 mL   100 units/mL

Novolin® **N**

NPH, Human Insulin
Isophane Suspension
(recombinant
DNA origin)

Novo Nordisk®
• Important: see insert
• To mix, shake carefully
• Keep in a cold place
• Avoid freezing

Novo Nordisk Inc.
Princeton, NJ 08540
1-800-727-6500
Manufactured by
Novo Nordisk A/S
DK-2880 Bagsvaerd
Denmark

Label 7 (NovoLog):

NovoLog®   NDC 0169-7501-11
List 750111

Insulin aspart Injection
(rDNA origin)

10 mL 100 units/mL (U-100)
Important: see insert
Keep in a cold place
Avoid freezing.
Rx only

Novo Nordisk Inc.
Princeton, NJ 08540
1-800-727-6500

Manufactured by
Novo Nordisk A/S
DK-2880 Bagsvaerd, Denmark

Label 8 (Humalog):

NDC 0002-7510-01   VL-7510
10 mL   100 units per mL

Humalog®

insulin lispro injection,
USP (rDNA origin)
Rx only   **U-100**

Lilly

For subcutaneous use.
See accompanying literature for dosage.
Eli Lilly and Company, Indianapolis, IN 46285, USA

Label 9 (Humulin R U-500):

℞   NDC 0002-8501-01

20 mL   **U-500**   HI-500
(Concentrated)

Humulin® R
REGULAR
insulin human injection, USP (rDNA origin)
500 units per mL

Lilly

Warning—High Potency
Not for Ordinary Use
IMPORTANT: SEE INSTRUCTIONS FOR USE.
Refrigerate. Do Not freeze.
Marketed by: Lilly USA, LLC
Indianapolis, IN 46285, USA

IMPORTANT:
SEE INSTRUCTIONS FOR USE.

10. Brand name _____

    Generic name _____

    Action time _____

    Concentration _____

    Syringe _____

U.S. Patents 5,656,722; 5,370,629; 5,509,905
Mfd by: **Aventis Pharma Deutschland GmbH**
D-65926 Frankfurt am Main Frankfurt, Germany
Mfd for: **Aventis Pharmaceuticals Inc.**
Kansas City, MO 64137
Made in Germany
©2003
www.aventis-us.com
50070004

NDC 0088-2220-33

Lantus®
insulin glargine (rDNA origin) injection
100units/mL
(U-100)

DO NOT MIX WITH OTHER INSULINS
USE ONLY IF SOLUTION IS CLEAR AND COLORLESS WITH NO PARTICLES VISIBLE
FOR SUBCUTANEOUS INJECTION ONLY
USE WITH U-100 SYRINGE ONLY

One 10mL Vial
✚*Aventis*

3 0088-2220-33 7

11. Describe the three syringes available to measure U-100 insulin. _____

    _____

12. What would be your preferred syringe choice to measure 35 units of U-100 insulin?

    _____

13. There are 60 units of U-100 insulin per _____ mL.

14. There are 125 units of U-500 insulin per _____ mL.

15. True or False? The 50-unit Lo-Dose U-100 insulin syringe is intended to measure U-50 insulin only. _____

Questions 16 through 18: Referring to the labels provided for each question, identify the heparin dosage indicated by the colored area of the syringe.

16. _____ units of heparin

NDC 63323-017-10   1710

HEPFLUSH®-10
(HEPARIN LOCK FLUSH SOLUTION, USP)
100 USP units per 10 mL
(10 USP units per mL)
(Derived from Porcine Intestinal Mucosa)
Rx only
Single Dose Vial

Sterile, Nonpyrogenic
Preservative Free
Discard unused portion.
For maintenance of patency of intravenous injection devices only, not for anticoagulant therapy. May alter the results of blood coagulation tests. Each mL contains: 10 USP Units heparin sodium; 9 mg sodium chloride; Water for Injection q.s. Hydrochloric acid and/or sodium hydroxide may have been added for pH adjustment.
Usual Dosage: See insert.
Use only if solution is clear and seal intact.
Store at 20° to 25°C (68° to 77°F) [see USP Controlled Room Temperature].
Fresenius Kabi USA, LLC
Schaumburg, IL 60173

401889E

LOT/EXP

3 63323-017-10 1

SAMPLE. NOT FOR HUMAN USE.

2 mL

17. _____ units of heparin

Heparin
Sodium Injection, USP
50,000
USP units per [5 mL]
(**10,000** USP units per mL)
For IV or SC use
Multi-Dose Vial
Rx only
◄APP

NOT FOR LOCK FLUSH

From Porcine Intestinal Mucosa
This container closure is not made from natural rubber latex.
Usual Dosage: See insert.
Use only if solution is clear and seal intact.
Store at 20° to 25°C (68° to 77°F) [see USP Controlled Room Temperature].
Fresenius Kabi USA, LLC
Schaumburg, IL 60173

401588I

LOT/EXP

3 63323-542-07 8

SAMPLE. NOT FOR HUMAN USE.

3 mL

18. _____ units of heparin

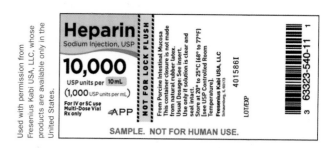

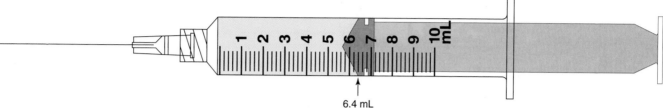

6.4 mL

Questions 19 through 22: You are asked to provide independent verification for high-alert drug dosages. As shown, your nurse colleague provides you with the drug order, labeled vial used to prepare the dosage, and the syringe filled with the dose amount. Determine if the drug drawn up is the correct dosage.

19. Order: Lantus U-100 insulin 67 units subcut daily at 0900

Correct dosage? Yes _____ No _____

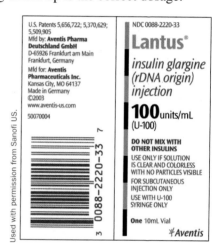

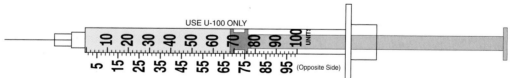

20. Order: Humulin-R regular U-100 insulin 15 units subcut stat

Correct dosage? Yes _____
No _____

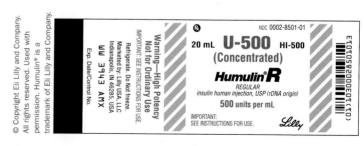

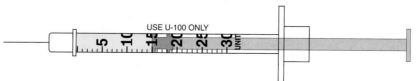

21. Order: Humulin 70/30 U-100 insulin
    23 units subcut daily at 0800

    Correct dosage? Yes _____

    No _____

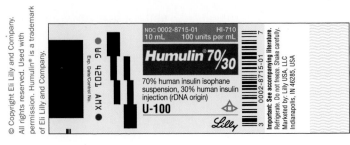

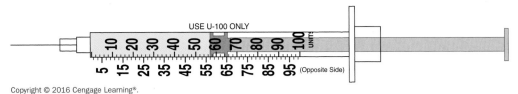

22. Order: Levemir U-100 insulin 57 units subcut
    daily at 0800

    Correct dosage? Yes _____

    No _____

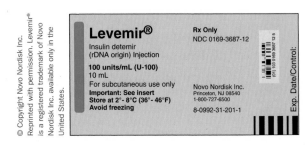

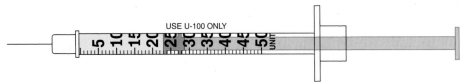

Questions 23 through 29: Draw an arrow on the syringe to identify the ordered dosages.

23. Order: heparin 7,200 units IV bolus
    stat prior to initiation of continuous
    heparin infusion

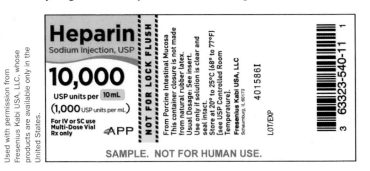

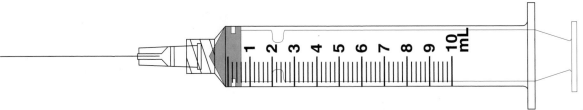

24. Order: heparin 4,000 units subcut 2 h
    prior to surgery

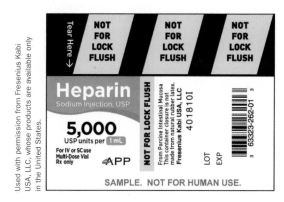

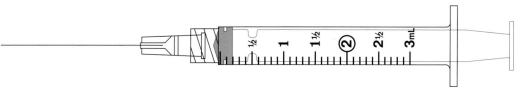

25. Order: D₅W 500 mL IV PB c̄ heparin
    50,000 units

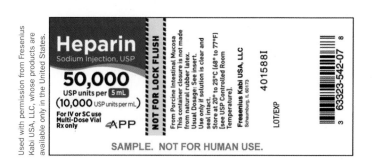

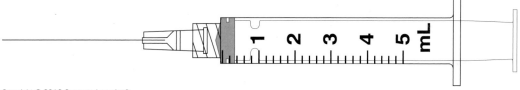

26. Order: Lantus U-100 insulin 66 units subcut daily at 0900

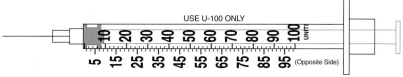

27. Order: Humalog U-100 insulin 16 units subcut stat

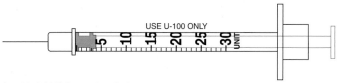

28. Order: Humulin R regular U-500 insulin 200 units subcut stat

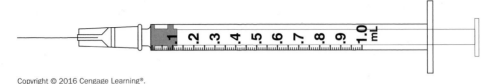

29. Order: Humulin R regular U-500 insulin 180 units subcut stat (for discharge teaching patient about home self-administration only)

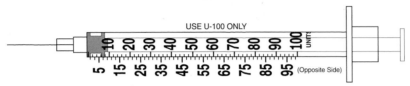

Questions 30–33: Draw arrows and label the dosage for each of the combination insulin orders to be measured in the same syringe. Label and measure the insulins in the correct order, indicating which insulin will be drawn up first.

30. Order: Novolin R regular U-100 insulin 21 units with Novolin N NPH U-100 insulin 15 units subcut stat

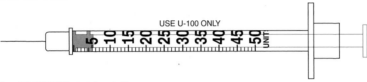

31. Order: Humulin R regular U-100 insulin 16 units with Humulin N NPH U-100 insulin 42 units subcut stat

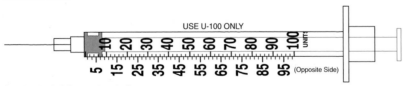

32. Order: Humulin R regular U-100 insulin 32 units with Humulin N NPH U-100 insulin 40 units subcut ā dinner

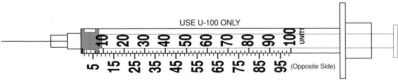

33. Order: Humulin R regular U-100 insulin 8 units with Humulin N NPH U-100 insulin 12 units subcut stat

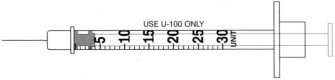

Questions 34 and 35: Identify the dose of insulin displayed in the dose window of the insulin pen.

34. _____ units of insulin

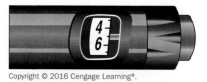

Copyright © 2016 Cengage Learning®.

35. _____ units of insulin

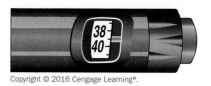

Copyright © 2016 Cengage Learning®.

Use the following medication order and insulin sliding scale to answer questions 36 through 40.

Order: insulin glulisine (Apidra) U-100 insulin subcut a.c. per sliding scale.

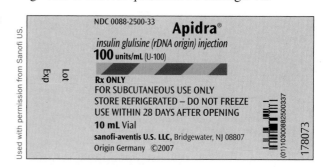

INSULIN SLIDING SCALE

Insulin Dose	Glucose Reading (mg/dL)*
No coverage	Glucose less than 160
2 units	160 to 220
4 units	221 to 280
6 units	281 to 340
8 units	341 to 400

*Glucose greater than 400: Hold insulin; call MD stat.

36. When will you check the patient's blood glucose level to determine the amount of insulin to give?

_____

37. At what range of blood glucose levels will you administer insulin? _____

38. The patient's blood glucose level before breakfast is 250 mg/dL. What should you do? _____

_____

39. The patient's blood glucose level before lunch is 150 mg/dL. How much insulin should you give now?

_____

40. The patient's blood glucose level before dinner is 410 mg/dL. What should you do now?

_____

After completing these problems, see pages 667–669 to check your answers.

SUMMARY

You are now prepared to solve many of the dosage calculations you will encounter in your health care career. Oral and parenteral drug orders, written in the forms presented thus far, account for a large percentage of prescriptions. You are aware that high-alert drugs account for a high percentage of drug errors and that extreme caution is required. You have learned to think through the process from order, to supply, to amount administered, and to apply the Three-Step Approach and the ratio-proportion method:

$$\frac{\text{Dosage on hand}}{\text{Amount on hand}} = \frac{\text{Dosage desired}}{\text{X Amount desired}}$$

Work the practice problems for Chapter 11. After completing the practice problems, you should feel comfortable and confident working dosage calculations. If not, seek additional instruction. Concentrate on accuracy. Remember: One error in dosage calculation can be a serious risk to your patient.

CLINICAL REASONING SKILLS

Although many parenteral medication solutions are supplied in unit-dose vials or ampules with concentrations based on the dosage per 1 mL, some multidose vials have 2 mL, 10 mL, or another total container volume as the quantity. Failing to identify the quantity of the supplied medication will result in an incorrect dose.

ERROR

Making the assumption that the dosage of the supplied medication was provided in a supply of 1 mL and failing to identify the correct volume to use as the *quantity* in the dosage calculation ratio-proportion

Possible Scenario

A patient experienced nausea and vomiting following abdominal surgery. The doctor ordered *droperidol 0.5 mg IV slow push q.4h p.r.n., nausea and vomiting.* The nurse selected the correct medication from the stock supply and set up and calculated the dosage calculation formula as follows.

Used with permission from Akorn, Inc.

NDC 11098-010-02   2 mL ampoule

INAPSINE®

(DROPERIDOL) INJECTION

5 mg/2 mL (2.5 mg/mL)

TAYLOR
PHARMACEUTICALS
Decatur, IL 62522
ADPADL   Rev. 3/00
LOT
EXP.

$$\frac{5 \text{ mg}}{1 \text{ mL}} \times \frac{0.5 \text{ mg}}{\text{X mL}}$$

$$5X = 0.5$$

$$\frac{5X}{5} = \frac{0.5}{5}$$

$$X = 0.1 \text{ mL} \qquad \textbf{INCORRECT}$$

Assuming the supplied concentration was 5 mg per mL, the nurse incorrectly set up the first ratio as $\frac{5 \text{ mg}}{1 \text{ mL}}$. The 2 mL single-dose ampule was actually labeled in large letters as 5 mg/2 mL and in smaller letters (2.5 mg/mL). The dose the nurse administered was 0.1 mL. The **correct** calculation should have been either of the following.

$$\frac{5 \text{ mg}}{2 \text{ mL}} \times \frac{0.5 \text{ mg}}{\text{X mL}}$$

$$5X = 1$$

$$\frac{5X}{5} = \frac{1}{5}$$

$$X = 0.2 \text{ mL}$$

or

$$\frac{2.5 \text{ mg}}{1 \text{ mL}} \times \frac{0.5 \text{ mg}}{\text{X mL}}$$

$$2.5X = 0.5$$

$$\frac{2.5X}{2.5} = \frac{0.5}{2.5}$$

$$X = 0.2 \text{ mL} \qquad \textbf{CORRECT}$$

The correct amount to be administered was 0.2 mL. The patient received half the ordered dose. The patient stopped vomiting but continued with a significant amount of nausea. The nurse medicated the patient again as soon as the p.r.n. medication was due, but the patient experienced unnecessary discomfort in the meantime.

Potential Outcome

The nurse may have picked up the error the next time the medication was administered, but chances are that the same mistake would be repeated. The patient might again not have adequate relief of nausea and remain in significant discomfort. Not realizing that the patient received an incorrect dose, the nurse might contact the physician to increase the ordered dose for this patient. When the next nurse assigned to this patient calculated the correct volume of the increased dose, the patient could then be given a dose that was considerably higher than administered previously. With the higher dose, possibly ordered unnecessarily, the patient would be at greater risk for side effects and adverse reactions, such as increased sedation, hypotension, or tachycardia.

Prevention

The supply concentration always involves two values used in the first ratio—the dosage strength expressed as the weight of the drug per a certain volume or capacity amount, in this case 5 mg per 2 mL or 2.5 mg/mL. Carefully read the label to be sure you understand and copy down the correct supply dosage when setting up the proportion. Although drug labels often express the dosage strength of the drug as per 1 mL, do not assume that this is the case. Always read the label for the exact supply dosage strength or concentration.

CLINICAL REASONING SKILLS

Many insulin errors occur when the nurse fails to clarify an incomplete order. Let's look at an example of an insulin error when the order did not include the type of insulin to be given.

ERROR

Failing to clarify an insulin order when the type of insulin is not specified

Possible Scenario

Suppose the physician who intended for a patient to receive NPH U-100 insulin wrote an insulin order this way:

| Humulin U-100 insulin 50 units subcut a.c. breakfast | **INCORRECT** |

Because the physician did not specify the type of insulin, the nurse assumed it was regular insulin and noted that on the medication administration record. Suppose the patient was given the regular U-100 insulin instead of the insulin intended by the physician. Several hours later, the patient develops signs of hypoglycemia (low blood glucose), including shakiness, tremors, confusion, and sweating.

| Humulin U-100 NPH insulin 50 units subcut a.c. breakfast | **CORRECT** |

Potential Outcome

A stat blood glucose would likely reveal a dangerously low glucose level. The patient would be given a glucose infusion to increase the blood sugar. The nurse may not realize the error until she and the doctor check the original order and find that the incomplete order was filled in by the nurse. When the doctor did not specify the type of insulin, the nurse assumed that the physician meant regular, which is short acting, when in fact intermediate-acting NPH insulin was desired.

Prevention

This error could have been avoided by remembering all the essential components of an insulin order: brand or generic name, type of insulin (such as regular or NPH), supply dosage, the amount to give in units, and the frequency. When you fill in an incomplete order, you are essentially practicing medicine without a license. This would be a clear malpractice incident. It does not make sense to put yourself and your patient in such jeopardy. A simple phone call would clarify the situation for everyone involved. Further, the nurse should have double-checked the dosage with another licensed practitioner. Had the nurse done so, the error could have been discovered prior to administration.

PRACTICE PROBLEMS—CHAPTER 11

Calculate the amount you will prepare for 1 dose. Indicate the syringe you will select to measure the medication.

1. Order: hydromorphone (Dilaudid) 4 mg slow IV push (over 10 min) q.4h p.r.n., severe pain

   Supply: hydromorphone 10 mg/mL

   Give: _____ mL   Select: _____ syringe

2. Order: morphine sulfate 15 mg slow IV push (over 5 min) stat

   Supply: morphine sulfate 10 mg/mL

   Give: _____ mL   Select: _____ syringe

3. Order: digoxin 0.6 mg slow IV push stat

   Supply: digoxin 500 mcg per 2 mL

   Give: _____ mL   Select: _____ syringe

4. Order: hydroxyzine 15 mg IM stat

   Supply: hydroxyzine 25 mg/mL

   Give: _____ mL   Select: _____ syringe

5. Order: clindamycin 300 mg IV PB q.i.d.

   Supply: clindamycin 0.6 g per 4 mL

   Give: _____ mL   Select: _____ syringe

6. Order: metoclopramide 50 mg added to 50 mL IV PB bag as one-time order to infuse over 30 min

   Supply: 30 mL single-dose vial metoclopramide 5 mg/mL

   Give: _____ mL   Select: _____ syringe

7. Order: hydroxyzine 40 mg IM q.4h p.r.n., agitation

   Supply: hydroxyzine 50 mg/mL

   Give: _____ mL   Select: _____ syringe

8. Order: **diazepam 5 mg IV q.4h p.r.n., agitation**

   Supply: diazepam 10 mg per 2 mL

   Give: _____ mL   Select: _____ syringe

9. Order: **glycopyrrolate 200 mcg IM 60 min pre-op**

   Supply: glycopyrrolate 0.2 mg/mL

   Give: _____ mL   Select: _____ syringe

10. Order: **phenytoin 280 mg IV q.8h**

    Supply: phenytoin 100 mg per 2 mL ampule

    Give: _____ mL   Select: _____ syringe

11. Order: **atropine 0.6 mg IM on call to O.R.**

    Supply: atropine 0.4 mg/mL

    Give: _____ mL   Select: _____ syringe

12. Order: **diazepam 3 mg IV stat**

    Supply: diazepam 10 mg per 2 mL

    Give: _____ mL   Select: _____ syringe

13. Order: **heparin 6,000 units subcut q.12h**

    Supply: heparin 10,000 units/mL vial

    Give: _____ mL   Select: _____ syringe

14. Order: **tobramycin sulfate 75 mg IV PB q.8h**

    Supply: tobramycin sulfate 40 mg/mL

    Give: _____ mL   Select: _____ syringe

15. Order: **morphine sulfate 6 mg slow IV push q.3h p.r.n., severe pain**

    Supply: morphine sulfate 10 mg/mL ampule

    Give: _____ mL   Select: _____ syringe

16. Order: **atropine 0.3 mg IM on call to O.R.**

    Supply: atropine 0.4 mg/mL

    Give: _____ mL   Select: _____ syringe

17. Order: **ketorolac 20 mg IV q.6h p.r.n., severe pain**

    Supply: ketorolac 30 mg/mL

    Give: _____ mL   Select: _____ syringe

18. Order: **gentamicin 40 mg IV q.8h**

    Supply: gentamicin 80 mg per 2 mL

    Give: _____ mL   Select: _____ syringe

19. Order: **hydromorphone 3 mg slow IV push (over 5–10 min) q.4h p.r.n., severe pain**

    Supply: hydromorphone 10 mg/mL

    Give: _____ mL   Select: _____ syringe

20. Order: **morphine sulfate 8 mg slow IV push q.4h p.r.n., severe pain**

    Supply: morphine sulfate 5 mg/mL

    Give: _____ mL   Select: _____ syringe

21. Order: **vitamin B$_{12}$ 0.75 mg IM daily**

    Supply: vitamin B$_{12}$ 1,000 mcg/mL

    Give: _____ mL   Select: _____ syringe

22. Order: **phytonadione 5 mg IM stat**

    Supply: phytonadione 10 mg/mL

    Give: _____ mL   Select: _____ syringe

23. Order: **promethazine 35 mg IM q.4h p.r.n., nausea and vomiting**

    Supply: promethazine 50 mg/mL

    Give: _____ mL   Select: _____ syringe

24. Order: **heparin 8,000 units subcut stat**

    Supply: heparin 10,000 units/mL

    Give: _____ mL   Select: _____ syringe

25. Order: **morphine sulfate 10 mg subcut q.4h p.r.n., severe pain**

    Supply: morphine sulfate 8 mg/mL

    Give: _____ mL   Select: _____ syringe

26. Order: **digoxin 0.4 mg IV stat**

    Supply: digoxin 500 mcg per 2 mL

    Give: _____ mL   Select: _____ syringe

27. Order: **furosemide 60 mg slow IV push (over 3 min) stat**

    Supply: furosemide 20 mg per 2 mL ampule

    Give: _____ mL   Select: _____ syringe

28. Order: **heparin 4,000 units subcut q.6h**

    Supply: heparin 5,000 units/mL

    Give: _____ mL   Select: _____ syringe

29. Order: **hydralazine 30 mg IV q.6h**

    Supply: hydralazine 20 mg/mL

    Give: _____ mL   Select: _____ syringe

30. Order: **verapamil 4 mg slow IV push (over 2 min) stat**

    Supply: verapamil 2.5 mg/mL

    Give: _____ mL   Select: _____ syringe

31. Order: **heparin 3,500 units subcut q.12h**

    Supply: heparin 5,000 units/mL

    Give: _____ mL   Select: _____ syringe

32. Order: **neostigmine 0.5 mg IM stat**

    Supply: 1 mg/mL

    Give: _____ mL   Select: _____ syringe

33. Order: **ciprofloxacin 100 mg added to 50 mL IV PB q.12h**

    Supply: ciprofloxacin 400 mg per 40 mL

    Give: _____ mL   Select: _____ syringe

34. Order: *Novolin R regular U-100 insulin 16 units subcut a.c.*

    Supply: Novolin R regular U-100 insulin, with standard 100-unit and Lo-Dose 30-unit U-100 insulin syringes

    Give: _____ units   Select: _____ syringe

35. Order: *Novolin N NPH U-100 insulin 25 units subcut ā breakfast*

    Supply: Novolin N NPH U-100 insulin with standard 100-unit and Lo-Dose 50-unit U-100 insulin syringes

    Give: _____ units   Select: _____ syringe

36. Order: *heparin 5,800 units IV bolus ASAP prior to initiation of continuous heparin infusion*

    Supply: heparin 1,000 units/mL 10 mL multidose vial

    Give: _____ mL   Select: _____ syringe

Calculate 1 dose of each of the drug orders numbered 37 through 48. Draw an arrow on the syringe indicating the calibration line that corresponds to the dose to be administered. Identify the letter of the medication label selected. The labels provided on pages 334–335 are the medications you have available. Indicate dosages that must be divided.

37. Order: *haloperidol decanoate 150 mg IM monthly*

    Give: _____ mL   Label: _____

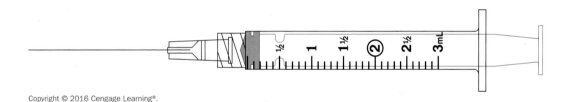

38. Order: *gentamicin 50 mg IV q.8h*

    Give: _____ mL   Label: _____

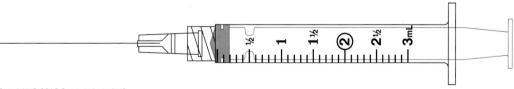

39. Order: *droperidol 1 mg IV stat*

    Give: _____ mL   Label: _____

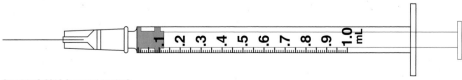

40. Order: **famotidine 15 mg IV stat**

Give: _____ mL   Label: _____

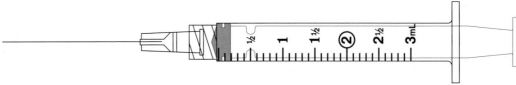

41. Order: **naloxone 0.2 mg IV stat**

Give: _____ mL   Label: _____

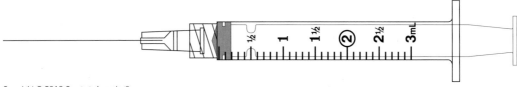

42. Order: **Humulin R regular U-100 insulin 22 units subcut stat**

Give: _____ units   Label: _____

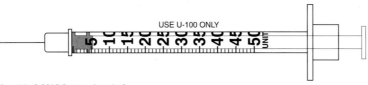

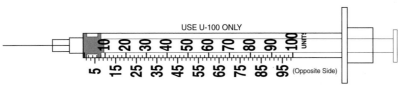

43. Order: **ketorolac 24 mg IV q.6h p.r.n., pain**

Give: _____ mL   Label: _____

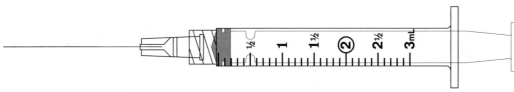

44. Order: **promethazine 15 mg IM q.4h p.r.n., nausea and vomiting**

    Give: _____ mL   Label: _____

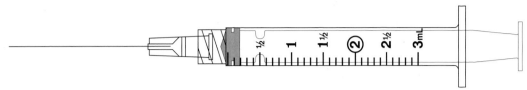

45. Order: **diltiazem 25 mg slow IV push (over 2 min) stat**

    Give: _____ mL   Label: _____

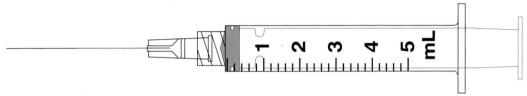

46. Order: **digoxin 0.125 mg IV daily × 7 days**

    Give: _____ mL   Label: _____

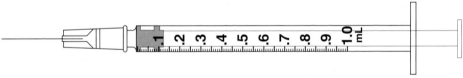

47. Order: **Novolin R regular U-100 insulin 32 units with Novolin N NPH U-100 insulin 54 units subcut ā breakfast**

    Give: _____ total units   Labels: _____

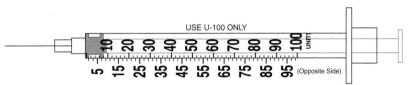

48. Order: **Novolin 70/30 U-100 insulin 46 units subcut ā dinner**

    Give: _____ units   Label: _____

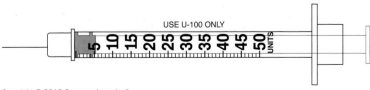

FAMOTIDINE INJECTION

20 mg/2 mL

Rx ONLY

NDC 55390-029-10

2 mL Single dose vial

FOR INTRAVENOUS USE ONLY AFTER DILUTION.

USUAL DOSAGE: See package insert.

Store at 2° to 8°C (36° to 46°F).

Manufactured for:
Bedford Laboratories™
Bedford, OH 44146   FAM-V03

A

NDC 63323-010-02   1002

GENTAMICIN

INJECTION, USP

equivalent to 40 mg/mL Gentamicin

80 mg/2 mL

For IM or IV Use.
Must be diluted for IV use.

2 mL Multiple Dose Vial

Sterile   Rx only

APP Pharmaceuticals, LLC
Schaumburg, IL 60173

401896D

LOT/EXP

63323-010-02

SAMPLE. NOT FOR HUMAN USE.

B

KETOROLAC
TROMETHAMINE
INJECTION USP

30 mg/mL
1 mL Vial

FOR IM OR IV USE ONLY

NDC 55390-481-01

1 mL Single-dose Vial

Protect from light.

Rx ONLY

Manufactured for:
Bedford Laboratories™
Bedford, OH 44146

KC-KRLVA03

C

Exp. Date/Control:

U-100   NDC 0169-1833-11

10 mL   100 units/mL

Novolin® R

Regular, Human Insulin Injection (recombinant DNA origin) USP

Novo Nordisk®
• **Important:** see insert
• Keep in a cold place
• Avoid freezing

Novo Nordisk Inc.
Princeton, NJ 08540
1-800-727-6500
Manufactured by
Novo Nordisk A/S
DK-2880 Bagsvaerd
Denmark

D

Exp. Date/Control:

U-100   NDC 0169-1837-11

10 mL   100 units/mL

Novolin® 70/30

70% NPH, Human Insulin Isophane Suspension and 30% Regular, Human Insulin Injection (recombinant DNA origin)

Novo Nordisk®
• **Important:** see insert
• To mix, shake carefully
• Keep in a cold place
• Avoid freezing

Novo Nordisk Inc.
Princeton, NJ 08540
1-800-727-6500
Manufactured by
Novo Nordisk A/S
DK-2880 Bagsvaerd
Denmark

E

NDC 0703-7021-03   Rx only

Haloperidol
Decanoate Injection

100 mg*/mL

***as haloperidol**

IM Use Only
1 mL Vial
Sterile
10 Vials

TEVA

*Each mL haloperidol decanoate injection, 100 mg/mL contains 141.04 mg haloperidol decanoate USP, equivalent to 100 mg haloperidol in a sesame oil vehicle, with 1.2% (w/v) benzyl alcohol as a preservative. **For Intramuscular Use Only.**
Usual Dosage: See package insert for full prescribing information.
The dose of haloperidol decanoate should be expressed in terms of its haloperidol content.
Store at 20° to 25°C (68° to 77°F)
[See USP Controlled Room Temperature].
Do not refrigerate or freeze.
PROTECT FROM LIGHT.
Retain in carton until contents are used.
Teva Pharmaceuticals USA
Sellersville, PA 18960   Rev. A 10/2011

Y10686

F

NDC 0703-2191-04   Rx only

Promethazine
Hydrochloride
Injection, USP

25 mg/mL

FOR DEEP INTRAMUSCULAR OR INTRAVENOUS USE

1 mL Single Dose Vials
25 Vials

TEVA

Each mL contains: Promethazine hydrochloride 25 mg, edetate disodium 0.1 mg, calcium chloride 0.04 mg, sodium metabisulfite 0.25 mg and phenol 5 mg in water for injection. pH 4.0–5.5; buffered with acetic acid-sodium acetate. Sealed under nitrogen.
Usual Dosage: See Package Insert.
PROTECT FROM LIGHT: Keep covered in carton until time of use.
Store at room temperature 20°–25°C (68°–77°F) [See USP Controlled Room Temperature].
Teva Pharmaceuticals USA
Sellersville, PA 18960
Rev. A 11/2011

Y10765

G

NDC 11098-010-01

INAPSINE®

(DROPERIDOL)
INJECTION

1 mL ampoule

2.5 mg/mL

TAYLOR
PHARMACEUTICALS
Decatur, IL 62522

ADPABL   Rev. 7/98

LOT

EXP.

H

Exp. Date/Control No.

NDC 0002-8215-01   HI-210

10 mL   100 units per mL

Humulin® R

REGULAR
insulin human injection,
USP (rDNA origin)

U-100

Important: See accompanying literature.
Refrigerate. Do not freeze.

Marketed by Lilly USA, LLC, Indianapolis, IN 46285, USA

Lilly

I

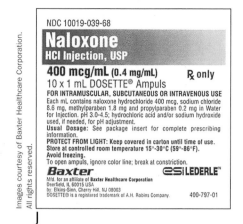

J

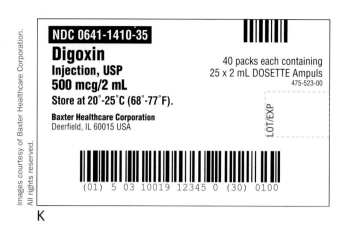

K

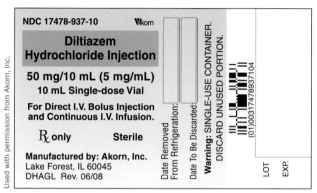

L

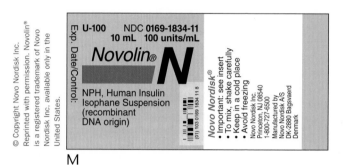

M

49. Describe the strategy you would implement to prevent this medication error.

Possible Scenario

Suppose the physician ordered Humulin R regular U-100 insulin 40 units c̄ Humulin N NPH U-100 insulin 20 units subcut a.c. breakfast. The nurse selected the vials of Humulin R and Humulin N U-100 insulin from the medication drawer and injected 40 units of air in the Humulin N vial and 20 units of air in the Humulin R vial, drew up 20 units of Humulin R, and then drew up 40 units of Humulin N.

Potential Outcome

The patient received the incorrect dosage of insulin because the nurse drew up 20 units of Humulin R and 40 units of Humulin N instead of the dosage that was ordered: 40 units of Humulin R and 20 units of Humulin N. Because the patient received too little short-acting insulin (one-half the amount ordered), the patient would likely show signs of hyperglycemia, such as urinary frequency, thirst, and potential visual changes. Not only would this patient feel uncomfortable at the time of the hyperglycemia, it would also be more difficult for the physician to get control of the patient's blood glucose levels in the future. Also, the increased dose of NPH insulin may put the patient at risk for hypoglycemia later in the day, and a high blood glucose level could increase the risk of infection.

Prevention

_____

_____

50. Describe the clinical reasoning you would use to prevent this medication error.

Possible Scenario

Suppose the physician ordered Novolog U-100 insulin 10 units subcut stat for a patient with a blood glucose of 300 mg/dL. The nurse selected the Novolog U-100 insulin from the patient's medication drawer and selected a 1 mL syringe to administer the dose. The nurse looked at the syringe for the

10-unit mark and was confused as to how much should be drawn up. The nurse finally decided to draw up 1 mL of insulin into the syringe, administered the dose, and then began to question whether the correct dosage was administered. The nurse called the supervisor for advice.

Potential Outcome

The patient would have received 10 times the correct dosage of insulin. Because this was a short-acting insulin, the patient would likely show signs of severe hypoglycemia, such as loss of consciousness, seizures, myocardial infarction, and potential death. There is substantial risk of harm for this patient.

Prevention

_____

_____

After completing these problems, see pages 669–672 to check your answers.

Be sure to use the online software for additional practice!

REFERENCES

American Diabetes Association. (2013). Standards of medical care in diabetes—2013. *Diabetes Care, 36,* Suppl 1S11-S66. doi:10.2337/dc13-S011

Cohen, H. (2007). Protecting patients from harm: Reduce the risk of high alert drugs. *Nursing 2007,* September 2007, 49–55.

Grissinger, M. (2010). Avoiding medication errors with insulin therapy. Recorded Program. Retrieved from http://www.schererclin.com/documents/scherer_avoiding_med_errors.pdf

Hahn, K. (2007). The top ten drug errors and how to prevent them. *Medscape Nurses Education.* Retrieved from http://www.medscape.org/viewarticle/556487

Institute for Safe Medication Practices. (2011). Key definitions for purposes of the 2011 ISMP medication safety self assessment for hospitals. Retrieved from http://www.ismp.org/selfassessments/Hospital/2011/definitions.pdf

Institute for Safe Medication Practices. (2013a). Important change with heparin labels. Retrieved from http://www.ismp.org/NAN/files/NAN-20130610.pdf

Institute for Safe Medication Practices. (2013b). ISMP *Medication Safety Alert,* Ongoing concern about insulin pen reuse shows hospitals need to consider transitioning away from them. Retrieved from http://www.ismp.org/newsletters/acutecare/showarticle.aspx?id=41

McCulloch, D. (2008). General principles of insulin therapy in diabetes mellitus. *Up to Date.* Section Editor: Nathan, D. Deputy Editor: Mulder, J. Last updated April 8, 2011; last literature review version 19.2, May 2011. Retrieved from http://www.uptodate.com/contents/general-principles-of-insulin-therapy-in-diabetes-mellitus?source=search_result&selectedTitle=1%7E150

Onufer, C. (2002). Could you be in danger? Insulin. The #1 drug error in hospitals. *Diabetes Health.* Retrieved from http://www.diabeteshealth.com/read/2002/11/01/3039/could-u-be-in-danger-insulin—the-1-drug-error-in-hospitals/

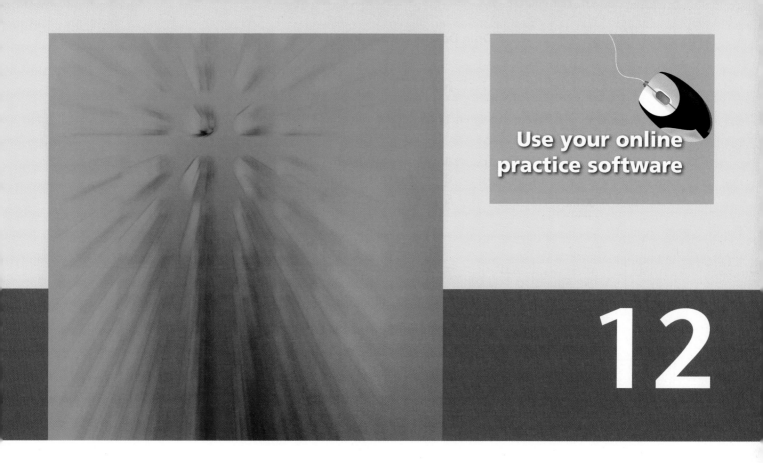

Reconstitution of Solutions

OBJECTIVES

Upon mastery of Chapter 12, you will be prepared to safely reconstitute and administer injectable and noninjectable solutions. To accomplish this, you will also be able to:

- Define and apply the terms *solvent (diluent), solute,* and *solution.*
- Reconstitute and label medications supplied in powder or dry form.
- Differentiate between varying directions for reconstitution and select the correct set to prepare the dosage ordered.
- Apply the Three-Step Approach to calculate accurate dosages.
- Calculate the amount of solute and solvent needed to prepare a desired strength and quantity of an irrigating solution or enteral feeding.

Some parenteral medications are supplied in powder form and must be mixed with water or some other liquid before administration. As more health care is provided in the home setting, nurses and other health care workers must dilute topical irrigants, soaks, and nutritional feedings. This process of mixing and diluting solutions is referred to as *reconstitution.*

The process of reconstitution is comparable to the preparation of hot chocolate from a powdered mix. By adding the correct amount of hot water (referred to as the *solvent* or *diluent*) to the package of powdered hot chocolate drink mix (referred to as the *solute*), you prepare a tasty, hot beverage (the mixture is called a *solution*).

The properties of solutions are important concepts to understand. Learn them well now, because we will apply them again when we examine intravenous solutions.

SOLUTION PROPERTIES

As you look at Figures 12-1 and 12-2a, let's define the terms of reconstitution.

FIGURE 12-1   Concentrated liquid solute: 50 milliliters of concentrated solute diluted with 50 milliliters of solvent make 100 milliliters of diluted solution

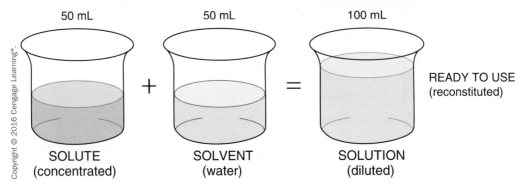

FIGURE 12-2(a)   Solid solute: The solid powder form of 500 mg of azithromycin (Zithromax) is reconstituted with 4.8 mL of sterile water as the diluent to make 5 mL of azithromycin (Zithromax) IV solution with the supply dosage of 100 mg/mL

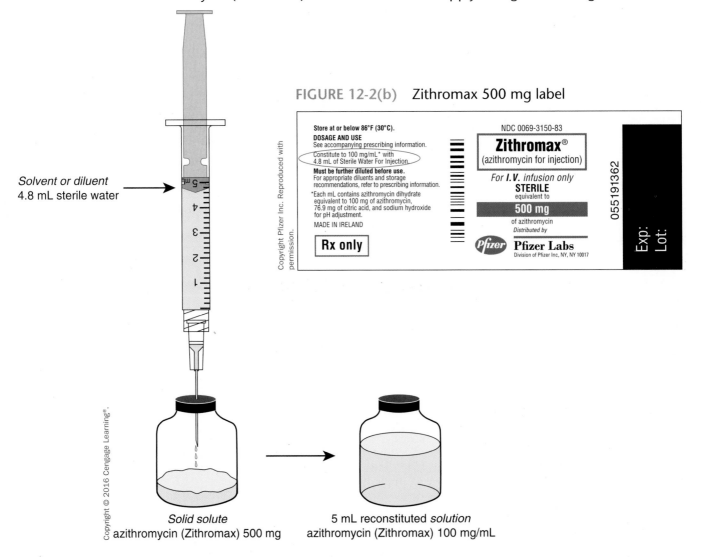

FIGURE 12-2(b)   Zithromax 500 mg label

Solvent or diluent
4.8 mL sterile water

Store at or below 86°F (30°C).
DOSAGE AND USE
See accompanying prescribing information.
Constitute to 100 mg/mL* with
4.8 mL of Sterile Water For Injection.
Must be further diluted before use.
For appropriate diluents and storage
recommendations, refer to prescribing information.
*Each mL contains azithromycin dihydrate
equivalent to 100 mg of azithromycin,
76.9 mg of citric acid, and sodium hydroxide
for pH adjustment.
MADE IN IRELAND

Rx only

NDC 0069-3150-83

Zithromax®
(azithromycin for injection)

For *I.V.* infusion only
STERILE
equivalent to
500 mg
of azithromycin
Distributed by
Pfizer **Pfizer Labs**
Division of Pfizer Inc, NY, NY 10017

055191362

Exp:
Lot:

Solid solute
azithromycin (Zithromax) 500 mg

5 mL reconstituted *solution*
azithromycin (Zithromax) 100 mg/mL

- *Solute*—a substance to be dissolved or diluted. It can be in solid or liquid form.
- *Solvent*—a substance (liquid) that dissolves another substance to prepare a solution. *Diluent* is a synonymous term.
- *Solution*—the mixture resulting from a solute plus a solvent.

To prepare a therapeutic solution, you will add a solvent or diluent (usually normal saline or water) to a solute (solid substance or concentrated stock solution) to obtain the required strength of a stated volume of a solution. This means that the solid substance or concentrate, called a *solute,* is diluted with a solvent to obtain a reconstituted solution of a weaker strength. However, the amount of the drug that was in the pure solute or concentrated stock solution still equals the amount of pure drug in the diluted solution. The solvent has simply been added to the solute, expanding the total volume.

Figure 12-1 shows that the amount of pure drug (solute) remains the same in the concentrated form and in the resulting solution. However, in the solution, notice that the solute is dispersed throughout the resulting weaker solution.

The *strength* of a solution, or *concentration,* was briefly discussed in Chapters 8 and 10. Solution strength indicates the ratio of solute to solvent. Consider how each of these substances—solute and solvent—contributes a certain number of parts to the total solution.

Look at the Zithromax 500 mg label (Figure 12-2b). The label directions indicate that 4.8 mL of sterile water (solvent) should be added to the powder (solid solute) to prepare the reconstituted solution. As the label indicates, the resulting supply dosage would be 100 mg of azithromycin (Zithromax) per 1 mL of solution.

Let's thoroughly examine the reconstitution of powdered injectable medications.

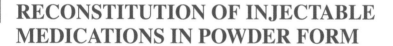

RECONSTITUTION OF INJECTABLE MEDICATIONS IN POWDER FORM

Some medications are unstable when stored in solution or liquid form. Thus, they are packaged in powdered form and must be dissolved, or reconstituted, by a liquid solvent, or diluent, and mixed thoroughly. Reconstitution is a necessary step in medication preparation to create a measurable and usable dosage form. The pharmacist often does this before dispensing liquid medications, for oral as well as parenteral routes. However, nurses need to understand reconstitution and know how to accomplish it. Some medications must be prepared by the nurse just prior to administration because they become unstable when stored in solution form.

CAUTION
Before reconstituting injectable drugs, read and follow the label or package insert directions carefully, including checking the drug and diluent expiration dates. Consult a pharmacist with any questions.

Let's look at the rules for reconstituting injectable medications from powder to liquid form. Follow these rules carefully to ensure that the patient receives the correct dosage of the intended solution.

RULE
When reconstituting injectable medications, you must determine both the type and the amount of diluent to be used.

Some powdered medications are packaged by the manufacturer with special diluents for reconstitution. Sterile water and 0.9% sodium chloride (normal saline) are most commonly used as

FIGURE 12-3   Reconstitution diluent for parenteral powdered drugs

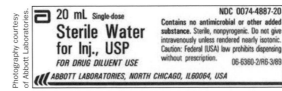

diluents in parenteral medications. Both sterile water (Figure 12-3) and normal saline are available *preservative-free* when intended for a single use only, as well as in *bacteriostatic* form with preservative when intended for more than one use. Carefully check the instructions, expiration date, and vial label for the appropriate diluent.

RULE

When reconstituting injectable medications, you must determine the volume in mL of diluent to be used for the route as ordered, then reconstitute the drug and note the resulting supply dosage on the vial.

Because many reconstituted parenteral medications can be administered either intramuscularly (IM) or intravenously (IV), it is essential to verify the route of administration before reconstituting the medication. Remember that the intramuscular volume of 3 mL or less per adult injection site (or 1 mL if deltoid site) is determined by the patient's age and condition and the intramuscular site selected. The directions take this into account by stating the minimum volume or quantity of diluent that should be added to the powdered drug for IM use. Often, the powdered drug itself adds volume to the solution. The powder displaces the liquid as it dissolves and increases the total resulting volume. The resulting volume of the reconstituted drug is usually given on the label. This resulting volume determines the liquid's concentration or supply dosage.

Look at the directions on the cefazolin label (Figure 12-4). It states, "To prepare solution add 2 mL sterile water for injection or 0.9% sodium chloride injection. Resulting solution contains approximate volume of 2.2 mL (225 mg per mL)." Notice that when 2 mL of diluent are added (Figure 12-4a) and the powder is dissolved, the bulk of the powder adds an additional 0.2 mL for a total solution of 2.2 mL (Figure 12-4b). (The amount of diluent added will vary with each medication.) Thus, the supply dosage available after reconstitution is *225 mg of cefazolin per mL of solution* (Figure 12-4c). Figure 12-4(d) demonstrates the reconstitution procedure for cefazolin 500 mg to fill the order of *cefazolin 225 mg IV q.6h.*

Single-dose vials contain only enough medication for one dose, and the resulting contents are administered after the powder is diluted. But in some cases the nurse also may dilute a powdered medication in a multiple-dose vial that will yield more than one dose. When this is the case, it is important to clearly label the vial after reconstitution. Labeling is discussed in the next section.

FIGURE 12-4   Cefazolin 500 mg powder: **(a)** Quantity of diluent; **(b)** Resulting total volume of solution; **(c)** Concentration of solution expressed per 1 mL

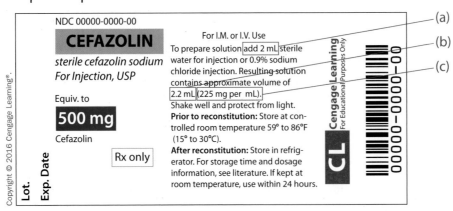

FIGURE 12-4(d)   Cefazolin reconstitution procedure to fill the order *cefazolin 225 mg IV q.6h*

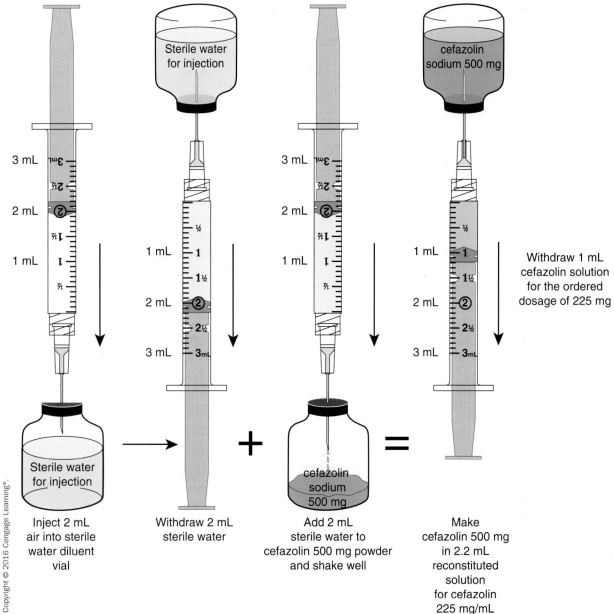

Inject 2 mL air into sterile water diluent vial

Withdraw 2 mL sterile water

Add 2 mL sterile water to cefazolin 500 mg powder and shake well

Make cefazolin 500 mg in 2.2 mL reconstituted solution for cefazolin 225 mg/mL

CAUTION

The quantity (volume) of the diluent may not be the same as the resulting quantity (volume) of the solution. To calculate the dose (amount to give), you must identify the concentration of the solution, which may be expressed either as the total dosage in the container per total quantity (resulting volume, such as 500 mg per 2.2 mL) or the dosage of medication per specified quantity (usually per 1 mL, such as 225 mg/mL).

TYPES OF RECONSTITUTED PARENTERAL SOLUTIONS

There are two types of reconstituted parenteral solutions: single strength and multiple strength. The simplest type to dilute is a *single-strength* solution. This type usually has the recommended dilution directions and resulting supply dosage printed on the label, as seen on the cefazolin 500 mg label in Figure 12-4 and the Zithromax label in Figure 12-2(b). Some medications have several directions for dilution that allow the nurse to select the best supply dosage. This is called a *multiple-strength* solution and requires even more careful reading of the instructions, such as on the Pfizerpen label shown in Figure 12-7 (page 345). Sometimes these directions for reconstitution are not included on the vial label (Figure 12-11c, page 354). You must consult the package insert or other printed instructions to ensure accurate dilution of the parenteral medication.

Let's look at some examples to clarify what the health care professional needs to do to correctly reconstitute and calculate dosages of parenteral medications supplied in powder form.

Single-Strength Solution

EXAMPLE 1 ▪

Order: *acyclovir 800 mg IV q.8h for 7 days*

Acyclovir (Zovirax) is an antiviral indicated for genital herpes infections, localized cutaneous herpes zoster infections (shingles), and chickenpox (varicella). It is supplied in capsules, tablets, suspension, powder for injection, solution for injection, cream, and ointment. Oral or topical medication is sufficient for most patients, but the intravenous route is used to treat serious infections in immunosuppressed patients. The powder for injection is given only by the intravenous injection route and is available as 500 mg/vial and 1,000 mg/vial for reconstitution. Depending on the type and severity of infection, intravenous dosages of 5 mg/kg to 10 mg/kg may be ordered for 7 to 21 days in a single dose or multiple doses. You will learn more about medication dosages based on body weight in Chapter 13, so for now, just consider the process you need to follow to administer the ordered dosage.

For this first example, you will administer the medication to a 175 lb hospitalized adult, recently treated with chemotherapy for cancer, who is diagnosed with a herpes zoster infection (shingles). You will retrieve the drug from the individual patient's unit-dose drawer (Figure 12-5).

FIGURE 12-5   Individual patient unit-dose drawer stocked with 24-hour supply of acyclovir

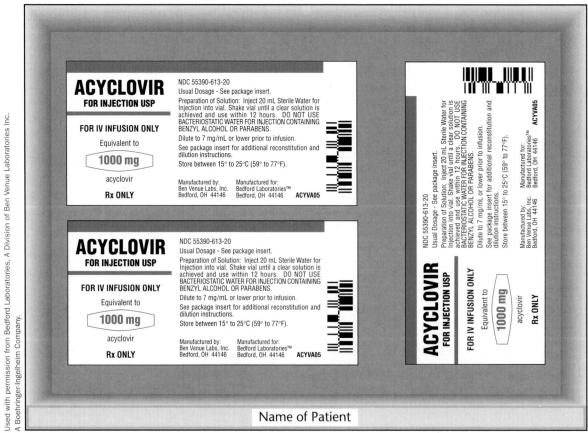

Carefully sort through and analyze the information provided on the label.

- First, how much and what type of diluent must you add? According to the directions on the label, you will *inject 20 mL of Sterile Water for Injection into vial.*

- Second, what is the resulting supply dosage or concentration? That information is not included on the label. You must read the package insert. According to the insert, when reconstituted with 20 mL of diluent the result is *a solution concentration of 50 mg acyclovir per mL.*

- Third, what is the resulting total volume of the reconstituted solution? The *total volume is 20 mL.* You know this because 1,000 mg divided by 20 mL equals 50 mg/mL which is the supply concentration. Therefore, in this example, the powder did not add any volume to the solution.

- Finally, to fill the order as prescribed, how many full doses are available in one vial? The order is for 800 mg, and the single-dose vial contains 1,000 mg. This is enough for *1 full dose,* but not enough for 2 full doses. Two doses would require 1,600 mg. You will remove 1 vial from the unit-dose drawer, leaving 2 vials for the 2 doses that remain to be given in the 24 hours.

After reconstitution, you are ready to apply the same Three-Step Approach to dosage calculation that you learned in Chapters 10 and 11.

Step 1   **Convert**   For the ordered dose of 800 mg, no conversion is necessary. The units are in the same system (metric) and the same size (mg).

Step 2   **Think**   The supply is 50 mg/mL. You want to give more than 1 mL. In fact, you want to give much more than 1 mL. Think of it another way. The total vial now has 1,000 mg in 20 mL. You want 800 mg, which is slightly less than 1,000 mg, so you will need slightly less than 20 mL.

Step 3   **Calculate** $\dfrac{\text{Dosage on hand}}{\text{Amount on hand}} = \dfrac{\text{Dosage desired}}{\text{X Amount desired}}$

$$\dfrac{50 \text{ mg}}{1 \text{ mL}} \diagup\!\!\!\!\diagdown \dfrac{800 \text{ mg}}{\text{X mL}}$$ Cross-multiply

$$50X = 800$$

$$\dfrac{50X}{50} = \dfrac{800}{50}$$ Simplify: Divide both sides of the equation by the number before the unknown X.

$$X = 16 \text{ mL}$$ Label the units to match the unknown X.

Give 16 mL of acyclovir reconstituted to 50 mg/mL, intravenously every 8 hours for 7 days.

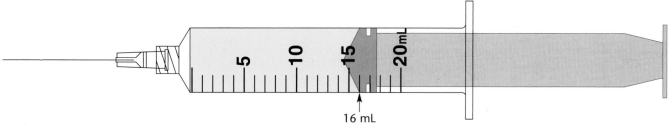

16 mL

This vial of acyclovir 1,000 mg contains only 1 full ordered dose of reconstituted drug. Any remaining medication is usually discarded. Because this vial provides only 1 dose, you will not have to label and store any of the reconstituted drug.

But how will you administer the intravenous medication? Even though it has been reconstituted according to directions, it is not yet ready for administration. According to the package insert, the *calculated dose should be removed and added to any appropriate intravenous solution at a volume selected for administration during each 1 hour infusion. Infusion concentrations of approximately 7 mg/mL or lower are recommended.* This means the amount measured in the syringe will be injected into an IV piggyback bag and timed to infuse slowly over an hour. This requires advanced skills, which you will learn in Chapter 15.

EXAMPLE 2 ■

Suppose the drug order reads *acyclovir 450 mg IV q.8h for 7 days.*

Using the same size vial of acyclovir and the same dilution instructions as in the previous example, you would now have 2 full doses of acyclovir, making this a *multiple-dose vial.* The supply is the same, 50 mg/mL.

$$\frac{\text{Dosage on hand}}{\text{Amount on hand}} = \frac{\text{Dosage desired}}{\text{X Amount desired}}$$

$$\frac{50 \text{ mg}}{1 \text{ mL}} \diagtimes \frac{450 \text{ mg}}{\text{X mL}} \qquad \text{Cross-multiply}$$

$$50\text{X} = 450$$

$$\frac{50\text{X}}{50} = \frac{450}{50} \qquad \text{Simplify: Divide both sides of the equation by the number before the unknown X.}$$

$$\text{X} = 9 \text{ mL} \qquad \text{Label the units to match the unknown X.}$$

Select a 10 mL syringe, and measure 9 mL of acyclovir reconstituted to 50 mg/mL.

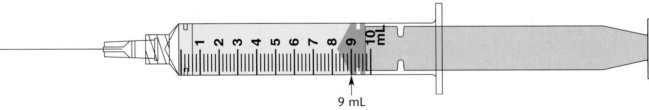

9 mL

RULE

When reconstituting multiple-dose injectable medications, verify the length of drug potency. Store the reconstituted drug appropriately with a reconstitution label attached.

If multiple doses result from the reconstitution of a powdered drug, the solution must be used in a timely manner. Because the drug potency (or stability) may be several hours to several days, check the drug label, package information sheet, or drug reference for how long the drug may be used after reconstitution. Store the drug appropriately at room temperature, or refrigerate as per the manufacturer's instructions. The package insert for acyclovir states, "Reconstituted solution should be used within 12 hours. Refrigeration of reconstituted solution may result in the formation of a precipitate which will redissolve at room temperature."

CAUTION

The length of potency is different from the expiration date. The expiration date is provided by the manufacturer on the label. It indicates the last date the drug may be reconstituted and used.

When you reconstitute or mix a multiple-dose vial of medication in powdered form, it is important that the vial be clearly labeled with the *date and time* of preparation, the strength or *supply dosage* you prepared, *length of potency, storage directions,* and your *initials.* Because the medication becomes unstable after storage for long periods, the date and time are especially important. Figure 12-6 shows the proper label for the acyclovir reconstituted to 50 mg/mL. Because there are 2 doses of reconstituted drug in this vial, and 2 doses will be administered 8 hours apart (now at 0800, then again at 1600), this drug may be stored for a second use in the patient's unit-dose drawer. While refrigeration is not required for acyclovir, if it is refrigerated the vial should stand at room temperature until precipitate dissolves prior to use.

FIGURE 12-6 Reconstitution label for acyclovir

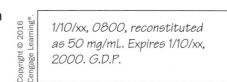

1/10/xx, 0800, reconstituted as 50 mg/mL. Expires 1/10/xx, 2000. G.D.P.

Multiple-Strength Solution

Some parenteral powdered medications have directions for preparing several different solution strengths to allow you to select a particular dosage strength. This results in a reasonable amount to be given to a particular patient.

EXAMPLE ▪

Let's consider the medication penicillin G potassium. It is supplied in a multi-dose vial as a sterile powder that must be reconstituted prior to administration by the IM or IV route. The drug is indicated for a wide variety of infections such as pneumococcal pneumonia, streptococcal pharyngitis, syphilis, and gonorrhea. The recommended dosage and frequency varies greatly depending on age, weight, and severity of infection. A newborn infant at risk for a streptococcal infection might receive 50,000 units/kg every 12 hours, whereas a large adult could be ordered 5 million units every 4 hours for a severe meningitis infection. Therefore, several different directions for reconstitution are necessary to allow for a reasonable volume to be administered.

Order: **penicillin G potassium 300,000 units IM stat**

For this example, you will administer the medication to an 83-year-old patient who weighs 110 lb. She was first seen as an outpatient by a family practice nurse practitioner. Preparations are being made for admission to a small community hospital for intravenous drug therapy, but prior to leaving the office the patient is to receive 1 dose of the medication by the IM route. The medication will be retrieved from the stock medication cabinet as shown in Figure 12-7.

FIGURE 12-7 Penicillin G potassium (Pfizerpen) label with 4 options for reconstitution

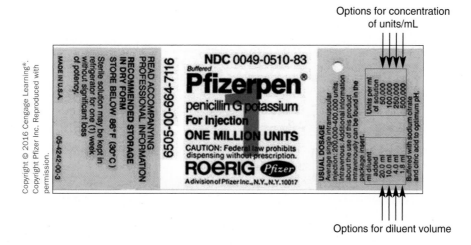

This vial contains a total of 1,000,000 units of penicillin. The reconstitution instructions are shown on the right side of the label. The instructions detail four different parenteral-solution supply dosages or concentrations that are determined by the added diluent volume. The left column provides a choice of suggested volumes of diluent. The right column indicates the final solution strength in units per mL. Let's look at each of the four instructions. Notice how these reconstituted concentrations differ and when each might be selected.

Add 20 mL Diluent

Refer to the first set of directions, which indicates to add 20 mL diluent to prepare 50,000 units per milliliter of solution. Is this a good choice for preparing the medication to fill the order for this patient? What do we know?

- First, to follow the first set of directions, how much and what type of diluent must you add? According to the directions, you will *add 20 mL of diluent.* (You must check the package insert to determine the type of diluent, because this information is not stated on the label. The package insert recommends: Water for Injection or Sterile Isotonic Sodium Chloride Solution for Parenteral Use.)

- Second, what is the concentration of the reconstituted penicillin? When adding 20 mL of diluent, the *supply dosage or concentration is 50,000 units/mL.*

- Third, what is the resulting total volume of this reconstituted solution? The *total volume is 20 mL.* You know this because the supply dosage is 50,000 units/mL or 1,000,000 units per 20 mL. The volume of diluent is large enough that the powder dissolves without adding any significant additional volume.

- Finally, how many full doses of penicillin as ordered are available in this vial? The vial contains 1,000,000 units, and the order is for 300,000 units. There are *3 full doses* (plus some extra) in this vial. If you choose this concentration, a reconstitution label would be required.

This means that when you add 20 mL of sterile diluent to this vial of powdered penicillin, the result is 1,000,000 units of penicillin in 20 mL of solution, with a concentration of 50,000 units per mL.

Apply the Three-Step Approach to dosage calculation.

Step 1	**Convert**	No conversion is necessary. When a medication is ordered in units, the supply used must also be in units.
Step 2	**Think**	The order is for 300,000 units and the supply is 50,000 units/mL. You want to give more than 1 mL. In fact, you want to give 6 times 1 mL.
Step 3	**Calculate**	$\dfrac{\text{Dosage on hand}}{\text{Amount on hand}} = \dfrac{\text{Dosage desired}}{\text{X Amount desired}}$

$$\frac{50,000 \text{ units}}{1 \text{ mL}} \diagdown\!\!\!\!\diagup \frac{300,000 \text{ units}}{\text{X mL}} \qquad \text{Cross-multiply}$$

$$50,000X = 300,000$$

$$\frac{50,000X}{50,000} = \frac{300,000}{50,000} \qquad \text{Simplify: Divide both sides of the equation by the number before the unknown X.}$$

$$X = 6 \text{ mL} \qquad \text{Label the units to match the unknown X.}$$

Because each dose is 6 mL and the total volume is 20 mL, 2 additional full doses would remain in the vial. However, this is an IM dose, and 3 mL is the maximum volume for a large adult muscle. This patient is an elderly person who only weighs 110 lb and may have less muscle mass. To safely administer this order using this concentration, you would need to inject the patient with three 2 mL syringes filled with 2 mL of penicillin each. Therefore, this is a poor choice of reconstitution instructions to prepare this order for this patient.

Add 10 mL Diluent

Refer to the second set of directions on the penicillin label, which indicates to add 10 mL of diluent for 100,000 units per mL of solution. Would this prepare an appropriate concentration to fill the order? What do we know?

- First, to correctly follow the second set of directions, how much and what type of diluent must you add? According to the directions, you will add *10 mL of diluent.* (You must check the package insert to determine the type of diluent, because this information is not stated on the label. The package insert recommends: Water for Injection or Sterile Isotonic Sodium Chloride Solution for Parenteral Use.)

- Second, what is the concentration of the reconstituted penicillin? When adding 10 mL of diluent, the *supply dosage or concentration is 100,000 units/mL.*

- Third, what is the resulting total volume of this reconstituted solution? The *total volume is 10 mL.* You know this because the supply dosage is 100,000 units/mL or 1,000,000 units per 10 mL. The solution volume is large enough that the powder does not add significant volume to the solution.

- Finally, how many full doses of penicillin as ordered are available in this vial? The vial contains 1,000,000 units, and the order is for 300,000 units. There are *3 full doses* (plus some extra) in this vial. If you select this set of instructions, you will need to add a reconstitution label to the vial after mixing.

This means that when you add 10 mL of sterile diluent to this vial of powdered penicillin, the result is 1,000,000 units of penicillin in 10 mL of solution with a concentration of 100,000 units per mL.

Apply the Three-Step Approach to dosage calculation.

Step 1	**Convert**	No conversion is necessary. When a medication is ordered in units, the supply used must also be in units.
Step 2	**Think**	The order is for 300,000 units and the supply is 100,000 units/mL. You want to give more than 1 mL. In fact, you want to give 3 times 1 mL.

Step 3   **Calculate**

$$\frac{\text{Dosage on hand}}{\text{Amount on hand}} = \frac{\text{Dosage desired}}{\text{X Amount desired}}$$

$$\frac{100{,}000 \text{ units}}{1 \text{ mL}} \diagup\hspace{-0.9em}\diagdown \frac{300{,}000 \text{ units}}{\text{X mL}} \qquad \text{Cross-multiply}$$

$$100{,}000\text{X} = 300{,}000$$

$$\frac{100{,}000\text{X}}{100{,}000} = \frac{300{,}000}{100{,}000} \qquad \text{Simplify: Divide both sides of the equation by the number before the unknown X.}$$

$$\text{X} = 3 \text{ mL} \qquad \text{Label the units to match the unknown X.}$$

Because each dose is 3 mL and the total volume is 10 mL, 2 additional full doses would remain. As an IM dose, 3 mL is the maximum volume for a large adult muscle. Although this generally is a safe volume and would require only one injection, remember this patient is elderly and only weighs 110 lb. Perhaps another concentration would result in a lesser volume that would be more readily absorbed.

Add 4 mL Diluent

Refer to the third set of directions on the penicillin label, which indicates to add 4 mL of diluent for 250,000 units per mL of solution. Would this prepare an appropriate concentration to fill the order?

What is different about this set of directions? Let's analyze the information provided on the label.

- First, to follow the third set of directions, how much and what type of diluent must you add? According to the directions, you will *add 4 mL of diluent.* (Remember that you must check the package insert to determine the type of diluent, because this information is not stated on the label. The package insert recommends: Water for Injection or Sterile Isotonic Sodium Chloride Solution for Parenteral Use.)

- Second, what is the supply dosage of the reconstituted penicillin? When adding 4 mL of diluent, the supply dosage is *250,000 units/mL.*

- Third, what is the resulting total volume of this reconstituted solution? The *total volume is 4 mL.* You know this because the supply dosage is 250,000 units/mL or 1,000,000 units per 4 mL. The powder does not add significant volume to the solution.

- Finally, how many full doses of penicillin are available in this vial? The vial contains 1,000,000 units, and the order is for 300,000 units. Regardless of the concentration, there are still *3 full doses* (plus some extra) in this vial. A reconstitution label would be needed.

This means that when you add 4 mL of sterile diluent to the vial of powdered penicillin, the result is 4 mL of solution with 250,000 units of penicillin per mL.

Calculate 1 dose.

Step 1	**Convert**	No conversion is necessary. When a medication is ordered in units, the supply used must also be in units.
Step 2	**Think**	The order is for 300,000 units and the supply is 250,000 units/mL. You want to give more than 1 mL but less than 2 mL.

Step 3   **Calculate**

$$\frac{\text{Dosage on hand}}{\text{Amount on hand}} = \frac{\text{Dosage desired}}{\text{X Amount desired}}$$

$$\frac{250{,}000 \text{ units}}{1 \text{ mL}} \bowtie \frac{300{,}000 \text{ units}}{\text{X mL}} \qquad \text{Cross-multiply}$$

$$250{,}000\text{X} = 300{,}000$$

$$\frac{250{,}000\text{X}}{250{,}000} = \frac{300{,}000}{250{,}000} \qquad \begin{array}{l}\text{Simplify: Divide both sides of the}\\ \text{equation by the number before the}\\ \text{unknown X.}\end{array}$$

$$\text{X} = 1.2 \text{ mL} \qquad \begin{array}{l}\text{Label the units to match the}\\ \text{unknown X.}\end{array}$$

Because each dose is 1.2 mL and the total volume is 4 mL, 2 additional full doses would remain. The dose volume of 1.2 mL is considerably less than the maximum volume for a large adult muscle. This concentration would result in a reasonable volume that would be readily absorbed by a small, elderly patient. This is a good choice of concentration instructions to use to prepare this order. However, is it now too concentrated? According to the package insert, the total volume of intramuscular injections *should* be kept small. Solutions in concentrations up to 100,000 units of penicillin per mL of diluent may be used with a minimum of discomfort, but greater concentrations of penicillin G per mL are physically possible and may be employed where therapy demands. Because a concentration of 250,000 units is needed to deliver this smaller injection, you should prepare the patient for potential soreness at the injection site.

Select a 3 mL syringe, and measure 1.2 mL of penicillin G potassium reconstituted to 250,000 units/mL.

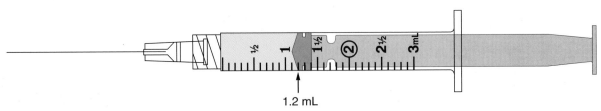

1.2 mL

CAUTION
The supply dosage of a reconstituted drug is an essential detail that the preparer must write on the multiple-dose vial label. Once a powdered drug is reconstituted, there is no way to verify how much diluent was actually added unless it is properly labeled.

Be sure to add a label to the reconstituted penicillin G potassium 250,000 units/mL vial (Figure 12-8).

FIGURE 12-8 Reconstitution label for penicillin G potassium 1,000,000 units with 4 mL diluent

1/30/xx, 0800, reconstituted as 250,000 units/mL. Expires 2/06/xx, 0800. Keep refrigerated. G.D.P.

Add 1.8 mL Diluent

The fourth set of directions instructs you to add 1.8 mL diluent for a solution concentration of 500,000 units/mL. Let's examine this information.

- First, to fulfill the fourth set of directions, how much and what type of diluent must you add? The directions state to *add 1.8 mL of diluent.* (You must check the package insert to determine the type of diluent, because this information is not stated on the label. The package insert recommends: Use Water for Injection or Sterile Isotonic Sodium Chloride Solution for Parenteral Use.)

- Second, what is the supply dosage of the reconstituted penicillin? When adding 1.8 mL of diluent, the supply dosage is *500,000 units/mL.*

- Third, what is the resulting total volume of this reconstituted solution? The *total volume is 2 mL.* You know this because the supply dosage is 500,000 units/mL or 1,000,000 units per 2 mL. The powder displaces 0.2 mL of the solution, causing the resulting total volume to be larger than the volume of diluent used. (Notice that this is the most concentrated, or the strongest, of the four concentrations.)

- Finally, how many full doses of penicillin are available in this vial? The vial contains 1,000,000 units, and the order is for 300,000 units. Notice that regardless of the concentration, there are *3 full doses* (plus some extra) in this vial. This reconstitution label will differ from the one in the previous example, because this is a different concentration.

Following the fourth set of directions, you add 1.8 mL of diluent to prepare 2 mL of solution with a resulting concentration of 500,000 units of penicillin in each 1 mL.

Calculate 1 dose.

Step 1 **Convert**   No conversion is necessary. When a medication is ordered in units, the supply used must also be in units.

Step 2 **Think**   The order is for 300,000 units and the supply is 500,000 units/mL. You want to give less than 1 mL.

Step 3 **Calculate**
$$\frac{\text{Dosage on hand}}{\text{Amount on hand}} = \frac{\text{Dosage desired}}{\text{X Amount desired}}$$

$$\frac{500,000 \text{ units}}{1 \text{ mL}} \diagup\!\!\!\!\diagdown \frac{300,000 \text{ units}}{\text{X mL}}$$ Cross-multiply

$$500,000\text{X} = 300,000$$

$$\frac{500,000\text{X}}{500,000} = \frac{300,000}{500,000}$$ Simplify: Divide both sides of the equation by the number before the unknown X.

$$\text{X} = 0.6 \text{ mL}$$ Label the units to match the unknown X.

Because each dose is 0.6 mL and the total volume is 2 mL, you would have enough for 2 additional full doses. This supply dosage would result in a reasonable volume for an IM injection for an infant, a small child, or anyone with wasted muscle mass. This volume would be acceptable to administer to this 83-year-old patient who weighs 110 lb. But remember, this concentration of 500,000 units/mL is twice as concentrated as the 250,000 units/mL dosage strength. While both strengths would be okay, the 250,000 units/mL concentration would be the preferred choice for this patient and would cause the least discomfort.

To administer this concentration, select a 3 mL syringe, and measure 0.6 mL of penicillin G potassium reconstituted to 500,000 units/mL.

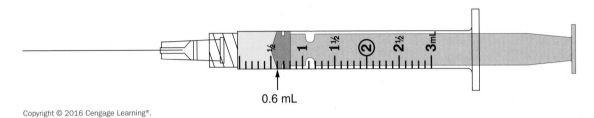

0.6 mL

Finally, add the label to the reconstituted penicillin G potassium 500,000 units/mL vial (Figure 12-9).

FIGURE 12-9 Reconstitution label for penicillin G potassium 1,000,000 units with 1.8 mL diluent

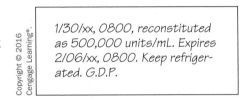

1/30/xx, 0800, reconstituted as 500,000 units/mL. Expires 2/06/xx, 0800. Keep refrigerated. G.D.P.

As you can see from these four possible reconstituted strengths, 3 full doses are available from this multiple-dose vial in each case. The added diluent volume is the vital factor that determines the resulting concentration. The *supply dosage* ultimately determines the *injectable volume per dose*.

MATH TIP
When multiple directions for diluting are given, the smaller the amount of diluent added, the greater or stronger the resulting solution concentration will be.

RECONSTITUTED PARENTERAL SOLUTIONS WITH VARIOUS ROUTES

A variety of drugs are labeled and packaged with reconstitution instructions. Some drugs are for IM use only and some are for IV use only, whereas others may be used for either. Some are even suitable for subcut, IM, or IV administration. Carefully check the route and related reconstitution directions. The following material gives examples of several types of directions that you will encounter.

Drugs With Injection Reconstitution Instructions for Either IM or IV

EXAMPLE ■

Order: *methylprednisolone 200 mg IV q.6h*

Methylprednisolone is a corticosteroid used to treat a wide variety of inflammatory or allergic conditions, such as rheumatoid arthritis, dermatologic diseases, status asthmaticus, autoimmune disorders, and adjunctive therapy of pneumonia. It may be administered orally in dosages of 4 to 48 mg/day, and intramuscularly or intravenously as methylprednisolone sodium succinate (Solu-Medrol) in doses of 40 to

250 mg q.4-6h for most uses. Methylprednisolone solution for injection is supplied in vials containing 40 mg, 125 mg, 500 mg, 1 g, and 2 g sterile powder requiring reconstitution.

For this example, you will administer the medication to a 54-year-old patient of average weight who has been admitted to the hospital medical unit with a diagnosis of pneumonia after being treated in the emergency department for asthmatic exacerbation. You will need to retrieve the correct medication from a matrix drawer in the automatic dispensing cabinet and reconstitute the solution. Consider the medication supply pictured (Figure 12-10).

FIGURE 12-10 Illustrated ADC matrix drawer with prepackaged cartons containing vials: **(a)** hydrocortisone sodium succinate 500 mg (Solu-Cortef); **(b)** hydrocortisone sodium succinate 1000 mg (Solu-Cortef); **(c)** methylprednisolone sodium succinate 500 mg (Solu-Medrol); **(d)** methylprednisolone sodium succinate 1 g (Solu-Medrol)

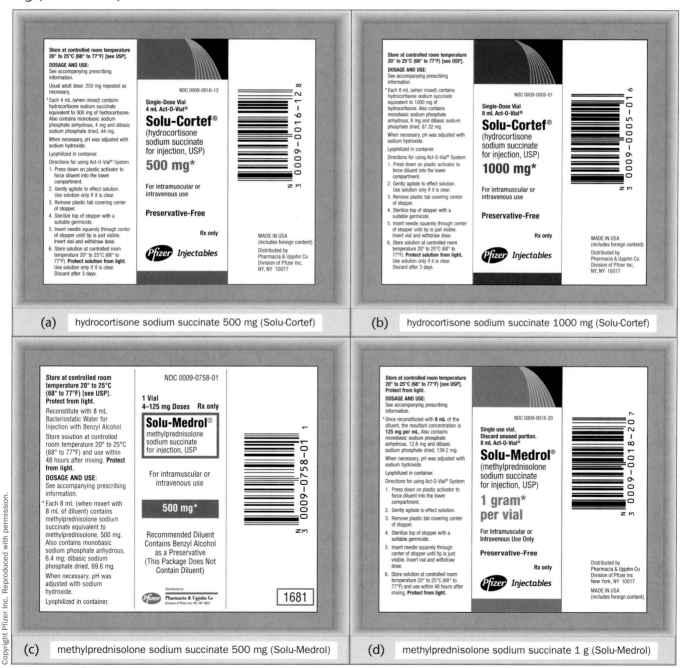

(a) hydrocortisone sodium succinate 500 mg (Solu-Cortef)

(b) hydrocortisone sodium succinate 1000 mg (Solu-Cortef)

(c) methylprednisolone sodium succinate 500 mg (Solu-Medrol)

(d) methylprednisolone sodium succinate 1 g (Solu-Medrol)

Which carton will you pick? First take care not to mistake Solu-Medrol, a brand name for methylprednisolone sodium succinate, with the look-alike/sound-alike drug Solu-Cortef, a brand name for hydrocortisone sodium succinate. They are both corticosteroids but are different drugs. The only correct choices are Figures 12-10(c) and 12-10(d). Remember, you will be administering this medication again in 6 hours. The labels indicate that the reconstituted drug can be stored for 48 hours. THINK: the ordered dose is 200 mg; therefore, the 500 mg vial will supply 2 full doses. However, the 1 g vial, which you know is equal to 1,000 mg, will supply 5 full doses, and could be completely used before the reconstituted solution needs to be discarded. Both supplies would be a correct choice. For this example, let's imagine you will be on duty long enough to administer 2 doses and choose to use the 500 mg vial.

The 500 mg supply of powdered methylprednisolone for IM or IV injection contains directions on the left side of the label that state, "Reconstitute with 8 mL Bacteriostatic Water for Injection with Benzyl Alcohol . . . Each 8 mL (when mixed with 8 mL of diluent) contains methylprednisolone sodium succinate equivalent to methylprednisolone, 500 mg." These instructions will apply to orders for either the intramuscular or intravenous route.

What do we know?

- First, to fill the order, how much and what type of diluent must you add? According to the directions, you will *reconstitute with 8 mL bacteriostatic water for injection with benzyl alcohol.*

- Second, what is the supply dosage of the reconstituted methylprednisolone? When adding 8 mL of diluent, the *supply dosage is 500 mg per 8 mL.*

- Third, what is the resulting total volume of this reconstituted solution? The *total volume is 8 mL.* Any amount that the powdered drug displaces in solution is insignificant and does not add volume. You know this because the instructions tell you that *each 8 mL contains methylprednisolone, 500 mg.*

- Finally, remember how many full doses of methylprednisolone are available in this vial. The vial contains 500 mg, and the order is for 200 mg. There are *2 full doses* in the vial (plus some extra). A reconstitution label is needed. The label indicates that the reconstituted drug can be stored for 48 hours.

This means that you have available a vial of 500 mg of methylprednisolone to which you will add 8 mL of diluent. The final yield of the solution is 500 mg per 8 mL, which is your supply dosage.
    Calculate 1 dose.

Step 1   **Convert**   For the ordered dose of 200 mg, no conversion is necessary. The units are in the same system (metric) and the same size (mg).

Step 2   **Think**   The order is for 200 mg and the supply is 500 mg per 8 mL. 200 mg is slightly less than $\frac{1}{2}$ of 500 mg; therefore, you want to give slightly less than 4 mL, which is $\frac{1}{2}$ of 8 mL.

Step 3   **Calculate** $\dfrac{\text{Dosage on hand}}{\text{Amount on hand}} = \dfrac{\text{Dosage desired}}{\text{X Amount desired}}$

$$\dfrac{500 \text{ mg}}{8 \text{ mL}} \diagup\!\!\!\!\diagdown \dfrac{200 \text{ mg}}{\text{X mL}}$$ Cross-multiply

$$500\text{X} = 1,600$$

$$\dfrac{500\text{X}}{500} = \dfrac{1,600}{500}$$ Simplify: Divide both sides of the equation by the number before the unknown X.

$$\text{X} = 3.2 \text{ mL}$$ Label the units to match the unknown X.

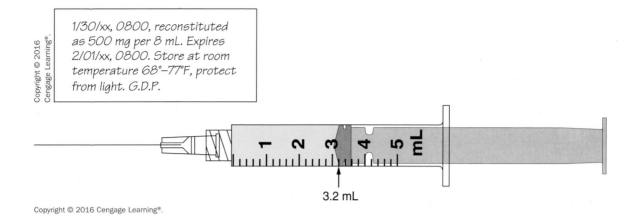

1/30/xx, 0800, reconstituted as 500 mg per 8 mL. Expires 2/01/xx, 0800. Store at room temperature 68°–77°F, protect from light. G.D.P.

3.2 mL

But how will you administer the intravenous medication? Even though it has been reconstituted according to directions, it is not yet ready for administration. According to the package insert, this preparation may be administered by intravenous injection or by intravenous infusion. When high-dose therapy is desired, Solu-Medrol should be administered intravenously over at least 30 minutes. This means when the dose is low, the 3.2 mL measured in the syringe may be slowly injected directly into the IV tubing, but with higher doses the measured amount should be further diluted by injecting into an IV piggyback bag and timed to infuse slowly over 30 minutes. This requires advanced skills, which you will learn in Chapter 15.

DRUGS WITH DIFFERENT IM AND IV RECONSTITUTION INSTRUCTIONS

Now let's consider a medication that has different reconstitution instructions for the IM and IV routes. The nurse must carefully check the route ordered and then follow the directions that correspond to that route. In such cases, it is important not to interchange the dilution instructions for IM and IV administrations.

EXAMPLE 1 ■

Order: **Rocephin 250 mg IM stat**

Rocephin is a brand name for ceftriaxone, a broad-spectrum cephalosporin antibiotic for intravenous or intramuscular administration. It is indicated for the treatment of infections by susceptible organisms, such as lower respiratory tract infections, acute bacterial otitis media, skin and skin structure infections, urinary tract infections, uncomplicated gonorrhea, pelvic inflammatory disease, bacterial septicemia, bone and joint infections, intra-abdominal infections, meningitis, and surgical prophylaxis. It is supplied as a powder for injection in vials containing 250 mg, 500 mg, 1 g, 2 g, and 10 g. For most infections the recommended dose is 0.5 mg to 1 g q.12h or 1 to 2 g q.2–4h, but for the treatment of uncomplicated gonococcal infections, a single intramuscular dose of 250 mg is recommended.

For this example, a 22-year-old patient seeks medical care at an urgent care facility with complaints of painful urination. He is diagnosed with gonococcal urethritis and will receive the one-time dose of Rocephin as ordered. The nurse recalls that Rocephin is a cephalosporin and begins with "cef" or "ceph" and searches for a 250 mg vial in the stock medication supply cabinet. The stock supply contains three cephalosporins side by side on the shelf (Figure 12-11).

The nurse thinks the correct medication is ceftriaxone (Figure 12-11c), but to be safe she does not rely on memory and verifies in a drug reference that ceftriaxone is the generic name for Rocephin. The nurse selects the 1 gram vial and makes a note to check with the office manager about stocking the medication

FIGURE 12-11   Illustrated stock medication cabinet with vials of **(a)** cefazolin; **(b)** cefepime; **(c)** ceftriaxone for reconstitution

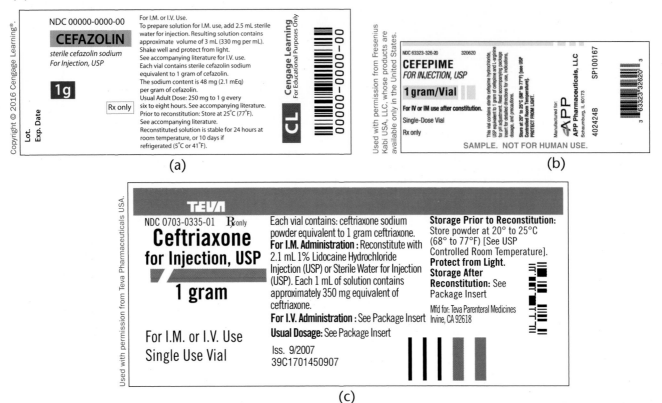

(a)   (b)

(c)

in smaller doses. Notice that the ceftriaxone has one set of instructions for IM use and another set for IV administration that can be found on the package insert. You will need to reconstitute the powdered medication with the IM instructions for this patient.

Supply: 1 g vial of powdered ceftriaxone with IM reconstitution directions on the label that state, "For IM Administration: Reconstitute with 2.1 mL 1% Lidocaine Hydrochloride Injection (USP) or Sterile Water for Injection (USP). Each 1 mL of solution contains approximately 350 mg equivalent of ceftriaxone."

■ First, to fill the order, how much and what type of diluent must you add? According to the directions, you will *add 2.1 mL of diluent.* Two diluents are recommended on the label: *1% lidocaine hydrochloride injection (USP) or sterile water for injection (USP).* Use sterile water for injection.

■ Second, what is the supply dosage of the reconstituted ceftriaxone? The resulting *supply dosage is 350 mg/mL.*

■ Third, what is the resulting total volume of this reconstituted solution? *The total volume is larger than the volume of the diluent.* We know this because the resulting supply dosage is 350 mg/mL or 1,050 mg per 3 mL. While 1,050 mg is approximately equal to the supplied dose of 1 g, 3 mL is considerably larger than 2.1 mL, the volume of the diluent. The solution volume is not sufficient to dilute the powder without adding additional volume. Therefore, you cannot use 2.1 mL as the volume for the supply dosage in your calculation.

■ Finally, how much ceftriaxone will remain in this vial? The vial contains 1 g or 1,000 mg. The order is for 250 mg. 750 mg will be left in the vial. According to the package insert, the *solution reconstituted with sterile water for injection is stable at room temperature for 24 hours and refrigerated for 3 days* (Figure 12-12). If the vial will be stored for a possible future use, a reconstitution label is needed.

This means that you have available a vial of 1 g of ceftriaxone to which you will add 2.1 mL of sterile water for injection as the diluent. The final yield of the solution has a volume greater than the amount of diluent, with a supply dosage of 350 mg/mL.

FIGURE 12-12 Package insert for ceftriaxone with storage information for intramuscular administration

Ceftriaxone for injection, USP *intramuscular* solutions remain stable (loss of potency less than 10%) for the following time periods:

Diluent	Concentration mg/mL	Storage Room Temp. (25°C)	Storage Refrigerated (4°C)
Sterile Water for injection	100 250, 350	2 days 24 hours	10 days 3 days
0.9% Sodium Chloride Solution	100 250, 350	2 days 24 hours	10 days 3 days
5% Dextrose Solution	100 250, 350	2 days 24 hours	10 days 3 days
Bacteriostatic Water + 0.9% Benzyl Alcohol	100 250, 350	24 hours 24 hours	10 days 3 days
1% Lidocaine Solution (without epinephrine)	100 250, 350	24 hours 24 hours	10 days 3 days

Step 1   Convert   For the ordered dose of 200 mg, no conversion is necessary. The units are in the same system (metric) and the same size (mg).

Step 2   Think   The order is for 250 mg and the supply is 350 mg/mL. You want to give less than 1 mL.

Step 3   Calculate $\dfrac{\text{Dosage on hand}}{\text{Amount on hand}} = \dfrac{\text{Dosage desired}}{\text{X Amount desired}}$

$$\frac{350 \text{ mg}}{1 \text{ mL}} \diagup\!\!\!\!\diagdown \frac{250 \text{ mg}}{\text{X mL}}$$ Cross-multiply

$$350\text{X} = 250$$

$$\frac{350\text{X}}{350} = \frac{250}{350}$$ Simplify: Divide both sides of the equation by the number before the unknown X.

$$\text{X} = 0.71 \text{ mL}$$ Label the units to match the unknown X.

1/30/xx, 0800, reconstituted as 350 mg/mL for IM use. Expires 2/2/xx, 0800. Keep refrigerated. G.D.P.

What syringe will you choose to administer the IM injection? You actually have two choices. Recall from Chapter 6 that critical medications in volumes less than 1 mL and other medications less than 0.5 mL should be measured in a 1 mL syringe with increments of hundredths. Because ceftriaxone is not listed as a high-alert drug (see Chapter 9, Figure 9-1) and the volume needed is greater than 0.5 mL, you may use either a 1 mL or 3 mL syringe.

If you choose to use a 1 mL syringe, draw up the exact amount of 0.71 mL. If the syringe comes prepackaged with a needle, it will likely be a smaller gauge and shorter length than what is needed for an IM injection. You may need to change the needle to the correct size.

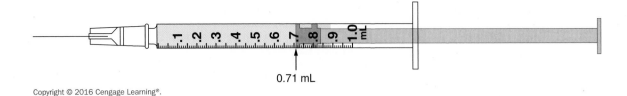

If you choose to use a 3 mL syringe, round 0.71 to 0.7 and draw up 0.7 mL.

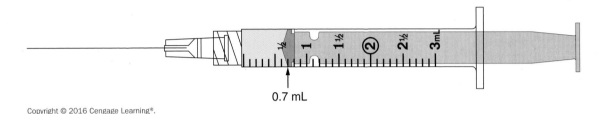

> ## CAUTION
>
> When using a 1 mL syringe prepackaged with a needle for an IM dose, you may need to change needles. Change needles *prior* to drawing up medication. Changing needles after the medication is measured may alter the actual dose of medication injected.

EXAMPLE 2 ■

Order: *ceftriaxone 400 mg IV q.12h*

In this example, your patient is an 82-year-old woman who has been admitted to the hospital from the long-term care center with a diagnosis of recurrent urinary tract infection. She was treated unsuccessfully twice with oral antibiotics but now will be receiving therapy with a cephalosporin by the intravenous route. Although a usual adult dose of ceftriaxone is 1 g per day in 2 divided doses, she will receive a slightly lower dose due to a history of renal impairment. The supply will be retrieved from an automated dispensing cabinet (ADC) (Figure 12-13).

FIGURE 12-13   Illustrated ADC matrix drawer with vials of ceftriaxone for reconstitution containing: **(a)** 250 mg; **(b)** 1 g; **(c)** 2 g

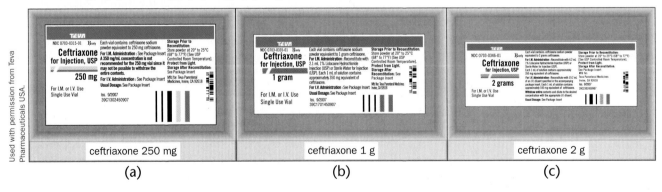

Which supply should you choose? If you select the 250 mg supply, you would need 2 vials to provide the 400 mg dosage. This would be the least convenient and more time-consuming choice. Both the 1 g and 2 g vials contain enough medication for the ordered dosage with more doses remaining. Recall from the previous example that after reconstitution ceftriaxone may be stored for 24 hours at room temperature and up to 3 days if refrigerated. Let's pick the 1 g vial, which will supply enough medication for two administration times.

FIGURE 12-14 Package insert information for ceftriaxone for injection IV administration

Intravenous Administration

Ceftriaxone for injection, USP should be administered intravenously by infusion over a period of 30 minutes. Concentrations between 10 mg/mL and 40 mg/mL are recommended; however, lower concentrations may be used if desired. Reconstitute vials with an appropriate IV diluent (see **COMPATIBILITY AND STABILITY**).

Vial Dosage Size	Amount of Diluent to be Added
250 mg	2.4 mL
500 mg	4.8 mL
1 g	9.6 mL
2 g	19.2 mL

After reconstitution, each 1 mL of solution contains approximately 100 mg equivalent of ceftriaxone. Withdraw entire contents and dilute to the desired concentration with the appropriate IV diluent.

- First, to fill the order, how much and what type of diluent must you add? According to the directions, you will *add 9.6 mL of appropriate IV diluent* to the 1 g vial (Figure 12-14). The package insert lists *sterile water for injection* as one of five appropriate IV diluents.

- Second, what is the supply dosage of the reconstituted ceftriaxone? The resulting *supply dosage is 100 mg/mL.*

- Third, what is the resulting total volume of this reconstituted solution? The *total volume is larger than the volume of the diluent*. We know this because the resulting supply dosage is 100 mg/mL or 1,000 mg per 10 mL. The solution volume is not sufficient to dilute the powder without adding additional volume. Therefore, you cannot use 9.6 mL, the volume of the diluent, in your calculation.

- Finally, how many full doses of ceftriaxone are available in this vial? The vial contains 1 g or 1,000 mg. The order is for 400 mg. There are *2 full doses* in the vial. According to the package insert, the *reconstituted solution is stable at room temperature for 24 hours and refrigerated for 3 days*. A reconstitution label is needed.

This means that you have available a vial of 1 g of ceftriaxone to which you will add 9.6 mL of diluent for IV administration. The final yield of the solution has a volume greater than the diluent with a supply dosage of 100 mg/mL. Most IV antibiotics are then further diluted in an approved IV solution and infused over a specified time period. You will learn more about this in Section 4.

Calculate 1 dose.

Step 1 Convert For the ordered dose of 400 mg, no conversion is necessary. The units are in the same system (metric) and the same size (mg).

Step 2 Think The order is for 400 mg and the supply is 100 mg/mL. You want to give more than 1 mL. In fact, you want to give 4 times this amount, or 4 mL.

Step 3 Calculate $\dfrac{\text{Dosage on hand}}{\text{Amount on hand}} = \dfrac{\text{Dosage desired}}{\text{X Amount desired}}$

$$\dfrac{100 \text{ mg}}{1 \text{ mL}} \bowtie \dfrac{400 \text{ mg}}{\text{X mL}}$$ Cross-multiply

$$100\text{X} = 400$$

$$\dfrac{100\text{X}}{100} = \dfrac{400}{100}$$ Simplify: Divide both sides of the equation by the number before the unknown X.

$$\text{X} = 4 \text{ mL}$$ Label the units to match the unknown X.

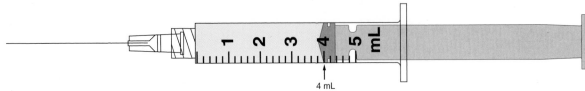

1/30/xx, 0800, reconstituted as 100 mg/mL for IV use. Expires 1/31/xx, 0800. Store at room temperature. G.D.P.

4 mL

Remember, even though it has been reconstituted according to directions, the ceftriaxone injection may not be ready yet for administration. How should you administer the intravenous medication? According to additional instructions in the package insert, the reconstituted solution may be further diluted in a 50–100 mL IV piggyback bag of compatible solution and administered over 10–30 minutes. You will learn more about this skill in Chapter 15.

Drugs With Instructions to "See Package Insert" for Dilution and Administration

Some labels only give the dosage strength contained in the vial and other minimal information that is insufficient to properly reconstitute or safely store the drug. To prepare the powdered medication, you must see the package insert. The following example demonstrates the use of the package insert for calculating the dosage.

EXAMPLE ▪

Order: amphotericin B 37.5 mg IV daily

Amphotericin B for Injection is an antifungal agent administered primarily to patients with progressive, potentially life-threatening fungal infections. The treatment is initiated with doses of 0.25 mg/kg/day with doses up to 1.5 mg/kg/day depending on the type of infection. For an average-size adult of 75 kg, the calculated dosage range would fall between 19 to 113 mg per day. Dosages must be individualized and adjusted according to the patient's tolerance. You will learn about calculating dosages based on body weight in Chapter 13.

For this example, blood cultures have revealed your patient has a systemic fungal infection requiring a highly effective antifungal therapy. This medication is not routinely stocked in the medical-surgical unit automated dispensing cabinet so the pharmacy has delivered an individual dose for your patient. The medication is packaged in a small carton (Figure 12-15a) with the package insert inside (Figure 12-15b).

FIGURE 12-15(a) Amphotericin B 50 mg label

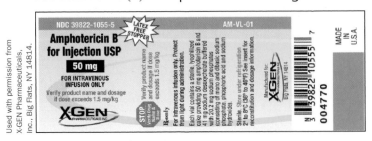

FIGURE 12-15(b)   Amphotericin B package insert reconstitution information

Preparation of Solutions

Reconstitute as follows: An initial concentrate of 5 mg amphotericin B per mL is first prepared by rapidly expressing 10 mL Sterile Water for Injection USP *without a bacteriostatic agent* directly into the lyophilized cake, using a sterile needle (minimum diameter: 20 gauge) and syringe. Shake the vial immediately until the colloidal solution is clear. The infusion solution, providing 0.1 mg amphotericin B per mL, is then obtained by further dilution (1:50) with 5% Dextrose Injection USP *of pH above 4.2.* The pH of each container of Dextrose Injection should be ascertained before use. Commercial Dextrose Injection usually has a pH above 4.2; however, if it is below 4.2, then 1 or 2 mL of buffer should be added to the Dextrose Injection before it is used to dilute the concentrated solution of amphotericin B. The recommended buffer has the following composition:

Dibasic sodium phosphate (anhydrous)	1.59 g
Monobasic sodium phosphate (anhydrous)	0.96 g
Water for Injection USP	qs 100.0 mL

- First, to fill the order, how much and what type of diluent must you add? For initial concentration, the directions advise you to *add 10 mL of sterile water for injection USP without a bacteriostatic agent.* Further, the directions state, "The infusion solution, providing 0.1 mg amphotericin B per mL, is then obtained by further dilution (1:50) with 5% Dextrose Injection USP of pH above 4.2." This means that before administration to the patient, the initial concentration of 5 mg/mL must be further diluted for infusion to 0.1 mg/mL or 1:50 concentration. (We will use the latter information after we calculate the dosage.)

- Second, what is the supply dosage of the reconstituted amphotericin B? When adding 10 mL of diluent, the *supply dosage is 5 mg/mL.*

- Third, what is the resulting total volume of this reconstituted solution? The *total volume is 10 mL.* You know this because the supply dosage is 5 mg/mL or 50 mg per 10 mL. The powder does not add significant volume to this solution.

- Finally, how many full doses of amphotericin B are available in this vial? The vial contains 50 mg, and the order is for 37.5 mg. There is enough for *1 full dose* (plus some extra) in the vial but not enough for 2 full doses. No reconstitution label is needed.

This means that you have available a vial of 50 mg of amphotericin B to which you will add 10 mL of diluent. The final yield of the solution is 5 mg/mL, which is your supply dosage.

Calculate 1 dose of the initial concentration (before further dilution).

Step 1	**Convert**	For the ordered dose of 37.5 mg, no conversion is necessary. The units are in the same system (metric) and the same size (mg).
Step 2	**Think**	The order is for 37.5 mg and the supply is 5 mg/mL. You want to give much more than 1 mL but less than 10 mL, which would be 10 times 5 mg or 50 mg.
Step 3	**Calculate**	$\dfrac{\text{Dosage on hand}}{\text{Amount on hand}} = \dfrac{\text{Dosage desired}}{\text{X Amount desired}}$

$$\frac{5 \text{ mg}}{1 \text{ mL}} \diagdown\!\!\!\!\diagup \frac{37.5 \text{ mg}}{\text{X mL}} \qquad \text{Cross-multiply}$$

$$5X = 37.5$$

$$\frac{5X}{5} = \frac{37.5}{5} \qquad \text{Simplify: Divide both sides of the equation by the number before the unknown X.}$$

$$X = 7.5 \text{ mL} \qquad \text{Label the units to match the unknown X.}$$

For the most accurate measurement, use both 3 mL and 5 mL syringes to measure the 7.5 mL dose.

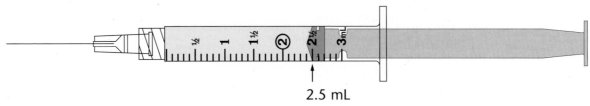

2.5 mL

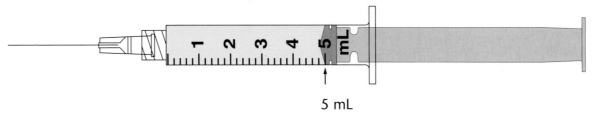

5 mL

Recall that the instructions indicate that further dilution of the initial concentration is required before administration: *The infusion solution, providing 0.1 mg amphotericin B per mL, is then obtained by further dilution (1:50) with 5% dextrose injection.* This may be accomplished by adding 49 mL of 5% dextrose and water injection to each 1 mL (5 mg) of amphotericin B solution. We have 7.5 mL of concentrated amphotericin solution to dilute; therefore, we need to add it to *7.5 × 49 = 367.5 or 368 mL* of IV solution before administering this drug intravenously.

Rapid intravenous infusion of amphotericin B has been associated with hypotension, hypokalemia, arrhythmias, and shock. Therefore, rapid infusion should be avoided. Intravenous infusion should be given over a period of approximately 2 to 6 hours. You will learn the skill of managing intravenous infusions in Chapter 15.

REMEMBER

It is the responsibility of the nurse or health care practitioner administering medications to be familiar with the action, therapeutic uses, recommended dosages, adverse and side effects, contraindications, and safe administration methods. Read package inserts and consult reputable drug references before preparing and administering medication.

QUICK REVIEW

- Check expiration dates of the drug and diluent before beginning reconstitution.

It is important that you remember the following points when reconstituting drugs.

- If any medicine remains for future use after reconstitution, clearly label:

    1. Date and time of preparation.
    2. Strength or concentration per volume.
    3. Potency expiration.
    4. Recommended storage.
    5. Your initials.

- Read all instructions carefully. If no instructions accompany the vial, confer with the pharmacist before proceeding.

- When reconstituting multiple-strength parenteral powders, select the dosage strength that is appropriate for the patient's age, size, and condition.

- Carefully select the correct reconstitution directions for IM or IV administration.

Review Set 26

For questions 1 through 10, let's focus only on the mathematical aspects of dosage calculation to reinforce the skill of reconstitution. These problems will present different medication orders for drugs that we have already worked with in the examples in this chapter. Use the labels provided for the supplied dosage, and draw an arrow on the syringe(s) for the correct dose amount. Select the preferred syringe, if more than one is provided. Prepare a reconstitution label, if needed.

1. Order: *acyclovir 0.5 g IV q.8h*

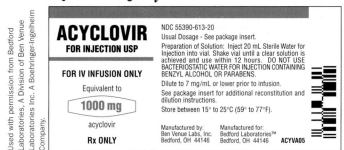

ACYCLOVIR
FOR INJECTION USP

FOR IV INFUSION ONLY

Equivalent to

1000 mg

acyclovir

Rx ONLY

NDC 55390-613-20
Usual Dosage - See package insert.
Preparation of Solution: Inject 20 mL Sterile Water for Injection into vial. Shake vial until a clear solution is achieved and use within 12 hours. DO NOT USE BACTERIOSTATIC WATER FOR INJECTION CONTAINING BENZYL ALCOHOL OR PARABENS.
Dilute to 7 mg/mL or lower prior to infusion.
See package insert for additional reconstitution and dilution instructions.
Store between 15° to 25°C (59° to 77°F).

Manufactured by: Manufactured for:
Ben Venue Labs, Inc.   Bedford Laboratories™
Bedford, OH 44146   Bedford, OH 44146   ACYVA05

Used with permission from Bedford Laboratories, A Division of Ben Venue Laboratories Inc. A Boehringer-Ingelheim Company.

According to the package insert, when mixed according to the instructions on the label, the resulting solution contains 50 mg acyclovir per mL. The reconstituted solution should be used within 12 hours. Refrigeration of reconstituted solution may result in the formation of a precipitate that will redissolve at room temperature.

Reconstitute with _____ mL diluent for a concentration of _____ mg/mL.

Give: _____ mL

How many full doses are available in this vial? _____ dose(s)

Prepare a reconstitution label for the remaining solution.

Reconstitution label

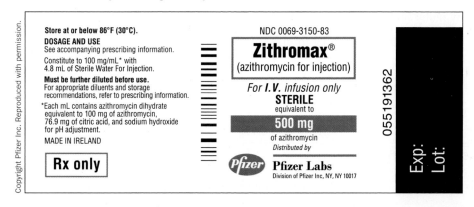

Copyright © 2016 Cengage Learning®.

2. Order: *azithromycin 0.5 g IV daily*

Store at or below 86°F (30°C).
DOSAGE AND USE
See accompanying prescribing information.
Constitute to 100 mg/mL* with
4.8 mL of Sterile Water For Injection.
Must be further diluted before use.
For appropriate diluents and storage
recommendations, refer to prescribing information.
*Each mL contains azithromycin dihydrate
equivalent to 100 mg of azithromycin,
76.9 mg of citric acid, and sodium hydroxide
for pH adjustment.
MADE IN IRELAND

Rx only

NDC 0069-3150-83

Zithromax®
(azithromycin for injection)

For *I.V.* infusion only
STERILE
equivalent to

500 mg
of azithromycin
Distributed by

Pfizer **Pfizer Labs**
Division of Pfizer Inc, NY, NY 10017

055191362

Exp:
Lot:

Copyright Pfizer Inc. Reproduced with permission.

Reconstitute with _____ mL diluent for a concentration of _____ mg/mL.

Give: _____ mL

How many full doses are available in this vial? _____ dose(s)

Does this reconstituted medication require a reconstitution label? _____

Explain: _____

3. Order: *penicillin G potassium 1,000,000 units IV q.6h*

Copyright Pfizer Inc. Reproduced with permission.	05-4243-32-6

SEE ACCOMPANYING
PRESCRIBING INFORMATION

**RECOMMENDED STORAGE
IN DRY FORM.**

Store below 86°F (30°C).

Sterile solution may be kept
in refrigerator for one (1)
week without significant loss
of potency.

6505-00-958-3305

Buffered

NDC 0049-0520-83
Rx only

Pfizerpen®
(penicillin G potassium)

5

For Injection

FIVE MILLION UNITS

Pfizer **Roerig**
Division of Pfizer Inc, NY, NY 10017

USUAL DOSAGE
Average single intramuscular injection:
200,000-400,000 units.
Intravenous: Additional information about
the use of this product intravenously can
be found in the package insert.

mL diluent added	Units per mL of solution
18.2 mL	250,000
8.2 mL	500,000
3.2 mL	1,000,000

Buffered with sodium citrate and citric acid
to optimum pH.

PATIENT: _____

ROOM NO: _____

DATE DILUTED: _____

Describe the three concentrations, and calculate the amount to give for each of the supply dosage concentrations.

Reconstitute with _____ mL diluent for a concentration of _____ units/mL.

Give: _____ mL

Reconstitute with _____ mL diluent for a concentration of _____ units/mL.

Give: _____ mL

Reconstitute with _____ mL diluent for a concentration of _____ units/mL.

Give: _____ mL

Indicate the concentration you would choose, and explain the rationale for your selection.

Select _____ units/mL and give _____ mL. Rationale: _____

_____

How many full doses are available in this vial? _____ dose(s)

Prepare a reconstitution label for the remaining solution.

[ ]

Reconstitution label

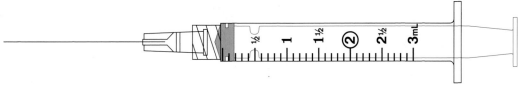

4. Order: **methylprednisolone 175 mg IV daily**

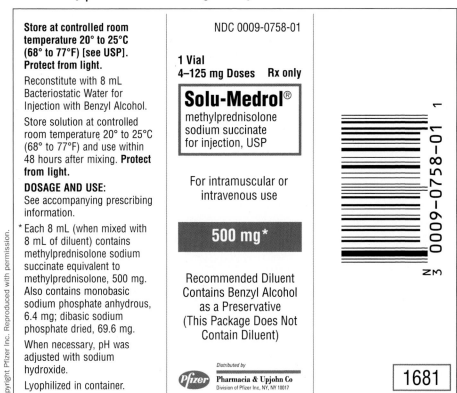

Store at controlled room temperature 20° to 25°C (68° to 77°F) [see USP]. Protect from light.

Reconstitute with 8 mL Bacteriostatic Water for Injection with Benzyl Alcohol.

Store solution at controlled room temperature 20° to 25°C (68° to 77°F) and use within 48 hours after mixing. **Protect from light.**

DOSAGE AND USE:
See accompanying prescribing information.

* Each 8 mL (when mixed with 8 mL of diluent) contains methylprednisolone sodium succinate equivalent to methylprednisolone, 500 mg. Also contains monobasic sodium phosphate anhydrous, 6.4 mg; dibasic sodium phosphate dried, 69.6 mg.

When necessary, pH was adjusted with sodium hydroxide.

Lyophilized in container.

Copyright Pfizer Inc. Reproduced with permission.

NDC 0009-0758-01

1 Vial
4–125 mg Doses   Rx only

Solu-Medrol®
methylprednisolone sodium succinate for injection, USP

For intramuscular or intravenous use

500 mg*

Recommended Diluent Contains Benzyl Alcohol as a Preservative (This Package Does Not Contain Diluent)

Distributed by
Pfizer **Pharmacia & Upjohn Co**
Division of Pfizer Inc, NY, NY 10017

1681

Reconstitute with _____ mL diluent for a concentration of _____ mg per _____ mL or _____ mg/mL.

Give: _____ mL

How many full doses are available in this vial? _____ dose(s)

Prepare a reconstitution label for the remaining solution.

Reconstitution label

5. Order: *penicillin G potassium 500,000 units IV q.6h*

NDC 0049-0510-83
Buffered
Pfizerpen®
penicillin G potassium
For Injection
ONE MILLION UNITS
CAUTION: Federal law prohibits dispensing without prescription.
ROERIG *Pfizer*
A division of Pfizer Inc., N.Y., N.Y. 10017

READ ACCOMPANYING PROFESSIONAL INFORMATION
RECOMMENDED STORAGE IN DRY FORM
STORE BELOW 86°F (30°C)
Sterile solution may be kept in refrigerator for one (1) week without significant loss of potency.
MADE IN U.S.A.
05-4242-00-3
6505-00-664-7116

Copyright Pfizer Inc. Reproduced with permission.

USUAL DOSAGE
Average single intramuscular injection: 200,000-400,000 units.
Intravenous: Additional information about the use of this product intravenously can be found in the package insert.

ml diluent added	Units per ml of solution
20.0 ml	50,000
10.0 ml	100,000
4.0 ml	250,000
1.8 ml	500,000

Buffered with sodium citrate and citric acid to optimum pH.

PATIENT:
ROOM NO.:
DATE DILUTED:

Describe the four concentrations, and calculate the amount to give for each of the supply dosage concentrations.

Reconstitute with _____ mL diluent for a concentration of _____ units/mL.

Give: _____ mL

Reconstitute with _____ mL diluent for a concentration of _____ units/mL.

Give: _____ mL

Reconstitute with _____ mL diluent for a concentration of _____ units/mL.

Give: _____ mL

Reconstitute with _____ mL diluent for a concentration of _____ units/mL.

Give: _____ mL

Indicate the concentration you would choose, and explain the rationale for your selection.

Select _____ units/mL and give _____ mL. Rationale: _____

_____

How many full doses are available in this vial? _____ dose(s)

Prepare a reconstitution label for the remaining solution.

Reconstitution label

6. Order: **methylprednisolone sodium succinate 24 mg slow IV push q.12h**

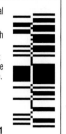

MethylPREDNISolone
Sodium Succinate
for Injection, USP

NDC 55390-209-10   Single Dose Vial
Reconstitute with 1.2 mL of
Bacteriostatic Water for Injection with
benzyl alcohol.

FOR IM OR IV USE

40 mg*

Rx ONLY
Recommended Diluent
Contains Benzyl Alcohol as a
Preservative.

*Each 1 mL (when mixed) contains:
Methylprednisolone sodium succinate
equiv. to 40 mg methylprednisolone.
Lyophilized in container.
Protect from light.
Manufactured for:
Bedford Laboratories™
Bedford, OH 44146   MPNL-V01

See package insert for complete product information.
Reconstitute with 1.2 mL of Bacteriostatic Water for Injection with benzyl alcohol.
*Each 1 mL (when mixed) contains: Methylprednisolone sodium succinate equivalent to 40 mg methylprednisolone; also 1.6 mg monobasic sodium phosphate anhydrous; 17.46 mg dibasic sodium phosphate dried; 25 mg lactose hydrous; 8.8 mg benzyl alcohol added as preservative.
When necessary, pH was adjusted with sodium hydroxide. Lyophilized in container.
Store at 20° to 25°C (68° to 77°F). See USP controlled room temperature. Use within 48 hours after mixing. Protect from light.

LOT
EXP

Manufactured by:
Ben Venue Labs, Inc.
Bedford, OH 44146

BEDFORD
LABORATORIES™

Manufactured for:
Bedford Laboratories™
Bedford, OH 44146

Reconstitute with _____ mL diluent for a concentration of _____ mg/mL.

Give: _____ mL

How many full doses are available in this vial? _____ dose(s)

Prepare a reconstitution label for the remaining solution.

Reconstitution label

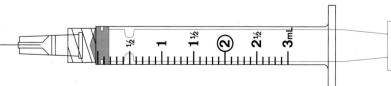

7. Order: *ceftriaxone 750 mg IV q.12h*

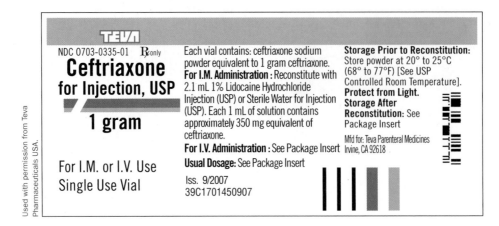

Used with permission from Teva Pharmaceuticals USA.

Package insert for ceftriaxone states, "Reconstituted solution is stable at room temperature for 24 hours and refrigerated for 3 days." Administration instructions:

Intravenous Administration

Ceftriaxone for injection, USP should be administered intravenously by infusion over a period of 30 minutes. Concentrations between 10 mg/mL and 40 mg/mL are recommended; however, lower concentrations may be used if desired. Reconstitute vials with an appropriate IV diluent (see **COMPATIBILITY AND STABILITY**).

Vial Dosage Size	Amount of Diluent to be Added
250 mg	2.4 mL
500 mg	4.8 mL
1 g	9.6 mL
2 g	19.2 mL

After reconstitution, each 1 mL of solution contains approximately 100 mg equivalent of ceftriaxone. Withdraw entire contents and dilute to the desired concentration with the appropriate IV diluent.

Used with permission from Teva Pharmaceuticals USA.

Reconstitute with _____ mL diluent for a concentration of _____ g per _____ mL or _____ mg/mL.

Give: _____ mL

How many full doses are available in this vial? _____ dose(s)

Will the drug remain potent to use all available doses? _____

Explain: _____

Prepare a reconstitution label for the remaining solution.

Reconstitution label

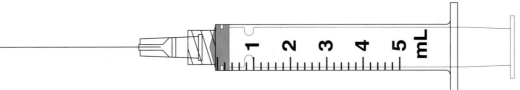

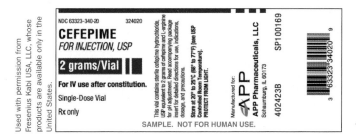

8. Order: *cefepime 1,500 mg IV q.12h in 100 mL D₅W (5% Dextrose and Water IV solution) IV PB*

Package insert states:

Administration

For intravenous infusion, constitute the 1 g, or 2 g vial, and add an appropriate quantity of the resulting solution to an IV container with one of the compatible IV fluids listed in the Compatibility and Stability subsection. THE RESULTING SOLUTION SHOULD BE ADMINISTERED OVER APPROXIMATELY 30 MINUTES.

Single-Dose Vials for Intravenous/Intramuscular Administration	Amount of Diluent to Be Added (mL)	Approximate Available Volume (mL)	Approximate Cefepime Concentration (mg/mL)
cefepime vial content			
1 g (IV)	10	11.3	100
1 g (IM)	2.4	3.6	280
2 g (IV)	10	12.5	160

Compatibility and Stability Intravenous: Cefepime is compatible at concentrations between 1 mg/mL and 40 mg/mL with the following IV infusion fluids: 0.9% Sodium Chloride Injection, 5% and 10% Dextrose Injection, M/6 Sodium Lactate Injection, 5% Dextrose and 0.9% Sodium Chloride Injection, Lactated Ringers and 5% Dextrose Injection, Normosol-R and Normosol-M in 5% Dextrose Injection. These solutions may be stored up to 24 hours at controlled room temperature 20°–25°C (68°–77°F) or 7 days in a refrigerator 2°–8°C (36°–46°F).

Reconstitute with _____ mL diluent for an initial concentration of _____ g per _____ mL or _____ mg/mL.

Give: _____ mL

How many full doses are available in this vial? _____ dose(s)

Prepare a reconstitution label for the remaining solution.

Reconstitution label

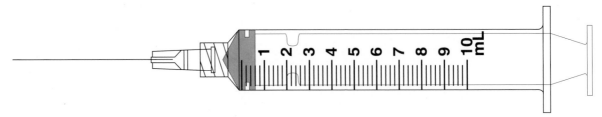

9. Order: *cephradine 250 mg IV q.6h*

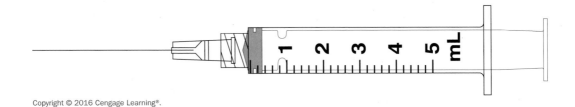

Reconstitute with _____ mL diluent for a concentration of _____ mg/mL.

Give: _____ mL

How many full doses are available in this vial? _____ dose(s)

10. Order: *cefazolin 250 mg IV q.6h*

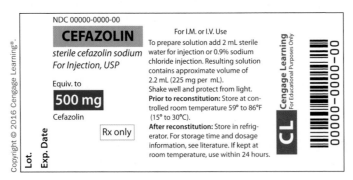

Reconstitute with _____ mL diluent for a concentration of _____ mg/mL.

Give: _____ mL

How many full doses are available in this vial? _____ dose(s)

Prepare a reconstitution label for the remaining solution.

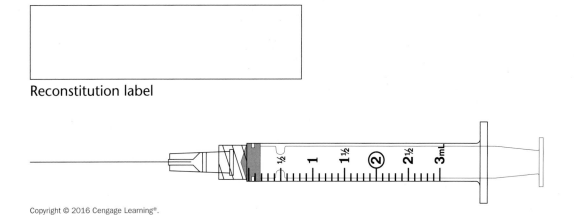

Reconstitution label

Questions 11 through 15 are medication-preparation simulations. You will utilize all aspects of safe dosage preparation and calculation of medications, including collecting data about the drug, selecting the supplied dosage, computing the amount to give, and measuring with equipment for medication administration. Refer to a nursing drug guide, such as the *Delmar Nurse's Drug Handbook,* to answer specific questions about the medication prior to administering.

11. An advanced oncology certified nurse (AOCN) is preparing to administer the ordered maintenance dose of cytarabine to a patient who weighs 100 kg. The setting is an outpatient clinic and the medication will be retrieved from a stock supply cabinet. The nurse will prepare the powder for reconstitution in a specially designated area.

    Order: **cytarabine 100 mg subcut q.1 week**

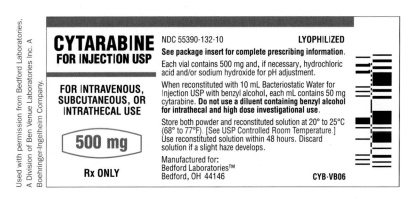

    a. For what condition(s) is cytarabine indicated? _____

    b. What dosage strengths of cytarabine may be supplied in powder for injection? _____

    _____

    c. By what parenteral routes may cytarabine be administered? _____

    d. What is the usual recommended adult maintenance dosage range when given by subcutaneous route? _____

    e. Reconstitute with _____ mL diluent for a concentration of _____ mg/mL.

    f. Give: _____ mL (Caution: maximum recommended subcut injection is 1 mL.)

    g. Cytarabine is designated as a high-alert medication. What additional precaution must be taken prior to administration? _____

h. Mark correct amount on the syringe(s):

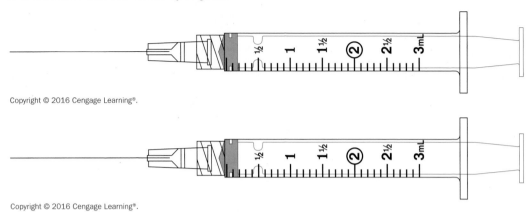

Copyright © 2016 Cengage Learning®.

Copyright © 2016 Cengage Learning®.

i. How many full doses are available in this vial? _____ dose(s)

j. Prepare a reconstitution label for the remaining solution.

Reconstitution label

12. A patient is admitted to the medical-surgical unit with an order for intravenous doxycycline to begin now and continue every 12 hours. You are planning to administer the first dose at 0900 and then schedule according to hospital routine at 2100 tonight and 0900 tomorrow. The ordered dose of the reconstituted powder will be drawn up in a syringe and further diluted in either a 100 mL or 200 mL IVPB bag for intermittent infusion. A 24-hour supply of the medication will be stocked by the pharmacy in the patient's unit-dose drawer as pictured below.

Order: *doxycycline 200 mg IVPB stat, then 50 mg IVPB q.12h*

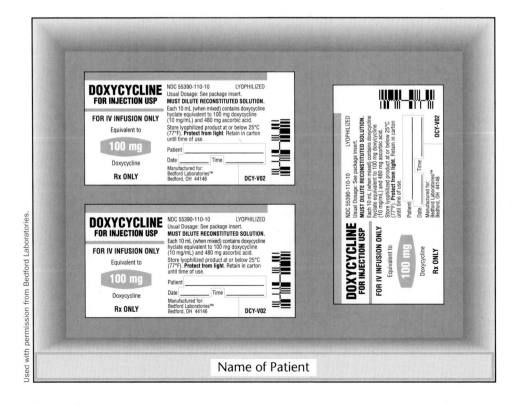

Name of Patient

a. For what condition(s) is doxycycline indicated? _____

b. What dosage strengths of doxycycline may be supplied in powder for injection? _____

_____

c. By what parenteral routes may doxycycline be administered? _____

d. What is the usual recommended adult dosage range for initial and daily doses?

_____

e. How many vials will be needed for the initial dose? _____

f. Reconstitute with _____ mL diluent for a concentration of _____ mg/10 mL or
_____ mg/mL.

g. Calculate the initial ordered dose to be administered at 0900. Add _____ mL of
reconstituted solution to 200 mL IVPB bag for continuous infusion.

h. Mark correct amount on the syringe(s):

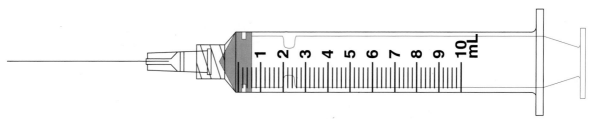

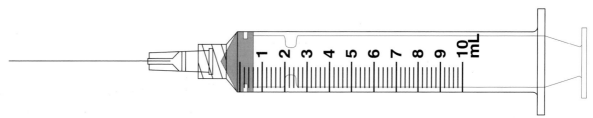

i. Calculate the second ordered dose to be administered at 2100. Add _____ mL of
reconstituted solution to 100 mL IVPB bag for continuous infusion.

j. Mark correct amount on the syringe(s):

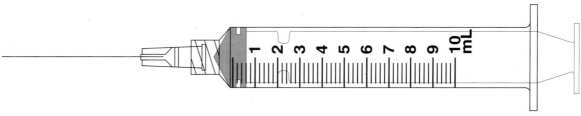

k. How many full doses are available in this vial? _____ dose(s)

l. The package insert states, "Reconstituted solutions may be stored up to 72 hours prior to start
of infusion if refrigerated and protected from sunlight and artificial light. Infusion must then
be completed within 12 hours. Solutions must be used within these time periods or discarded."
Prepare a reconstitution label for the remaining solution.

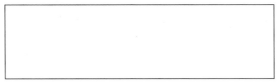

Reconstitution label

Questions 13 through 15: For these problems, imagine you are working on a hospital medical-surgical unit and you are administering routine scheduled medications to three different patients. The medications are stored in powdered form and require reconstitution prior to administration. They will be retrieved from the automated dispensing cabinet as pictured.

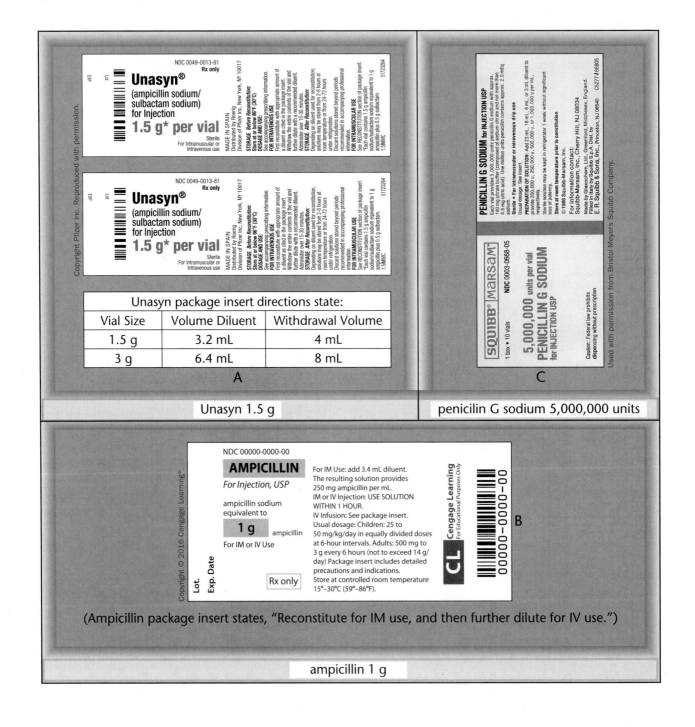

Unasyn package insert directions state:		
Vial Size	Volume Diluent	Withdrawal Volume
1.5 g	3.2 mL	4 mL
3 g	6.4 mL	8 mL

A

Unasyn 1.5 g

C

penicilin G sodium 5,000,000 units

(Ampicillin package insert states, "Reconstitute for IM use, and then further dilute for IV use.")

ampicillin 1 g

13. Order: ampicillin 750 mg IV q.6h

    a. For what condition(s) is ampicillin indicated? _____

    b. What dosage strengths of ampicillin may be supplied in powder for injection? _____

    _____

    c. By what parenteral routes may ampicillin be administered? _____

    d. What is the usual recommended adult dosage? _____

    _____

    e. Indicate the letter of the vial you will select from the ADC to use: _____.

    f. Reconstitute with _____ mL diluent for a concentration of _____ mg/mL.

    g. Add _____ mL of reconstituted solution to 100 mL IVPB bag for continuous infusion.

    h. Mark correct amount on the syringe(s):

    i. How many full doses are available in this vial? _____ dose(s)

    j. Does this reconstituted medication require a reconstitution label? _____

    Explain: _____

14. Order: penicillin G sodium 1,500,000 units IV q. 12h

    a. For what condition(s) is penicillin G sodium indicated?

    _____

    b. What dosage strengths of penicillin G sodium may be supplied in powder for injection?

    _____

    c. By what parenteral routes may penicillin G sodium be administered? _____

    _____

    d. What is the usual recommended dosage range for initial and daily doses? _____

    _____

    e. Indicate the letter of the vial you will select from the ADC to use: _____

    f. Describe the four concentrations, and calculate the amount to give for each of the supply
       dosage concentrations.

    Reconstitute with _____ mL diluent for a concentration of _____ units/mL.

    Give: _____ mL

    Reconstitute with _____ mL diluent for a concentration of _____ units/mL.

    Give: _____ mL

    Reconstitute with _____ mL diluent for a concentration of _____ units/mL.

    Give: _____ mL

    Reconstitute with _____ mL diluent for a concentration of _____ units/mL.

    Give: _____ mL

g. Indicate the concentration you would choose to add to 100 mL IVPB bag for continuous infusion and explain the rationale for your selection.

Select _____ units/mL and give _____ mL. Rationale: _____

_____

h. Mark correct amount on the syringe(s):

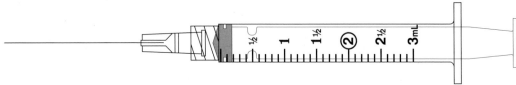

i. How many full doses are available in this vial? _____ dose(s)

j. Prepare a reconstitution label for the remaining solution.

[reconstitution label box]

Reconstitution label

15. Order: Unasyn 2 g IV q.6h

a. For what condition(s) is Unasyn indicated? _____

b. What are the generic names and doses of the two drugs combined in the supplied vial of Unasyn?_____

c. What dosage strengths of Unasyn may be supplied in powder for injection? _____

_____

d. By what parenteral routes may Unasyn be administered? _____

e. What is the usual recommended dosage range for Unasyn? _____

_____

f. Indicate the letter of the vial you will select: _____

g. How many vials will be needed for 1 dose?_____

h. Reconstitute with _____ mL diluent for a concentration of _____ g per _____ mL.

i. Draw up _____ mL of reconstituted solution from first vial and _____ mL from second vial to add to 100 mL IVPB bag for continuous infusion.

j. Mark correct amount on the syringe(s):

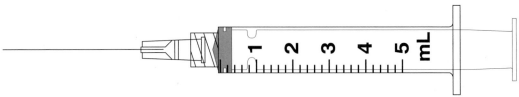

k. Which of the manufactured supply dosages would be preferred to administer this dose? _____

l. Prepare a reconstitution label for the remaining solution.

Reconstitution label

After completing these problems, see pages 673–680 to check your answers.

RECONSTITUTION OF NONINJECTABLE SOLUTIONS

Now let's look at reconstitution of noninjectable solutions such as nutritional formulas and irrigating solutions. In most cases, the nurse or health care professional must dilute a liquid concentrate (solute) with water or saline (solvent) to make a weaker solution.

Solution Concentration

An important concept for understanding solution concentration or strength is that the amount of solvent used to decrease the total concentration is determined by the desired final strength of the solution. The *less* solvent added, the *more concentrated* the final solution strength; the *more* solvent added, the *less concentrated* the final solution strength. Think of orange juice concentrate as a way to illustrate this concept. The directions call for three cans of water to be added to one can of orange juice concentrate. The result is "reconstituted juice," a ready-to-drink beverage. If you like a stronger orange taste, you might add only two cans of water, making it a *more* concentrated juice; but you get *less total volume* to drink. If you have several people wanting to drink orange juice, you might choose to add four cans of water to the final total volume. You get *more* volume, but the orange juice is *less* concentrated; therefore, it is more dilute, because you have increased the water (solvent) content. Note that in either case, the amount of orange juice concentrate in the final solution is the same.

Medical notation to express the strength of a solution uses either a ratio, a percent, or a fraction. The fraction is the preferred form, because it is easily applied in calculations and helps explain the ratio of solute to total solution. Recall that a ratio or percent can also be expressed as a fraction.

RULE

When the strength of a solution made from a liquid concentrate is expressed as a fraction:

- The numerator of the fraction is the number of parts of solute.

- The denominator of the fraction is the total number of parts of total solution.

- The difference between the denominator (final solution) and the numerator (parts of solute) is the number of parts of solvent.

Let's describe some solutions made from liquid concentrates.

EXAMPLE 1 ■

$\frac{1}{4}$ **strength reconstituted orange juice** made from canned frozen concentrate

$\frac{1}{4}$ strength $= \dfrac{1 \text{ part (can) of frozen orange juice concentrate}}{4 \text{ parts (cans) of total reconstituted orange juice}}$

- 1 part (can) frozen orange juice concentrate (*solute,* numerator)

- 4 parts (cans) of total reconstituted orange juice (*solution,* denominator)

- $4 - 1 = 3$ parts (cans) of water (*solvent*)

Three cans of water added to 1 can frozen orange juice concentrate makes 4 cans of a final reconstituted orange juice solution. The resulting $\frac{1}{4}$ strength reconstituted orange juice is comparable to the strength of fresh juice.

EXAMPLE 2 ■

$\frac{1}{3}$ **strength nutritional formula**

- 1 part concentrate formula as the solute

- 3 parts of total solution

- $3 - 1 = 2$ parts solvent (water)

Therefore, 1 can of nutritional formula concentrate and 2 cans of water make a $\frac{1}{3}$ strength nutritional formula.

Calculating Solutions

To prepare a prescribed solution of a certain strength from a solute, you can apply a formula similar to the one you learned for calculating dosages.

RULE

To prepare solutions,

1. Apply ratio-proportion to find the amount of solute (X)

   Ratio for desired solution strength $= \dfrac{\text{X Amount of solute}}{\text{Quantity of desired solution}}$

2. Quantity of desired solution − Amount of solute = Amount of solvent

The unknown X you are solving for is the quantity or amount of solute you will need to add to the solvent to prepare the desired solution. Let's look at how this rule is applied in health care.

TOPICAL SOLUTIONS AND IRRIGANTS

Topical or irrigating solutions may be mixed from powders, salts, or liquid concentrates. Asepsis in mixing, storage, and use is essential. Liquids can quickly harbor microorganisms. Our focus here is to review the essentials of reconstitution, but nurses and other health care professionals need to be alert at all times to the chain of infection.

Most often, nurses and other health care professionals will further dilute ready-to-use solutions, which are called *full-strength* or stock solutions, to create a less concentrated liquid. Consider the desired solution strength as well as the final volume needed for the task.

EXAMPLE 1 ■

Hydrogen peroxide, which is usually available full strength as a 3% solution, can be drying to the skin and should not be directly applied undiluted. For use as a topical antiseptic, the therapeutic protocol is to reconstitute hydrogen peroxide to $\frac{1}{2}$ strength, with normal saline used as the solvent. You decide to make 4 fluid ounces that can be kept in a sterile container at the patient's bedside for traction pin care.

Step 1	**Convert**	No conversion is necessary.

Step 2   **Think**   The fraction represents the desired solution strength: $\frac{1}{2}$ strength means 1 part solute (hydrogen peroxide) to 2 total parts solution. The amount of solvent is $2 - 1 = 1$ part saline. Because you need 4 fl oz of solution, you estimate that you will need $\frac{1}{2}$ of it as solute and $\frac{1}{2}$ of it as solvent, or 2 fl oz hydrogen peroxide and 2 fl oz saline to make a total of 4 fl oz of $\frac{1}{2}$ strength hydrogen peroxide.

Step 3   **Calculate**   Remember that $\frac{1}{2}$ strength $= \frac{1 \text{ part solute}}{2 \text{ parts total solution}}$. Here, the desired solution strength is $\frac{1}{2}$. The quantity of solution desired is 4 fl oz. You want to know how much solute (X fl oz) you will need.

$$\frac{1}{2} \diagdown\!\!\!\diagup \frac{\text{X fl oz (solute)}}{\text{4 fl oz (solution)}}$$

$$2X = 4$$

$$\frac{2X}{2} = \frac{4}{2}$$

$$X = 2 \text{ fl oz (solute)}$$

The quantity of solute (full-strength hydrogen peroxide) you will need to prepare the desired solution $\left(4 \text{ fl oz of } \frac{1}{2} \text{ strength hydrogen peroxide}\right)$ is represented by X (2 fl oz). The amount of solvent is 4 fl oz − 2 fl oz = 2 fl oz. If you add 2 fl oz of full-strength hydrogen peroxide (solute) to 2 fl oz of normal saline (solvent), you will prepare 4 fl oz of a $\frac{1}{2}$ strength hydrogen peroxide topical antiseptic.

EXAMPLE 2 ■

Suppose a physician orders a patient's wound irrigated with $\frac{2}{3}$ strength hydrogen peroxide in normal saline solution q.4h while awake. You will need 60 mL per irrigation and will do three irrigations during your 12-hour shift. You will need to prepare 60 mL × 3 irrigations = 180 mL total solution. How much stock hydrogen peroxide and normal saline will you need?

Step 1	**Convert**	No conversion is necessary.

Step 2   **Think**   You want to make $\frac{2}{3}$ strength, which means 2 parts solute (concentrated hydrogen peroxide) to 3 total parts solution. The amount of solvent is $3 - 2 = 1$ part saline. Because you need 180 mL of solution, you estimate that you will need $\frac{2}{3}$ of it as solute $\left(\frac{2}{3} \times 180 \text{ mL} = 120 \text{ mL}\right)$ and $\frac{1}{3}$ of it as solvent $\left(\frac{1}{3} \times 180 \text{ mL} = 60 \text{ mL}\right)$.

Step 3   **Calculate** $\frac{2}{3} \diagdown\!\!\!\diagup \frac{\text{X mL (solute)}}{\text{180 mL (solution)}}$

$$3X = 360$$

$$\frac{3X}{3} = \frac{360}{3}$$

$$X = 120 \text{ mL (solute)}$$

120 mL is the quantity of solute (hydrogen peroxide) that you will need to prepare the desired solution (180 mL of $\frac{2}{3}$ strength). Because you want to make a total of 180 mL of solution for wound irrigation, the amount of solvent you will need is 180 mL − 120 mL = 60 mL of normal saline. Therefore, to make 180 mL of $\frac{2}{3}$ strength hydrogen peroxide, mix 120 mL full-strength hydrogen peroxide and 60 mL normal saline.

ORAL AND ENTERAL FEEDINGS

The principles of reconstitution are frequently applied to nutritional liquids for children and adults with special needs. Premature infants require increased calories for growth yet cannot take large volumes of fluid. Children who suffer from intestinal malabsorption require incremental changes as their bodies adjust to more-concentrated formulas. Adults, especially the elderly, also experience nutritional problems that can be remedied with liquid nutrition. Prepared solutions that are taken orally or through feeding tubes are usually available and ready to use from manufacturers. Nutritional solutions may also be mixed from powders or liquid concentrates. Figure 12-16 shows examples of the three forms of one nutritional formula. Directions on the label detail how much water should be added to the powdered form or liquid concentrate. Nutritionists provide further expertise in creating complex solutions for special patient needs.

As mentioned previously, health care professionals must be alert at all times to the chain of infection. Asepsis in mixing, storage, and use of nutritional liquids is essential. Because they contain sugars, such liquids have an increased risk for contamination during preparation and spoilage during storage and use. These are important concepts to teach a patient's family members.

FIGURE 12-16   Nutritional formulas

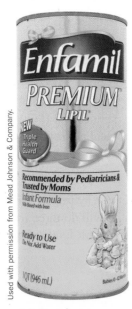
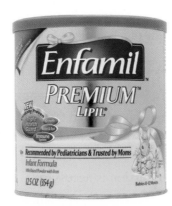
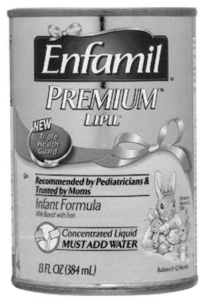

(a) Ready to use   (b) Powder for reconstitution   (c) Concentrated liquid for reconstitution

Diluting Ready-to-Use Nutritional Liquids

Ready-to-use nutritional liquids are those solutions that are normally administered directly from the container without any further dilution. Most ready-to-use formulas contain 20 calories per fluid ounce and are used for children and adults. The manufacturer balances the solute (nutrition) and solvent (water) to create a balanced full-strength solution. However, some children and adults require less than full-strength formula for a short period to normalize intestinal absorption. Nutritional formulas are diluted with sterile water or tap water for oral use. Consult the facility policy regarding the use of tap water to reconstitute nutritional formulas. Let's look at a few typical examples.

EXAMPLE 1 ■

A physician orders **Ensure $\frac{1}{4}$ strength 120 mL q.2h via NG tube X 3 feedings** for a patient who is recovering from gastric surgery. Available are 4 and 8 fl oz cans of Ensure ready-to-use formula. Let's calculate conversion for both supply sizes.

Step 1	**Convert**	Approximate equivalent: 1 fl oz = 30 mL

$$\frac{1 \text{ fl oz}}{30 \text{ mL}} \diagdown\!\!\!\diagup \frac{4 \text{ fl oz}}{X \text{ mL}} \qquad\qquad \frac{1 \text{ fl oz}}{30 \text{ mL}} \diagdown\!\!\!\diagup \frac{8 \text{ fl oz}}{X \text{ mL}}$$

X = 120 mL (per 4 fl oz can)   X = 240 mL (per 8 fl oz can)

Step 2	**Think**	You need 120 mL total reconstituted formula for each of 3 feedings. This is a total of 120 mL × 3 = 360 mL. But you must dilute the full-strength formula to $\frac{1}{4}$ strength. You know that $\frac{1}{4}$ strength means 1 part formula to 4 parts solution. The solvent needed is 4 − 1 = 3 parts water. You will need $\frac{1}{4}$ of the solution as solute ($\frac{1}{4}$ × 360 mL = 90 mL) and $\frac{3}{4}$ of the solution as solvent ($\frac{3}{4}$ × 360 mL = 270 mL). Therefore, if you mix 90 mL of full-strength formula with 270 mL of water, you will have 360 mL of $\frac{1}{4}$ strength formula.

Step 3	**Calculate**	$\frac{1}{4} \diagup\!\!\!\diagdown \frac{X \text{ mL}}{360 \text{ mL}}$

$$4X = 360$$

$$\frac{4X}{4} = \frac{360}{4}$$

X = 90 mL (full-strength Ensure)

You need 90 mL of the formula (solute). Use 90 mL from the 4 fl oz can, because it contains 120 mL. (You will have 30 mL left over.) The amount of solvent needed is 360 mL − 90 mL = 270 mL water. Add 270 mL water to 90 mL of full-strength Ensure to make a total of 360 mL of $\frac{1}{4}$ strength Ensure. You now have enough for 3 full feedings. Administer 120 mL to the patient for each feeding.

EXAMPLE 2 ■

The physician orders **800 mL of $\frac{3}{4}$ strength Sustacal through a gastrostomy tube over 8 hours** to supplement a patient while he sleeps. Sustacal ready-to-use formula comes in 10 fl oz cans.

Step 1	**Convert**	Approximate equivalent: 1 fl oz = 30 mL

$$\frac{1 \text{ fl oz}}{30 \text{ mL}} \diagdown\!\!\!\diagup \frac{10 \text{ fl oz}}{30 \text{ mL}}$$

X = 300 mL (per 10 fl oz can)

Step 2	**Think**	The ordered solution strength is $\frac{3}{4}$. This means 3 parts solute to 4 total parts in solution. You know that $\frac{3}{4}$ of the 800 mL will be solute, or full-strength Sustacal ($\frac{3}{4}$ × 800 mL = 600 mL), and $\frac{1}{4}$ of the solution will be solvent, or water ($\frac{1}{4}$ × 800 mL = 200 mL). This proportion of solute to solvent will reconstitute the Sustacal to the required $\frac{3}{4}$ strength and total volume of 800 mL.

Step 3	**Calculate**	$\frac{3}{4} \diagup\!\!\!\diagdown \frac{X \text{ mL}}{800 \text{ mL}}$

$$4X = 2,400$$

$$\frac{4X}{4} = \frac{2,400}{4}$$

X = 600 mL (full-strength Sustacal)

You need 600 mL of the formula (solute). Because the 10 fl oz can contains 300 mL, you will need 2 cans (600 mL) to prepare the $\frac{3}{4}$ strength Sustacal as ordered. The amount of solvent needed is 800 mL − 600 mL = 200 mL water. Add 200 mL water to 600 mL (or 2 cans) of full-strength Sustacal to make a total of 800 mL of $\frac{3}{4}$ strength Sustacal for the full feeding.

QUICK REVIEW

- *Solute*—a concentrated or solid substance to be dissolved or diluted.

- *Solvent*—or diluent, a liquid substance that dissolves another substance to prepare a solution.

- *Solution*—the resulting mixture of a solute plus a solvent.

- When a fraction expresses the strength of a desired solution to be made from a liquid concentrate:

  - The *numerator* of the fraction is the number of parts of *solute*.

  - The *denominator* of the fraction is the total number of parts of *solution*.

  - The *difference between the denominator and the numerator* is the number of parts of *solvent*.

- To prepare solutions:

  1. Ratio for desired solution strength $= \dfrac{\text{X Amount of solute}}{\text{Quantity of desired solution}}$

  2. Quantity of desired solution − Amount of solute = Amount of solvent

Review Set 27

Explain how you would prepare each of the following solutions, using liquid stock hydrogen peroxide as the solute and saline as the solvent.

1. 480 mL of $\frac{1}{3}$ strength for wound irrigation _____

2. 4 fl oz of $\frac{1}{4}$ strength for skin cleansing _____

3. 240 mL of $\frac{3}{4}$ strength for skeletal pin care _____

4. 16 fl oz of $\frac{1}{2}$ strength for wound care _____

Explain how you would prepare each of the following from ready-to-use nutritional formulas for the specified time period. Note which supply would require the least waste of unused formula.

5. Order: $\frac{1}{3}$ strength Ensure 900 mL via NG tube over 9 h

   Supply: Ensure 4, 8, and 12 fl oz cans _____

6. Order: $\frac{1}{4}$ strength Isomil 4 fl oz p.o. q.4 h for 24 h

   Supply: Isomil 3, 6, and 12 fl oz cans _____

7. Order: $\frac{2}{3}$ strength Sustacal 300 mL p.o. q.i.d.

   Supply: Sustacal 5 and 10 fl oz cans _____

8. Order: $\frac{1}{2}$ strength Ensure 26 fl oz via gastrostomy tube over 5 h

   Supply: 4, 8, and 12 fl oz cans _____

9. Order: $\frac{1}{2}$ strength Sustacal 250 mL p.o. q.i.d.

   Supply: Sustacal 5 and 10 fl oz cans _____

10. Order: $\frac{3}{4}$ strength Isomil 8 fl oz p.o. q.4 h for 24 h

   Supply: Isomil 3, 6, and 12 fl oz cans _____

11. Order: $\frac{2}{3}$ strength Ensure 6 fl oz via gastrostomy tube over 2 h

   Supply: Ensure 4, 8, and 12 fl oz cans _____

12. Order: $\frac{1}{4}$ strength Ensure 16 fl oz via NG tube over 6 h

   Supply: Ensure 4, 8, and 12 fl oz cans _____

After completing these problems, see pages 680–681 to check your answers.

CLINICAL REASONING SKILLS

Often, when reconstituting a medication, the powdered drug itself adds volume to the solution. In this case, the resulting volume will be greater than the volume of the diluent used to prepare the solution. Care must be taken to verify the actual volume of the reconstituted solution or the dose administered may be incorrect.

ERROR

Misinterpreting the reconstitution instructions on the label of a powdered drug and incorrectly calculating a dose of medication using the volume of the diluent added as the amount on hand in the dosage calculation formula

Possible Scenario

An adult patient has an order for *penicillin G potassium 1,000,000 units IM q.6h.* The supply of penicillin G potassium was stored in powdered form, and the nurse needed to reconstitute the powder to solution. The nurse first determined what would be an appropriate solution concentration and circled the reconstitution instructions. The drug was labeled as pictured below.

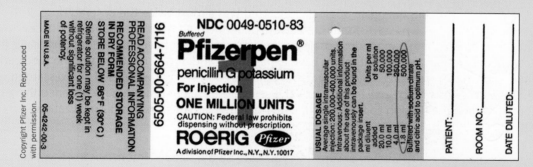

After adding 1.8 mL of the recommended diluent, the nurse set up the dosage calculation as:

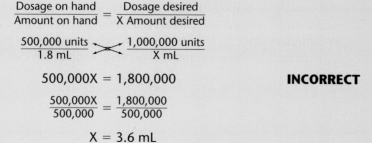

$$\frac{\text{Dosage on hand}}{\text{Amount on hand}} = \frac{\text{Dosage desired}}{\text{X Amount desired}}$$

$$\frac{500,000 \text{ units}}{1.8 \text{ mL}} \diagdown \frac{1,000,000 \text{ units}}{\text{X mL}}$$

$$500,000\text{X} = 1,800,000 \qquad\qquad \textbf{INCORRECT}$$

$$\frac{500,000\text{X}}{500,000} = \frac{1,800,000}{500,000}$$

$$\text{X} = 3.6 \text{ mL}$$

The calculated volume exceeded the maximum amount for an intramuscular injection. Because this was the most concentrated solution recommended, the nurse decided the medication would need to be divided into two syringes, each containing 1.8 mL. There was not enough solution in one vial, so the nurse mixed up two vials. Prior to the nurse administering the two intramuscular injections, the patient questioned why he was getting two injections when every other time the nurses only gave him one injection. The nurse returned to the medication room and asked another nurse to verify the calculation. The second nurse pointed out that the solution strengths were provided in units per mL as printed on the top of the right column of the label. There were actually 500,000 units in 1 mL, not in 1.8 mL, which was the volume of the diluent. The **correct** calculation and reconstitution label should have been:

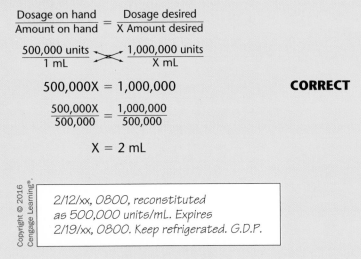

$$\frac{\text{Dosage on hand}}{\text{Amount on hand}} = \frac{\text{Dosage desired}}{\text{X Amount desired}}$$

$$\frac{500{,}000 \text{ units}}{1 \text{ mL}} \diagup\!\!\!\!\diagdown \frac{1{,}000{,}000 \text{ units}}{\text{X mL}}$$

$$500{,}000\text{X} = 1{,}000{,}000 \qquad\qquad \textbf{CORRECT}$$

$$\frac{500{,}000\text{X}}{500{,}000} = \frac{1{,}000{,}000}{500{,}000}$$

$$\text{X} = 2 \text{ mL}$$

> 2/12/xx, 0800, reconstituted
> as 500,000 units/mL. Expires
> 2/19/xx, 0800. Keep refrigerated. G.D.P.

The nurse now recognized the mistake. There was exactly enough solution left in one vial to add to a syringe containing 1.8 mL to make the required volume of 2 mL. The other medication and syringe were discarded. The nurse then administered the correct dose to the patient in one intramuscular injection.

Potential Outcome

The dose of penicillin the nurse originally prepared was almost twice the ordered dose. If two intramuscular injections were administered, the patient would have experienced unnecessary discomfort. Receiving 1 extra dose of penicillin likely would not have had serious physical consequences, but the patient might have experienced additional side effects of the medication if additional doses were given. An extra vial of penicillin and syringe were used and discarded, adding unnecessary costs to the patient or hospital. Further, the incident might have lessened the patient's confidence in the nursing care provided, causing increased stress to this hospitalization.

Prevention

Always read the entire label to ensure that you have all the needed information. The nurse made an error in this case by only reading the last line of the reconstitution instructions. The error could also have been avoided if the nurse stopped to ask, "Does this make sense?" The total quantity of the powdered penicillin G potassium in the vial was 1,000,000 units, which was the ordered dosage. The nurse should have recognized the calculation error when the incorrect calculated dose required an additional vial to be reconstituted. Ultimately, a mistake was avoided because the nurse listened to the patient. An educated, informed patient is one more way medication errors can be prevented.

CLINICAL REASONING SKILLS

Errors in formula dilution occur when the nurse fails to correctly calculate the amount of solute and solvent needed for the required solution strength.

ERROR

Incorrect calculation of solute and solvent

Possible Scenario

Suppose the physician ordered $\frac{1}{3}$ strength Isomil 90 mL p.o. q.3h for 4 feedings for an infant recovering from gastroenteritis. The concentration will be increased after these feedings. The nurse knows she will give all four feedings during her 12-hour shift, so she makes up 360 mL of formula. She takes a 3 fl oz bottle of ready-to-use Isomil and adds three 3 fl oz bottles of water for oral use. She thinks, "One-third means one bottle of formula and three bottles of water. The amount I need even works out!"

Potential Outcome

What the nurse has actually mixed is a $\frac{1}{4}$ strength solution. Because the infant is getting a more dilute solution than intended, the amount of water to solute is increased and the incremental tolerance of more concentrated formula could be jeopardized. Thinking that the child is tolerating $\frac{1}{3}$ strength, the physician might increase it to $\frac{2}{3}$ strength, and the infant may have problems digesting this more concentrated formula. His progress could be slowed or even set back.

Prevention

The nurse should have thought through the meaning of the terms of a solution. If so, she would have recognized that $\frac{1}{3}$ strength means 1 part solute (formula) to 3 total parts of solution with 2 parts water, not 1 part formula to 3 parts water. She should have applied the calculation formula or ratio-proportion to determine the amount of solute (full-strength Isomil) needed and the amount of solvent (water) to add. If she did not know how to prepare the formula, she should have conferred with another nurse or called the pharmacy or dietary services for assistance. Never guess. Think and calculate with accuracy.

PRACTICE PROBLEMS—CHAPTER 12

Calculate the amount you will prepare for 1 dose. Indicate the syringe you will select to measure the medication.

1. Order: Zosyn 2.5 g IV q.8h

   Supply: 3.375 g vial of Zosyn powder for injection

   Directions: Reconstitute Zosyn with 5 mL of a diluent from the list for a total solution volume of 5 mL.

   The concentration is _____ g per _____ mL.

   Give: _____ mL

   Select: _____ syringe

2. Order: *ampicillin 500 mg IV q.6h*

   Supply: ampicillin 500 mg vial of powder for injection

   Directions: Reconstitute with 1.7 mL diluent for a concentration of 250 mg/mL (and then further dilute for IV use as instructed).

   Give: _____ mL

   Select: _____ syringe

3. Order: *cefazolin 500 mg IV q.6h*

   Supply: cefazolin 1 g vial of powder for injection

   Directions: Reconstitute with 2.5 mL diluent to yield 3 mL with a concentration of 330 mg/mL.

   Give: _____ mL

   Select: _____ syringe

4. Order: *ceftriaxone 900 mg IV q.12h in 50 mL 5% Dextrose and Water IV solution*

   Supply: ceftriaxone 1 g vial of powder for injection

   Package insert states: For IV administration, reconstitute with 9.6 mL diluent to the vial for a concentration of 100 mg/mL.

   Give: _____ mL

   How many full doses are available in this vial? _____

   Select: _____ syringe

5. Order: *cefepime 500 mg IV q.12h*

   Supply: cefepime 1 g vial of powder for injection

   Directions: Reconstitute with 2.4 mL diluent for an approximate available volume of 3.6 mL and a concentration of 280 mg/mL.

   Give: _____ mL

   Select: _____ syringe

   How many full doses are available in this vial? _____ dose(s)

   Prepare a reconstitution label for the remaining solution. The drug is stable for up to 7 days refrigerated and 24 hours at controlled room temperature.

   ```
   ┌─────────────────────────────┐
   │                             │
   │                             │
   │                             │
   │                             │
   └─────────────────────────────┘
   ```
   Reconstitution label

6. Order: *Synercid 375 mg IV q.8h*

   Supply: Synercid 500 mg vial of powder for injection

   Directions: Reconstitute with 5 mL sterile water for a concentration of 100 mg/mL.

   Give: _____ mL

   Select: _____ syringe

   How many full doses are available in this vial? _____ dose(s)

Calculate 1 dose of each of the drug orders numbered 7 through 15. The labels shown on pages 386–389 are the medications that you have available. Indicate which syringe you would select to measure the dose to be administered. Specify if a reconstitution label is required for multiple-dose vials.

7. Order: *cefazolin 300 mg IV q.8h*

   Reconstitute with _____ mL diluent for a concentration of _____ mg/mL and give _____ mL.

   Select: _____ syringe

   How many full doses are available in this vial? _____ dose(s)

   Is a reconstitution label required? _____

8. Order: *methylprednisolone sodium succinate 200 mg IV q.6h*

   Reconstitute with _____ mL diluent for a concentration of _____ mg per _____ mL or _____ mg/mL and give _____ mL.

   Select: _____ syringe

   How many full doses are available in this vial? _____ dose(s)

   Is a reconstitution label required? _____

9. Order: *ceftriaxone 1.25 g IV q.12h*

   Reconstitute with _____ mL diluent for a concentration of _____ mg/mL and give _____ mL.

   Select: _____ syringe

   How many full doses are available in this vial? _____ dose(s)

   Is a reconstitution label required? _____

10. Order: *penicillin G sodium 500,000 units IM q.12h*

    If smallest volume for injection is desired, reconstitute with _____ mL diluent for a concentration of _____ units/mL and give _____ mL.

    Select: _____ syringe

    How many full doses are available in this vial? _____ dose(s)

    Is a reconstitution label required? _____

11. Order: *ceftriaxone 200 mg IM q.12h*

    Reconstitute with _____ mL diluent for a concentration of _____ mg/mL and give _____ mL.

    Select: _____ syringe

    How many full doses are available in this vial? _____ dose(s)

    Is a reconstitution label required? _____

12. Order: *cefpodoxime 200 mg p.o. q.12h*

    Reconstitute with _____ mL diluent for a concentration of _____ mg/mL and give _____ mL.

    How many full doses are available in this bottle? _____ dose(s)

    Is a reconstitution label required? _____

13. Order: *cefazolin 400 mg IV q.6h*

Reconstitute with _____ mL diluent for a concentration of _____ mg/mL and give _____ mL.

Select: _____ syringe

How many full doses are available in this vial? _____ dose(s)

Is a reconstitution label required? _____

14. Order: *penicillin G potassium 2,000,000 units IM q.8h*

Reconstitute with _____ mL diluent for a concentration of _____ units/mL and give _____ mL.

Select: _____ syringe

How many full doses are available in this vial? _____ dose(s)

Is a reconstitution label required? _____

15. Order: *penicillin G potassium 1,000,000 units IM q.8h*

Reconstitute with _____ mL diluent for a concentration of _____ units/mL and give _____ mL.

Select: _____ syringe

How many full doses are available in this vial? _____ dose(s)

Is a reconstitution label required? _____

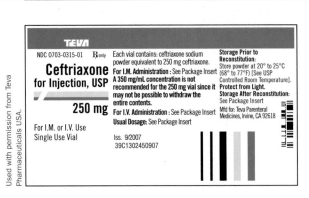

SQUIBB® MARSAM™

1 box • 10 vials   NDC 0003-0668-05

5,000,000 units per vial
PENICILLIN G SODIUM
for INJECTION USP

Caution: Federal law prohibits dispensing without prescription

PENICILLIN G SODIUM for INJECTION USP

Each vial provides 5,000,000 units penicillin G sodium with approx. 140 mg citrate buffer (composed of sodium citrate and not more than 4.6 mg citric acid). One million units penicillin contains approx. 2.0 mEq sodium.

Sterile • For intramuscular or intravenous drip use
Usual dosage: See insert
PREPARATION OF SOLUTION: Add 23 mL, 18 mL, 8 mL, or 3 mL diluent to provide 200,000 u, 250,000 u, 500,000 u, or 1,000,000 u per mL, respectively.
Sterile solution may be kept in refrigerator 1 week without significant loss of potency.
Store at room temperature prior to constitution
© 1986 Squibb-Marsam, Inc.

For information contact:
Squibb-Marsam, Inc., Cherry Hill, NJ 08034

Made by Glaxochem, Ltd., Greenford, Middlesex, England.
Filled in Italy by Squibb S.p.A. Dist. by
E. R. Squibb & Sons, Inc., Princeton, NJ 08540   C5277 / 66805

TEVA

NDC 0703-0315-01   ℞only
Ceftriaxone
for Injection, USP

250 mg

For I.M. or I.V. Use
Single Use Vial

Each vial contains: ceftriaxone sodium powder equivalent to 250 mg ceftriaxone.
For I.M. Administration : See Package Insert
A 350 mg/mL concentration is not recommended for the 250 mg vial since it may not be possible to withdraw the entire contents.
For I.V. Administration : See Package Insert
Usual Dosage: See Package Insert

Iss. 9/2007
39C1302450907

Storage Prior to Reconstitution:
Store powder at 20° to 25°C (68° to 77°F) [See USP Controlled Room Temperature].
Protect from Light.
Storage After Reconstitution:
See Package Insert

Mfd for: Teva Parenteral Medicines, Irvine, CA 92618

Package insert states:

Intravenous Administration

Ceftriaxone for injection, USP should be administered intravenously by infusion over a period of 30 minutes. Concentrations between 10 mg/mL and 40 mg/mL are recommended; however, lower concentrations may be used if desired. Reconstitute vials with an appropriate IV diluent. After reconstitution, each 1 mL of solution contains approximately 100 mg equivalent of ceftriaxone. Withdraw entire contents and dilute to the desired concentration with the appropriate IV diluent.

Vial Dosage Size	Amount of Diluent to Be Added
250 mg	2.4 mL
500 mg	4.8 mL
1 g	9.6 mL
2 g	19.2 mL

Intramuscular Administration: Reconstitute ceftriaxone for injection powder with the appropriate diluent. Inject diluent into vial, shake vial thoroughly to form solution. Withdraw entire contents of vial into syringe to equal total labeled dose.

After reconstitution, each 1 mL of solution contains approximately 250 mg or 350 mg equivalent of ceftriaxone according to the amount of diluent indicated below. If required, more dilute solutions could be utilized. A 350 mg/mL concentration is not recommended for the 250 mg vial because it may not be possible to withdraw the entire contents.

| Vial Dosage Size | Amount of Diluent to Be Added | |
	250 mg/mL	350 mg/mL
250 mg	0.9 mL	
500 mg	1.8 mL	1.0 mL
1 g	3.6 mL	2.1 mL
2 g	7.2 mL	4.2 mL

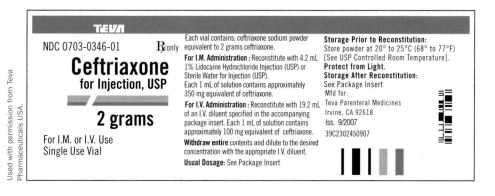

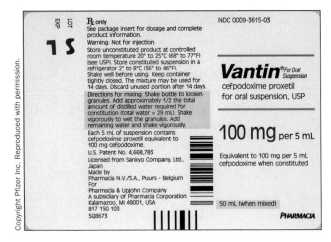

Rx only
See package insert for dosage and complete product information.
Warning: Not for injection
Store unconstituted product at controlled room temperature 20° to 25°C (68° to 77°F) [see USP]. Store constituted suspension in a refrigerator 2° to 8°C (36° to 46°F). Shake well before using. Keep container tightly closed. The mixture may be used for 14 days. Discard unused portion after 14 days.
Directions for mixing: Shake bottle to loosen granules. Add approximately 1/2 the total amount of distilled water required for constitution (total water = 29 mL). Shake vigorously to wet the granules. Add remaining water and shake vigorously.
Each 5 mL of suspension contains cefpodoxime proxetil equivalent to 100 mg cefpodoxime.
U.S. Patent No. 4,668,783
Licensed from Sankyo Company, Ltd., Japan
Made by
Pharmacia N.V./S.A., Puurs - Belgium
For
Pharmacia & Upjohn Co
A subsidiary of Pharmacia Corporation
Kalamazoo, MI 49001, USA
817 150 103
5Q8673

NDC 0009-3615-03

Vantin®For Oral Suspension
cefpodoxime proxetil
for oral suspension, USP

100 mg per 5 mL

Equivalent to 100 mg per 5 mL
cefpodoxime when constituted

50 mL (when mixed)

PHARMACIA

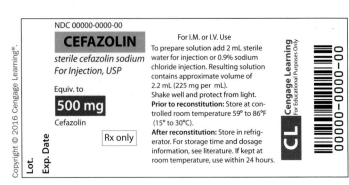

NDC 00000-0000-00

CEFAZOLIN
sterile cefazolin sodium
For Injection, USP

Equiv. to

500 mg
Cefazolin

Rx only

For I.M. or I.V. Use
To prepare solution add 2 mL sterile water for injection or 0.9% sodium chloride injection. Resulting solution contains approximate volume of 2.2 mL (225 mg per mL).
Shake well and protect from light.
Prior to reconstitution: Store at controlled room temperature 59° to 86°F (15° to 30°C).
After reconstitution: Store in refrigerator. For storage time and dosage information, see literature. If kept at room temperature, use within 24 hours.

Lot.
Exp. Date

CL Cengage Learning For Educational Purposes Only

00000-0000-00

Store at controlled room temperature 20° to 25°C (68° to 77°F) [see USP]. Protect from light.

Reconstitute with 8 mL Bacteriostatic Water for Injection with Benzyl Alcohol.

Store solution at controlled room temperature 20° to 25°C (68° to 77°F) and use within 48 hours after mixing. **Protect from light.**

DOSAGE AND USE:
See accompanying prescribing information.

* Each 8 mL (when mixed with 8 mL of diluent) contains methylprednisolone sodium succinate equivalent to methylprednisolone, 500 mg. Also contains monobasic sodium phosphate anhydrous, 6.4 mg; dibasic sodium phosphate dried, 69.6 mg.

When necessary, pH was adjusted with sodium hydroxide.

Lyophilized in container.

NDC 0009-0758-01

1 Vial
4–125 mg Doses   Rx only

Solu-Medrol®
methylprednisolone
sodium succinate
for injection, USP

For intramuscular or
intravenous use

500 mg*

Recommended Diluent
Contains Benzyl Alcohol
as a Preservative
(This Package Does Not
Contain Diluent)

Distributed by
Pfizer **Pharmacia & Upjohn Co**
Division of Pfizer Inc, NY, NY 10017

3 0009-0758-01 1

1681

05-4243-32-6

SEE ACCOMPANYING
PRESCRIBING INFORMATION

**RECOMMENDED STORAGE
IN DRY FORM.**

Store below 86°F (30°C).

Sterile solution may be kept in refrigerator for one (1) week without significant loss of potency.

6505-00-958-3305

Buffered
NDC 0049-0520-83
Rx only

Pfizerpen®
(penicillin G potassium)

For Injection
FIVE MILLION UNITS

5

Pfizer **Roerig**
Division of Pfizer Inc, NY, NY 10017

USUAL DOSAGE
Average single intramuscular injection: 200,000-400,000 units.
Intravenous: Additional information about the use of this product intravenously can be found in the package insert.

mL diluent added	Units per mL of solution
18.2 mL	250,000
8.2 mL	500,000
3.2 mL	1,000,000

Buffered with sodium citrate and citric acid to optimum pH.

PATIENT: _____

ROOM NO: _____

DATE DILUTED: _____

Explain how you would prepare each of the following hydrogen peroxide (solute) and normal saline (solvent) irrigation orders:

16. 16 fl oz of $\frac{1}{8}$ strength solution _____

17. 320 mL of $\frac{3}{8}$ strength solution _____

18. 80 mL of $\frac{5}{8}$ strength solution _____

19. 18 fl oz of $\frac{2}{3}$ strength solution _____

20. 1 pt of $\frac{7}{8}$ strength solution _____

21. 1 L of $\frac{1}{4}$ strength solution _____

Explain how you would prepare each of the following from ready-to-use nutritional formulas for the specified time period. Note how many cans or bottles of supply are needed and how much unused formula would remain from the used supply.

22. Order: $\frac{1}{4}$ strength Enfamil 12 mL via NG tube q.h. for 10h

Supply: Enfamil 3 fl oz bottles

_____

23. Order: $\frac{3}{4}$ strength Sustacal 360 mL over 4h via gastrostomy tube

Supply: Sustacal 10 fl oz cans

_____

24. Order: $\frac{2}{3}$ strength Ensure. Give 90 mL q.h. for 5h via NG tube.

Supply: Ensure 8 fl oz cans

_____

25. Order: $\frac{3}{8}$ strength Enfamil. Three patients need 32 fl oz of the $\frac{3}{8}$ strength Enfamil for one feeding each.

Supply: Enfamil 6 fl oz bottles

_____

26. Order: $\frac{1}{8}$ strength Ensure. Give 160 mL stat via NG tube.

Supply: Ensure 4 fl oz cans

_____

27. Order: $\frac{1}{2}$ strength Ensure 55 mL hourly for 10h via gastrostomy tube

Supply: Ensure 12 fl oz cans

_____

The nurse is making up $\frac{1}{4}$ **strength Enfamil formula** for several infants in the nursery.

28. If 8 fl oz cans of ready-to-use Enfamil are available, how many cans of formula will be needed to make 48 fl oz of reconstituted $\frac{1}{4}$ strength Enfamil? _____ can(s)

29. How many fl oz of water will be added to the Enfamil in question 28 to correctly reconstitute the $\frac{1}{4}$ strength Enfamil? _____ fl oz

30. Describe the strategy you would implement to prevent this medication error.

Possible Scenario

Suppose a physician ordered **penicillin G potassium 1,000,000 units IM stat** for a patient with a severe staph infection. Look at the label of the medication on hand.

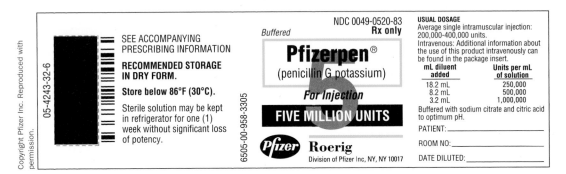

The nurse, in a hurry to give the medication stat, selected the first concentration given on the label: 250,000 units/mL. Next, the nurse calculated the dosage using ratio-proportion.

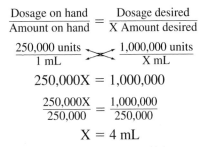

$$\frac{\text{Dosage on hand}}{\text{Amount on hand}} = \frac{\text{Dosage desired}}{\text{X Amount desired}}$$

$$\frac{250,000 \text{ units}}{1 \text{ mL}} \diagdown \frac{1,000,000 \text{ units}}{\text{X mL}}$$

$$250,000\text{X} = 1,000,000$$

$$\frac{250,000\text{X}}{250,000} = \frac{1,000,000}{250,000}$$

$$\text{X} = 4 \text{ mL}$$

The nurse added 18.2 mL diluent to the vial and drew up 4 mL of medication. It was not until the nurse drew up the 4 mL that the error was recognized. The nurse realized that 4 mL IM should not be administered in one injection site. The nurse called the pharmacy for another vial of penicillin G potassium and prepared the dose again, using 3.2 mL of diluent for a concentration of 1,000,000 units/mL. To give 1,000,000 units, the nurse easily calculated to give 1 mL, which was a safe volume of medication for IM injection in adults.

Potential Outcome

If the nurse had selected a 5 mL syringe and changed the needle appropriate for an IM injection to give 4 mL in one injection, the patient would likely have developed an abscess at the site. A 4 mL dose is an excessive volume of medication to administer into the muscle. The patient's hospital stay would likely have been lengthened. Further, the nurse and the hospital may have faced a malpractice suit. The alternative would have been to divide the dose into two injections. Although the patient would have safely received the correct dosage, to give two injections when only one was necessary would have been poor nursing judgment.

Prevention

_____

_____

After completing these problems, see pages 681–683 to check your answers.

Be sure to use the online software for additional practice!

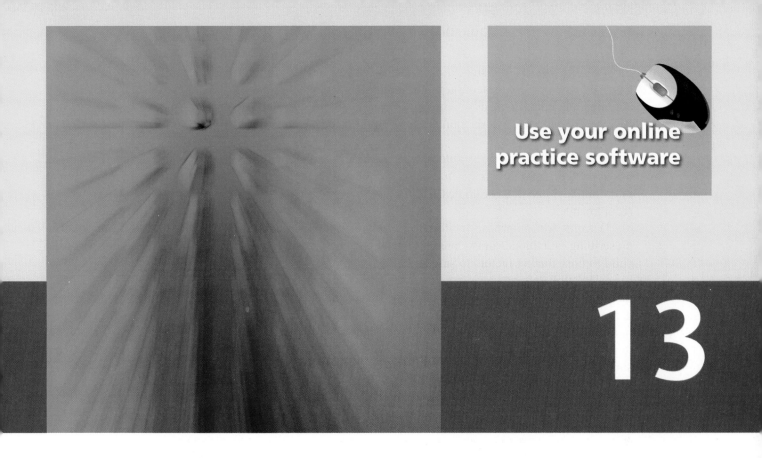

Use your online practice software

13

Pediatric and Adult Dosages Based on Body Weight

OBJECTIVES

Upon mastery of Chapter 13, you will be able to calculate drug dosages based on body weight and verify the safety of medication orders. To accomplish this, you will also be able to:

- Convert pounds to kilograms.
- Consult a reputable drug resource to calculate the recommended safe dosage per kilogram of body weight.
- Compare the ordered dosage with the recommended safe dosage.
- Determine whether the ordered dosage is safe to administer.
- Apply body weight dosage calculations to patients across the life span.

Only a licensed physician, dentist, physician assistant, or nurse practitioner (in some states) may prescribe the dosage of medications. However, before administering a drug, the nurse should know if the ordered dosage is safe. This is important for all patients, but it is of the utmost importance for infants, children, frail elderly, and critically ill adults.

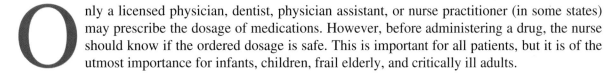

CAUTION
Those who administer drugs to patients are legally responsible for recognizing incorrect and unsafe dosages and for alerting the prescribing practitioner.

The one who administers a drug is just as responsible for the patient's safety as the one who prescribes it. For the protection of the patient and yourself, you must familiarize yourself with the recommended dosage of drugs or consult a reputable drug reference, such as the *package insert* that accompanies the drug or the annual drug guide of the American Hospital Formulary Service, *AHFS Drug Information.*

Standard adult dosage is determined by the drug manufacturer. Dosage is usually recommended based on the requirements of an average-weight adult. Frequently, an adult range is given, listing a minimum and maximum safe dosage, allowing the nurse to simply compare what is ordered to what is recommended.

Dosages for infants and children are based on their unique and changing body differences. The prescribing practitioner must consider the weight, height, body surface area, age, and condition of the child as contributing factors to safe and effective medication dosages. The two methods currently used for calculating safe pediatric dosages are *body weight* (such as mg/kg) and *body surface area* (BSA, measured in square meters, m^2). The body weight method is more common in pediatric situations and is emphasized in this chapter. The BSA method is based on both weight and height. It is used primarily in oncology and critical care situations. BSA is discussed in Chapter 16. Although used most frequently in pediatrics, both the body weight and BSA methods are also used for adults, especially in critical care situations. The calculations are the same.

ADMINISTERING MEDICATIONS TO CHILDREN

Numerically, the infant's or child's dosage appears smaller, but proportionally, pediatric dosages are frequently much larger per kilogram of body weight than the usual adult dosage. Infants—birth to 1 year—have a greater percentage of body water and a decreased ability to absorb water-soluble drugs, necessitating dosages of oral and some parenteral drugs that are proportionally higher than do those given to persons of larger size. Children—ages 1 to 12 years—metabolize drugs more readily than do adults, necessitating higher dosages. Both infants and children, however, are growing, and their organ systems are still maturing. Immature physiological processes related to absorption, distribution, metabolism, and excretion put them continuously at risk for overdose, toxic reactions, and even death. Adolescents—ages 13 to 18 years—are often erroneously thought of as adults because of their body weight (greater than 110 pounds or 50 kilograms) and mature physical appearance. In fact, they should still be regarded as physiologically immature, with unpredictable growth spurts and hormonal surges. Drug therapy for the pediatric population is further complicated because little detailed pharmacologic research has been done on children and adolescents. The infant or child, therefore, must be frequently evaluated for desired clinical responses to medications, and serum drug levels are needed to help adjust some drug dosages. It is important to remember that administration of an incorrect dosage to adult patients is dangerous, but with a child, the risk is even greater. Therefore, using a reputable drug reference to verify safe pediatric dosages is a critical health care skill.

A well-written drug reference developed especially for pediatric clinicians is the *Pediatric and Neonatal Dosage Handbook* (Taketomo, 2014). There is also a variety of pocket-size pediatric drug handbooks; the classic is *The Harriet Lane Handbook* (Johns Hopkins Hospital, Engorn, & Flerlage, 2015).

CONVERTING POUNDS TO KILOGRAMS

The body weight method uses calculations based on the person's weight in kilograms. Recall that the pounds-to-kilograms conversion was introduced in Chapter 4.

REMEMBER

1 kg = 2.2 lb and 1 lb = 16 oz
Simply stated, weight in pounds is approximately twice (slightly more) than the metric weight in kg; or weight in kg is approximately $\frac{1}{2}$ (slightly less) than the weight in pounds. You can estimate weight in kg by halving the weight in lb.

MATH TIP

When converting pounds to kilograms, round kilogram weight to one decimal place (tenths).

EXAMPLE 1 ■

Convert 45 lb to kg

Approximate equivalent: 1 kg = 2.2 lb

THINK: $\frac{1}{2}$ of 45 = approximately 23 (answer will be slightly less)

$$\frac{1 \text{ kg}}{2.2 \text{ lb}} \times \frac{\text{X kg}}{45 \text{ lb}}$$

$$2.2X = 45$$

$$\frac{2.2X}{2.2} = \frac{45}{2.2}$$

$$X = 20.45 \text{ kg} = 20.5 \text{ kg}$$

EXAMPLE 2 ■

Convert 10 lb 12 oz to kg

Approximate equivalents: 1 kg = 2.2 lb
1 lb = 16 oz

First convert ounces to pounds.

$$\frac{1 \text{ lb}}{16 \text{ oz}} \times \frac{\text{X lb}}{12 \text{ oz}}$$

$$16X = 12$$

$$\frac{16X}{16} = \frac{12}{16}$$

$$X = \frac{3}{4} \text{ lb}$$

Now you know that 10 lb 12 oz = $10\frac{3}{4}$ lb

Now you are ready to convert $10\frac{3}{4}$ lb to kg. Because you are converting to the metric system, your answer must be in decimals.

Think: $\frac{1}{2}$ of $10\frac{3}{4}$ = approximately 5

$$10\frac{3}{4} = 10.75$$

$$\frac{1 \text{ kg}}{2.2 \text{ lb}} \times \frac{\text{X kg}}{10.75 \text{ lb}}$$

$$2.2X = 10.75$$

$$\frac{2.2X}{2.2} = \frac{10.75}{2.2}$$

$$X = 4.88 \text{ kg} = 4.9 \text{ kg}$$

BODY WEIGHT METHOD FOR CALCULATING SAFE PEDIATRIC DOSAGE

The most common method of prescribing and administering the therapeutic amount of medication for a child is to calculate the amount of drug according to the child's body weight in **kilograms.** The nurse then compares the child's ordered dosage to the recommended safe dosage from a reputable drug resource before administering the medication. The intent is to ensure that the ordered dosage is safe and effective before calculating the amount to give and administering the dose to the patient.

RULE

To verify safe pediatric dosage recommended by body weight:

1. Convert the child's weight from pounds to kilograms (rounded to tenths).

2. Calculate the safe dosage in mg/kg or mcg/kg (rounded to tenths) for a child of this weight, as recommended by a reputable drug reference: **multiply mg/kg by child's weight in kg.**

3. Compare the ordered dosage to the recommended dosage, and decide if the dosage is safe.

4. If safe, calculate the amount to give and administer the dose; if the dosage seems unsafe, consult with the prescribing practitioner before administering the drug.

Note: The dosage per kg may be mg/kg, mcg/kg, g/kg, mEq/kg, unit/kg, milliunit/kg, etc.

For each pediatric medication order, you must ask yourself, "Is this dosage safe?" Let's work through some examples.

Single-Dosage Drugs

Single-dosage drugs are intended to be given once or p.r.n. Dosage ordered by the body weight method is based on **mg/kg/dose, calculated by multiplying the recommended mg/kg by the patient's kg weight for each dose.**

EXAMPLE ▪

Order: morphine sulfate 1.8 mg IM stat

Morphine sulfate is an opioid analgesic given for moderate to severe pain. It may be administered by the oral, rectal, subcutaneous, intramuscular, intravenous, and epidural routes. The usual starting dosage in opioid-naive patients (patients who have not received morphine before) is 0.05 mg/kg q.3–4h. The solution for injection is supplied in many concentrations such as 5 mg/mL, 8 mg/mL, 10 mg/mL, and 15 mg/mL, just to name a few. Morphine is a high-alert drug that may result in respiratory depression. A second nurse should independently check the original order, dosage calculations, and IV pump settings.

In this scenario, you are working in the urgent care clinic and have just received a 10-year-old child with a suspected fracture of his wrist due to a skateboard accident. He is crying and rates his pain as a 7 on a 0 to 10-point scale. His mother claims that his weight is 79 lb.

Before administering the pain medication, you will need to get an accurate weight and determine if the ordered dosage is safe. His weight on the bedside scale is 79 lb.

1. **Convert lb to kg.** Approximate equivalent: 1 kg = 2.2 lb

   THINK: $\frac{1}{2}$ of 79 = approximately 40 (answer will be slightly less)

   $$\frac{1 \text{ kg}}{2.2 \text{ lb}} \diagdown \frac{X \text{ kg}}{79 \text{ lb}}$$

   $$2.2X = 79$$

   $$\frac{2.2X}{2.2} = \frac{79}{2.2}$$

   $$X = 35.90 \text{ kg} = 35.9 \text{ kg}$$

2. **Calculate mg/kg as recommended by a reputable drug resource.** A reputable drug resource indicates that the usual IM dosage may be initiated at 0.05 mg/kg/dose.

   Use ratio-proportion to calculate how many mg per dose of the medication should be ordered.

   For each dose: Ratio for recommended mg/kg = Ratio for desired mg/kg

   $$\frac{0.05 \text{ mg}}{1 \text{ kg}} \diagdown \frac{X \text{ mg}}{35.9 \text{ kg}}$$

   $$X = 0.05 \times 35.9$$

   $$X = 1.79 \text{ mg} = 1.8 \text{ mg (per dose)}$$

   Or, you can simply multiply mg/kg/dose by the child's weight in kg.

   Per dose: 0.05 mg/k̶g̶/dose × 35.9 k̶g̶ = 1.79 mg/dose = 1.8 mg/dose

---

MATH TIP
Notice that the kg unit of measurement cancels out, leaving the unit as mg/dose.

$\frac{\text{mg/k̶g̶}}{\text{dose}} \times \text{k̶g̶} = \text{mg/dose}$

or

$\text{mg/k̶g̶/dose} \times \text{k̶g̶} = \text{mg/dose}$

---

3. **Decide if the dosage is safe by comparing ordered and recommended dosages.** For this child's weight, 1.8 mg is the recommended dosage, and 1.8 mg is the ordered dosage. Yes, the dosage is safe.

   Morphine is a Schedule II controlled substance, so you will retrieve it from the double-locked medication supply cabinet as illustrated in Figure 13-1.

   Which supply will you choose? The order is for 1.8 mg, slightly less than 2 mg, but do not select the drug in Figure 13-1a. Hydromorphone sounds a lot like morphine and is also an opioid analgesic, but it is much more potent, meaning it is effective at a much lower dosage. Hydromorphone and morphine are look-alike/sound-alike (LASA) drugs. Mix-up errors have resulted in death. Spelling HYDROmorphone with Tall Man letters will help prevent this type of error.

   Either morphine vial would provide less than 1 mL for injection of this dose but using a concentration of 10 mg/mL (Figure 13-1c) would require a very small amount to measure in the syringe. Let's choose 5 mg/mL (Figure 13-1b).

FIGURE 13-1 Illustrated locked medication cabinet with controlled substances (opioid narcotics)

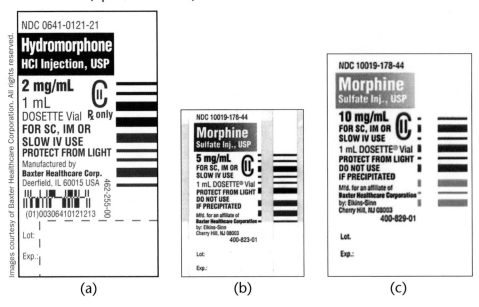

(a)   (b)   (c)

4. **Calculate 1 dose.** Apply the Three-Step Approach to dosage calculation.

Step 1   **Convert**   For the ordered dosage of 1.8 mg, no conversion is necessary. The units are in the same system (metric) and the same size (mg).

Step 2   **Think**   You want to give less than 1 mL. Estimate that you want to give less than 0.5 mL.

Step 3   **Calculate**

$$\frac{\text{Dosage on hand}}{\text{Amount on hand}} = \frac{\text{Dosage desired}}{\text{X Amount desired}}$$

$$\frac{5\ \text{mg}}{1\ \text{mL}} \diagdown\!\!\!\!\diagup \frac{1.8\ \text{mg}}{\text{X mL}}$$

$$5X = 1.8$$

$$\frac{5X}{5} = \frac{1.8}{5}$$

$$X = 0.36\ \text{mL}$$

This is a small-volume child's dose. Measure 0.36 mL in a 1 mL syringe. Route is IM. You may need to change the needle.

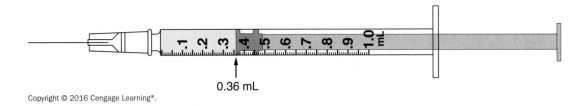

0.36 mL

Take caution; you're not finished. Remember that morphine sulfate is a controlled substance. You are only withdrawing 0.36 mL, which will leave 0.64 mL remaining. You can't just discard what is left over. All the solution must be accounted for and documented. Ask another nurse to witness you wasting the remainder according to agency policy and cosign the record.

Single-Dosage-Range Drugs

Some single-dosage medications indicate a minimum and maximum range, or a safe dosage range.

EXAMPLE 1 ■

Order: **midazolam 1.5 mg IM X 1 dose 30 minutes prior to MRI**

Midazolam is in the pharmacologic class benzodiazepines, and is used for preprocedural sedation and anxiolysis in pediatric patients. Procedures that are not painful but induce anxiety or require the child to remain still are frequently performed with sedation. The drug may be administered orally or intramuscularly, 30 to 60 minutes prior to the procedure. The usual *oral* dosage for children is 0.25 to 0.5 mg/kg, and may require up to 1 mg/kg but the dosage should not exceed 20 mg/dose. The usual *IM* dosage is less, 0.1 to 0.15 mg/kg up to 0.5 mg/kg but not to exceed 10 mg/dose. It is supplied for injection in concentrations of 1 mg/mL and 5 mg/mL and as cherry-flavored oral syrup with 2 mg/mL dosage strength. Midazolam is a high-alert medication. Overdose may result in serious harm or death. Ordered dosages should be expressed in milligrams, not by volume (mL or tsp). A second nurse should independently check the original order and dosage calculations.

For this scenario, you are working on a busy pediatric inpatient unit. Two of your assigned patients are scheduled to be transported to the radiology department for magnetic resonance imaging (MRI). The equipment creates a loud noise that may frighten young children so preprocedural sedation is ordered. You receive a call from radiology requesting that you premedicate the first scheduled patient, a 9-month-old infant who weighs 22 lb.

You need to determine if this dosage is safe prior to administration.

1. **Convert lb to kg.** Approximate equivalent: 1 kg = 2.2 lb

   THINK: $\frac{1}{2}$ of 22 = 11 (answer will be slightly less)

$$\frac{1 \text{ kg}}{2.2 \text{ lb}} \diagup\!\!\!\!\diagdown \frac{X \text{ kg}}{22 \text{ lb}}$$

$$2.2X = 22$$

$$\frac{2.2 \, X}{2.2} = \frac{22}{2.2}$$

$$X = 10 \text{ kg}$$

2. **Calculate recommended dosage.** Notice that the recommended IM dosage is represented as a range of "0.1 to 0.15 mg/kg" for dosing flexibility. Calculate the minimum and maximum safe dosage range.

   Use ratio-proportion to calculate mg/kg range for each dose.

   Ratio for minimum recommended mg/kg = Ratio for minimum desired mg/kg

$$\frac{0.1 \text{ mg}}{1 \text{ kg}} \diagup\!\!\!\!\diagdown \frac{X \text{ mg}}{10 \text{ kg}}$$

$$X = 0.1 \times 10$$

$$X = 1 \text{ mg (per dose)}$$

   Ratio for maximum recommended mg/kg = Ratio for maximum desired mg/kg

$$\frac{0.15 \text{ mg}}{1 \text{ kg}} \diagup\!\!\!\!\diagdown \frac{X \text{ mg}}{10 \text{ kg}}$$

$$X = 0.15 \times 10$$

$$X = 1.5 \text{ mg (per dose)}$$

   Or, you can simply multiply mg/kg/dose × the child's weight in kg.

   Minimum per dose: 0.1 mg/kg/dose × 10 kg = 1 mg/dose

   Maximum per dose: 0.15 mg/kg/dose × 10 kg = 1.5 mg/dose

3. **Decide if the ordered dosage is safe.** The recommended dosage range for this child is 1 mg to 1.5 mg, and the ordered dosage of 1.5 mg is within this range. Yes, the ordered dosage is safe.

You will retrieve the medication from the automated dispensing cabinet (ADC) matrix drawer illustrated in Figure 13-2.

FIGURE 13-2   Illustrated automatic dispensing cabinet (ADC) matrix drawer with four supply dosages of midazolam

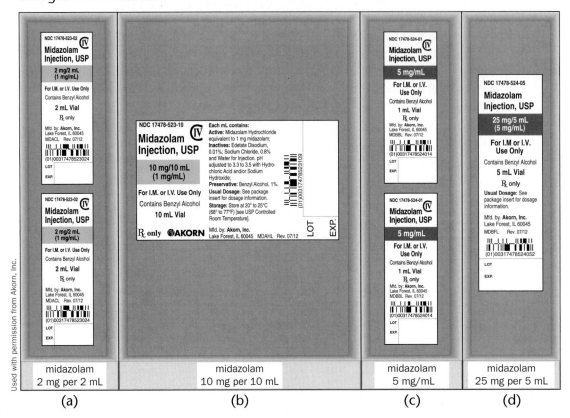

There are four different supply dosages for midazolam in the ADC (Figure 13-2). Which supply will you choose? The order is for 1.5 mg, slightly less than 2 mg. The vial with 2 mg per 2 mL (Figure 13-2a) initially seems to be the best one, but remember, you are giving an IM injection to a 9-month-old infant. The safe volume for an intramuscular injection in an infant is between 0.5 mL and 1 mL. If you pick this vial, you would be giving too much volume (1.5 mL) for this size muscle. Now look at label (b), 10 mg per 10 mL or 1 mg/mL. Compare what is stated in the parenthesis on labels (a) and (b). They are the same concentration, so the volume calculated will be the same for both vials. Vial (b) will not work either. Now look at the remaining two labels (c) and (d). Notice that they both also have the same concentration (5 mg/mL) except vial (d) is just a larger container (25 mg per 5 mL). You only need 1.5 mg, so let's choose vial (c).

4. **Calculate 1 dose.** Apply the Three-Step Approach to dosage calculation.

Step 1   **Convert**   For the ordered dosage of 1.5 mg, no conversion is necessary. The units are in the same system (metric) and the same size (mg).

Step 2   **Think**   The supply provides 5 mg in 1 mL. You want to give 1.5 mg, which is less than $\frac{1}{2}$ of 5 mg, so you estimate that you will need less than $\frac{1}{2}$ of a mL, or less than 0.5 mL.

Step 3 Calculate $\dfrac{\text{Dosage on hand}}{\text{Amount on hand}} = \dfrac{\text{Dosage desired}}{\text{X Amount desired}}$

$$\dfrac{5 \text{ mg}}{1 \text{ mL}} \diagdown\!\!\!\!\diagup \dfrac{1.5 \text{ mg}}{\text{X mL}}$$

$$5\text{X} = 1.5$$

$$\dfrac{5\text{X}}{5} = \dfrac{1.5}{5}$$

$$\text{X} = 0.3 \text{ mL}$$

This is a small-volume child's dose. Measure it in a 1 mL syringe. Route is IM. You may need to change the needle.

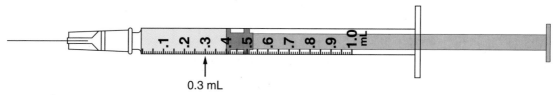

0.3 mL

EXAMPLE 2 ■

Order: midazolam 6 mg IM X 1 dose 30 minutes prior to MRI

Two hours later, you receive another call from radiology requesting that you premedicate the second scheduled patient, a 7-year-old child who weighs 55 lb.

You need to determine if this dosage is safe prior to administration. Remember that the recommended IM dosage is 0.1 to 0.15 mg/kg up to 0.5 mg/kg but not to exceed 10 mg/dose.

1. **Convert lb to kg.** Approximate equivalent: 1 kg = 2.2 lb

   THINK: $\frac{1}{2}$ of 55 = $27\frac{1}{2}$ (answer will be slightly less)

   $$\dfrac{1 \text{ kg}}{2.2 \text{ lb}} \diagdown\!\!\!\!\diagup \dfrac{\text{X kg}}{55 \text{ lb}}$$

   $$2.2\text{X} = 55$$

   $$\dfrac{2.2\text{X}}{2.2} = \dfrac{55}{2.2}$$

   $$\text{X} = 25 \text{ kg}$$

2. **Calculate recommended dosage.**

   Multiply mg/kg/dose × the child's weight in kg.

   Minimum per dose: 0.1 mg/kg/dose × 25 kg = 2.5 mg

   Maximum per dose: 0.15 mg/kg/dose × 25 kg = 3.75 mg

3. **Decide if the ordered dosage is safe.** The recommended IM dosage range for this child is 2.5 mg to 3.75 mg, and the ordered dosage of 6 mg is NOT within this range; it is higher. Remember, the reference states the dosage may go up to 0.5 mg/kg IM if it doesn't exceed 10 mg/dose. Let's calculate the highest limit. Highest limit per dose: 0.5 mg/kg/dose × 25 kg = 12.5 mg

   Check again. The highest limit calculated for this child's weight is 12.5 mg but the most he would be allowed to receive is 10 mg. The ordered dosage of 6 mg is only just a little bit more than $\frac{1}{2}$ that dosage. Yes, this dosage is more than the usual IM range but does not exceed the highest limit.

Look again at the supply of midazolam in the automated dispensing cabinet (ADC) matrix drawer (Figure 13-2). Will you choose the same vial (c)? The total dosage in the vial is 5 mg and you need 6 mg. You could use the larger 25 mg vial (d) but then you would discard 19 mg. A better choice would be to choose two of the 5 mg vials.

4. **Calculate 1 dose.** Apply the Three-Step Approach to dosage calculation.

| Step 1 | **Convert** | For the ordered dosage of 6 mg, no conversion is necessary. The units are in the same system (metric) and the same size (mg). |

| Step 2 | **Think** | You want to give 6 mg, which is just slightly more than 5 mg. There are 5 mg in 1 mL, so you want to give slightly more than 1 mL. |

Step 3   **Calculate**

$$\frac{\text{Dosage on hand}}{\text{Amount on hand}} = \frac{\text{Dosage desired}}{\text{X Amount desired}}$$

$$\frac{5\ \text{mg}}{1\ \text{mL}} \diagdown \diagup \frac{6\ \text{mg}}{\text{X mL}}$$

$$5X = 6$$

$$\frac{5X}{5} = \frac{6}{5}$$

$$X = 1.2\ \text{mL}$$

An injection of 1.2 mL in a large muscle of a 55 lb child is reasonable. Measure 1.2 mL in a 3 mL syringe.

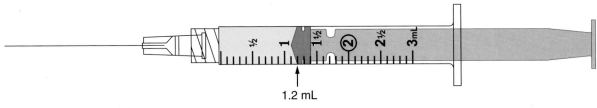

1.2 mL

CAUTION

Compare the previous two examples. The infant received 1.5 mg in a dose volume of 0.3 mL and the school-age child received 6 mg in a dose volume of 1.2 mL. Children's weights and drug dosages vary greatly and orders must be individualized for every child. Do not guess if an ordered dosage is safe or base your decision on a dosage given previously to another child. Calculate every order to determine safe dosage before administering any medication to a child.

Routine or Round-the-Clock Drugs

Routine or round-the-clock drugs are intended to produce a continuous effect on the body over 24 hours. They are recommended as a *total daily dosage:* **mg/kg/day to be divided into some number of individual doses,** such as "3 divided doses," "4 divided doses," "divided doses every 8 hours," and so on. "Three divided doses" means that the drug total daily dosage is divided equally and is administered three times per day, either t.i.d. or q.8h depending on the medication and order. Likewise, "4 divided doses" means that the total daily drug dosage is divided equally and administered four times per day either q.i.d. or q.6h depending on the medication and order. Recommendations such as "divided doses every 8 hours" specify that the total daily drug dosage should be divided equally and administered q.8h.

EXAMPLE ■

Order: *Cefaclor 100 mg p.o. t.i.d.*

Cefaclor is a second-generation cephalosporin, a broad-spectrum anti-infective used to treat a variety of infections. It is used in adults and children and administered only by the oral route. It is supplied in 250 mg and 500 mg capsules; 125 mg, 187 mg, 250 mg, and 375 mg chewable tablets; 375 mg and 500 mg extended-release tablets; and 125 mg per 5 mL, 187 mg per 5 mL, 250 mg per 5 mL, and

375 mg per 5 mL strawberry-flavored oral suspension. The usual dosage is sometimes included on the label for convenience, but this will not be as detailed as the information for recommended dosage in a drug guide or package insert. For this scenario, you are working on a pediatric unit caring for a child who weighs $33\frac{1}{2}$ lb. After 3 days of treatment with cefoxitin (an intravenous cephalosporin) 200 mg IVPB q.6h, the medication is changed to cefaclor, an oral cephalosporin, in preparation for discharge to home. Notice, the oral dosage ordered is less than the IV dosage that the child has been receiving. The two medications are similar but are not identical, so the nurse will need to determine if the new order is a recommended dosage. The pharmacy mixed the oral suspension and delivered it to the unit (Figure 13-3).

FIGURE 13-3   Cefaclor 125 mg/5 mL label

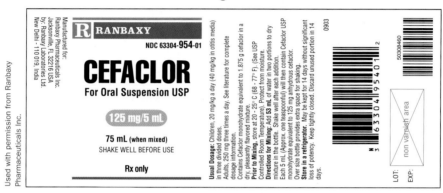

You need to determine if this dosage is safe prior to administration.

1. **Convert lb to kg.** Approximate equivalent: 1 kg = 2.2 lb

   THINK: $\frac{1}{2}$ of 33 = approximately 17 (answer will be slightly less)

   Represent $33\frac{1}{2}$ as 33.5, because you are converting lb to kg (metric measure), and the answer must be a decimal number.

   $$\frac{1 \text{ kg}}{2.2 \text{ lb}} \times \frac{X \text{ kg}}{33.5 \text{ lb}}$$

   $$2.2X = 33.5$$

   $$\frac{2.2X}{2.2} = \frac{33.5}{2.2}$$

   $$X = 15.22 \text{ kg} = 15.2 \text{ kg}$$

2. **Calculate recommended dosage.** Figure 13-3 shows the recommended dosage on the drug label, "Usual dose—Children, 20 mg/kg a day . . . in three divided doses." First calculate the total daily dosage using ratio-proportion or simply multiply: 20 mg/kg/day × 15.2 kg = 304 mg/day. Then, divide this total daily dosage into 3 doses: 304 mg ÷ 3 doses = 101.33 mg/dose = 101.3 mg/dose.

3. **Decide if the ordered dosage is safe.** Yes, the ordered dosage is safe because this is an *oral* dose and 100 mg is a *reasonably safe* dosage for a 101.3 mg recommended single dosage.

4. **Calculate 1 dose.** Apply the Three-Step Approach to dosage calculation.

Step 1   **Convert**   For the ordered dosage of 100 mg, no conversion is necessary. The units are in the same system (metric) and the same size (mg).

Step 2   **Think**   You want to give 100 mg, which is slightly less than 125 mg. Estimate that because there are 125 mg in 5 mL, you want to give slightly less than 5 mL.

Step 3   **Calculate** $\dfrac{\text{Dosage on hand}}{\text{Amount on hand}} = \dfrac{\text{Dosage desired}}{\text{X Amount desired}}$

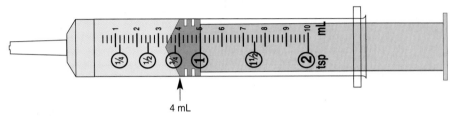

$$\frac{125 \text{ mg}}{5 \text{ mL}} \times \frac{100 \text{ mg}}{\text{X mL}}$$

$$125\text{X} = 500$$

$$\frac{125\text{X}}{125} = \frac{500}{125}$$

$$\text{X} = 4 \text{ mL}$$

4 mL

In preparation for discharge, the nurse plans to provide medication administration teaching to the parent by explaining the dose volume of the ordered dosage and demonstrating the proper technique using an oral syringe. Can you see where a potential medication error might occur? The hospital pharmacy has supplied a concentration of 125 mg per 5 mL. Recall that there are many concentration variations for cefaclor. The outpatient pharmacy the parent uses may not stock all four available concentrations. Suppose the outpatient pharmacy dispenses a concentration of 250 mg per 5 mL. THINK: 250 mg per 5 mL is twice as concentrated as 125 mg per 5 mL; therefore, the same volume of 4 mL of the dispensed medication will be twice the ordered dosage. Include in your discharge teaching that medication dosages should always be referred to by dosage strength, not by dose volume, and the pharmacist may answer any concerns about the prescription instructions.

CAUTION

Medications that are commonly administered to children will be supplied in a variety of dosage concentrations due the wide range of ordered dosages based on age and weight. To prevent medication errors, always refer to the ordered dosage strength, not the ordered dose volume. Contact the prescriber to verify any medications ordered by volume that do not include the supply concentration.

Daily-Dosage-Range Drugs

Many medications are recommended by a minimum and maximum mg/kg range per day, to be divided into some number of doses. They are given in divided doses round the clock for a total daily dosage.

EXAMPLE ▪

Order: *amoxicillin 200 mg p.o. q.8h*

Amoxicillin is an anti-infective in the pharmacologic class, aminopenicillins. It is used in the treatment of skin and skin structure infections, otitis media, sinusitis, respiratory infections, genitourinary infections, and endocarditis prophylaxis. For most infections, the oral dosage for adults is 250 to 500 mg q.8h or 500 to 875 mg q.12h (not to exceed 2 to 3 g/day). For children greater than 3 months old, the oral dosage is 25 to 50 mg/kg/day in divided doses q.8h or 25 to 50 mg/kg/day in individual doses q.12h. For infants less than 3 months old, the oral dosage is 20 to 30 mg/kg/day in divided doses q.12h. It is supplied in chewable tablets, tablets, extended-release tablets, capsules, suspension (pediatric drops), and powder for oral suspension. The reconstituted powder for oral suspension will supply concentrations of 125 mg per 5 mL, 200 mg per 5 mL, 250 mg per 5 mL, and 400 mg per 5 mL. As you can see, the recommended dosage varies considerably based on age and weight, which would explain the need for so many choices of supplied concentrations.

For this scenario, an experienced medical-surgical nurse who recently transferred to the pediatric unit in a community hospital is preparing to administer the ordered medication to a 22 lb, 16-month-old child being treated for otitis media (inner ear infection). You need to determine if this dosage is safe prior to administration. The pharmacy mixed the oral suspension and delivered it to the unit (Figure 13-4). Note, for convenience, the average dosage range for children is provided on the label. This varies slightly from the information included in the drug reference, but let's use the label information for our calculations.

FIGURE 13-4 Amoxicillin 250 mg per 5 mL label

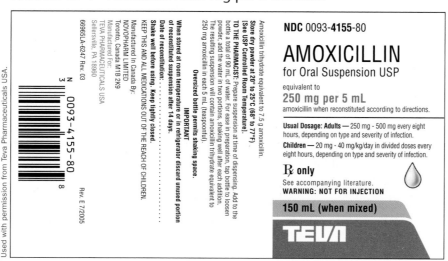

1. **Convert lb to kg.** Approximate equivalent: 1 kg = 2.2 lb

   THINK: $\frac{1}{2}$ of 22 = 11 (answer will be slightly less)

$$\frac{1 \text{ kg}}{2.2 \text{ lb}} \diagdown \frac{X \text{ kg}}{22 \text{ lb}}$$

$$2.2X = 22$$

$$\frac{2.2X}{2.2} = \frac{22}{2.2}$$

$$X = 10 \text{ kg}$$

2. **Calculate recommended dosage.** Look at the label for amoxicillin (Figure 13-4). It describes the recommended dosage for children as "20 mg – 40 mg/kg/day in divided doses every eight hours . . . ," which results in 3 doses in 24 hours.

   Calculate the minimum and maximum daily dosage using ratio-proportion, or simply multiply mg/kg/day × the child's weight in kg then divide by the number of doses per day.

   Minimum total daily dosage: 20 mg/kg/day × 10 kg = 200 mg/day

   Minimum dosage for each single dose: 200 mg ÷ 3 doses = 66.66 mg/dose = 66.7 mg/dose

   Maximum total daily dosage: 40 mg/kg/day × 10 kg = 400 mg/day

   Maximum dosage for each single dose: 400 mg ÷ 3 doses = 133.33 mg/dose = 133.3 mg/dose

   The single-dosage range for this child is 66.7 to 133.3 mg/dose.

3. **Decide if the ordered dosage is safe.** The ordered dosage is 200 mg, and the allowable, safe dosage is 66.7 to 133.3 mg/dose. No, according to the information on the drug label, this dosage is too high and is not safe.

4. **You will need to contact the prescriber to discuss the order.**

Before contacting the prescriber, let's repeat our calculations using the more detailed recommendations provided in the drug reference. You can save yourself a calculation step with the following shortcut, based on the total daily dosage. According to the drug reference, the total allowable dosage for children greater than 3 months of age is 25 to 50 mg/kg/day in divided doses q.8h.

Calculate recommended minimum and maximum daily dosage range for *this* child.

You know that the total daily dosage is divided into 3 doses in 24 hours.

Minimum total daily dosage: 25 mg/kg/day × 10 kg = 250 mg/day

Maximum total daily dosage: 50 mg/kg/day × 10 kg = 500 mg/day

Daily dosage per this order: 200 mg/dose × 3 doses/day = 600 mg/day

Decide if the ordered daily dosage is safe. The ordered daily dosage is 600 mg, and the allowable safe daily dosage according to the drug reference is 250 to 500 mg/day. We have confirmation that the dosage ordered is too high and is not safe. It could result in serious harm to the child, including renal damage, especially if this is continued for the full course of therapy. Further, the nurse who administered the dosage would be liable for any patient harm. The nurse should contact the prescriber to discuss the concern about the ordered dosage.

Had the nurse relied on previous experience with adult patients, the ordered dosage would not have seemed excessive compared to the usual adult dosage of 250 to 500 mg q.8h. Fortunately, the nurse in this scenario took the time to calculate the recommended dosage based on this child's age and weight.

CAUTION

Recommended children's dosages vary considerably from usual adult dosages based on age and weight. Do not rely on previous experience with adults to determine the safe dosage range for children. Always calculate the dosage for each child based on current age and weight.

Daily-Dosage-Range Drugs With Maximum Daily Allowance

Some medications have a range of mg/kg/day recommended, with a maximum allowable total amount per day also specified.

EXAMPLE ■

Order: *cefazolin 1.5 g IV q.8h*

Cefazolin is an anti-infective belonging to the pharmacologic class of first-generation cephalosporins. It is used to treat skin and skin structure infections (including burn wounds), pneumonia, urinary tract infections, bone and joint infections, and septicemia ranging in seriousness from mild to severe. The usual adult dosage for mild infections is 250 to 500 mg q.8h and for moderate to severe infections it is 500 mg to 2 g q.6–8h with a maximum total daily dosage of 12 g/day. The recommended dosage for children and infants greater than 1 month old is 16.7 to 33.3 mg/kg q.8h with a maximum total daily dosage of 6 g/day.

This means that regardless of how much the child weighs, the maximum safe allowance of this drug is 6 g per 24 hours. For this scenario, the nurse is preparing to administer the ordered cefazolin to a 92 lb, 14-year-old patient with a serious joint infection. The nurse is concerned that the ordered dosage may be too high because it falls within the usual dosage range for an adult. Before calling the prescriber for clarification, the nurse needs to determine if this dosage is safe.

1. **Convert lb to kg.** Approximate equivalent: 1 kg = 2.2 lb

   THINK: $\frac{1}{2}$ of 92 = approximately 46 (answer will be slightly less)

   $$\frac{1 \text{ kg}}{2.2 \text{ lb}} \times \frac{X \text{ kg}}{92}$$

   $$2.2X = 92$$

   $$\frac{2.2X}{2.2} = \frac{92}{2.2}$$

   $$X = 41.81 \text{ kg} = 41.8 \text{ kg}$$

2. **Calculate recommended dosage.**

   Minimum mg/kg/dose: 16.7 mg/kg/dose × 41.8 kg = 698.06 or 698 mg/dose

   Maximum mg/kg/dose: 33.3 mg/kg/dose × 41.8 kg = 1391.94 or 1,392 mg/dose

   Total ordered dose per day: 1.5 g/dose × 3 doses/day = 4.5 g/day

3. **Decide if the dosage is safe.** The ordered dosage of 1.5 g exceeds the recommended maximum mg/kg/dose of 1,392 mg (1.392 g). Yet, the total ordered dosage per day of 4.5 g is lower than the maximum allowable total daily dosage of 6 g. Based on the mg/kg recommendations in the drug resource available to the nurse, the ordered q.8h dosage is too high even though it does not exceed the overall maximum daily dosage. The prescriber may have based the ordered dosage on current evidence for practice not yet published in the nursing drug guide.

4. **Contact the prescriber to discuss the order.**

Underdosage

Underdosage, as well as overdosage, can be a hazard. If the medication is necessary for the treatment or comfort of the patient, then giving too little can be just as hazardous as giving too much. Dosage that is less than the recommended therapeutic amount is also considered unsafe, because it may be ineffective.

EXAMPLE ■

Order: *ibuprofen 40 mg p.o. q.6h p.r.n., temp 101.6°F and above*

Ibuprofen is a nonopioid analgesic. In addition to treating mild to moderate pain, it is also classified as an antipyretic and used to reduce fever. The recommended oral dosage to treat pain in infants and children is 4 to 10 mg/kg/dose q.6–8h, but the dosage range recommended to treat fever is slightly different. As an antipyretic the recommended range is 5 mg/kg for temperatures less than 102.5°F (39.17°C) or 10 mg/kg for higher temperatures q.4–6h, not to exceed 40 mg/kg/day. In this scenario the nurse is caring for a $17\frac{1}{2}$ lb, 7-month-old child. The child experienced a febrile seizure at home and was admitted to the hospital pediatric unit with a diagnosis of otitis media (inner ear infection). The nurse reviewed the hospital record, which showed an initial temperature of 103.2°F in the emergency department, and serial temperatures at 4-hour intervals of 101.9°F and 102.6°F after transfer to the unit despite the child receiving two doses of ibuprofen. Concerned that the child is not receiving adequate antipyretic therapy, the nurse calculates the recommended dosage range.

1. **Convert lb to kg.** Approximate equivalent: 1 kg = 2.2 lb

    THINK: $\frac{1}{2}$ of $17\frac{1}{2}$ = approximately 9 (answer will be slightly less)

    Represent $17\frac{1}{2}$ as 17.5, because you are converting lb to kg; kg is a metric unit measured in decimals.

    $$\frac{1 \text{ kg}}{2.2 \text{ lb}} \diagup\!\!\!\diagdown \frac{X \text{ kg}}{17.5 \text{ lb}}$$

    $$2.2X = 17.5$$

    $$\frac{2.2X}{2.2} = \frac{17.5}{2.2}$$

    $$X = 17.95 \text{ kg} = 8 \text{ kg}$$

2. **Calculate recommended dosage.** The minimum dosage of 5 mg/kg is recommended for temperatures less than 102.5°F and the maximum dosage of 10 mg/kg is recommended for higher temperatures. Calculate the minimum and maximum safe dosage range.

    Multiply mg/kg/dose × the child's weight in kg

    Minimum per dose: 5 mg/kg/dose × 8 kg = 40 mg/dose

    Maximum per dose: 10 mg/kg/dose × 8 kg = 80 mg/dose

3. **Decide if the dosage is safe.** The dosage ordered is the recommended dosage for temperatures lower than 102.5°F but the antipyretic therapy has been ineffective. A higher dosage is indicated now that the temperature is again over 102.5°F, but if the child receives the 10 mg/kg/dose every 4 hours the maximum daily dosage of 40 mg/kg will be reached after only 4 doses.

4. **Contact the physician.** In preparation for the call to the physician, the nurse prepares a concise report including a description of the situation, background information, an assessment of what the problem is, and plans to recommend that the child be given a one-time dose of ibuprofen 80 mg now but continue the 40 mg dose as long as the temperature does not exceed 102.5°F. The physician agrees and revises the order to ibuprofen 80 mg p.o. q.6h p.r.n., fever greater than 102.5°F and ibuprofen 40 mg p.o. q.4h p.r.n., fever 101.6° to 102.5°F. Underdosage with an antipyretic may result in serious complications of hyperthermia. Likewise, consider how underdosage with an antibiotic may prolong an infection and underdosage of a pain reliever may be inadequate to effectively treat the patient's pain, delaying recovery.

REMEMBER

The information in the drug reference provides important details related to specific use of medications and appropriate dosages for certain age groups, to provide safe, therapeutic dosing. Both the physician and nurse must work together to ensure accurate and safe dosages that are within the recommended parameters as stated by the manufacturer on the label, in a drug insert, or in a reputable drug reference.

CAUTION

Many over-the-counter preparations, such as fever reducers and cold preparations, have printed dosing instructions that show the recommended child dose per pound (Figure 13-5). Manufacturers understand that most parents in the United States measure their child's weight in pounds and are most familiar with household measurement. The recommended dosage for at-home administration is often measured in teaspoons. Recall that pounds and teaspoons are primarily used for measurement in the home setting. In the clinical setting, you should measure body weight in kg and calculate dosage by the body weight method, using recommended dosage in mg/kg, not mg/lb.

FIGURE 13-5 Label with dosage instructions per pound

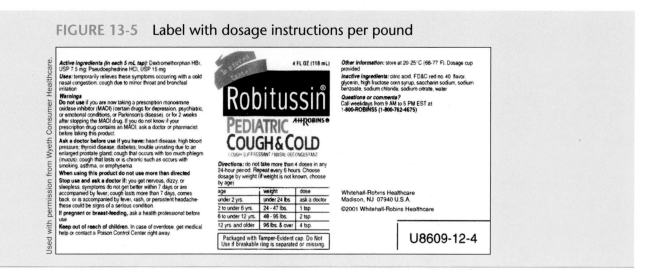

COMBINATION DRUGS

Some medications contain two drugs combined into one solution or suspension. To calculate the safe dosage of these medications, the nurse should consult a pediatric drug reference. When combination drugs are referred to by brand name, they may be ordered by the amount to give or dose volume of the concentration desired.

EXAMPLE 1 ▪

Order: *co-trimoxazole 40/200 suspension 7.5 mL p.o. q.12h*

Co-trimoxazole 40/200 suspension is a combination drug containing trimethoprim (TMP) 40 mg and sulfamethoxazole (SMX) 200 mg in 5 mL oral suspension. It is an anti-infective drug used to treat bronchitis, gastroenteritis, otitis media, urinary tract infections, and pneumocystis carinii pneumonia. It is given by both oral and IV routes. The tablets are supplied in dosages of 20 mg TMP/100 mg SMX, 80 mg TMP/400 mg SMX, and double strength—160 mg TMP/800 mg SMX. The oral suspension is only supplied in one dosage strength—40 mg TMP/200 mg SMX per 5 mL (Figure 13-6).

FIGURE 13-6 Co-trimoxazole 40/200 oral suspension

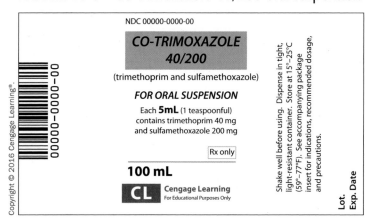

Let's consider the ratio of TMP/ SMX in each supplied form: 20:100, 80:400, 160:800, or 40:200. Do you see a pattern? It may be clearer to view the ratios as fractions and reduce to lowest terms.

$$\underset{5}{\cancel{\dfrac{20}{100}}}, \underset{5}{\cancel{\dfrac{80}{400}}}, \underset{5}{\cancel{\dfrac{160}{800}}}, \underset{5}{\cancel{\dfrac{40}{200}}}$$ All are ratios of 1 mg TMP to 5 mg SMX.

Because they are manufactured in ratios with safe dosages of both drug components, if the order is safe for one drug it will also be safe for the other. The recommended dosages of co-trimoxazole are expressed only by the TMP component. For mild to moderate infections, the usual IV or oral dosage is 6 to 12 mg TMP/kg/day divided q.12h, and for serious infections it is 15 to 20 mg TMP/kg/day divided q.6–8h.

Determine if the volume ordered will deliver a safe dosage for a 22 lb patient.

1. **Convert lb to kg.** Approximate equivalent: 1 kg = 2.2 lb

   THINK: $\frac{1}{2}$ of 22 = 11 (answer will be slightly less)

   $$\frac{1 \text{ kg}}{2.2 \text{ lb}} \times \frac{X \text{ kg}}{22 \text{ lb}}$$

   $$2.2X = 22$$

   $$\frac{2.2X}{2.2} = \frac{22}{2.2}$$

   $$X = 10 \text{ kg}$$

2. **Calculate the safe dosage for the TMP range.**

   TMP minimum daily dosage: 6 mg/kg/day × 10 kg = 60 mg/day

   Divided into 2 doses/day: 60 mg ÷ 2 doses = 30 mg/dose

   TMP maximum daily dosage: 12 mg/kg/day × 10 kg = 120 mg/day

   Divided into 2 doses/day: 120 mg ÷ 2 doses = 60 mg/dose

3. **Calculate the volume of medication for the dosage range.**

   Minimum dose volume: $\dfrac{\text{Dosage on hand}}{\text{Amount on hand}} = \dfrac{\text{Dosage desired}}{\text{X Amount desired}}$

   $$\frac{40 \text{ mg}}{5 \text{ mL}} \times \frac{30 \text{ mg}}{X \text{ mL}}$$

   $$40X = 150$$

   $$\frac{40X}{40} = \frac{150}{40}$$

   $$X = 3.75 \text{ mL, minimum per dose}$$

   Maximum dose volume: $\dfrac{\text{Dosage on hand}}{\text{Amount on hand}} = \dfrac{\text{Dosage desired}}{\text{X Amount desired}}$

   $$\frac{40 \text{ mg}}{5 \text{ mL}} \times \frac{60 \text{ mg}}{X \text{ mL}}$$

   $$40X = 300$$

   $$\frac{40X}{40} = \frac{300}{40}$$

   $$X = 7.5 \text{ mL, maximum per dose}$$

4. **Decide if the dose volume is safe.** Because the physician ordered 7.5 mL, the dosage falls within the safe range and it is a safe dose.

   What dosage of TMP did the physician actually order per dose for this child?

   Use ratio-proportion: Ratio for dosage on hand = Ratio for desired dosage

   Notice that the unknown X is now in the numerator; but the known ratio is still on the left and the unknown ratio is on the right. You are not calculating the amount of dose volume to give (mL desired); you are calculating the dosage (X) to determine if the dosage ordered is safe.

$$\frac{\text{Dosage on hand}}{\text{Amount on hand}} = \frac{\text{X Dosage desired}}{\text{Amount desired}}$$

$$\frac{40\text{ mg}}{5\text{ mL}} \diagup\!\!\!\diagdown \frac{\text{X mg}}{7.5\text{ mL}}$$ The unknown "X" is the desired dosage.

$$5X = 300$$

$$\frac{5X}{5} = \frac{300}{5}$$

$$X = 60\text{ mg}$$

The patient receives 60 mg of TMP in each 7.5 mL dose.

This is the dosage of TMP you would give in one 7.5 mL dose, which matches the upper limit of the safe dosage range.

Compare the number of possible supplied concentrations for co-trimoxazole suspension to the available supply of cefaclor suspension (Figure 13-3, p. 401). Notice that the ordered dosage is expressed in the volume but it also includes the concentration of co-trimoxazole suspension, even though it is only supplied in 40 mg TMP/200 mg SMX. Generally, oral suspensions should be ordered by dosage strength, not dose volume. Consider the confusion and potential for error if cefaclor, with the multiple supplied concentrations, was ordered by the volume alone.

CAUTION

Frequently, oral suspensions are supplied in multiple concentrations. Single drugs should be ordered by dosage strength. Combination drugs may be ordered by dose volume but to avoid medication error, the order must also include the supplied concentration.

EXAMPLE 2 ■

Order: *Tylenol and codeine suspension 7.5 mL (acetaminophen 120 mg with codeine 12 mg per 5 mL) p.o. stat and then q.4h p.r.n., pain*

Tylenol and codeine suspension is a combination of a nonopioid analgesic and an opioid analgesic used in the management of mild to moderate pain. Opioids may have serious consequences, especially in infants and children. Overdosage of acetaminophen has resulted in liver damage. Determining the safe dosage prior to administration is imperative. The recommended dosage for children under 12 years of age is 0.5 to 1 mg codeine/kg/dose every 4 to 6 hours as needed and 10 to 15 mg acetaminophen/kg/dose every 4 to 6 hours as needed. The maximum daily dosage of acetaminophen is 90 mg/kg but is not to exceed 2.6 g acetaminophen/24 hours. In this scenario a 42 lb, 5-year-old child is experiencing pain after having two teeth repaired. The pediatric oral surgeon has ordered 1 dose of the analgesic to be given immediately and has written a prescription for the nurse to provide to the parent for home use. Determine if the initial dosage is safe and if the maximum safe daily dosage of acetaminophen will be exceeded if the child receives the p.r.n. dose every 4 hours.

1. **Convert lb to kg.** Approximate equivalent: 1 kg = 2.2 lb

   THINK: $\frac{1}{2}$ of 42 = 21 (answer will be slightly less)

$$\frac{1\text{ kg}}{2.2\text{ lb}} \diagup\!\!\!\diagdown \frac{\text{X kg}}{42\text{ lb}}$$

$$2.2X = 42$$

$$\frac{2.2X}{2.2} = \frac{42}{2.2}$$

$$X = 19.09\text{ kg} = 19.1\text{ kg}$$

2. **Calculate the safe dosage range for the codeine.**

   codeine minimum per dose: 0.5 mg/kg/dose $\times$ 19.1 kg = 9.55 mg/dose = 9.6 mg/dose

   codeine maximum per dose: 1 mg/kg/dose $\times$ 19.1 kg = 19.1 mg/dose

3. **Calculate the dose volume of medication for the minimum and maximum dosage.**

   Minimum dose volume: $\dfrac{\text{Dosage on hand}}{\text{Amount on hand}} = \dfrac{\text{Dosage desired}}{\text{X Amount desired}}$

   $$\dfrac{12\text{ mg}}{5\text{ mL}} \bowtie \dfrac{9.6\text{ mg}}{\text{X mL}}$$

   $$12\text{X} = 48$$

   $$\dfrac{12\text{X}}{12} = \dfrac{48}{12}$$

   $$\text{X} = 4\text{ mL, minimum per dose}$$

   Maximum dose volume: $\dfrac{\text{Dosage on hand}}{\text{Amount on hand}} = \dfrac{\text{Dosage desired}}{\text{X Amount desired}}$

   $$\dfrac{12\text{ mg}}{5\text{ mL}} \bowtie \dfrac{19.1\text{ mg}}{\text{X mL}}$$

   $$12\text{X} = 95.5$$

   $$\dfrac{12\text{X}}{12} = \dfrac{95.5}{12}$$

   $$\text{X} = 7.95\text{ mL} = 8\text{ mL, maximum per dose}$$

4. **Decide if the dose volume is safe.** The ordered dosage is within the safe recommended range of 4 mL to 8 mL.

5. **Calculate the safe maximum daily dosage of acetaminophen.**

   Acetaminophen maximum per day: 90 mg/kg $\times$ 19.1 kg = 1,719 mg (per day)

6. **Calculate the dose volume of the maximum safe daily dosage of acetaminophen.**

   $$\dfrac{180\text{ mg}}{5\text{ mL}} \bowtie \dfrac{1,719\text{ mg}}{\text{X mL}}$$

   $$180\text{X} = 8,595$$

   $$\dfrac{180\text{X}}{180} = \dfrac{8,595}{180}$$

   $$\text{X} = 47.75\text{ mL} \qquad \text{Safe daily volume of acetaminophen}$$

7. **Determine the potential total dose volume of acetaminophen, if administered q.4h (6 times daily).**

   7.5 mL/dose $\times$ 6 doses = 45 mL

8. **Decide if the total daily dose volume of acetaminophen is safe.** The total volume of 45 mL is slightly lower than the maximum safe daily dose volume of 47.75 mL. The child may receive the ordered dosage of pain medication q.4h without exceeding the maximum daily dosage of acetaminophen.

Be sure to take the time to double-check pediatric dosage. The health care provider who administers the medication has the last opportunity to ensure safe drug therapy.

ADULT DOSAGES BASED ON BODY WEIGHT

Some adult dosage recommendations are based on body weight too, although less frequently than for children. The information you learned about calculating and verifying children's body weight dosages can be applied to adults. It is important that you become familiar and comfortable with reading labels, drug inserts, and drug reference books to understand the drugs you are administering and to check any order that appears questionable.

EXAMPLE ▪

Order: *gentamicin 100 mg IV q.8h*

Gentamicin is an anti-infective drug, classified as an aminoglycoside, used primarily to treat serious infections, but may be used for less serious infections when penicillin or other less toxic drugs are contraindicated. Many regimens are used, but due to the high risk of ototoxicity (involving the ear) or nephrotoxicity (involving the kidney), most involve dosages adjusted on the basis of blood level monitoring and assessment of renal function. The traditional dosage for IM or IV in adults is a loading dose of 2 mg/kg then 1 to 1.7 mg/kg q.8h (up to 6 mg/kg/day in 3 divided doses). If once-daily dosing is employed, the usual dosage is 5 mg/kg q.24h. Prior to administration, doses should be further diluted to a concentration of 10 mg/mL and infused slowly over 30 minutes to 2 hours. Following the initial loading dose, subsequent doses/intervals are based on blood level monitoring and renal function assessment for patients with renal impairment. The blood peak level for gentamicin should not exceed 10 mcg/mL. The solution for injection is available in concentrations of 10 mg/mL and 40 mg/mL (Figure 13-7). For this scenario the nurse is preparing to administer the fifth scheduled dose of gentamicin to an 82-year-old adult with bacterial septicemia who weighs 150 lb.

FIGURE 13-7   Gentamicin 80 mg/2 mL label

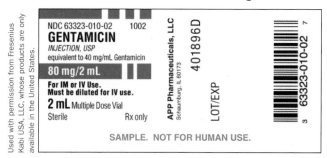

Determine if this dosage is safe.

1. **Convert lb to kg**. Approximate equivalent: 1 kg = 2.2 lb

   THINK: $\frac{1}{2}$ of 150 = 75 (answer will be slightly less)

   $$\frac{1 \text{ kg}}{2.2 \text{ lb}} \diagdown\diagup \frac{X \text{ kg}}{150 \text{ lb}}$$

   $$2.2X = 150$$

   $$\frac{2.2X}{2.2} = \frac{150}{2.2}$$

   $$X = 68.18 \text{ kg} = 68.2 \text{ kg}$$

2. **Calculate the recommended dosage range.**

   Minimum per dose: 1 mg/kg/dose × 68.2 kg = 68.2 mg/dose

   Maximum per dose: 1.7 mg/kg/dose × 68.2 kg = 115.9 mg/dose

3. **Decide if the dosage is safe.** The ordered dosage of gentamicin 100 mg given intravenously every 8 hours is within the recommended range and is safe. The nurse may proceed to administer the medication.

Calculate the amount to give for 1 dose.

Step 1   **Convert**   No conversion needed.

Step 2   **Think**   100 mg is a little larger than 80 mg, so you want to give a little more than 2 mL.

Step 3   **Calculate** $\dfrac{80 \text{ mg}}{2 \text{ mL}} \bowtie \dfrac{100 \text{ mg}}{X \text{ mL}}$

$$80X = 200$$

$$\frac{80X}{80} = \frac{200}{80}$$

$$X = 2.5 \text{ mL, given intravenously every 8 hours}$$

The medication is not yet ready for administration. According to administration guidelines, it must be further diluted to a concentration of 10 mg/mL and infused slowly over 30 minutes to 2 hours. The nurse will inject the 2.5 mL into a piggyback IV bag and use an IV tubing set to administer the medication. You will learn about this skill in Chapter 15.

Seven hours later, the nurse notices that the order has been changed to **gentamicin 80 mg IV q.8h**. Prior to the next scheduled administration, the nurse will need to determine if the new order is in the recommended range. Based on previous calculations, the 80 mg dosage still falls within the safe range. Curious about the reason for the decreased dosage, the nurse checks the recent lab work and finds the blood peak level of gentamicin was 12 mcg/mL that morning. Realizing that decreased renal function due to the aging process may place the 82-year-old patient at greater risk for toxicities, the nurse decides to carefully assess for signs of injury to the ears or kidneys.

QUICK REVIEW
To use the body weight method to verify the safety of pediatric and adult dosages:

- Convert body weight from pounds and ounces to kilograms: 1 kg = 2.2 lb; 1 lb = 16 oz.
- Calculate the recommended safe dosage in mg/kg.
- Compare the ordered dosage with the recommended dosage to decide if the dosage is safe.
- If the dosage is safe, calculate the amount to give for 1 dose; if not safe, notify the prescriber.
- Combination drugs are ordered by dose volume. Check a reputable drug reference to be sure the dose ordered contains the safe amount of each drug as recommended.

Review Set 28

For questions 1 through 10, let's focus only on the mathematical aspects of dosage calculation to reinforce the body weight approach to determining safe dosages.

1. Order: **dicloxacillin sodium 125 mg p.o. q.6h** for a child who weighs 55 lb. The recommended dosage of dicloxacillin sodium for children weighing less than 40 kg is 12.5 to 25 mg/kg/day p.o. in equally divided doses q.6h for moderate to severe infections.

Child's weight: _____ kg

Recommended minimum daily dosage for this child: _____ mg/day

Recommended minimum single dosage for this child: _____ mg/dose

Recommended maximum daily dosage for this child: _____ mg/day

Recommended maximum single dosage for this child: _____ mg/dose

Is the dosage ordered safe? _____

2. Dicloxacillin sodium is available as an oral suspension of 62.5 mg per 5 mL. If the dosage ordered in question 1 is safe, give _____ mL. If not safe, explain why and describe what you should do. _____

_____

3. Order: **chloramphenicol 55 mg IV q.12h** for an 8-day-old infant who weighs 2,200 g. The recommended dosage of chloramphenicol for neonates less than 2 kg is 25 mg/kg once daily, and for neonates more than 2 kg and older than 7 days of age is 50 mg/kg/day divided q.12h.

Child's weight: _____ kg

Recommended daily dosage for this child: _____ mg/day

Recommended single dosage for this child: _____ mg/dose

Is the dosage ordered safe? _____

4. Chloramphenicol is available as a solution for injection of 1 g per 10 mL. If the dosage ordered in question 3 is safe, give _____ mL. If not safe, explain why and describe what you should do. _____

_____

5. Order: **cefixime 120 mg p.o. daily** for a child who weighs 33 lb. The recommended dosage of cefixime for children who weigh less than 50 kg is 8 mg/kg p.o. once daily or 4 mg/kg q.12h.

Child's weight: _____ kg

Recommended single dosage for this child: _____ mg/dose

Is the dosage ordered safe? _____

6. Cefixime is available as a suspension of 100 mg per 5 mL in a 50 mL bottle. If the dosage ordered in question 5 is safe, give _____ mL. If not safe, explain why and describe what you should do. _____

_____

How many full doses are available in the bottle of cefixime? _____ dose(s)

7. Order: **acetaminophen 480 mg p.o. q.4h p.r.n., temperature 101.6°F or greater.** The child's weight is 32 kg. The recommended child's dosage of acetaminophen is 10 to 15 mg/kg/dose p.o. q.4h p.r.n. for fever.

Recommended minimum single dosage for this child: _____ mg/dose

Recommended maximum single dosage for this child: _____ mg/dose

Is the dosage ordered safe? _____

8. Acetaminophen is available as a suspension of 160 mg per 5 mL. If the dosage ordered in question 7 is safe, give _____ mL. If not safe, explain why and describe what you should do.

_____

_____

9. Order: *cephalexin 125 mg p.o. q.6h* for a child who weighs 44 lb. The recommended pediatric dosage of cephalexin is 25 to 50 mg/kg/day in 4 equally divided doses.

   Child's weight: _____ kg

   Recommended minimum daily dosage for this child: _____ mg/day

   Recommended minimum single dosage for this child: _____ mg/dose

   Recommended maximum daily dosage for this child: _____ mg/day

   Recommended maximum single dosage for this child: _____ mg/dose

   Is the dosage ordered safe? _____

10. Cephalexin is available in a suspension of 125 mg per 5 mL. If the dosage ordered in question 9 is safe, give _____ mL. If not safe, explain why and describe what you should do.

   _____

   _____

The labels provided represent the drugs available to answer questions 11 through 20. Verify safe dosages, indicate the amount to give, and draw an arrow on the accompanying measuring device. Explain unsafe dosages and describe the appropriate action to take.

11. Order: *kanamycin sulfate 34 mg IV q.8h* for an infant who weighs 7 lb 8 oz. The recommended dosage of kanamycin sulfate for adults and children is 15 mg/kg/day in 2 or 3 equal doses, not to exceed 1.5 g/day.

   Infant's weight: _____ kg

   Recommended daily dosage for this infant: _____ mg/day

   Recommended single dosage for this infant: _____ mg/dose

   Is the dosage ordered safe?

   _____

NDC 0015-3512-20
EQUIVALENT TO   NSN 6505-00-926-9202
75 mg KANAMYCIN per 2 mL
KANTREX®
Kanamycin Sulfate Injection, USP
Pediatric Injection
FOR I.M. OR I.V. USE
CAUTION: Federal law prohibits dispensing without prescription.

0.09% sodium bisulfite added as an antioxidant, buffered with 0.33% sodium citrate. • Adjusted to pH 4.5 with H_2SO_4. • Kantrex Pediatric Injection should not be physically mixed with other anti-bacterial agents.
READ ACCOMPANYING CIRCULAR
Distributed by APOTHECON®
A Bristol-Myers Squibb Co.
Princeton, NJ 08540
Made in USA   3512200RL-1

MAXIMUM DOSE: 15 MG/KG/DAY

Cont:
Exp. Date:

12. If the dosage ordered in question 11 is safe, give _____ mL. If not safe, explain why and describe what you should do. _____

   _____

13. Order: *co-trimoxazole suspension 7.5 mL of trimethoprim 40 mg per 5 mL p.o. q.12h* for a child who weighs 15 kg and has a urinary tract infection. The recommended dosage of co-trimoxazole (trimethoprim and sulfamethoxazole) for such infections in children is based on the trimethoprim at 8 mg/kg/day in 2 equal doses.

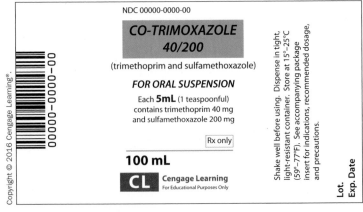

NDC 00000-0000-00

CO-TRIMOXAZOLE 40/200
(trimethoprim and sulfamethoxazole)

FOR ORAL SUSPENSION

Each **5mL** (1 teaspoonful) contains trimethoprim 40 mg and sulfamethoxazole 200 mg

Rx only

100 mL

CL **Cengage Learning**
For Educational Purposes Only

Shake well before using. Dispense in tight, light-resistant container. Store at 15°–25°C (59°–77°F). See accompanying package insert for indications, recommended dosage, and precautions.

Lot.
Exp. Date

Recommended daily trimethoprim dosage for this child: _____ mg/day

Recommended single trimethoprim dosage for this child: _____ mg/dose

Recommended single dose for this child: _____ mL/dose

Is the dose ordered safe? _____

14. If the dose ordered in question 13 is safe, give _____ mL. If not safe, explain why and describe what you should do. _____

_____

The dose ordered is equivalent to _____ teaspoons.

Copyright © 2016 Cengage Learning®.

15. Order: **ampicillin 400 mg IM q.6h** for a 10-year-old child who weighs 72 lb. Recommended dosage: See label.

    Child's weight: _____ kg

    Recommended minimum daily dosage for this child: _____ mg/day

    Recommended minimum single dosage for this child: _____ mg/dose

NDC 00000-0000-00

AMPICILLIN

For Injection, USP

ampicillin sodium equivalent to

500 mg ampicillin

For IM or IV Use

Rx only

Lot.
Exp. Date

For IM Use: add 1.7 mL diluent. The resulting solution provides 250 mg ampicillin per mL. IM or IV Injection: USE SOLUTION WITHIN 1 HOUR. IV Infusion: See package insert. Usual dosage: Children: 25 to 50 mg/kg/day in equally divided doses at 6-hour intervals. Adults: 500 mg to 3 g every 6 hours (not to exceed 14 g/day). Package insert includes detailed precautions and indications. Store at controlled room temperature 15°–30°C (59°–86°F).

Cengage Learning
For Educational Purposes Only

CL

00000-0000-00

Copyright © 2016 Cengage Learning®.

Recommended maximum daily dosage for this child: _____ mg/day

Recommended maximum single dosage for this child: _____ mg/dose

Is the dosage ordered safe? _____

16. If the dosage ordered in question 15 is safe, give _____ mL. If not safe, explain why and describe what you should do. _____

_____

Copyright © 2016 Cengage Learning®.

17. Order: **amoxicillin oral suspension 100 mg p.o. q.8h** for a child who weighs 39 lb. Recommended dosage: See label.

    Child's weight: _____ kg

    Recommended minimum daily dosage for this child: _____ mg/day

    Recommended minimum single dosage for this child: _____ mg/dose

Recommended maximum daily dosage for this child: _____ mg/day

Recommended maximum single dosage for this child: _____ mg/dose

Is the dosage ordered safe? _____

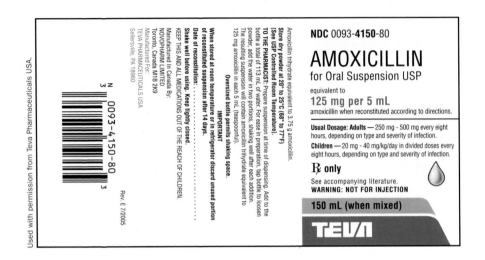

18. If the dosage ordered in question 17 is safe, give _____ mL. If not safe, explain why and describe what you should do. _____

_____

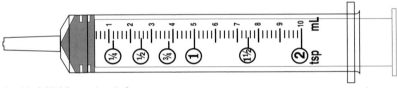

Copyright © 2016 Cengage Learning®.

19. Order: **Terramycin 100 mg IM q.8h** for a 9-year-old child who weighs 55 lb. Recommended pediatric dosage: See label.

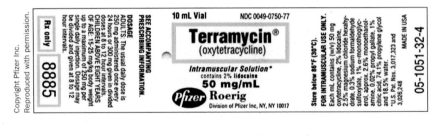

Child's weight: _____ kg

Recommended minimum daily dosage for this child: _____ mg/day

Recommended minimum single dosage for this child: _____ mg/dose

Recommended maximum daily dosage for this child: _____ mg/day

Recommended maximum single dosage for this child: _____ mg/dose

Is the dosage ordered safe? _____

20. If the dosage ordered in question 19 is safe, give _____ mL. If not safe, explain why and describe what you should do. _____

_____

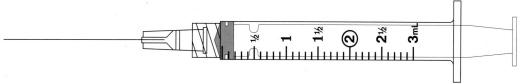

Questions 21 through 24: You are caring for a 3-year-old child, weighing 30 lb, who is receiving chemotherapy known to cause nausea and vomiting. The antiemetic, granisetron, will be administered prior to chemotherapy for prevention, and following chemotherapy for treatment, of nausea and vomiting. The recommended IV dosage for children 2 to 16 years is 10 mcg/kg within 30 min prior to chemotherapy or 20 to 40 mcg/kg/day once or divided twice daily.

Used with permission from Fresenius Kabi USA, LLC, whose products are only available in the United States.	NDC 63323-317-01 361701 **GRANISETRON** **HYDROCHLORIDE** *INJECTION* **0.1 mg/mL** **For IV use only** Rx only **1 mL** Single-Use Vial APP Pharmaceuticals, LLC Schaumburg, IL 60173 402323A LOT/EXP 63323-317-01 SAMPLE. NOT FOR HUMAN USE.

21. Order: granisetron 136 mcg direct IV, 30 minutes prior to chemotherapy

    Child's weight: _____ kg

    Is the dosage ordered safe? _____

22. If the dosage ordered in question 21 is safe, give _____ mL. If not safe, explain why and describe what you should do.

    _____

    _____

23. Order: granisetron 170 mcg direct IV q.12h p.r.n., nausea/vomiting

    Recommended minimum daily dosage for this child: _____ mcg/day

    Recommended minimum single dosage for this child: _____ mcg/dose

    Recommended maximum daily dosage for this child: _____ mcg/day

    Recommended maximum single dosage for this child: _____ mcg/dose

    Is the dosage ordered safe? _____

24. If the dosage ordered in question 23 is safe, give _____ mL. If not safe, explain why and describe what you should do.

    _____

    _____

For questions 25 through 30, the medications will be retrieved from an automated dispensing cabinet (ADC) matrix drawer, as illustrated, to administer a variety of different orders. Utilize all aspects of safe dosage calculation of medication, including collecting data about the drug, selecting the supply dosage, computing the dosage, and measuring with equipment for medication administration. Refer to a nursing drug guide, such as the *Delmar Nurse's Drug Handbook,* to answer specific questions about the medication prior to administering.

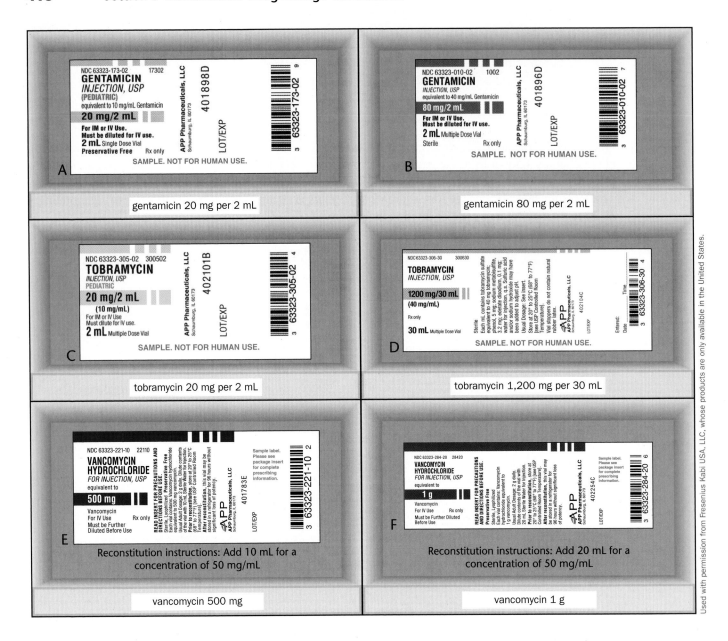

A   gentamicin 20 mg per 2 mL

B   gentamicin 80 mg per 2 mL

C   tobramycin 20 mg per 2 mL

D   tobramycin 1,200 mg per 30 mL

E   Reconstitution instructions: Add 10 mL for a concentration of 50 mg/mL

vancomycin 500 mg

F   Reconstitution instructions: Add 20 mL for a concentration of 50 mg/mL

vancomycin 1 g

25. Order: **tobramycin 375 mg IV q.24h** for 56-year-old patient weighing 200 lb

For what condition(s) is tobramycin indicated? _____

What dosage strengths of tobramycin may be supplied in solution for injection? _____

_____

By what parenteral routes may tobramycin be administered? _____

What is the usual recommended adult dosage range? _____

Recommended minimum single dosage for this patient: _____ mg/dose

Recommended maximum single dosage for this patient: _____ mg/dose

Is the dosage ordered safe? _____

26. Identify the letter of the label showing the supplied dosage strength that you will use to calculate 1 dose. _____

    If the dosage ordered in question 25 is safe, give _____ mL.

    If not safe, explain why and describe what you should do.

    _____

    _____

    Select the appropriate syringe and mark the correct amount:

27. Order: **gentamicin 12 mg IV q.8h** for 2-month-old patient weighing $10\frac{1}{2}$ lb

    For what condition(s) is gentamicin indicated? _____

    What dosage strengths of gentamicin may be supplied in solution for injection? _____

    _____

    By what parenteral routes may gentamicin be administered? _____

    What is the usual recommended infant dosage? _____

    Recommended single dosage for this infant: _____ mg/dose

    Is the dosage ordered safe? _____

28. Identify the letter of the label showing the supplied dosage strength that you will use to calculate 1 dose. _____

    If the dosage ordered in question 27 is safe, give _____ mL.

    If not safe, explain why and describe what you should do.

    _____

    _____

    Select the appropriate syringe and mark the correct amount:

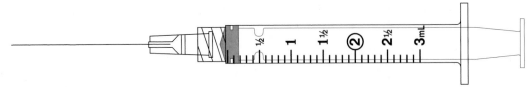

29. Order: *vancomycin 660 mg IV q.6h* for 3-year-old child weighing 36 lb

    For what condition(s) is vancomycin indicated? _____

    What dosage strengths of vancomycin may be supplied in solution for injection? _____

    _____

    By what parenteral routes may vancomycin be administered? _____

    What is the usual recommended child dosage range? _____

    Recommended daily dosage for this child: _____ mg/day

    Recommended single q.6h dosage for this child: _____ mg/dose

    Recommended single q.8h dosage for this child: _____ mg/dose

    Is the dosage ordered safe? _____

30. Identify the letter of the label showing the supplied dosage strength that you will use to calculate 1 dose. _____

    If the dosage ordered in question 29 is safe, give _____ mL.

    If not safe, explain why and describe what you should do.

    _____

    _____

    Select the appropriate syringe and mark the correct amount:

    After completing these problems, see pages 683–687 to check your answers.

| CLINICAL REASONING SKILLS | Medication errors in pediatrics often occur when the nurse fails to properly identify the child before administering the dose. |

ERROR

Failing to identify the child before administering a medication

Possible Scenario

Suppose the physician ordered *ampicillin 500 mg IV q.6h* for a child with pneumonia. The nurse calculated the dosage to be safe, checked to be sure the child had no allergies, and prepared the medication. The child had been assigned to a semiprivate room. The nurse entered the room and noted only one child in the room and administered the IV ampicillin to that child, without checking the identification of the child. Within an hour of the administered ampicillin, the child began to break out in hives and had signs of respiratory distress. The nurse asked the child's mother, "Does Johnny have any known allergies?" The mother replied, "This is James, not Johnny, and yes, James is allergic to penicillin. His roommate, Johnny, is in the playroom." At this point, the nurse realized that the ampicillin was given to the wrong child, who was allergic to penicillin.

Potential Outcome

James's physician would have been notified, and he would likely have ordered epinephrine subcut stat (given for anaphylactic reactions), steroids, and an antihistamine, followed by close monitoring of the child. Anaphylactic reactions can range from mild to severe. Ampicillin is a derivative of penicillin and would not have been prescribed for a child such as James.

Prevention

This error could easily have been avoided had the nurse remembered the cardinal rule of *identifying the patient* before administering *any* medication. Children are mobile, and you cannot assume the identity of a child simply because he or she is in a particular room. The correct method of identifying the child is to check the wrist or ankle band and compare it to the medication administration record with the child's name and ID number. Remember: The first of the *Six Rights* of medication administration is the *right patient*.

| CLINICAL REASONING SKILLS | When the recommended dosage of a medication is given with a low and high range, the minimum and maximum dosages must be calculated to determine the safety of a drug order. This is the only way to ensure that the drug to be administered is not an overdose or an underdose. |

ERROR

Calculating only the maximum recommended dose of an ordered medication to determine safety

Possible Scenario

The physician ordered *tobramycin 9.5 mg IV q.8h* for a 2-week-old infant who weighed 11 lb and who had a serious infection. The recommended dosage for children and infants greater than 1 week old is 1.5 to 1.9 mg/kg q.6h or 2 to 2.5 mg/kg q.8h. The nurse calculated a safe dosage range prior to administering what would be the third dose of this medication, although it was administered two previous times by other nurses. First, the nurse correctly converted the infant's weight from pounds to kilograms using ratio-proportion.

$$\frac{1 \text{ kg}}{2.2 \text{ lb}} \diagdown \frac{X \text{ kg}}{11 \text{ lb}}$$

$$2.2X = 11 \text{ lb}$$

$$\frac{2.2}{2.2} = \frac{11}{2.2}$$

$$X = 5 \text{ kg}$$

Then, the nurse correctly calculated the minimum and maximum recommended dosages by multiplying the recommended dosage by the infant's weight.

Minimum single q.8h dose: 2 mg/kg × 5 kg = 10 mg
Maximum single q.8h dose: 2.5 mg/kg × 5 kg = 12.5 mg

The nurse recognized that the ordered dose fell below the minimum recommended dose for tobramycin to be administered every 8 hours. Considering the serious infection the infant had, the nurse doubted that the physician planned to give such a low dose and contacted the physician for clarification. The physician realized that the dose was mistakenly calculated according to the q.12h recommendation and wrote a new order.

Potential Outcome

The first 2 dosages of tobramycin fell slightly below the minimum recommended dose for the frequency ordered. This situation was discussed with the nurse manager of the pediatric unit along with the other two staff nurses involved. One staff nurse admitted to administering medication occasionally without actually calculating a safe dose if it looked like it was the correct dose. The other nurse always checked to see that ordered medications were not overdoses but didn't usually worry about checking for underdoses. The nurse manager was alarmed by such lax in following safety protocols and emphasized the importance of always verifying dosages on pediatric patients, especially infants. The manager followed up with the Education department to schedule follow up training. In this situation, the mistake was caught early and corrected but could have caused significant harm to the infant by inadequately treating a severe infection.

Prevention

When reading drug reference guides, make sure you read all the dosage recommendations thoroughly. It is easy to see how, when in a hurry, a physician or nurse might have misinterpreted the drug reference information and thought that it read 1.5 to 1.9 mg/kg q.8h. Don't hurry or take shortcuts when administering medications. Always calculate the minimum and maximum recommended doses when a dosage range is given.

PRACTICE PROBLEMS—CHAPTER 13

For questions 1 through 8, convert the following weights to kilograms. Round to one decimal place.

1. 12 lb = _____ kg

2. 8 lb 4 oz = _____ kg

3. 1,570 g = _____ kg

4. 2,300 g = _____ kg

5. 34 lb = _____ kg

6. 6 lb 10 oz = _____ kg

7. 52 lb = _____ kg

8. 890 g = _____ kg

9. The recommended dosage of tobramycin for adults with serious infections that are not life threatening is 3 mg/kg/day in 3 equally divided doses q.8h. What should you expect the total daily dosage of tobramycin to be for an adult with a serious infection who weighs 80 kg?
_____ mg/day

10. What should you expect a single dosage of tobramycin to be for the adult described in question 9?
_____ mg/dose

The labels provided represent the drugs available to answer questions 11 through 42. Verify safe dosages, indicate the amount to give, and draw an arrow on the accompanying measuring device. Explain unsafe dosages and describe the appropriate action to take.

11. Order: *gentamicin 40 mg IV q.8h* for a child who weighs 43 lb. The recommended dosage for children is 2 to 2.5 mg/kg q.8h.

    Child's weight: _____ kg

    Recommended minimum single dosage for this child: _____ mg/dose

    Recommended maximum single dosage for this child: _____ mg/dose

    Is the ordered dosage safe? _____

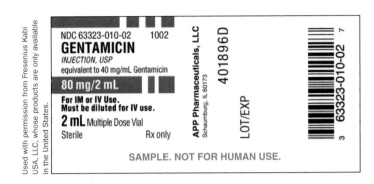

12. If the dosage ordered in question 11 is safe, give _____ mL. If not safe, explain why and describe what you should do. _____

    _____

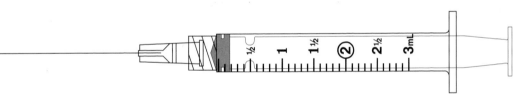

13. Order: *furosemide oral solution 10 mg p.o. b.i.d.* for a child who weighs 16 lb. The recommended pediatric dosage is 0.5 to 2 mg/kg b.i.d.

    Child's weight: _____ kg

    Recommended minimum single dosage for this child: _____ mg/dose

    Recommended maximum single dosage for this child: _____ mg/dose

    Is the ordered dosage safe? _____

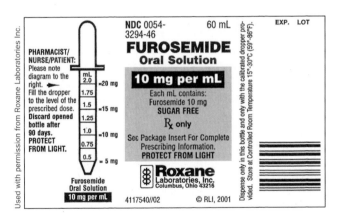

14. If the dosage ordered in question 13 is safe, give _____ mL. If not safe, explain why and describe what you should do. _____

    _____

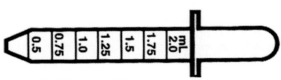

15. Order: *carbamazepine 150 mg p.o. b.i.d.* for a child who is 5 years old and weighs 40 lb. The recommended dosage for children under 6 years of age is 10 to 20 mg/kg/day in 2 to 4 divided doses per day, not to exceed 400 mg/day.

Child's weight: _____ kg

Recommended minimum daily dosage for this child: _____ mg/day

Recommended minimum single dosage for this child: _____ mg/dose

Recommended maximum daily dosage for this child: _____ mg/day

Recommended maximum single dosage for this child: _____ mg/dose

Is the dosage ordered safe? _____

16. If the dosage ordered in question 15 is safe, give _____ mL. If not safe, explain why and describe what you should do. _____

NDC 0078-0508-83

Tegretol®

carbamazepine USP

Suspension

100 mg/5 mL

IMPORTANT: Shake well before using.

Each 5 mL contains 100 mg carbamazepine USP.

©Novartis

450 mL

Dispense in tight, light-resistant container (USP).

Rx only

☋ **NOVARTIS**

Used by permission of Novartis AG.

Keep this and all drugs out of the reach of children.
Dosage: See package insert.
Do not store above 30°C (86°F).
Manufactured by:
Patheon Whitby Inc.
Whitby Ontario Canada
L1N 5Z5
Distributed by:
Novartis Pharmaceuticals Corporation
East Hanover, New Jersey 07936
3685-11-07A

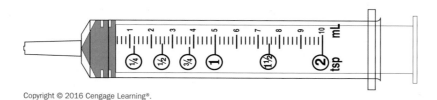

Copyright © 2016 Cengage Learning®.

17. Order: *Depakene 150 mg p.o. b.i.d.* for a child who is 10 years old and weighs 64 lb. The recommended dosage for adults and children 10 years and older is 10 to 15 mg/kg/day up to a maximum of 60 mg/kg/day. If the total daily dosage exceeds 250 mg, divide the dose.

Child's weight: _____ kg

Recommended minimum daily dosage for this child: _____ mg/day

Recommended minimum single dosage for this child: _____ mg/dose

Recommended maximum daily dosage for this child: _____ mg/day

Recommended maximum single dosage for this child: _____ mg/dose

Is the dosage ordered safe? _____

Do not accept if band on cap is broken or missing.

Each 5 mL contains equivalent of 250 mg valproic acid as the sodium salt.

See enclosure for prescribing information.

©Abbott

Abbott Laboratories
North Chicago,
IL60064, U.S.A.
Exp.
Lot

Used with permission from Abbott Laboratories.

NDC 0074-5682-16
16 fl oz Syrup

DEPAKENE®

VALPROIC ACID
SYRUP, USP

**250 mg
per 5 mL**

☐ Caution: Federal (U.S.A.) law prohibits dispensing without prescription.

6505-01-094-9241

Dispense in the original container or a glass, USP tight container.

Store below 86°F (30°C).

0074568216

02-7538-2/R12

18. If the dosage ordered in question 17 is safe, give _____ mL. If not safe, explain why and describe what you should do. _____

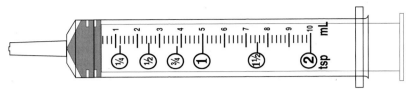

Copyright © 2016 Cengage Learning®.

19. Order: **penicillin G sodium 125,000 units IV daily** for an infant who weighs 2,500 g. The recommended dosage for infants is 50,000 units/kg/day in a single dose.

   Child's weight: _____ kg

   Recommended daily dosage for this child: _____ units/day

   Recommended single dosage for this child: _____ units/dose

   Is the ordered dosage safe? _____

SQUIBB® MARSAM™

1 box • 10 vials   NDC 0003-0668-05

5,000,000 units per vial
PENICILLIN G SODIUM
for INJECTION USP

Caution: Federal law prohibits
dispensing without prescription

PENICILLIN G SODIUM for INJECTION USP

Each vial provides 5,000,000 units penicillin G sodium with approx.
140 mg citrate buffer (composed of sodium citrate and not more than
4.6 mg citric acid). One million units penicillin contains approx. 2.0 mEq
sodium.
Sterile • For intramuscular or intravenous drip use
Usual dosage: See insert
PREPARATION OF SOLUTION: Add 23 mL, 18 mL, 8 mL, or 3 mL diluent to
provide 200,000 u, 250,000 u, 500,000 u, or 1,000,000 u per mL,
respectively.
Sterile solution may be kept in refrigerator 1 week without significant
loss of potency.
Store at room temperature prior to constitution
© 1986 Squibb-Marsam, Inc.
For information contact:
Squibb-Marsam, Inc., Cherry Hill, NJ 08034
Made by Glaxochem, Ltd., Greenford, Middlesex, England.
Filled in Italy by Squibb S.p.A. Dist. by
E. R. Squibb & Sons, Inc., Princeton, NJ 08540   C5277 / 66805

20. If the dosage ordered in question 19 is safe, reconstitute with _____ mL diluent for a total solution volume of _____ mL with a concentration of _____ units/mL.

   Give _____ mL. If not safe, explain why and describe what you should do. _____

   _____

Copyright © 2016 Cengage Learning®.

21. Order: **amoxicillin oral suspension 150 mg p.o. q.8h** for a child who weighs 41 lb. Recommended dosage: See label.

   Child's weight: _____ kg

   Recommended minimum daily dosage for this child: _____ mg/day

   Recommended minimum single dosage for this child: _____ mg/dose

   Recommended maximum daily dosage for this child: _____ mg/day

   Recommended maximum single dosage for this child: _____ mg/dose

   Is the dosage ordered safe? _____

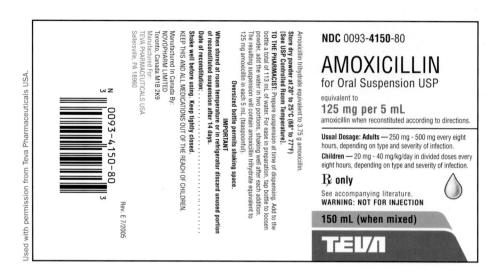

22. If the dosage ordered in question 21 is safe, give _____ mL. If not safe, explain why and describe what you should do. _____

_____

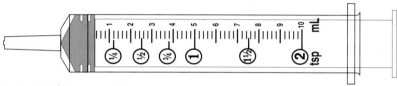

Copyright © 2016 Cengage Learning®.

23. Order: *cefaclor oral suspension 187 mg p.o. q.8h* for a child with otitis media who weighs $30\frac{1}{2}$ lb. Recommended dosage: See label.

Child's weight: _____ kg

Recommended daily dosage for this child: _____ mg/day

Recommended single dosage for this child: _____ mg/dose

Is the dosage ordered safe? _____

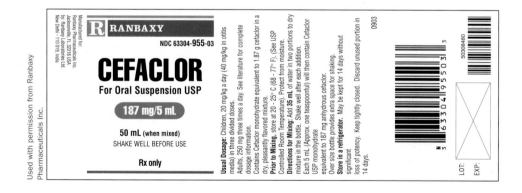

24. If the dosage ordered in question 23 is safe, give _____ mL. If not safe, explain why and describe what you should do. _____

_____

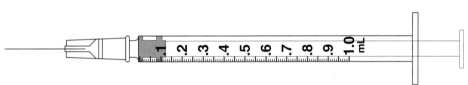

25. Order: **Narcan 100 mcg subcut stat** for a child who weighs 22 lb.
    Recommended pediatric dosage: 0.01 mg/kg/dose.

    Child's weight: _____ kg

    Recommended single dosage for this child: _____ mg/dose

    Is the dosage ordered safe? _____

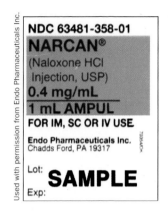

NDC 63481-358-01

NARCAN®
(Naloxone HCl
Injection, USP)
0.4 mg/mL
1 mL AMPUL
FOR IM, SC OR IV USE

Endo Pharmaceuticals Inc.
Chadds Ford, PA 19317

Lot:
SAMPLE
Exp:

26. If the dosage ordered in question 25 is safe, give _____ mL. If not safe, explain why and
    describe what you should do.

    _____

    _____

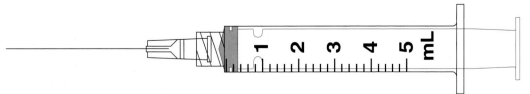

27. Order: **tobramycin 35 mg IV q.8h**
    for a child who weighs 14 kg. The
    recommended pediatric dosage of
    tobramycin is 2 to 2.5 mg/kg q.8h or
    1.5 to 1.9 mg/kg q.6h.

    Recommended minimum single dosage
    for this child: _____ mg/dose

    Recommended maximum single dos-
    age for this child: _____ mg/dose

    Is the dosage ordered safe? _____

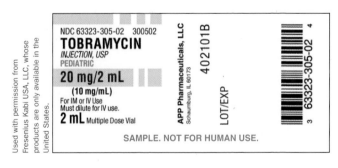

NDC 63323-305-02   300502

TOBRAMYCIN
INJECTION, USP
PEDIATRIC

20 mg/2 mL
(10 mg/mL)
For IM or IV Use
Must dilute for IV use.
2 mL Multiple Dose Vial

402101B

LOT/EXP

SAMPLE. NOT FOR HUMAN USE.

28. If the dosage ordered in question 27 is safe, give _____ mL. If not safe, explain why and
    describe what you should do. _____

    _____

29. Order: **ceftriaxone 1 g IV q.12h** for a child with a serious infection who weighs 20 lb. The recommended pediatric dosage of ceftriaxone is a total daily dosage of 50 to 75 mg/kg given once a day (or in equally divided doses twice a day), not to exceed 2 g/day.

    Supply: ceftriaxone 1 g per 50 mL single-dose container

    Child's weight: _____ kg

    Recommended minimum daily dosage for this child: _____ mg/day

    Recommended minimum single dosage for this child: _____ mg/dose

    Recommended maximum daily dosage for this child: _____ mg/day

    Recommended maximum single dosage for this child: _____ mg/dose

    Is the dosage ordered safe? _____

30. If the dosage ordered in question 29 is safe, give _____ mL. If not safe, explain why and describe what you should do. _____

    _____

31. Order: **Robinul 50 mcg IM 60 minutes pre-op** for a child who weighs 11.4 kg. The recommended pediatric preanesthesia dosage of Robinul (glycopyrrolate) is 0.002 mg/lb of body weight given intramuscularly.

    NDC 60977-155-63
    Robinul Injectable
    (Glycopyrrolate Injection, USP) ℞ only
    0.2 mg/mL NOT FOR USE IN NEWBORNS
    FOR INTRAMUSCULAR
    OR INTRAVENOUS ADMINISTRATION
    20 mL Multiple Dose Vial
    Baxter
    Manufactured by
    Baxter Healthcare Corporation
    Deerfield, IL 60015 USA

    Water for Injection, USP q.s./Benzyl Alcohol, NF (preservative) 0.9%. pH adjusted, when necessary, with hydrochloric acid and/or sodium hydroxide.
    Usual Dosage:
    See accompanying descriptive literature. Store at 20°C-25°C (68°F-77°F) [See USP Controlled Room Temperature].
    462-182-00

    VOID

    Child's weight: _____ lb

    Recommended single dosage for this child: _____ mg/dose

    Is the dosage ordered safe? _____

32. If the dosage ordered in question 31 is safe, give _____ mL. If not safe, explain why and describe what you should do. _____

33. Order: **ceftriaxone 600 mg IV q.12h** for a 6-month-old infant with a serious infection who weighs 18 lb. For the treatment of serious miscellaneous infections other than meningitis, the recommended total daily dosage of ceftriaxone for pediatric patients is 50 to 75 mg/kg given in divided doses every 12 hours. The total daily dose should not exceed 2 grams.

    Infant's weight: _____ kg

    The total daily dosage ordered for this infant: _____ mg/day or _____ g/day

    Recommended minimum single dosage for this infant: _____ mg/dose

    Recommended maximum single dosage for this infant: _____ mg/dose

    Is the dosage ordered safe? _____

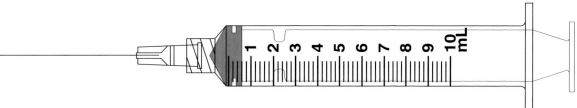

Package Insert for IV: "Add 9.6 mL to 1 g vial. After reconstitution, each 1 mL of solution contains approximately 100 mg equivalent of ceftriaxone."

34. If the dosage ordered in question 33 is safe, reconstitute with _____ mL diluent for a total solution volume of _____ mL with a concentration of _____ mg/mL. Give _____ mL. If not safe, explain why and describe what you should do. _____

_____

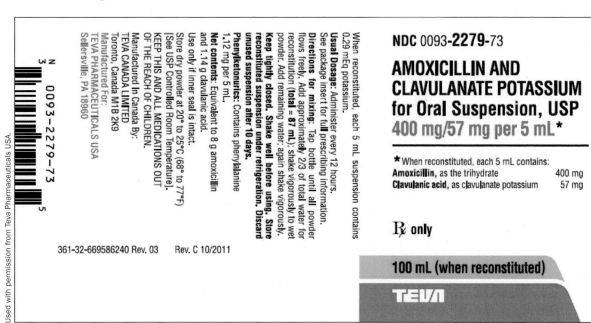

Copyright © 2016 Cengage Learning®.

35. Order: *amoxicillin/clavulanate 200 mg p.o. q.12h* for a 5-year-old child who weighs 45 lb. The recommended dosage of this combination drug is based on the amoxicillin at 25 mg/kg/day in divided doses q.12h or 20 mg/kg/day in divided doses q.8h.

Child's weight: _____ kg

Recommended daily dosage for this child: _____ mg/day

Recommended single dosage for this child: _____ mg/dose

Is the dosage ordered safe? _____

36. If the dosage ordered in question 35 is safe, give _____ mL. If not safe, explain why and describe what you should do. _____

_____

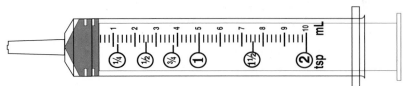

37. Order: *cefaclor oral suspension 75 mg p.o. t.i.d.* for a child with an upper respiratory infection who weighs 18 lb. Recommended dosage: See label.

Child's weight: _____ kg

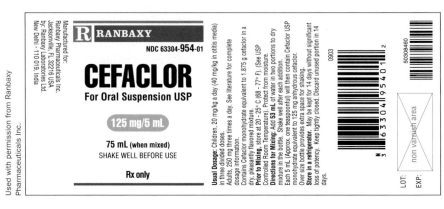

Recommended daily dosage for this child: _____ mg/day

Recommended single dosage for this child: _____ mg/dose

Is the dosage ordered safe? _____

38. If the dosage ordered in question 37 is safe, give _____ mL. If not safe, explain why and describe what you should do.

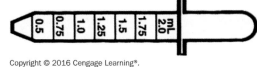

_____

_____

39. Order: *Vantin 100 mg p.o. q.i.d. × 10 days* for a 4-year-old child with tonsillitis who weighs 45 lb. Recommended dosage for children 5 months to 12 years: 5 mg/kg (maximum of 100 mg/dose) q.12h (maximum daily dosage: 200 mg) for 5 to 10 days.

Child's weight: _____ kg

Recommended daily dosage for this child: _____ mg/day

The total daily dosage ordered for this child: _____ mg/day

Is the dosage ordered safe? _____

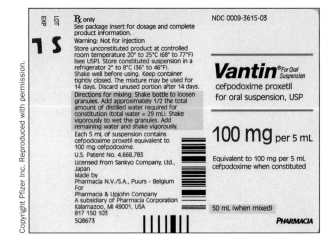

40. If the dosage ordered in question 39 is safe, give _____ mL. If not safe, explain why and describe what you should do. _____

_____

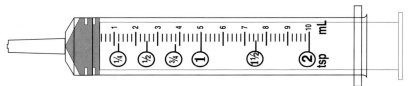

41. Order: *Biaxin*
    175 mg p.o. q.12h
    for a child who
    weighs 51 lb.
    Recommended
    pediatric dosage:
    See label.

    Child's weight:
    _____ kg

    Recommended daily
    dosage for this child:
    _____ mg/day

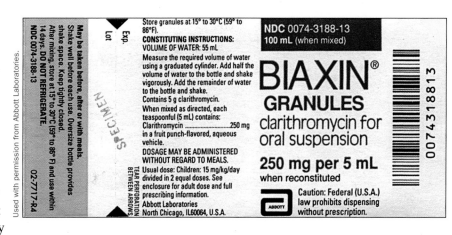

    Recommended single dosage for this child: _____ mg/dose

    Is the dosage ordered safe? _____

42. If the dosage ordered in question 41 is safe, give _____ mL. If not safe, explain why and
    describe what you should do. _____

    _____

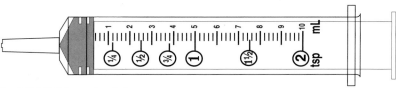

Questions 43 through 48 ask you to apply the steps on your own to determine safe dosages, just as you
would do in the clinical setting. Calculate the amount to give and mark an arrow on the measuring device,
or explain unsafe dosages and describe the appropriate action. Note if a reconstitution label is required
(see question 49).

43. Order: *methylprednisolone 10 mg IV q.6h* for a child who weighs 95 lb. Recommended pediatric
    dosage: Not less than 0.5 mg/kg/day.

    If the dosage ordered is safe, give _____ mL. If not safe, explain why and describe what you
    should do. _____

    _____

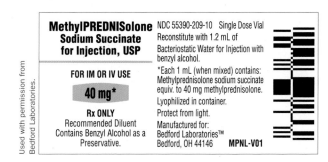

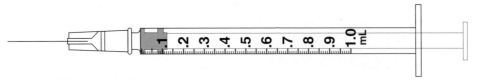

44. Order: **albuterol 1.4 mg p.o. t.i.d.** for a 2-year-old child who weighs 31 lb. Recommended pediatric dosage: 0.1 mg/kg, not to exceed 2 mg t.i.d.

    If the dosage ordered is safe, give _____ mL. If not safe, explain why and describe what you should do. _____

    _____

    _____

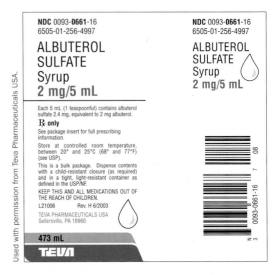

NDC 0093-**0661**-16
6505-01-256-4997

ALBUTEROL SULFATE
Syrup
2 mg/5 mL

Each 5 mL (1 teaspoonful) contains albuterol sulfate 2.4 mg, equivalent to 2 mg albuterol.

℞ only

See package insert for full prescribing information.

Store at controlled room temperature, between 20° and 25°C (68° and 77°F) (see USP).

This is a bulk package. Dispense contents with a child-resistant closure (as required) and in a tight, light-resistant container as defined in the USP/NF.

KEEP THIS AND ALL MEDICATIONS OUT OF THE REACH OF CHILDREN.

L21006   Rev. H 6/2003

TEVA PHARMACEUTICALS USA
Sellersville, PA 18960

473 mL

TEVA

NDC 0093-**0661**-16
6505-01-256-4997

ALBUTEROL SULFATE
Syrup
2 mg/5 mL

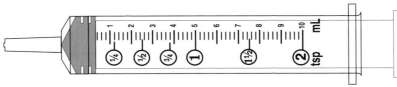

45. Order: **penicillin G potassium 450,000 units IV q.6h** for a child with a streptococcal infection who weighs 12 kg. Recommended pediatric dosage for streptococcal infections is 150,000 units/kg/day given in equal doses q.4 to 6h.

    If the dosage ordered is safe, reconstitute to a dosage supply of _____ units/mL and give _____ mL. If not safe, explain why and describe what you should do. _____

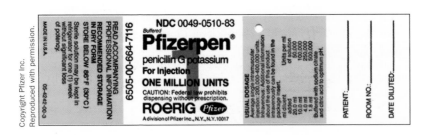

NDC 0049-0510-83

Buffered
Pfizerpen®
penicillin G potassium
For Injection
ONE MILLION UNITS

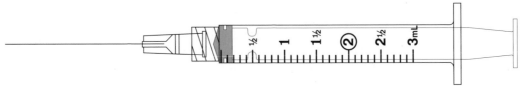

46. Order: **clonazepam 1 mg p.o. b.i.d.** for a 9-year-old child on initial therapy who weighs 56 lb. The recommended initial pediatric dosage of clonazepam for children up to 10 years or 30 kg is 0.01 to 0.03 mg/kg/day in 2 to 3 divided doses up to a maximum of 0.05 mg/kg/day.

If the dosage ordered is safe, give _____ tablet(s). If not safe, explain why and describe what you should do. _____

_____

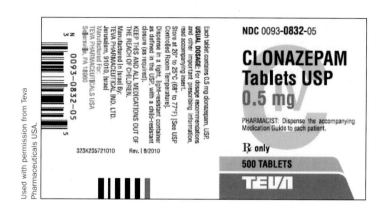

47. Order: **morphine sulfate 1 mg IM stat** for a child who weighs 18 lb. Recommended pediatric dosage: IM or subcut dosage may be initiated at 0.05 mg/kg/dose.

If the dosage ordered is safe, give _____ mL. If not safe, explain why and describe what you should do. _____

_____

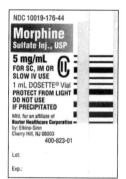

Images courtesy of Baxter Healthcare Corporation. All rights reserved.

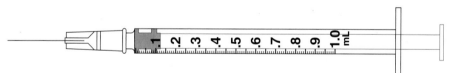

48. Order: **cefazolin 250 mg IM q.8h** for a 3-year-old child who weighs 35 lb. The recommended pediatric dosage of cefazolin sodium for children over 1 month: 25 to 50 mg/kg/day in 3 to 4 divided doses.

If the dosage ordered is safe, give _____ mL. If not safe, explain why and describe what you should do. _____

_____

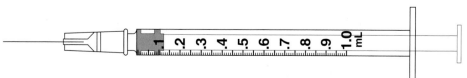

49. Refer to questions 43 through 48. Identify which drugs require a reconstitution label.

_____

_____

50. Describe the clinical reasoning you would use to prevent this medication error.

Possible Scenario

Suppose that the family practice resident ordered **tobramycin 110 mg IV q.8h** for a child with cystic fibrosis who weighs 10 kg. The pediatric reference guide states that the safe dosage of tobramycin for a child with severe infections is 7.5 mg/kg/day in 3 equally divided doses. The nurse received five admissions the evening of this order and neglected to calculate the safe dosage of the medication. The pharmacist prepared and labeled the medication in a syringe, and the nurse administered the first dose of the medication. An hour later, the resident arrived on the pediatric unit and inquired if the nurse had given the first dose. When the nurse confirmed that she had, the resident replied with concern, "I just realized that I ordered an adult dose of tobramycin. I had hoped that you hadn't given the medication yet."

Potential Outcome

The resident's next step would likely have been to discontinue the tobramycin and order a stat tobramycin level. The level would most likely have been elevated, and the child would have required close monitoring for renal damage and hearing loss.

Prevention

_____

_____

After completing these problems, see pages 687–693 to check your answers.

▣ Be sure to use the online software for additional practice!

REFERENCES

Johns Hopkins Hospital, Engorn, B, & Flerlage, J. (2015). *The Harriet Lane handbook* (20th ed.). Philadelphia: Saunders—Elsevier.

Taketomo, C. K. (2014). *Pediatric and Neonatal dosage handbook* (20th ed.). Cleveland, OH: LEXI-COMP.

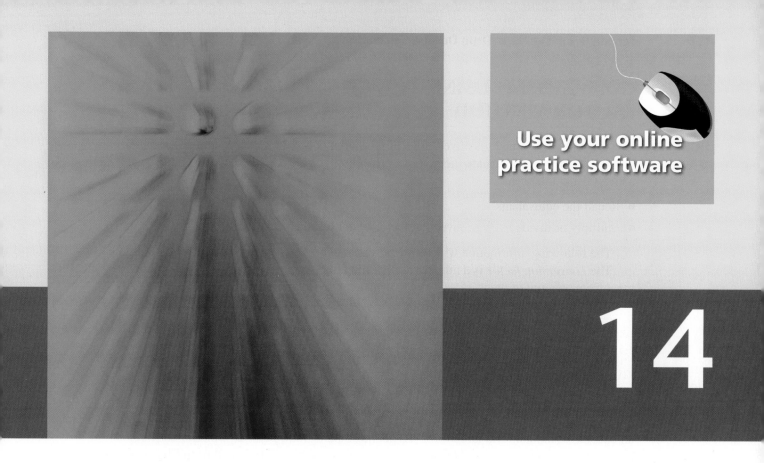

14

Alternative Dosage Calculation Methods: Formula and Dimensional Analysis

OBJECTIVES

Upon mastery of Chapter 14, you will be able to calculate the dosages of drugs using either the formula or dimensional analysis methods. To accomplish this, you will also be able to:

- Convert all units of measurement to the same system and same size units using the conversion factor method.
- Estimate the reasonable amount of the drug to be administered.
- Use the formula $\frac{D}{H} \times Q = X$ to calculate drug dosage.
- Solve both unit of measurement conversion and dosage calculation using dimensional analysis.

Y ou may prefer to calculate drug dosages by the formula method or dimensional analysis method. They are presented here as an alternative to the ratio-proportion method found in Chapters 10 to 13.

Try all three methods: *ratio-proportion, formula,* and *dimensional analysis.* Choose the one that is easiest and most logical to you.

CONVERTING USING THE CONVERSION FACTOR METHOD

In Chapter 4 you learned to convert units of measurement to the same system and same-size units using ratio-proportion. An alternate method of performing conversions is the conversion factor method. To convert using this method:

- Recall the equivalents.
- Multiply or divide by the conversion factor or equivalent.

The following information will help you remember when to multiply and when to divide.

The *conversion factor* is a number used with either multiplication or division to change a measurement from one unit of measurement to its *equivalent* in another unit of measurement.

RULE

To convert from a larger to a smaller unit of measurement, multiply by the conversion factor.

THINK: "*Larger* unit is going down to a *smaller* unit, so you will multiply." Larger ↓ Smaller → Multiply (×)

Stop and think about this. You know this is true because it takes *more* parts of a *smaller* unit to make an equivalent amount of a larger unit. To get *more* parts, *multiply*. Most metric conversions for dosage calculations are simply derived by multiplying or dividing by 1,000. Recall from Chapter 4 that multiplying by 1,000 is the same as moving the decimal point three places to the right.

EXAMPLE 1 ■

How many grams are equivalent to 3.5 kg?

You know that in metric measurement, 1 kg = 1,000 g. It takes 1,000 of the gram units to equal 1 of the kilogram units. Grams are smaller than kilograms; therefore, more are needed to make an equivalent amount. THINK: Larger ↓ Smaller → Multiply (×). The conversion factor for kilograms to grams is *1,000 g/kg*. Multiply by the conversion factor or move the decimal 3 places to the right.

kilograms (larger unit) × conversion factor (g/kg) = grams (smaller unit)

3.5 kg × 1,000 g/kg = 3,500 g; or 3.500. = 3,500 g

3.5 kg = 3,500 g

EXAMPLE 2 ■

Convert: 450 mcg to mg

Known equivalent: 1 mg = 1,000 mcg; therefore, conversion factor is 1,000 mcg/mg.

Smaller ↑ Larger → (÷)

Conversion factor: *1,000 mcg/mg*

450 mcg ÷ 1,000 mcg/mg = 450 mcg × 1 mg/1,000 mcg = 0.45 mg; or .450. = 0.45 mg

EXAMPLE 3 ■

Convert: 10 mL to t

Known approximate equivalent: 1 t = 5 mL; therefore, conversion factor is 5 mL/t.

Smaller ↑ Larger → (÷)

Conversion factor: *5 mL/t*

10 mL ÷ 5 mL/t = 10 mL × 1 t/5 mL = 2 t

EXAMPLE 4 ■

Convert: 150 lb to kg

Known approximate equivalent: 1 kg = 2.2 lb; therefore, conversion factor is 2.2 lb/kg.

Smaller ↑ Larger → Divide (÷)

Conversion factor: *2.2 lb/kg*

150 lb ÷ 2.2 lb/kg = 150 lb × 1 kg/2.2 lb = 68.18 kg = 68.2 kg

QUICK REVIEW

Use the conversion factor method to convert from one unit of measurement to another.

- Recall the equivalents.

- Identify the conversion factor.

- MULTIPLY by the conversion factor to convert to a smaller unit.
  THINK: Larger ↓ Smaller → Multiply (×)

- DIVIDE by the conversion factor to convert to a larger unit.
  THINK: Smaller ↑ Larger → Divide (÷)

- Most metric conversions in dosage calculations are derived by multiplying or dividing by 1,000.

Review Set 29

For questions # 1–15, use the conversion factor method to convert each of the following amounts to the unit indicated. Indicate the equivalent used in the conversion.

Equivalent   Equivalent

1. 50 mL = _____ L _____   8. 2.5 mL = _____ t _____

2. 300 g = _____ kg _____   9. 0.6 kg = _____ g _____

3. 84 lb = _____ kg _____   10. 7.5 cm = _____ in _____

4. 75 mL = _____ fl oz _____   11. 16 g = _____ mg _____

5. 750 mL = _____ L _____   12. 15 mL = _____ fl oz _____

6. 1½ fl oz = _____ mL _____   13. 3 oz = _____ lb _____

7. 625 mcg = _____ mg _____   14. 2 qt = _____ L _____

15. 15 kg = _____ lb _____

16. The medicine order states to administer a potassium chloride supplement added to at least 150 mL of juice. How many fluid ounces of juice should you pour? _____ fl oz

17. A child should have 5 mL of liquid Children's Tylenol (acetaminophen) every 4 hours as needed for fever above 100°F. To relate these instructions to the child's mother, you may advise her to give her child _____ teaspoon(s) of Tylenol per dose.

18. The doctor advises his patient to drink at least 2,000 mL of fluid per day. The patient should have approximately _____ 8 fl oz glasses of water per day.

19. A child needs 15 mL of a drug. How many teaspoonsful should he receive? _____ t

20. A doctor has ordered 250 mcg of digoxin. This is equivalent to how many milligrams? _____ mg

After completing these problems, see page 693 to check your answers.
For more practice, rework Review Sets 13 and 14 in Chapter 4 using the conversion factor method.

USING THE FORMULA METHOD TO CALCULATE DOSAGES

You can substitute the formula method for ratio-proportion in Step 3 of the *Three-Step Approach to Dosage Calculations.*

REMEMBER

Three-Step Approach to Dosage Calculations

Step 1	**Convert**	Ensure that all measurements are in the same system of measurement and the same size unit of measurement. If not, convert before proceeding.
Step 2	**Think**	Estimate what is a *reasonable amount* of the drug to administer.
Step 3	**Calculate**	Apply the formula: $\frac{D}{H} \times Q = X$

$$\frac{D \text{ (desired)}}{H \text{ (have)}} \times Q \text{ (quantity)} = X \text{ (amount)}$$

In this formula, *D* represents the *desired* dosage or the dosage ordered. You will find this in the doctor's or the health care practitioner's order. *H* represents the dosage you *have* on hand per a *quantity*, *Q*. Both *H* and *Q* constitute the *supply dosage* found on the label of the drug available. *X* is the unknown and represents the amount of the supply dosage form you want to give, such as *number of tablets* or *mL* of the drug available. Most of the time, *Q* is per 1 tablet or capsule, or per 1 mL; but this is not always the case. Always identify and insert *Q* in the formula.

EXAMPLE 1 ■

Order: gentamicin 60 mg IV q.8h

Supply: gentamicin 80 mg per 2 mL

Step 1	**Convert**	No conversion is necessary.
Step 2	**Think**	You want to give less than 2 mL; in fact, you want to give $\frac{60}{80}$ of 2 mL, or $\frac{3}{4}$ of 2 mL.
Step 3	**Calculate**	$\frac{D \text{ (desired)}}{H \text{ (have)}} \times Q \text{ (quantity)} = X \text{ (amount)}$

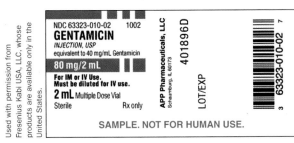

$$\frac{D}{H} \times Q = \frac{\overset{3}{\cancel{60 \text{ mg}}}}{\underset{4}{\cancel{80 \text{ mg}}}} \times 2 \text{ mL} = \frac{6}{4} \text{ mL} = 1.5 \text{ mL}$$

Give 1.5 mL intravenously every 8 hours.

EXAMPLE 2 ■

Order: Ritalin 10 mg p.o. daily

Supply: Ritalin 5 mg tablets

Step 1	**Convert**	No conversion is necessary.
Step 2	**Think**	You want to give more than 1 tablet. In fact, you want to give 2 times more, or 2 tablets.
Step 3	**Calculate**	$\frac{D}{H} \times Q = \frac{\overset{2}{\cancel{10 \text{ mg}}}}{\underset{1}{\cancel{5 \text{ mg}}}} \times 1 \text{ tab} = 2 \text{ tab}$

Give 2 tablets orally daily.

EXAMPLE 3 ■

Order: *Lopid 0.6 g p.o. b.i.d.*

Supply: Lopid 600 mg tablets

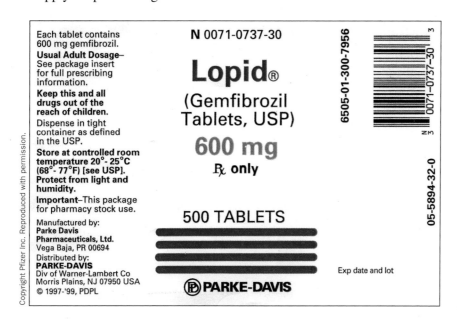

Step 1   **Convert**   Equivalent 1 g = 1,000 mg

Larger ↓ Smaller → Multiply (×); or move decimal 3 places to the right

Conversion factor: *1,000 mg/g*

0.6 g̶ × 1,000 mg/g̶ = 600 mg; or 0.600. = 600 mg

Step 2   **Think**   You want to give 600 mg, and each tablet supplies 600 mg. It is obvious that you want to give 1 tablet.

Step 3   **Calculate** $\dfrac{D}{H} \times Q = \dfrac{600\ \text{mg}}{600\ \text{mg}} \times 1\ \text{tab} = 1\ \text{tab}$

Give 1 tablet orally twice daily.

EXAMPLE 4 ■

Order: *clindamycin 0.6 g IV q.12h*

Supply: clindamycin 150 mg/mL

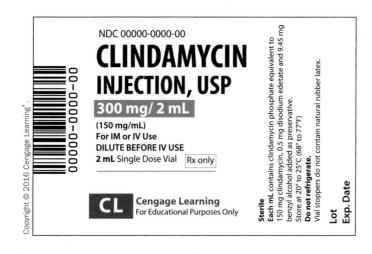

Step 1   **Convert**   Equivalent 1 g = 1,000 mg

Larger ↓ Smaller → Multiply (×); or move decimal 3 places to the right

The conversion factor is *1,000 mg/g.*

0.6 g̸ × 1,000 mg/g̸ = 600 mg; or 0.600. = 600 mg

Step 2   **Think**   You want to give more than 2 mL. In fact, you want 2 times 2 mL, or 4 mL.

Step 3   **Calculate** $\frac{D}{H} \times Q = \frac{\overset{4}{600 \text{ mg}}}{\underset{1}{150 \text{ mg}}} \times 1 \text{ mL} = \frac{4}{1} \text{ mL} = 4 \text{ mL}$

Give 4 mL intravenously every 12 hours.

QUICK REVIEW

When calculating dosages using the formula method:

Step 1   **Convert**   To units of the same system and the same size.

Step 2   **Think**   Estimate for a reasonable amount to give.

Step 3   **Calculate** $\frac{D}{H} \times Q = X$

$$\frac{D \text{ (desired)}}{H \text{ (have)}} \times Q \text{ (quantity)} = X \text{ (amount)}$$

- Drug dosages cannot be accurately calculated until all units of measurement are in the same system and the same size.

- Always **convert** first, then **think** or reason for the logical answer before you finally **calculate**.

- For most dosage calculation problems, convert to the smaller size unit. Example: g → mg

- Consider the reasonableness of the calculated amount to give. Example: You would question giving more than 3 tablets or capsules per dose for oral administration.

Review Set 30

Use the formula method to calculate the amount you will prepare for each dose.

1. Order: **Premarin 1.25 mg p.o. daily**

   Supply: Premarin 0.625 mg tablets

   Give: _____ tablet(s)

2. Order: **cimetidine 150 mg p.o. q.i.d. c̄ meals & bedtime**

   Supply: cimetidine liquid 300 mg per 5 mL

   Give: _____ mL

3. Order: **thiamine 80 mg IM stat**

   Supply: thiamine 100 mg/mL

   Give: _____ mL

4. Order: **ketorolac 20 mg IV q.6h p.r.n., pain**

   Supply: ketorolac 15 mg/mL

   Give: _____ mL

5. Order: **lithium 450 mg p.o. t.i.d.**

   Supply: lithium 300 mg per 5 mL

   Give: _____ mL

6. Order: **Ativan 2.4 mg IM bedtime p.r.n., anxiety**

   Supply: Ativan 4 mg/mL

   Give: _____ mL

7. Order: **prednisone 7.5 mg p.o. daily**

   Supply: prednisone 5 mg (scored) tablets

   Give: _____ tablet(s)

8. Order: **hydrochlorothiazide 30 mg p.o. b.i.d.**

   Supply: hydrochlorothiazide 50 mg per 5 mL

   Give: _____ mL

9. Order: **theophylline 160 mg p.o. q.6h**

    Supply: theophylline 80 mg per 15 mL

    Give: _____ mL

10. Order: **Tofranil 20 mg IM bedtime**

    Supply: Tofranil 25 mg per 2 mL

    Give: _____ mL

11. Order: **Indocin 15 mg p.o. t.i.d.**

    Supply: Indocin Suspension 25 mg per 5 mL

    Give: _____ mL

12. Order: **Ativan 2 mg IM 2 h pre-op**

    Supply: Ativan 4 mg/mL

    Give: _____ mL

13. Order: **phenobarbital 37.5 mg p.o. t.i.d.**

    Supply: phenobarbital 15 mg scored tablets

    Give: _____ tablet(s)

14. Order: **Diabinese 125 mg p.o. daily**

    Supply: Diabinese 100 mg or 250 mg tablets

    Select: _____ mg

    Give: _____ tablet(s)

15. Order: **chlorpromazine 60 mg IM stat**

    Supply: chlorpromazine 25 mg/mL

    Give: _____ mL

16. Order: **Synthroid 0.15 mg p.o. daily**

    Supply: Synthroid 75 mcg tablets

    Give: _____ tablet(s)

17. Order: **Elixophyllin elixir 96 mg p.o. q.6h**

    Supply: Elixophyllin elixir 80 mg per 15 mL

    Give: _____ mL

18. Order: **Solu-Medrol 100 mg IV q.6h**

    Supply: Solu-Medrol 80 mg/mL

    Give: _____ mL

19. Order: **fluphenazine elixir 8 mg p.o. q.8h**

    Supply: fluphenazine elixir 2.5 mg per 5 mL

    Give: _____ mL

20. Order: **Trimox 350 mg p.o. q.8h**

    Supply: Trimox 250 mg per 5 mL

    Give: _____ mL

After completing these problems, see pages 693–694 to check your answers.

USING DIMENSIONAL ANALYSIS TO CALCULATE DOSAGES

You may prefer to use dimensional analysis as an alternative to either the formula method or ratio-proportion method for calculating drug doses. When using the dimensional analysis method, you are not required to memorize formulas, and the conversion step, if needed, is part of the calculation.

You should practice with all methods and then select the method that is the easiest and most logical for you. Regardless of which method you prefer, you will have to master knowledge of common equivalents (such as 1 g = 1,000 mg, 1 mg = 1,000 mcg, 1 L = 1,000 mL, 1 in = 2.5 cm, 1 kg = 2.2 lb).

When using dimensional analysis, you must first determine the unit of measure (tablets, capsules, mL, etc.) that you seek to administer. This is determined by the medication order and the unit provided by the pharmacy.

If a medication is dispensed as a tablet, you would administer 1 tablet, a portion of a tablet, or multiple tablets. If a medication is dispensed as an oral or injection solution, you would usually administer milliliters (mL) of the liquid. The unit of what is to be administered will be on the left side of your equation.

RULE

Step 1   **Determine units desired**   For dimensional analysis, first write the unknown X and unit of measure desired on the left side of the equation, followed by an equal sign (=).

X (unknown quantity) is written first, followed by the **unit of measure** and then by an equal sign (=). For example,

X tablet =

or

X mL =

EXAMPLE ■

The prescriber orders *digoxin 0.125 mg p.o. daily.* Digoxin 250 mcg (0.25 mg) **tablets** are provided by the pharmacy.

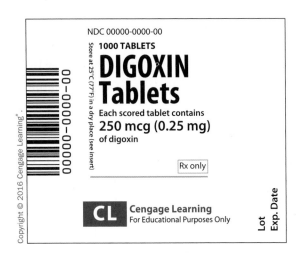

After review of the order and after receiving the medication in tablet form from the pharmacy, you determine that the unit to be administered is a **tablet.** However, the amount to administer is still unknown (**X**). The left side of your equation is ready.

X tablet =

RULE		
Step 2	**Think**	Carefully consider the reasonable amount of the drug that should be administered.

Once you have determined the unit of measure (tablet or mL) that you seek to administer, you must determine the reasonable amount of medication that must be prepared for administration.

In Step 1, you determined that the units are tablets and X tablet is set up to the left of the equal sign. In Step 2, you must consider the reasonable amount of the drug. You must decide whether you are going to administer 1 tablet, a portion of a tablet, or multiple tablets.

Because the pharmacy provided digoxin 0.25 mg tablets, logically you recognize that the reasonable amount will be less than 1 tablet, because 0.125 mg (the ordered dosage) is less than 0.25 mg (the dosage provided). In fact, you know that 0.125 is $\frac{1}{2}$ of 0.25, so you reason that you will give $\frac{1}{2}$ tablet.

RULE		
Step 3	**Calculate**	Set up the remainder of your dimensional analysis equation to include all necessary *desired dosage* ratio factors.

Now, you must continue to build your equation to determine the unknown amount (X) of tablets for the dose to administer. The right side of your equation will include all information required to arrive at X.

To determine the unknown (X) amount of tablets to prepare for administration, you must consider the strength and units (supply dosage) dispensed by the pharmacy. A 0.25 mg tablet of digoxin was dispensed. Therefore, you have available 0.25 mg per tablet, or 0.25 mg/1 tablet.

In this example, 0.25 mg/1 tablet is the same as 1 tablet/0.25 mg. Normally, it does not matter if the tablet is the numerator or denominator, because 1 tablet is truly 0.25 mg of the drug digoxin that was dispensed. However, the correct ratio to use in your calculations is determined as you continue to build your equation.

To determine whether to use 1 tablet/0.25 mg or 0.25 mg/1 tablet, you must look at the units to the left of your equal sign.

X tablet =

X tablets is the same as X tablets/1. Tablet is the numerator; 1 is the denominator. This is the *amount-to-give ratio.*

$$\frac{X \text{ tablet}}{1} =$$

MATH TIP
Dividing or multiplying a number by 1 does not change its value.

Because tablet is in the numerator on the left side of the equal sign, you must match it with tablet in the numerator on the right side of the equal sign. Therefore, you will choose **1 tablet/0.25 mg.** This is the *supply-dosage ratio.*

$$\frac{X \text{ tablet}}{1} = \frac{1 \text{ tablet}}{0.25 \text{ mg}}$$

RULE
For dimensional analysis, the units in the numerator on the left of the equal sign are the same units that are placed in the numerator of the first ratio factor on the right side of the equation.

CAUTION   THIS IS INCORRECT

$$\frac{X \text{ tablet}}{1} = \frac{0.25 \text{ mg}}{1 \text{ tablet}}$$

THIS IS INCORRECT, because tablets do not appear in the numerator on the left and right sides of the equation.

Let's continue; you have not completed setting up this problem. You need one more ratio factor. Because you are looking only for the number of tablets to administer, you must cancel all other units so that only tablet remains in the numerator as a unit of measure on the right side of the equation. The remaining information available to you is the dosage ordered by the physician for the nurse to administer. In this example, it is *digoxin 0.125 mg.*

You know that digoxin 0.125 mg is the same as digoxin 0.125 mg/1 because dividing or multiplying a number by 1 does not change its value. Therefore, **0.125 mg/1** is added to the equation, with mg in the numerator of the second ratio factor so that mg will cancel out, leaving the amount of tablets to administer to the patient. This is the *ordered-dosage ratio.*

RULE
When multiplying fractions, if the units in a numerator and the units in a denominator are the same, they cancel each other out.

$$\begin{array}{ccc} \text{Amount-} & \text{Supply-} & \text{Ordered-} \\ \text{to-Give} = & \text{Dosage} \times & \text{Dosage} \\ \text{Ratio} & \text{Ratio} & \text{Ratio} \end{array}$$

$$\frac{\text{X tablet}}{1} = \frac{\text{1 tablet}}{\text{0.25 mg}} \times \frac{\textbf{0.125 mg}}{\textbf{1}}$$

$$\frac{\text{X tablet}}{1} = \frac{\text{1 tablet}}{\text{0.25 \cancel{mg}}} \times \frac{\text{0.125 \cancel{mg}}}{1}$$

MATH TIP
When using dimensional analysis and after all cancellations have been made, only the units of measure to be administered remain (such as tablet or mL).

CAUTION   **THIS IS INCORRECT**

$$\frac{\text{X tablet}}{1} = \frac{\text{1 tablet}}{\text{0.25 mg}} \times \frac{1}{\text{0.125 mg}}$$

THIS IS INCORRECT, because **mg** does not appear in the numerator and the denominator on the right side of the equation. Therefore, **mg** cannot be cancelled out.

As you look at the correct equation and after all units are cancelled, only **tablet** (the unit of measure to administer) remains on the right side of the equation.

$$\frac{\text{X tablet}}{1} = \frac{\textbf{1 tablet}}{\text{0.25 \cancel{mg}}} \times \frac{\text{0.125 \cancel{mg}}}{1}$$

Now eliminate everything that was cancelled out, and calculate for the **amount of tablets** to give.

$$\frac{\text{X tablet}}{1} = \frac{0.125}{0.25} \text{ tablet} = \textbf{0.5 tablet}$$

X tablet = 0.5 tablet = $\frac{1}{2}$ tablet

You will administer $\frac{1}{2}$ of a 0.25 mg tablet of digoxin to provide 0.125 mg of the drug.
Let's consider more examples.

CAUTION
Remember: Before dividing a full tablet or caplet, you must know whether the formulation provided by the pharmacy may be split. The effect of a drug will be altered if it is split when the drug is provided as an extended-release (ER or XL), sustained-release (SR), delayed-release, or enteric-coated formulation.

CAUTION

If you calculate that a partial *capsule* of medication is to be administered, first stop and think, "Does this make sense?" Recalculate. If you are certain the calculation is correct, you should consult the pharmacist or prescriber for clarification and further direction, because capsules are not formulated to be divided.

EXAMPLE 1 ■

The drug order is for **Lopressor 50 mg p.o. q.12h**. The pharmacy dispenses Lopressor 25 mg tablets.

Step 1	**Determine units**	tablet (tab)
Step 2	**Think**	50 mg ordered
		25 mg tab supplied
		Dose will be greater than 1 tab. You will give 2 tab.
Step 3	**Calculate**	$\dfrac{X\ \text{tab}}{1} = \dfrac{1\ \text{tab}}{25\ \cancel{\text{mg}}} \times \dfrac{50\ \cancel{\text{mg}}}{1} = \dfrac{50}{25}\ \text{tab} = 2\ \text{tab}$

EXAMPLE 2 ■

Order: **Tylenol 240 mg p.o. q.4h p.r.n., pain**

Supply: Tylenol (acetaminophen) 160 mg chewable, scored tablets

Step 1	**Determine units**	tab
Step 2	**Think**	240 mg ordered
		160 mg tab supplied
		Dose will be more than 1 tab but less than 2 tab.
Step 3	**Calculate**	$\dfrac{X\ \text{tab}}{1} = \dfrac{1\ \text{tab}}{160\ \cancel{\text{mg}}} \times \dfrac{240\ \cancel{\text{mg}}}{1} = \dfrac{240}{160}\ \text{tab} = 1.5\ \text{tab} = 1\frac{1}{2}\ \text{tab}$

EXAMPLE 3 ■

Order: **cephalexin suspension 250 mg p.o. q.6h**

Supply: cephalexin 100 mg/mL

Step 1	**Determine units**	mL
Step 2	**Think**	250 mg ordered
		100 mg/mL supplied
		Dose will be greater than 1 mL and even greater than 2 mL.
Step 3	**Calculate**	$\dfrac{X\ \text{mL}}{1} = \dfrac{1\ \text{mL}}{100\ \cancel{\text{mg}}} \times \dfrac{250\ \cancel{\text{mg}}}{1} = \dfrac{250}{100}\ \text{mL} = 2.5\ \text{mL}$

Dimensional analysis is a unique method of calculation, because converting units of measurement can be included in the calculation on the right side of the equation. Let's consider calculating the proper dose to administer when the ordered units and the supplied units are **not** the same. All calculations and conversions necessary to arrive at your answer will still be included on the right side of the equal sign.

When you correctly set up your equation in dimensional analysis so that all units cancel except for the one you seek (amount to give), you will not be required to memorize formulas or acronyms. In both the formula and ratio-proportion methods, conversions are completed initially and as a separate step. In dimensional analysis, this is not necessary.

For example, the prescriber orders Lanoxin (digoxin) 125 mcg p.o. q.AM. The pharmacy supplies Lanoxin 0.125 mg tablets.

REMEMBER

When using dimensional analysis and after all cancellations have been made, only the units desired remain (such as tablet or mL).

Order: Lanoxin 125 mcg

Supply: Lanoxin 0.125 mg tab

Step 1	**Determine units**	tab

Step 2   **Think**   125 mcg ordered

0.125 mg supplied

1 mg = 1,000 mcg

Step 3   **Calculate**   Include the *conversion factor* in the right side of the equation as the second ratio, and then add the ordered dosage as the final ratio. Set it up so that all units cancel except the desired unit (tab). Notice that a pair of mg units and a pair of mcg units cancel.

Amount-to-Give Ratio	=	Supply-Dosage Ratio	×	Conversion-Factor Ratio	×	Ordered-Dosage Ratio

$$\frac{X \text{ tab}}{1} = \frac{1 \text{ tab}}{0.125 \text{ mg}} \times \frac{1 \text{ mg}}{1{,}000 \text{ mcg}} \times \frac{125 \text{ mcg}}{1} = \frac{125}{125} \text{ tab} = 1 \text{ tab}$$

CAUTION   **THIS IS INCORRECT**

$$\frac{X \text{ tab}}{1} = \frac{1 \text{ tab}}{0.125 \text{ mg}} \times \frac{1{,}000 \text{ mcg}}{1 \text{ mg}} \times \frac{1}{125 \text{ mcg}}$$

THIS IS INCORRECT. All units cannot be cancelled out, because mg does not appear in the numerator and the denominator. It appears twice in the denominator. If you continued with this calculation, your result would be 64 tablets instead of 1. Think about the magnitude of such an error. Your common sense should alert you that this is wrong.

As you continue to practice dimensional analysis, you realize that you can set up the problems without the added step of placing a 1 under X tablets on the left or under the ordered dosage on the right side of the equation. Consider the same Lanoxin example.

EXAMPLE ▪

$$\mathbf{X\ tab} = \frac{1 \text{ tab}}{0.125 \text{ mg}} \times \frac{1 \text{ mg}}{1{,}000 \text{ mcg}} \times \mathbf{125\ mcg} = 1 \text{ tab}$$

Let's practice this shortened method of dimensional analysis with more examples.

EXAMPLE 1 ▪

Order: *potassium chloride 30 mEq p.o. daily*

Supply: potassium chloride 20 mEq per 15 mL

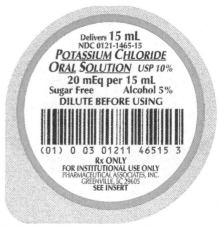

Step 1	**Determine units**	mL

Step 2	**Think**	You will administer more than 15 mL, because the dosage ordered (30 mEq) is greater than that which is supplied in 15 mL (20 mEq).

Step 3   **Calculate** $X \text{ mL} = \frac{15 \text{ mL}}{20 \text{ mEq}} \times 30 \text{ mEq}$

$= \frac{450}{20} \text{ mL} = 22.5 \text{ mL}$

Used with permission from Pharmaceutical Associates, Inc.

EXAMPLE 2 ▪

Order: *oxycodone HCl 15 mg p.o. q.4h p.r.n., pain*

Supply: oxycodone hydrochloride oral concentrated solution 20 mg/mL

Step 1	**Determine units**	mL

Step 2	**Think**	20 mg in 1 mL
		15 mg is less than 20 mg.
		Dose will be less than 1 mL.

Step 3   **Calculate** $X \text{ mL} = \frac{1 \text{ mL}}{20 \text{ mg}} \times 15 \text{ mg} = \frac{15}{20} \text{ mL} = 0.75 \text{ mL}$

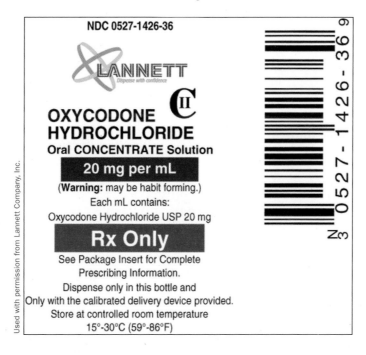

Used with permission from Lannett Company, Inc.

CAUTION

This is a concentrated medication and a small oral dose. It is necessary to administer the exact dose prescribed to avoid medication over- or underdosing. If a delivery device is supplied with the medication, it must be used. If a delivery device is not supplied, you must clearly label the oral syringe so that the medication is not inadvertently administered by the parenteral route.

EXAMPLE 3 ■

Order: terbutaline sulfate 10 mg
p.o. t.i.d.

Supply: terbutaline sulfate
5 mg tab

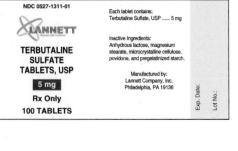

Step 1	**Determine units**	tab
Step 2	**Think**	5 mg in 1 tab

10 mg is more than 5 mg.

Dose will be more than 1 tab. You want to give 2 tab.

Step 3	**Calculate**	$X \text{ tab} = \frac{1 \text{ tab}}{5 \text{ mg}} \times 10 \text{ mg} = \frac{10}{5} \text{ tab} = 2 \text{ tab}$

EXAMPLE 4 ■

Order: haloperidol decanoate 0.25 g
IM monthly

Supply: haloperidol decanoate injection
100 mg/mL

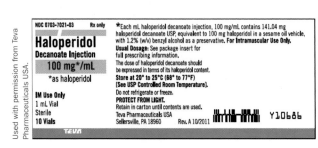

Step 1	**Determine units**	mL
Step 2	**Think**	100 mg in 1 mL

1 g = 1,000 mg

Dose will be more than 1 mL.

Step 3	**Calculate**	$X \text{ mL} = \frac{1 \text{ mL}}{100 \text{ mg}} \times \frac{1,000 \text{ mg}}{1 \text{ g}} \times 0.25 \text{ g} = \frac{250 \text{ mL}}{100} = 2.5 \text{ mL}$

EXAMPLE 5 ■

Order: dexamethasone 3 mg IV q.6h

Supply: dexamethasone sodium phosphate
injection 4 mg/mL

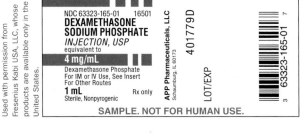

Step 1	**Determine units**	mL
Step 2	**Think**	4 mg in 1 mL

3 mg is less than 4 mg.

Dose will be less than 1 mL.

Step 3	**Calculate**	$X \text{ mL} = \frac{1 \text{ mL}}{4 \text{ mg}} \times 3 \text{ mg} = \frac{3}{4} \text{ mL} = 0.75 \text{ mL}$

EXAMPLE 6 ■

Order: levothyroxine 0.075 mg p.o. a.c. breakfast

Supply: Synthroid (levothyroxine) 25 mcg tablets

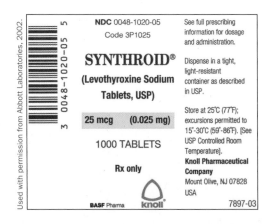

Step 1	**Determine units**	tab
Step 2	**Think**	Give more than 1 tab; in fact, you will give 3 tab.
Step 3	**Calculate**	X tab =

$$\frac{1 \text{ tab}}{25 \text{ mcg}} \times \frac{1,000 \text{ mcg}}{1 \text{ mg}} \times 0.075 \text{ mg} = \frac{75}{25} \text{ tab} = 3 \text{ tab}$$

EXAMPLE 7 ■

Order: *penicillin G potassium 1.2 million units IM daily*

Supply: penicillin G potassium vial with 5 million units to be reconstituted

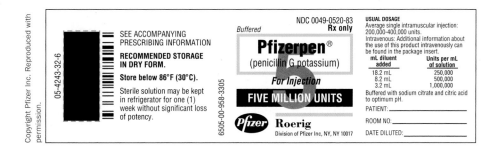

Step 1	**Determine units**	mL
Step 2	**Think**	Maximum IM dose volume to be administered to an adult patient is 3 mL. You choose to dilute with 8.2 mL of diluent. Per the label, the concentration is now 500,000 units/mL. You will give more than 1 mL to administer 1,200,000 units, or 1.2 million units.
Step 3	**Calculate**	$X \text{ mL} = \dfrac{1 \text{ mL}}{500,000 \text{ units}} \times 1,200,000 \text{ units} = \dfrac{1,200,000}{500,000} \text{ mL} = 2.4 \text{ mL}$

You can also add additional ratios to the right side of the equation to account for additional factors relevant to the patient and required conversions. Examples 8–10 demonstrate dimensional analysis dosage calculations for orders based on body weight (such as mg/kg). Refer to Chapter 13 for more information about medications ordered and recommended according to body weight.

EXAMPLE 8 ■

An elderly patient weighs 50 kg and is diagnosed with methicillin-resistant *Staphylococcus aureas* (MRSA) pneumonia.

Order: *vancomycin 15 mg/kg IV q.12h*

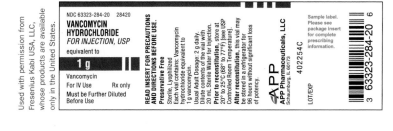

Supply: vancomycin 1 g diluted with 20 mL of sterile water for injection

Step 1	**Determine units**	mL
Step 2	**Think**	You will need to calculate the dosage for a patient who weighs 50 kg by including an *ordered-dosage/kg ratio* and a *body-weight ratio*.
		1 g = 1,000 mg
		Supply dosage is 1 g per 20 mL.
Step 3	**Calculate**	Set up the calculation to include all the ratio factors needed to calculate the dose so that g, mg, and kg all cancel, leaving mL.

Amount-to-Give Ratio	=	Supply-Dosage Ratio	×	Conversion-Factor Ratio	×	Ordered-Dosage/kg Ratio	×	Body-Weight Ratio

$$X \text{ mL} = \frac{20 \text{ mL}}{1 \text{ g}} \times \frac{1 \text{ g}}{1,000 \text{ mg}} \times \frac{15 \text{ mg}}{1 \text{ kg}} \times 50 \text{ kg} = \frac{20 \times 1 \times 15 \times 50}{1 \times 1,000 \times 1} \text{ mL}$$

$$= \frac{15,000}{1,000} \text{ mL} = 15 \text{ mL}$$

EXAMPLE 9 ■

An adolescent burn patient weighs 99 lb.

Order: *vancomycin 10 mg/kg IV q.8h*

Supply: vancomycin 500 mg diluted with 10 mL sterile water for injection

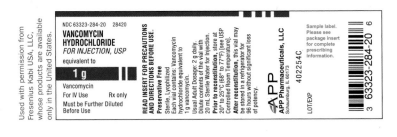

Step 1	**Determine units**	mL
Step 2	**Think**	You will need to calculate the dosage for a patient who weighs 99 lb. To calculate the ordered dosage, you must add a conversion-factor ratio to convert the patient's weight to kg.

$$1 \text{ kg} = 2.2 \text{ lb}$$

Supply dosage is 500 mg per 10 mL.

Step 3	**Calculate**	Set up the calculation to include all the ratio factors needed to calculate the dose so that mg, lb, and kg all cancel, leaving mL remaining.

Amount-to-Give Ratio	=	Supply-Dosage Ratio	×	Ordered-Dosage/kg Ratio	×	Conversion-Factor Ratio	×	Body-Weight Ratio

$$X \text{ mL} = \frac{10 \text{ mL}}{500 \text{ mg}} \times \frac{10 \text{ mg}}{1 \text{ kg}} \times \frac{1 \text{ kg}}{2.2 \text{ lb}} \times 99 \text{ lb} = \frac{10 \times 10 \times 1 \times 99}{500 \times 1 \times 2.2} \text{ mL} = \frac{9{,}900}{1{,}100} \text{ mL} = 9 \text{ mL}$$

The key to dimensional analysis is to think carefully about all the ratio factors required and to be careful setting up the ratios for your calculations so that all units cancel except the unit of the unknown (X) amount to give. Let's examine one final example that requires two conversions: supply dosage and weight.

EXAMPLE 10 ■

A patient diagnosed with MRSA bacteremia weighs 143 lb.

Order: *vancomycin 15 mg/kg IV q.12h*

Supply: vancomycin 1 g diluted with 20 mL of sterile water for injection

Step 1	**Determine units**	mL
Step 2	**Think**	You will need to calculate the dosage for a patient who weighs 143 lb.

$$1 \text{ kg} = 2.2 \text{ lb}$$

Supply dosage is 1 g per 20 mL.

$$1 \text{ g} = 1{,}000 \text{ mg}$$

Step 3	**Calculate**	Set up the calculation to include all the ratio factors needed to calculate the dose so that g, mg, lb, and kg all cancel, leaving mL.

Amount-to-Give Ratio	=	Supply-Dosage Ratio	×	Conversion-Factor Ratio	×	Ordered-Dosage/kg Ratio	×	Conversion-Factor Ratio	×	Body-Weight Ratio

$$X \text{ mL} = \frac{20 \text{ mL}}{1 \text{ g}} \times \frac{1 \text{ g}}{1{,}000 \text{ mg}} \times \frac{15 \text{ mg}}{1 \text{ kg}} \times \frac{1 \text{ kg}}{2.2 \text{ lb}} \times 143 \text{ lb} = \frac{20 \times 1 \times 15 \times 1 \times 143}{1 \times 1{,}000 \times 1 \times 2.2} \text{ mL}$$

$$= \frac{42{,}900}{2{,}200} \text{ mL} = 19.5 \text{ mL}$$

QUICK REVIEW

When calculating dosages using dimensional analysis:

Step 1	**Determine units desired**	X units = left side of the equation
Step 2	**Think**	Carefully consider the reasonable amount of the drug to give.
Step 3	**Calculate**	Set up the remainder of the dimensional analysis equation to include all necessary *desired-dosage* ratio factors.

- When using dimensional analysis, you must first determine the units of the medication you seek to administer: tablets, mL, etc.

- The unknown and units are placed on the left side of the equal sign: X tablets =

- The units in the numerator on the left of the equal sign are the same units that are placed in the numerator of the first ratio on the right side of the equation.

- All conversions are entered into the right side of the equation.

- When the units in a numerator and the units in a denominator are the same, they cancel each other out.

- When using dimensional analysis and after all cancellations have been made, only the units (tablets, mL, etc.) of the dose to administer remain.

- Always determine units, then think or reason for the logical answer. Set up your equation of ratio factors to cancel units, leaving the one you want to give, and calculate.

Review Set 31

Use dimensional analysis to calculate the amount you will prepare for each dose.

1. Order: **heparin 5,000 units subcut stat**

   Supply: heparin 10,000 units/mL

   Give: _____ mL

2. Order: **ketorolac 45 mg IV q.6h p.r.n., pain**

   Supply: ketorolac 15 mg/mL

   Give: _____ mL

3. Order: **phenytoin sodium 15 mg/kg slowly IV drip stat** (patient weighs 250 lb)

   Supply: phenytoin sodium 250 mg per 5 mL

   Give: _____ mL

4. Order: **hydroxyzine pamoate 60 mg p.o. q.4h p.r.n., nausea**

   Supply: hydroxyzine pamoate 25 mg per 5 mL

   Give: _____ mL

5. Order: **Keflex 0.5 g p.o. q.12h**

   Supply: Keflex (cephalexin) 250 mg per 5 mL

   Give: _____ mL

6. Order: **Depakene 0.01 g/kg p.o. q.12h** (patient weighs 143 lb)

   Supply: Depakene (valproic acid) 250 mg per 5 mL

   Give: _____ mL

7. Order: **DiaBeta 3.75 mg p.o. a.c. breakfast daily**

   Supply: DiaBeta (glyburide) 2.5 mg scored tablets

   Give: _____ tab

8. Order: **Lopressor 100 mg p.o. daily**

   Supply: Lopressor (metoprolol tartrate) 50 mg tablets

   Give: _____ tab

9. Order: **Lasix 20 mg per GT b.i.d.**

   Supply: Lasix (furosemide) 10 mg/mL

   Give: _____ mL

10. Order: **potassium chloride 24 mEq p.o. daily**

    Supply: Micro-K (potassium chloride) 8 mEq/tablet

    Give: _____ tab

11. Order: **Robinul 4 mcg/kg IM 1 h preop**
    (patient weighs 185 lb)

    Supply: Robinul (glycopyrrolate) 0.2 mg/mL

    Give: _____ mL

12. Order: **Epogen 150 units/kg subcut 3x/week**
    (patient weighs 133 lb)

    Supply: Epogen (epoetin alfa) 10,000 units/mL

    Give: _____ mL

13. Order: **morphine 50 mcg/kg subcut q.4h
    p.r.n., pain** (patient weighs 27 lb)

    Supply: morphine 2 mg/mL

    Give: _____ mL

14. Order: **albuterol sulfate 3 mg p.o. t.i.d.**

    Supply: albuterol sulfate syrup 2 mg
    per 5 mL

    Give: _____ mL

15. Order: **octreotide 150 mcg subcut t.i.d.**

    Supply: Sandostatin (octreotide) 0.2 mg/mL

    Give: _____ mL

16. Order: **phenobarbital 120 mg via GT daily**

    Supply: phenobarbital 20 mg/mL

    Give: _____ mL

17. Order: **midazolam 80 mcg/kg IM stat**
    (patient weighs 80 kg)

    Supply: midazolam 2 mg/mL

    Give: _____ mL

18. Order: **hydroxyzine hydrochloride 60 mg IM
    on call to OR**

    Supply: hydroxyzine hydrochloride
    50 mg/mL

    Give: _____ mL

19. Order: **cefaclor 990 mg/day total, divided
    p.o. q.8h**

    Supply: cefaclor 375 mg per 5 mL

    Give: _____ mL (per dose)

20. Order: **tobramycin 62 mg IV q.8h**

    Supply: tobramycin sulfate 20 mg per 2 mL

    Give: _____ mL

After completing these problems, see page 694 to check your answers.

For more practice, recalculate the amount you will prepare for each dose in Review Sets 22 through 28, using the formula and dimensional analysis methods.

CLINICAL REASONING SKILLS

Medications supplied in solution form are labeled with the concentration of the supplied dosage. Errors may occur if the nurse fails to check the quantity of the concentration prior to calculating the dose.

ERROR

Failing to check the concentration carefully on the label and assuming that the quantity of the supply dosage is per 1 mL

Possible Scenario

A patient experienced a generalized seizure at work and was medicated with an anticonvulsant and hospitalized for observation overnight. The patient began to seize again, this time the episodes occurring continuously, and an order was given to treat for status epilepticus with *diazepam 5 mg IV stat*. The nurse removed a vial labeled with diazepam 10 mg from the ADC cubby. Assuming that there was 10 mg per mL, the nurse calculated the dose using the formula method calculation as follows:

$$\frac{D}{H} \times Q \text{ (quantity)} = \frac{10 \text{ mg}}{5 \text{ mg}} \times 1 \text{ mL} = 0.5 \text{ mL} \qquad \textbf{INCORRECT}$$

The nurse administered 0.5 mL of the medication and placed the opened vial on the bedside table. The seizure did not stop, and after 10 minutes the physician ordered a second 5 mg dose. The nurse used the same vial and removed the solution remaining, expecting to have only enough for one more 0.5 mL dose. The nurse was surprised to find that there was actually 1.5 mL remaining in the 2 mL vial. After examining the vial more carefully, the nurse realized that the vial contained 2 mL total volume of diazepam and the concentration was clearly marked as 10 mg per 2 mL. Realizing the previous calculation error, the nurse recalculated the dose as follows:

$$\frac{D}{H} \times Q \text{ (quantity)} = \frac{5 \text{ mg}}{10 \text{ mg}} \times 2 \text{ mL} = \frac{10}{10 \text{ mL}} = 1 \text{ mL} \qquad \textbf{CORRECT}$$

The nurse then administered the correct amount of 1 mL for the second 5 mg dose. A few minutes later, the patient's seizures started to subside.

Potential Outcome

Due to a calculation error, the patient received a subtherapeutic dose of medication in a medical emergency. If the nurse had not recognized the error, the patient might have received additional inadequate doses of diazepam and the seizures might have lasted a significantly longer period of time. The longer the continuous seizure activity persists, the greater the risk for neurological damage.

Prevention

Many solutions supplied in ampules and vials have a dose concentration expressed per 1 mL. Nurses may become so accustomed to this that eventually they fail to look closely at the information provided on the labels. Use care reading the labels of all medications, even those you administer frequently. Medications supplied by different pharmaceutical companies may be prepared with different concentrations. When using the dosage calculation formula, always check for the Q (quantity of dosage concentration). Don't assume it is per 1 mL.

CLINICAL REASONING SKILLS

Medication errors will occur if the right side of the equation is set up improperly when using the dimensional analysis method for dosage calculations.

ERROR

All ratios necessary to arrive at the desired units are not entered correctly into the dimensional analysis equation

Possible Scenario

The physician ordered *erythromycin ethylsuccinate 20 mg/kg p.o. once prior to a dental procedure* for a child who weighed 45 lb. Six hours after the procedure, the child would receive an additional dosage of 10 mg/kg. The nurse who prepared the initial dose obtained erythromycin ethylsuccinate 200 mg per 5 mL from the pharmacy. The nurse calculated the dose using dimensional analysis and incorrectly set up the problem this way:

$$X \text{ mL} = \frac{5 \text{ mL}}{200 \text{ mg}} \times \frac{20 \text{ mg}}{1 \text{ kg}} \times 45 \text{ lb} = 22.5 \text{ mL} \qquad \textbf{INCORRECT}$$

The nurse who had prepared the drug was having a difficult time administering it to the child, who was experiencing a significant amount of oral pain. When the nurse requested the assistance of another nurse, the second nurse questioned the amount of drug measured in a plastic medicine cup that was being given as the prophylactic therapy before the dental procedure. At this point, the two nurses recalculated the dosage together and the correct dose was prepared.

Potential Outcome

Although doses as high as 30 to 50 mg/kg/day of erythromycin are given to children, the specific dose is determined by the severity of the infection. This child, who did not have a diagnosed infection, would have received a dosage approximately double that which was ordered by the physician and then approximately another double dosage of the drug ordered to be administered again 6 hours later. Improper administration of antibiotics has been attributed to bacterial mutations and development of strains of bacteria that are resistant to many antibiotics.

Prevention

This type of calculation error occurred because the nurse set up the dimensional analysis problem incorrectly. Not all necessary calculations were entered into the right side of the equation. The problem should have been set up and calculated this way:

$$X \text{ mL} = \frac{5 \text{ mL}}{200 \text{ mg}} \times \frac{20 \text{ mg}}{1 \text{ kg}} \times \frac{1 \text{ kg}}{2.2 \text{ lb}} \times 45 \text{ lb} = 10.2 \text{ mL} \quad \textbf{CORRECT}$$

Remember: All units of measure must cancel out, leaving only the unit you seek to give—in this case, mL. The nurse should have noticed that both mL and lb were remaining in the incorrect equation. That would have been a clue to double-check the calculation. It is important to think carefully before you begin your calculations, to determine all the ratios necessary and the proper way to set up the dimensional analysis equation.

PRACTICE PROBLEMS—CHAPTER 14

Calculate the amount to prepare 1 dose, using both the formula and dimensional analysis methods.

1. Order: lactulose 30 g in 100 mL fluid p.r. t.i.d.

   Supply: lactulose 3.33 g per 5 mL

   Give: _____ mL in 100 mL

2. Order: penicillin G potassium 500,000 units IM q.i.d.

   Supply: penicillin G potassium 5,000,000 units per 20 mL

   Give: _____ mL

3. Order: Keflex 100 mg p.o. q.i.d.

   Supply: Keflex oral suspension 250 mg per 5 mL

   Give: _____ mL

4. Order: amoxicillin 125 mg p.o. q.i.d.

   Supply: amoxicillin 250 mg per 5 mL

   NOTE: You are giving home-care instructions.

   Give: _____ t

5. Order: Benadryl 25 mg IM stat

   Supply: Benadryl 10 mg/mL

   Give: _____ mL

6. Order: diphenhydramine 40 mg p.o. stat

   Supply: diphenhydramine 12.5 mg per 5 mL

   Give: _____ mL

7. Order: penicillin G potassium 350,000 units IM b.i.d.

    Supply: penicillin G potassium 500,000 units per 2 mL

    Give: _____ mL

8. Order: Valium 3.5 mg IM q.6h p.r.n., anxiety

    Supply: Valium 10 mg per 2 mL

    Give: _____ mL

9. Order: tobramycin sulfate 90 mg IV q.8h

    Supply: tobramycin sulfate 80 mg per 2 mL

    Give: _____ mL

10. Order: heparin 2,500 units subcut b.i.d.

    Supply: heparin 20,000 units/mL

    Give: _____ mL

11. Order: Compazine 8 mg IM q.6h p.r.n., nausea

    Supply: Compazine 10 mg per 2 mL

    Give: _____ mL

12. Order: gentamicin 60 mg IV q.6h

    Supply: gentamicin 80 mg per 2 mL

    Give: _____ mL

13. Order: piperacillin 500 mg IV b.i.d.

    Supply: piperacillin 1 g per 2.5 mL

    Give: _____ mL

14. Order: Nilstat Oral Suspension 250,000 units p.o. q.i.d.

    Supply: Nilstat Oral Suspension 100,000 units/mL

    Give: _____ mL

15. Order: erythromycin estolate 80 mg p.o. q.4h

    Supply: erythromycin estolate 250 mg per 5 mL

    Give: _____ mL

16. Order: potassium chloride 10 mEq p.o. stat

    Supply: potassium chloride 20 mEq per 15 mL

    Give: _____ mL

17. Order: nafcillin 400 mg IV q.6h

    Supply: nafcillin 1 g per 4 mL

    Give: _____ mL

18. Order: Synthroid 150 mcg p.o. daily

    Supply: Synthroid 0.075 mg tablets

    Give: _____ tablet(s)

19. Order: amoxicillin 400 mg p.o. q.8h

    Supply: amoxicillin 250 mg per 5 mL

    Give: _____ mL

20. Order: **phenytoin 225 mg IV stat**

    Supply: phenytoin 50 mg/mL

    Give: _____ mL

21. Order: **Elixophyllin 160 mg p.o. q.6h**

    Supply: Elixophyllin 80 mg per 15 mL

    Give: _____ mL

22. Order: **chlorpromazine 35 mg IM stat**

    Supply: chlorpromazine 25 mg/mL

    Give: _____ mL

23. Order: **oxycodone hydrochloride 8 mg p.o. q.4h p.r.n., pain**

    Supply: oxycodone hydrochloride 20 mg/mL

    Add: _____ mL

24. Order: **promethazine 25 mg via NG tube h.s.**

    Supply: promethazine 6.25 mg per 5 mL

    Give: _____ mL

25. Order: **cefaclor 300 mg p.o. t.i.d.**

    Supply: cefaclor 125 mg per 5 mL

    Give: _____ mL

26. Describe the clinical reasoning you would use to prevent this medication error.

    Possible Scenario
    The physician ordered **Amoxil 50 mg p.o. q.i.d.** for a child with an upper respiratory infection. Amoxil is supplied in an oral suspension with 125 mg per 5 mL. The nurse calculated the dose this way:

    $$\frac{D}{H} \times Q = \frac{125 \text{ mg}}{50 \text{ mg}} \times 5 \text{ mL} = \frac{625}{50} \text{ mL} = 12.5 \text{ mL} \qquad \textbf{INCORRECT}$$

    Give 12.5 mL orally four times a day.

    Potential Outcome
    The patient received a large overdose and should have received only 2 mL. The child would likely develop complications from overdosage of amoxicillin. When the physician was notified of the error, she would likely have ordered the medication to be discontinued and had extra blood lab work done. An incident report would be filed and the family would be notified of the error.

    Prevention

    _____

    _____

After completing these problems, see pages 694–695 to check your answers.

🖱 Be sure to use the online software for additional practice!

SECTION 3 SELF-EVALUATION

Chapter 10—Oral Dosage of Drugs

T he following labels (A–N) represent the drugs you have available for the orders in questions 1 through 10. Select the correct label and identify the corresponding letter for filling these medication orders. Calculate the amount to give.

1. Order: Neurontin 0.2 g p.o. daily

   Select label _____ and give _____ capsule(s)

2. Order: atomoxetine 40 mg p.o. daily

   Select label _____ and give _____ capsule(s)

3. Order: Ritalin 10 mg p.o. t.i.d.

   Select label _____ and give _____ tablet(s)

4. Order: valproic acid 100 mg p.o. b.i.d.

   Select label _____ and give _____ mL

5. Order: potassium chloride 16 mEq p.o. daily

   Select label _____ and give _____ mL

6. Order: nitroglycerin 13 mg p.o. t.i.d.

   Select label _____ and give _____ capsule(s)

7. Order: Synthroid 0.05 mg p.o. daily

   Select label _____ and give _____ tablet(s)

8. Order: codeine 45 mg p.o. q.6h p.r.n., cough

   Select label _____ and give _____ tablet(s)

9. Order: furosemide 12.5 mg p.o. b.i.d.

   Select label _____ and give _____ mL

10. Order: albuterol sulfate 3 mg p.o. t.i.d.

    Select label _____ and give _____ mL

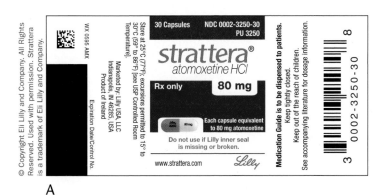

A

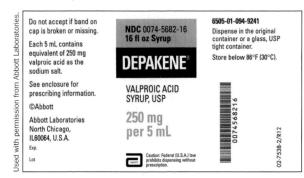

B

C

Store at controlled room temperature 15°- 30ºC (59°- 86°F).

DOSAGE AND USE
See package insert for full prescribing information.

Each capsule contains 100 mg of gabapentin.

Manufactured by:
Pfizer Pharmaceuticals Ltd.
Vega Baja, PR 00694

NDC 0071-0803-24
100 Capsules   **Rx only**

Neurontin®   (100)
(gabapentin) capsules

100 mg

Distributed by
Pfizer **Parke-Davis**
Division of Pfizer Inc, NY, NY 10017

7700

0 0071-0803-24 4
05-5810-32-4

D

N 3 58177-006-03 6

Each extended-release capsule contains:

Nitroglycerin. . . . . 9 mg

KEEP THIS AND ALL DRUGS OUT OF THE REACH OF CHILDREN.

NDC 58177-006-03

Nitroglycerin

Extended-release Capsules

9 mg

60 Capsules

Dispense in a tight container as defined in the USP/NF.

Store at controlled room temperature 15°-30°C (59°-86°F).

USUAL DOSAGE: See package insert for dosage, including nitrate-free intervals.

℞ Only

Manufactured by
Time-Caps Labs Inc. for
ETHEX Corporation
St. Louis, MO 63043-2413

P2062-7 6/98

ETHEX ETHEX ETHEX ETHEX ETHEX

E

3 0048-1020-05 5

NDC 0048-1020-05
Code 3P1025

SYNTHROID®

(Levothyroxine Sodium Tablets, USP)

25 mcg   **(0.025 mg)**

1000 TABLETS

Rx only

BASF Pharma   *knoll*

See full prescribing information for dosage and administration.

Dispense in a tight, light-resistant container as described in USP.

Store at 25°C (77°F); excursions permitted to 15°-30°C (59°-86°F). [See USP Controlled Room Temperature].

Knoll Pharmaceutical Company
Mount Olive, NJ 07828
USA

7897-03

F

WW 8736 AMX

Marketed by: Lilly USA, LLC
Indianapolis, IN 46285, USA
Product of Ireland

Expiration Date/Control No.

Store at 25°C (77°F); excursions permitted to 15° to 30°C (59° to 86°F) [see USP Controlled Room Temperature].

30 Capsules   NDC 0002-3229-30
           PU 3229

strattera®
atomoxetine HCl

Rx only   **40 mg**

Each capsule equivalent to 40 mg atomoxetine

Do not use if Lilly inner seal is missing or broken.

www.strattera.com   *Lilly*

Medication Guide is to be dispensed to patients.
Keep tightly closed.
Keep out of the reach of children.
See accompanying literature for dosage information.

3 0002-3229-30 4

G

N 3 0078-0439-05 3

EXP.
LOT

NDC 0078-0439-05

Ritalin® HCl
methylphenidate HCl USP   (C II)

5 mg

100 tablets   **Rx only**

ψ **NOVARTIS**

Dosage: See package insert.
Store at 25°C (77°F); excursions permitted to 15-30°C (59-86°F) [see USP Controlled Room Temperature].
Protect from light.
Dispense in tight, light-resistant container (USP).

Novartis Pharmaceuticals Corporation
East Hanover, New Jersey 07936 ©Novartis

5000090

H

Delivers **15 mL**
NDC 0121-1465-15
POTASSIUM CHLORIDE
ORAL SOLUTION USP 10%
20 mEq per 15 mL
Sugar Free   Alcohol 5%
DILUTE BEFORE USING

(01) 0 03 01211 46515 3

Rx ONLY
FOR INSTITUTIONAL USE ONLY
PHARMACEUTICAL ASSOCIATES, INC.
GREENVILLE, SC 29605
SEE INSERT

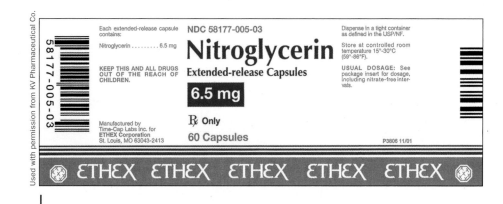

Each extended-release capsule
contains:

Nitroglycerin . . . . 6.5 mg

KEEP THIS AND ALL DRUGS
OUT OF THE REACH OF
CHILDREN.

Manufactured by
Time-Cap Labs Inc. for
ETHEX Corporation
St. Louis, MO 63043-2413

NDC 58177-005-03

Nitroglycerin

Extended-release Capsules

6.5 mg

℞ Only

60 Capsules

Dispense in a tight container
as defined in the USP/NF.

Store at controlled room
temperature 15°-30°C
(59°-86°F).

USUAL DOSAGE: See
package insert for dosage,
including nitrate-free intervals.

P3806 11/01

ETHEX   ETHEX   ETHEX   ETHEX   ETHEX

I

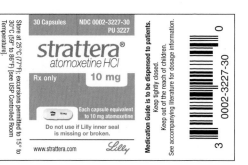

WW 8705 AMX

Store at 25°C (77°F); excursions permitted to 15° to
30°C (59° to 86°F) [see USP Controlled Room
Temperature]

30 Capsules   NDC 0002-3227-30
                 PU 3227

strattera®
atomoxetine HCl

Rx only   **10 mg**

Eli Lilly and Company
Indianapolis, IN 46285, USA
Product of Ireland

Expiration Date/Control No.

Each capsule equivalent
to 10 mg atomoxetine

Do not use if Lilly inner seal
is missing or broken.

www.strattera.com   *Lilly*

Medication Guide is to be dispensed to patients.
Keep tightly closed.
Keep out of the reach of children.
See accompanying literature for dosage information.

0002-3227-30

J

See Package Insert for
Complete Prescribing Information.

Store at Controlled Room Temperature
15°-30°C (59°-86°F).

PROTECT FROM MOISTURE.

Dispense in a well-closed container
as defined in the USP/NF.

TABLETS IDENTIFIED 54 783

(Side One) ⊝⊝ (Side Two)

DO NOT USE UNLESS TABLETS
CARRY THIS IDENTIFICATION

NDC 0054-
4156-25   100 Tablets   EXP. LOT

30 mg   ⓒ
CODEINE
Sulfate
Tablets USP

Each tablet contains
Codeine Sulfate 30 mg
℞ only.

☒ **Roxane**
Laboratories, Inc.
Columbus, Ohio 43216

4151001
039
© RLI, 1999

0054-4156-25

K

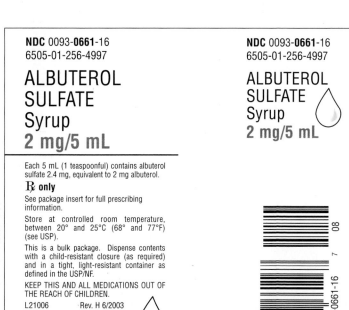

NDC 0093-**0661**-16
6505-01-256-4997

ALBUTEROL SULFATE
Syrup

2 mg/5 mL

Each 5 mL (1 teaspoonful) contains albuterol
sulfate 2.4 mg, equivalent to 2 mg albuterol.

℞ only

See package insert for full prescribing
information.

Store at controlled room temperature,
between 20° and 25°C (68° and 77°F)
(see USP).

This is a bulk package. Dispense contents
with a child-resistant closure (as required)
and in a tight, light-resistant container as
defined in the USP/NF.

KEEP THIS AND ALL MEDICATIONS OUT OF
THE REACH OF CHILDREN.

L21006   Rev. H 6/2003

TEVA PHARMACEUTICALS USA
Sellersville, PA 18960

473 mL

TEVA

NDC 0093-**0661**-16
6505-01-256-4997

ALBUTEROL SULFATE
Syrup

2 mg/5 mL

0093-0661-16

L

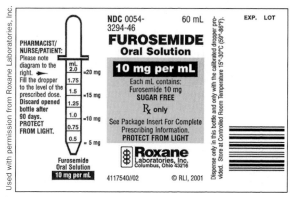

PHARMACIST/
NURSE/PATIENT:
Please note
diagram to the
right.
Fill the dropper
to the level of the
prescribed dose.
Discard opened
bottle after
90 days.
PROTECT
FROM LIGHT.

mL
2.0
1.75 — =20 mg
1.5
1.25 — =15 mg
1.0
0.75 — =10 mg
0.5 — = 5 mg

Furosemide
Oral Solution
10 mg per mL

NDC 0054-
3294-46   60 mL   EXP. LOT

FUROSEMIDE
Oral Solution

10 mg per mL

Each mL contains:
Furosemide 10 mg
SUGAR FREE

℞ only

See Package Insert For Complete
Prescribing Information.
PROTECT FROM LIGHT

☒ **Roxane**
Laboratories, Inc.
Columbus, Ohio 43216

4117540//02   © RLI, 2001

Dispense only in this bottle and only with the calibrated dropper provided. Store at Controlled Room Temperature 15°-30°C (59°-86°F).

M

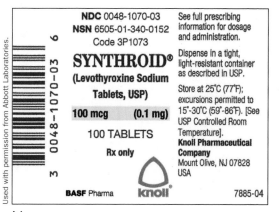

0048-1070-03

NDC 0048-1070-03
NSN 6505-01-340-0152
Code 3P1073

SYNTHROID®
(Levothyroxine Sodium
Tablets, USP)

100 mcg   **(0.1 mg)**

100 TABLETS

Rx only

BASF Pharma   knoll®

See full prescribing
information for dosage
and administration.

Dispense in a tight,
light-resistant container
as described in USP.

Store at 25°C (77°F);
excursions permitted to
15°-30°C (59°-86°F). [See
USP Controlled Room
Temperature].

**Knoll Pharmaceutical
Company**
Mount Olive, NJ 07828
USA

7885-04

N

Chapter 11—Parenteral Dosage of Drugs

The following labels (A–H) represent the drugs you have available for the orders in questions 11 through 18. Select the correct label and identify the corresponding letter for filling these parenteral medication orders. Calculate the amount to give.

11. Order: *clindamycin 0.6 g IV q.12h*

Select label _____ and give _____ mL

12. Order: *phenytoin 175 mg IV stat*

Select label _____ and give _____ mL

13. Order: *epinephrine 200 mcg subcut stat*

Select label _____ and give _____ mL

14. Order: *famotidine 20 mg IV at bedtime*

Select label _____ and give _____ mL

15. Order: *gentamicin 60 mg IV q.8h*

Select label _____ and give _____ mL

16. Order: *heparin 750 units subcut stat*

Select label _____ and give _____ mL

17. Order: *morphine 7.5 mg subcut q.4h p.r.n., pain*

Select label _____ and give _____ mL

18. Order: *Narcan 0.3 mg IM stat*

Select label _____ and give _____ mL

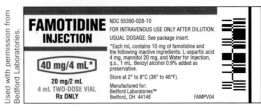

FAMOTIDINE INJECTION

NDC 55390-028-10
FOR INTRAVENOUS USE ONLY AFTER DILUTION.
USUAL DOSAGE: See package insert.

40 mg/4 mL*

*Each mL contains 10 mg of famotidine and the following inactive ingredients: L-aspartic acid 4 mg, mannitol 20 mg, and Water for Injection, q.s., 1 mL. Benzyl alcohol 0.9% added as preservative.
Store at 2° to 8°C (36° to 46°F).

20 mg/2 mL
4 mL TWO-DOSE VIAL
Rx ONLY

Manufactured for:
Bedford Laboratories™
Bedford, OH 44146   FAMPV04

A

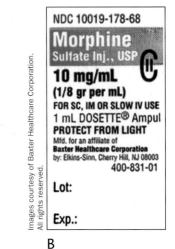

NDC 10019-178-68

Morphine
Sulfate Inj., USP

10 mg/mL
(1/8 gr per mL)
FOR SC, IM OR SLOW IV USE
1 mL DOSETTE® Ampul
PROTECT FROM LIGHT
Mfd. for an affiliate of
Baxter Healthcare Corporation
by: Elkins-Sinn, Cherry Hill, NJ 08003
400-831-01

Lot:

Exp.:

B

Dosage—See package insert.

℞ only

Manufactured by:
Parkedale Pharmaceuticals, Inc.
Rochester, MI 48307

For:
PARKE-DAVIS
Div of Warner-Lambert Co
Morris Plains, NJ 07950 USA

N 0071-4475-45
STERI-VIAL®
Dilantin®
(Phenytoin Sodium Injection, USP)
ready/mixed

250 mg in 5 mL
5 mL

Do not exceed 50 mg/minute IV IM/IV (no infusion)

© 1997-'98, Warner-Lambert Co.

4475G233

C

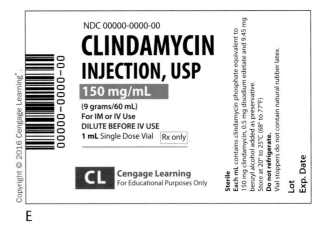

NDC 00000-0000-00

CLINDAMYCIN INJECTION, USP

150 mg/mL
(9 grams/60 mL)
For IM or IV Use
DILUTE BEFORE IV USE
1 mL Single Dose Vial Rx only

CL **Cengage Learning**
For Educational Purposes Only

Sterile
Each mL contains clindamycin phosphate equivalent to 150 mg clindamycin, 0.5 mg disodium edetate and 9.45 mg benzyl alcohol added as preservative.
Store at 20° to 25°C (68° to 77°F).
Do not refrigerate.
Vial stoppers do not contain natural rubber latex.
Lot
Exp. Date

E

NDC 63323-010-02 1002
GENTAMICIN
INJECTION, USP
equivalent to 40 mg/mL Gentamicin
80 mg/2 mL
For IM or IV Use.
Must be diluted for IV use.
2 mL Multiple Dose Vial
Sterile   Rx only

APP Pharmaceuticals, LLC
Schaumburg, IL 60173

401896D

LOT/EXP

3 63323-010-02 7

SAMPLE. NOT FOR HUMAN USE.

D

Tear Here →

NOT FOR LOCK FLUSH   NOT FOR LOCK FLUSH   NOT FOR LOCK FLUSH

Heparin
Sodium Injection, USP

1,000
USP units per **1mL**
For IV or SC use
Multi-Dose Vial
Rx only   ✦APP

NOT FOR LOCK FLUSH

From Porcine Intestinal Mucosa
This container closure is not made from natural rubber latex.
Fresenius Kabi USA, LLC

401805J

LOT
EXP

3 63323-540-01 2

SAMPLE. NOT FOR HUMAN USE.

F

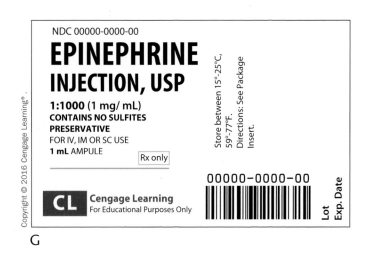

G

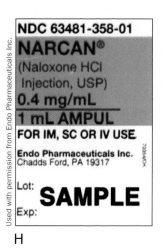

H

For questions 19 and 20, select and mark the amount to give on the correct syringe.

19. Order: Humulin-N NPH U-100 insulin 48 units subcut 30 min ā breakfast

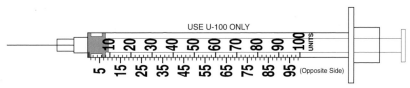

Copyright © 2016 Cengage Learning®.

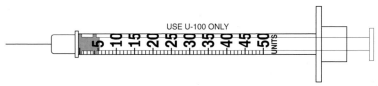

Copyright © 2016 Cengage Learning®.

20. Order: Novolin R regular U-100 insulin 12 units c̄ Novolin N NPH U-100 insulin 28 units subcut 30 min ā dinner

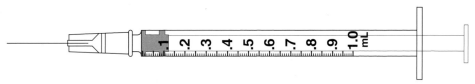

Copyright © 2016 Cengage Learning®.

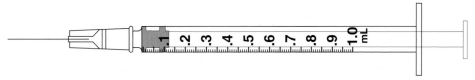

Copyright © 2016 Cengage Learning®.

Chapter 12—Reconstitution of Solutions

For questions 21 through 26, specify the amount of diluent to add and the resulting solution concentration. Calculate the amount to give, and indicate the dose with an arrow on the accompanying syringe. Finally, make a reconstitution label, if required.

21. Order: Zithromax 500 mg IV daily

Reconstitute with _____ mL diluent for a total solution volume of _____ mL with a concentration of _____ mg/mL.

Give: _____ mL

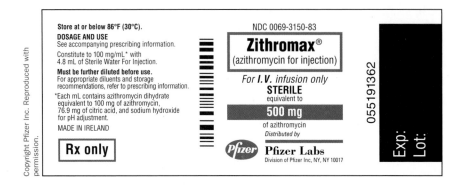

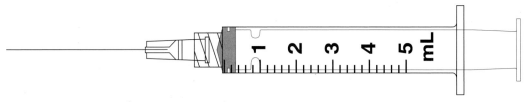

22. Order: vancomycin 400 mg IV q.6h

Reconstitute with _____ mL diluent for a total solution volume of _____ mL with a concentration of _____ mg/ _____ mL.

Give: _____ mL. There is/are _____ full dose(s) available in this vial.

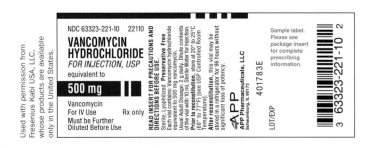

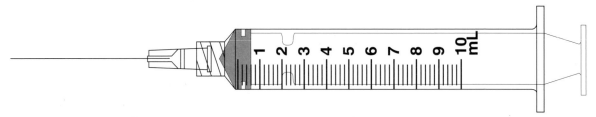

23. Order: *ceftriaxone 150 mg IV q.12h*

Reconstitute with _____ mL diluent for a total solution volume of _____ mL with a concentration of _____ mg/mL.

Give: _____ mL

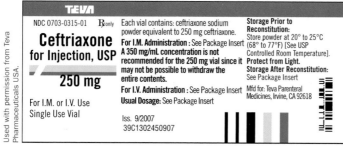

Package insert instructions for IV administration:
Add 2.4 mL diluent to 250 mg vial. After reconstitution, each 1 mL of solution contains approximately 100 mg equivalent of ceftriaxone. Reconstituted solution is stable at room temperature for 24 hours and refrigerated for 3 days.

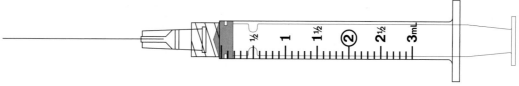

24. Order: *cefazolin 750 mg IM q.8h*

Reconstitute with _____ mL diluent for a total solution volume of _____ mL with a concentration of _____ mg/mL.

Give: _____ mL

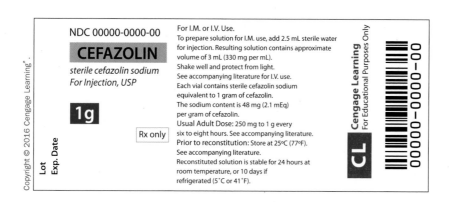

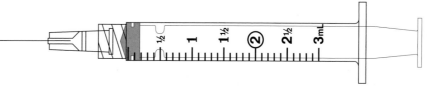

25. Order: *Solu-Medrol 250 mg IV q.6h*

    Reconstitute with _____ mL diluent for a total solution volume of _____ mL with a concentration of _____ mg/mL.

    Give: _____ mL. There are _____ full doses available in this vial.

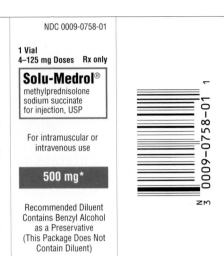

Store at controlled room temperature 20° to 25°C (68° to 77°F) [see USP]. **Protect from light.**

Reconstitute with 8 mL Bacteriostatic Water for Injection with Benzyl Alcohol.

Store solution at controlled room temperature 20° to 25°C (68° to 77°F) and use within 48 hours after mixing. **Protect from light.**

DOSAGE AND USE:
See accompanying prescribing information.

* Each 8 mL (when mixed with 8 mL of diluent) contains methylprednisolone sodium succinate equivalent to methylprednisolone, 500 mg. Also contains monobasic sodium phosphate anhydrous, 6.4 mg; dibasic sodium phosphate dried, 69.6 mg. When necessary, pH was adjusted with sodium hydroxide. Lyophilized in container.

NDC 0009-0758-01

1 Vial
4–125 mg Doses   Rx only

Solu-Medrol®
methylprednisolone sodium succinate
for injection, USP

For intramuscular or intravenous use

500 mg*

Recommended Diluent Contains Benzyl Alcohol as a Preservative (This Package Does Not Contain Diluent)

Distributed by
Pfizer **Pharmacia & Upjohn Co**
Division of Pfizer Inc, NY, NY 10017

1681

0009-0758-01 1

Copyright Pfizer Inc. Reproduced with permission.

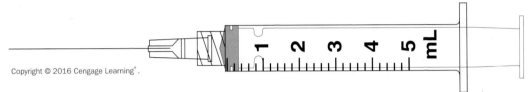

Copyright © 2016 Cengage Learning®.

26. Order: *Vantin 100 mg p.o. q.12h*

    Reconstitute with _____ mL diluent for a total solution volume of _____ mL with a concentration of _____ mg per _____ mL or _____ mg/mL.

    Give: _____ mL

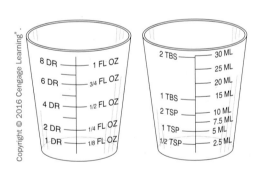

Copyright © 2016 Cengage Learning®.

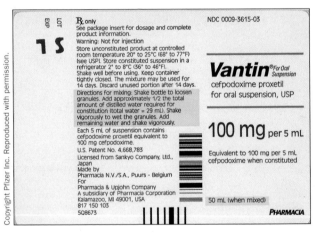

Copyright Pfizer Inc. Reproduced with permission.

R only
See package insert for dosage and complete product information.
Warning: Not for injection
Store unconstituted product at controlled room temperature 20° to 25°C (68° to 77°F) [see USP]. Store constituted suspension in a refrigerator 2° to 8°C (36° to 46°F). Shake well before using. Keep container tightly closed. The mixture may be used for 14 days. Discard unused portion after 14 days.
Directions for mixing: Shake bottle to loosen granules. Add approximately 1/2 the total amount of distilled water required for constitution (total water = 29 mL). Shake vigorously to wet the granules. Add remaining water and shake vigorously.
Each 5 mL of suspension contains cefpodoxime proxetil equivalent to 100 mg cefpodoxime.
U.S. Patent No. 4,668,783
Licensed from Sankyo Company, Ltd., Japan
Made by
Pharmacia N.V./S.A., Puurs - Belgium
For
Pharmacia & Upjohn Company
A subsidiary of Pharmacia Corporation
Kalamazoo, MI 49001, USA
817 150 103
5Q8673

NDC 0009-3615-03

Vantin® *For Oral Suspension*
cefpodoxime proxetil
for oral suspension, USP

100 mg per 5 mL

Equivalent to 100 mg per 5 mL cefpodoxime when constituted

50 mL (when mixed)

PHARMACIA

27. How many full doses are available of the medication supplied for question 26? _____ dose(s)

28. Will the medication supplied expire before it is used up for the order in question 26? _____
    Explain: _____

Prepare the following therapeutic solutions.

29. Order: *360 mL of $\frac{1}{3}$ strength hydrogen peroxide diluted with normal saline*

    Supply: 60 mL bottles of stock hydrogen peroxide solution

    Add _____ mL solute and _____ mL solvent.

30. Order: *240 mL $\frac{3}{4}$ strength Ensure*

    Supply: 8 fl oz can of Ensure

    Add _____ mL Ensure and _____ mL water.

Refer to the following order for questions 31 and 32.

Order: *Give $\frac{2}{3}$ strength Ensure 240 mL via NG tube q.3h*

Supply: Ready-to-use Ensure 8 fl oz can and sterile water

31. How much sterile water would you add to the 8 fl oz can of Ensure? _____ mL

32. How many complete feedings would this make? _____ feeding(s)

Use the following information to answer questions 33 and 34.

You will prepare formula to feed nine infants in the nursery. Each infant has an order for **4 fl oz** of $\frac{1}{2}$ **strength Isomil formula q.3h.** You have 8 fl oz cans of ready-to-use Isomil and sterile water.

33. How many cans of formula will you need to open to prepare the reconstituted formula for all nine infants for one feeding each? _____ can(s)

34. How many mL of sterile water will you add to the Isomil to reconstitute the formula for one feeding for all nine infants? _____ mL

Chapter 13—Pediatric and Adult Dosages Based on Body Weight

Calculate and assess the safety of the following dosage. Mark safe dosage on the measuring device supplied.

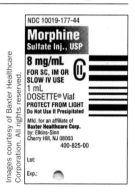

35. Order: **morphine 6 mg subcut q.4h p.r.n., severe pain** for a child who weighs 67 lb. Recommended pediatric dosage: 100 to 200 mcg/kg q.4h, up to a maximum of 15 mg/dose.

    If the dosage ordered is safe, give _____ mL. If not safe, explain why and describe what you should do. _____

    _____

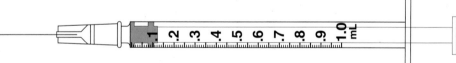

36. Order: **amoxicillin 75 mg p.o. q.8h** for a 15 lb child. Recommended dosage: See label.

    If the dosage ordered is safe, reconstitute with _____ mL diluent for a total solution volume of _____ mL and a concentration of _____ mg/mL and give _____ mL. If not safe, explain why and describe what you should do. _____

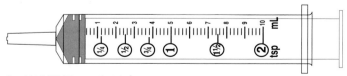

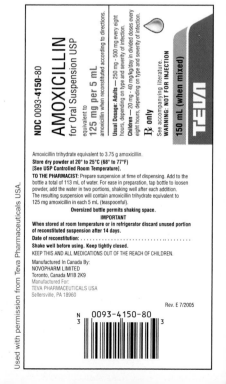

37. Order: *phenytoin 100 mg IV t.i.d.* for a child who weighs 20 kg. Recommended pediatric dosage: 5 mg/kg/day in 2 to 3 divided doses. If the dosage ordered is safe, give _____ mL. If not safe, explain why and describe what you should do. _____

_____

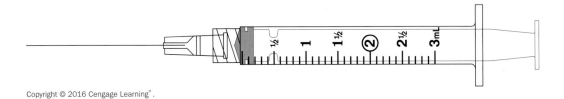

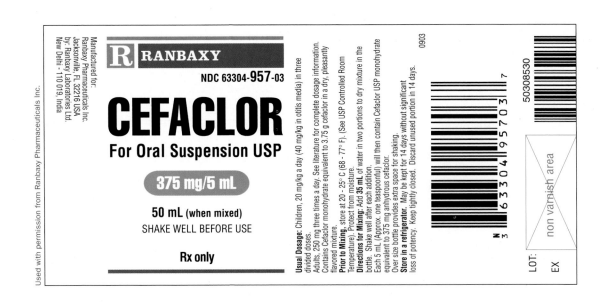

38. Order: *cefaclor 187 mg p.o. q.i.d.* for a child with otitis media who weighs 16 lb. Recommended dosage: See label.

   If the dosage ordered is safe, reconstitute with _____ mL diluent for a total solution volume of _____ mL and a concentration of _____ mg/mL. Give _____ mL. If not safe, explain why and describe what you should do. _____

_____

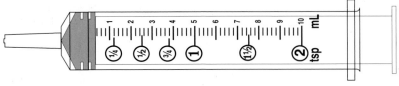

39. a) Order: **Kantrex 60 mg IV q.8h** for a child who weighs 16 lb. The recommended dosage of Kantrex for adults and children is 15 mg/kg/day in 2 to 3 divided doses, not to exceed 1.5 g/day.

    If the ordered dosage is safe, give _____ mL. If not safe, explain why and describe what you should do. _____

    _____

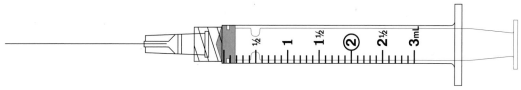

Copyright © 2016 Cengage Learning®.

    b) Refer to the recommended dosage of Kantrex given in question 39(a). What would you expect the single q.8h dosage of Kantrex to be for an adult who weighs 275 lb?

    _____ mg/dose

40. Describe the clinical reasoning you would use to prevent this medication error.

    Possible Scenario

    The physician ordered **amoxicillin 50 mg p.o. q.i.d.** for a child with an upper respiratory infection. Amoxicillin is supplied in an oral suspension with 125 mg per 5 mL. The nurse calculated the dose this way:

    $$\frac{50 \text{ mg}}{5 \text{ ml}} = \frac{125 \text{ mg}}{X \text{ mL}}$$

    $50X = 625$ **INCORRECT**

    $$\frac{50X}{50} = \frac{625}{50}$$

    $X = 12.5$ mL

    Potential Outcome

    The patient received a large overdose and should have received only 2 mL. The child would likely develop complications from the overdose of amoxicillin. When the physician was notified of the error, she would likely have ordered the medication discontinued and had extra blood lab work done. An incident report would be filed and the family would be notified of the error.

    Prevention

    _____

    _____

Chapter 14—Alternative Dosage Calculation Methods: Formula and Dimensional Analysis

Use the conversion factor method in questions 41 through 44 to convert each of the following amounts to the unit indicated. Indicate the approximate equivalent used in the conversion.

	Equivalent		**Equivalent**
41. 15 mg = _____ g _____		43. 625 mcg = _____ mg _____	
42. 115 lb = _____ kg _____		44. 0.3 g = _____ mg _____	

You are to prepare medicines for patients assigned to your medication cart. The following labels represent the drugs you have available for questions 45 through 50. Use both the formula and dimensional analysis methods to calculate the dosages.

45. Order: methotrexate 175 mg IV stat

Give: _____ mL

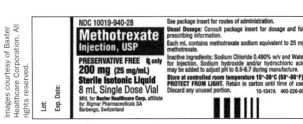

46. Order: famotidine 15 mg IV bolus stat

Give: _____ mL

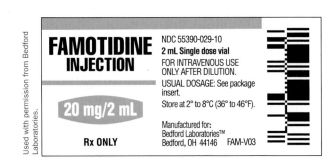

47. Order: vancomycin hydrochloride
500 mg IV q.6h

Give: _____ mL

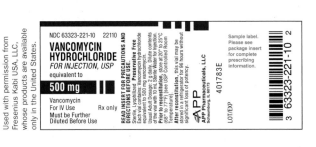

48. Order: Nitrostat 600 mcg SL p.r.n., angina

Give: _____ tablet(s)

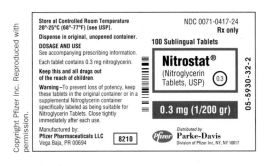

49. Order: metoclopramide 15 mg IV q.3h × 3 doses

    Give: _____ mL

50. Order: levothyroxine 0.15 mg IV daily

    Give: _____ mL

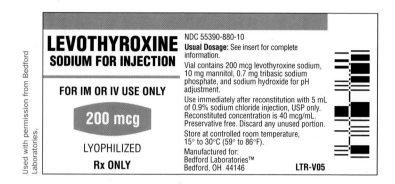

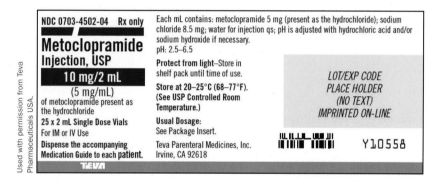

Section 3 Board Examination Practice

To obtain licensure, you will be required to pass a board examination. The following problems represent the various types of items on the NCLEX-RN® (National Council Licensure Examination for Registered Nurses) and NCLEX-PN® (National Council Licensure Examination for Practical Nurses) exams. Whether you will be taking one of these board examinations or one from another licensure board, alternate test items such as these are good practice. For additional practice, go to the online practice software that accompanies this text to respond to more interactive test items, including those using the calculator tool.

51. **NCLEX** *Fill-in-the-Blank* **Item**

    To administer U-500 insulin in the hospital setting, you will use a _____ syringe.

    Answer: _____

52. **NCLEX** *Multiple-Response* **Item**

    Before administering medications, the nurse should be sure the drug given is safe and accurate. Which of the following is/are part of safe clinical practice for medication administration? (Place a check mark beside all that apply.)

    Answer:

    a. Gather information about the drug.   _____

    b. Retrieve the right drug in the correct supply dosage. _____

    c. Estimate the reasonable amount to give.   _____

    d. Calculate the correct dose amount to give.   _____

53. **NCLEX** *Exhibit* **Item**

Order: potassium chloride 40 mEq p.o. daily

Supply dosage: Look at the label pictured.

How much potassium chloride will you prepare for the correct dose? (Place a check mark beside the correct answer.)

Answer:

a. 1/2 fl oz _____

b. 15 mL _____

c. 1 fl oz _____

d. 5 mL _____

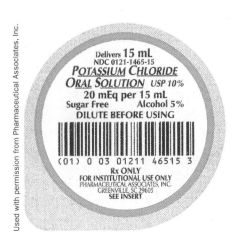

54. **NCLEX** *Drag-and-Drop / Ordered-Response* **Item**

Copy the tasks from the box onto the list in the proper sequence to *safely reconstitute an antibiotic powder with 2 mL diluent in order to administer 1 mL of the reconstituted drug.*

Answer:

Add 2 mL sterile water to the antibiotic powder.
Inject 2 mL air into the vial of sterile water.
Mix the powder and sterile water.
Withdraw 1 mL antibiotic solution.
Withdraw 2 mL sterile water.
Gather information about the drug.

_____

_____

_____

_____

_____

_____

55. **NCLEX** *Hot Box* **Item**

Identify the letter of the ratio factor of the dimensional analysis calculation that is set up **incorrectly,** resulting in the incorrect answer.

Order: ampicillin 12.5 mg/kg IV PB q.6h

Supply: 0.5 g per 2 mL

Child's weight: 45 lb

$$\text{X mL} = \frac{0.5\ g}{2\ mL} \times \frac{1\ g}{1,000\ mg} \times \frac{12.5\ mg}{1\ kg} \times \frac{1\ kg}{2.2\ lb} \times 45\ lb = \frac{281.25}{4,400}\ mL = 0.063\ mL = 0.06\ mL$$
     A   B   C   D   E   F

(The correct answer is 1 mL. This dose, if given for several days, could result in a more serious infection because of a calculation error and a hazardous underdosage.)

After completing these problems, see pages 695–700 to check your answers. Give yourself 1.8 points for each correct answer.

Perfect score = 100   My score = _____

Minimum mastery score = 86 (48 correct)

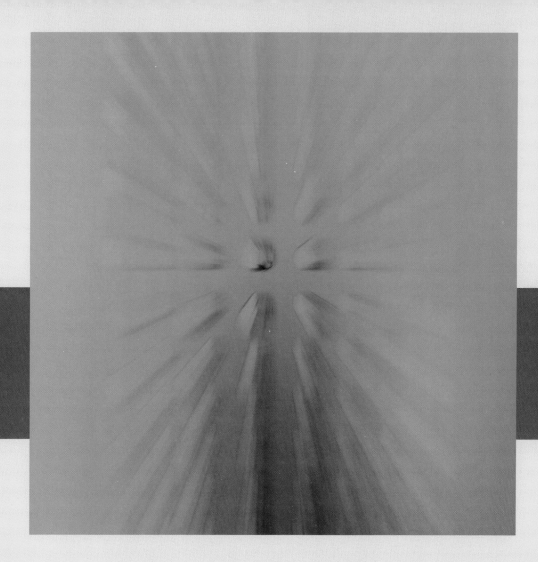

Advanced Calculations

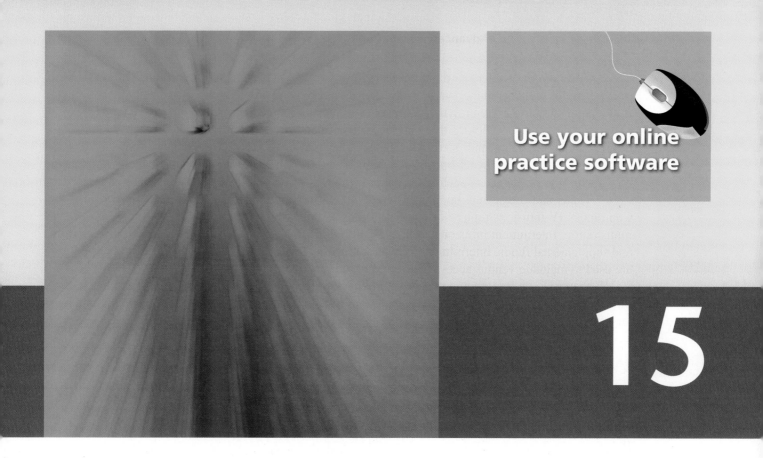

Intravenous Solutions, Equipment, and Calculations

OBJECTIVES

Upon mastery of Chapter 15, you will be able to calculate intravenous (IV) solution flow rates for electronic or manual infusion systems. To accomplish this, you will also be able to:

■ Identify common IV solutions and equipment.

■ Calculate the amount of specific components in common IV fluids.

■ Define the following terms: IV, peripheral line, central line, primary IV, secondary IV, saline/heparin locks, IV piggyback (IV PB), and IV push.

■ Calculate milliliters per hour: mL/h.

■ Recognize the calibration, or drop factor, in gtt/mL, as stated on the IV tubing package.

■ Apply the formula method to calculate IV flow rate in gtt/min:

$$\frac{\text{V (volume)}}{\text{T (time in min)}} \times \text{C (drop factor calibration)} = \text{R (rate of flow)}$$

■ Apply the shortcut method to calculate IV flow rate in gtt/min:

$$\frac{\text{mL/h}}{\text{Drop factor constant}} = \text{gtt/min}$$

■ Recalculate the flow rate when the IV is off schedule.

■ Verify infusion rate of dial-flow controllers.

■ Calculate small-volume IV PB.

■ Calculate rate for IV push medications.

■ Calculate IV infusion time.

■ Calculate IV infusion volume.

Intravenous (IV) refers to the administration of fluids, nutrients, and medication through a vein. IV fluids are ordered for a variety of reasons. They may be ordered for replacement of lost fluids, to maintain fluid and electrolyte balance, or to administer IV medications. *Replacement fluids* are often ordered because of losses that may occur from hemorrhage, vomiting, or diarrhea. *Maintenance fluids* sustain normal fluid and electrolyte balance. They may be used for the patient who is not yet depleted but is beginning to show symptoms of depletion. They may also be ordered for the patient who has the potential to become depleted, such as the patient who is allowed nothing by mouth (NPO) for surgery.

IV fluids and drugs may be administered by two methods: *continuous* and *intermittent* infusion. Continuous IV infusions replace or maintain fluids and electrolytes and serve as a vehicle for drug administration. Intermittent infusions, such as IV PB and IV push, are used for IV administration of drugs and supplemental fluids. Intermittent peripheral infusion devices, also known as saline or heparin locks, are used to maintain venous access without continuous fluid infusion.

IV therapy is an important and challenging nursing responsibility. This chapter covers the essential information and presents step-by-step calculations to help you gain a thorough understanding and mastery of this subject. Let's begin by analyzing IV solutions.

IV SOLUTIONS

IV solutions are ordered by a physician or prescribing practitioner; however, they are administered and monitored by the nurse. It is the responsibility of the nurse to ensure that the correct IV fluid is administered to the correct patient at the prescribed rate, following the same Six Rights for medication administration. IV fluids can be supplied in plastic solution bags or glass bottles, with the volume of the IV fluid container typically varying from 50 mL to 1,000 mL. Some IV bags may contain even more than 1,000 mL. Solutions used for total parenteral nutrition usually contain 2,000 mL or more in a single bag. The IV solution bag or bottle will be labeled with the exact components and amount of the IV solution. Health care practitioners often use abbreviations when communicating about the IV solution. Therefore, it is important for the nurse to know the common IV solution components and the solution concentration strengths represented by such abbreviations.

Solution Components

Glucose (dextrose), water, saline (sodium chloride, or NaCl), and selected electrolytes and salts are found in IV fluids. Dextrose and sodium chloride are the two most common solute components. Learn the following common IV component abbreviations.

REMEMBER

COMMON IV COMPONENT ABBREVIATIONS

Abbreviation	Solution Component
D	Dextrose
W	Water
S	Saline
NS	Normal saline (0.9% NaCl)
NaCl	Sodium chloride
RL	Ringer's lactate
LR	Lactated Ringer's

Solution Strength

The abbreviation letters indicate the solution components, and the numbers indicate the solution strength or concentration of the components (as shown in the examples that follow, such as D_5W). The numbers may be written as subscripts in the medical order.

FIGURE 15-1   IV solution label: D$_5$W

LOT   EXP

⊙   ⊙   NDC 0338-0017-04   **2B0064**   **1**

5% Dextrose Injection USP

2

3

1000 mL

EACH 100 mL CONTAINS   5 g DEXTROSE HYDROUS USP
pH 4.0 (3.2 TO 6.5)   OSMOLARITY 252 mOsmol/L (CALC)
STERILE   NONPYROGENIC   SINGLE DOSE CONTAINER   ADDITIVES
MAY BE INCOMPATIBLE   CONSULT WITH PHARMACIST IF AVAILABLE
WHEN INTRODUCING ADDITIVES USE ASEPTIC TECHNIQUE   MIX
THOROUGHLY   DO NOT STORE   DOSAGE   INTRAVENOUSLY AS
DIRECTED BY A PHYSICIAN   SEE DIRECTIONS   CAUTIONS   SQUEEZE
AND INSPECT INNER BAG WHICH MAINTAINS PRODUCT STERILITY
DISCARD IF LEAKS ARE FOUND   MUST NOT BE USED IN SERIES
CONNECTIONS   DO NOT ADMINISTER SIMULTANEOUSLY WITH BLOOD
DO NOT USE UNLESS SOLUTION IS CLEAR   FEDERAL (USA) LAW
PROHIBITS DISPENSING WITHOUT PRESCRIPTION   STORE UNIT IN
MOISTURE BARRIER OVERWRAP AT ROOM TEMPERATURE
(25ºC/77ºF) UNTIL READY TO USE   AVOID EXCESSIVE HEAT   SEE
INSERT

4

5

6

7

Baxter
BAXTER HEALTHCARE CORPORATION   Viaflex® CONTAINER
DEERFIELD IL 60015 USA   PL 146® PLASTIC
MADE IN USA   FOR PRODUCT INFORMATION   ♳
                        CALL 1-800-933-0303   v

8

⊙   ⊙   **9**

FIGURE 15-2   IV solution label: D$_5$LR

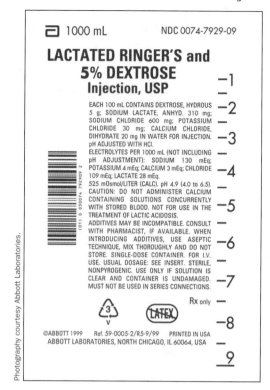

EXAMPLE 1 ■

Suppose an order includes D$_5$W. This abbreviation means *dextrose 5% in water* and is supplied as 5% Dextrose Injection, as in Figure 15-1. This means that the solution strength of the solute (dextrose) is 5%. The solvent is water. Recall from Chapter 8 that parenteral solutions expressed in a percent indicate X g per 100 mL. Read the IV bag label and notice that *each 100 mL contains 5 g dextrose.*

EXAMPLE 2 ■

Suppose a nurse writes D$_5$LR in the nurse's notes. This abbreviation means *dextrose 5% in Lactated Ringer's* and is supplied as Lactated Ringer's and 5% Dextrose Injection, as in Figure 15-2.

EXAMPLE 3 ■

An order states D$_5$NS 1,000 mL IV q.8h. This order means *administer 1,000 mL 5% dextrose in normal saline intravenously every 8 hours* and is supplied as 5% Dextrose and 0.9% Sodium Chloride (NaCl), as in Figure 15-3. *Normal saline* is the common term for 0.9% NaCl, because it has the same concentration of sodium chloride normally present in the blood. Another name is *physiologic saline.* The concentration of sodium chloride in normal saline is 0.9 g (or 900 mg) per 100 mL of solution.

Another common saline IV concentration is 0.45% NaCl, as in Figure 15-4. Notice that 0.45% NaCl is half the strength of 0.9% NaCl, which is normal saline. Thus, it is usually written as $\frac{1}{2}$ NS for half normal saline. Another saline solution strength is 0.225% NaCl (abbreviated as $\frac{1}{4}$ NS).

The goal of intravenous therapy, achieved through fluid infusion, is to maintain or regain fluid and electrolyte balance. When dextrose or saline *(solute)* is diluted in water for injection *(solvent)*, the result is *an IV solution* that can be administered to maintain or approximate the normal blood plasma. Blood or serum concentration is described in terms of *tonicity* or *osmolarity* and is measured in milliOsmols per

FIGURE 15-3   IV solution label: D₅NS

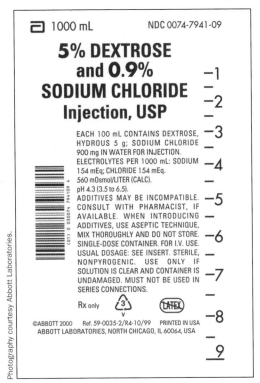

FIGURE 15-4   IV solution label: 0.45% NaCl

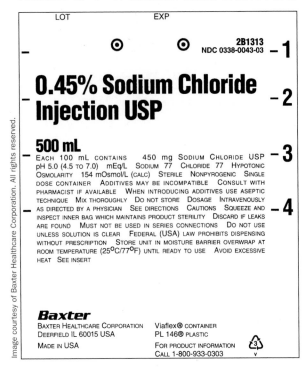

liter, or mOsm/L. IV fluids are concentrated and classified as *isotonic* (the same tonicity or osmolarity as blood and other body serums), *hypotonic* (lower tonicity or osmolarity than blood and other body serums), or *hypertonic* (higher tonicity or osmolarity than blood and other body serums). Normal saline (0.9% NaCl, or physiologic saline) is an isotonic solution. The osmolarity of a manufactured solution is detailed on the printed label. Look for the mOsm/L in the fine print under the solution name in Figures 15-1 through 15-4.

Figure 15-5 compares the three solution concentrations to normal serum osmolarity. Parenteral therapy is determined by unique patient needs, and these basic factors must be considered when ordering and infusing IV solutions.

FIGURE 15-5   Comparison of IV solution concentrations by osmolarity

Normal Serum Osmolarity (Normal Average Tonicity—All Ages) 280–320 mOsm/L

Hypotonic (<250 mOsm/L)	**Isotonic** (250–375 mOsm/L)	**Hypertonic** (>375 mOsm/L)
Solvent exceeds solute—used to dilute excess serum electrolytes, as in hyperglycemia	*Solvent and solutes are balanced*—used to expand volume and maintain normal tonicity	*Solutes exceed solvent*—used to correct electrolyte imbalances, as in loss from excess vomiting and diarrhea
Example of IV solution: *0.45% Saline (154 mOsm/L)*	Examples of IV solution: *0.9% Saline (308 mOsm/L) Lactated Ringer's (273 mOsm/L) 5% Dextrose in Water (252 mOsm/L)*	Examples of IV solution: *5% Dextrose and 0.9% NaCl (560 mOsm/L) 5% Dextrose and Lactated Ringer's (525 mOsm/L)*

Solution Additives

Electrolytes also may be added to the basic IV fluid. Potassium chloride (KCl) is a common IV additive and is measured in *milliequivalents* (mEq). The order is usually written to indicate the amount of milliequivalents per liter (1,000 mL) to be added to the IV fluid.

EXAMPLE ■

The physician orders D₅NS 1,000 mL IV c̄ 20 mEq KCl/L q.8h. This means to infuse 1,000 mL 5% dextrose and 0.9% sodium chloride IV solution, with 20 milliequivalents potassium chloride added per liter every 8 hours.

QUICK REVIEW

■ Pay close attention to IV abbreviations: *letters* indicate the solution components, and *numbers* indicate the concentration or solution strength.

■ Dextrose and sodium chloride (NaCl) are common IV solutes.

■ Solution strength expressed as a percent (%) indicates the number of g per 100 mL.

■ Normal saline is 0.9% sodium chloride: 0.9 g NaCl per 100 mL solution.

■ IV solution tonicity, or osmolarity, is measured in mOsm/L.

■ D₅W and normal saline are common isotonic solutions.

Review Set 32

For each of the following IV solutions labeled A through H:

a. Specify the *letter* of the illustration corresponding to the fluid abbreviation.

b. List the *solute(s)* of each solution, and identify the *strength (g/mL)* of each solute.

c. Identify the *osmolarity (mOsm/L)* of each solution.

d. Identify the *tonicity (isotonic, hypotonic,* or *hypertonic)* of each solution.

	a. Letter of matching illustration	b. Solutes and strength	c. Osmolarity (mOsm/L)	d. Tonicity
1. NS	_____	_____	_____	_____
2. D₅W	_____	_____	_____	_____
3. D₅NS	_____	_____	_____	_____
4. D₅ ½NS	_____	_____	_____	_____
5. D₅ ¼NS	_____	_____	_____	_____
6. D₅LR	_____	_____	_____	_____
7. D₅ ½NS c̄ 20 mEq KCl/L	_____	_____	_____	_____
8. ½NS	_____	_____	_____	_____

After completing these problems, see page 701 to check your answers.

◰ 500 mL   NDC 0074-7924-03

5% DEXTROSE and
0.225% SODIUM CHLORIDE
Injection, USP

—1

EACH 100 mL CONTAINS DEXTROSE, HYDROUS 5 g;
SODIUM CHLORIDE 225 mg IN WATER FOR INJECTION.
ELECTROLYTES PER 1000 mL: SODIUM 38.5 mEq; —2
CHLORIDE 38.5 mEq.
329 mOsmol/LITER (CALC).   pH 4.3 (3.5 to 6.5).
ADDITIVES MAY BE INCOMPATIBLE. CONSULT WITH
PHARMACIST, IF AVAILABLE. WHEN INTRODUCING
ADDITIVES, USE ASEPTIC TECHNIQUE, MIX —3
THOROUGHLY AND DO NOT STORE. SINGLE-DOSE
CONTAINER. FOR I.V. USE. USUAL DOSAGE: SEE
INSERT. STERILE, NONPYROGENIC. USE ONLY IF
SOLUTION IS CLEAR AND CONTAINER IS UNDAMAGED.
MUST NOT BE USED IN SERIES CONNECTIONS.

Rx only   ♲(3)   (LATEX)   —4

©ABBOTT 2000   v Ref. 59-0023-2/R4-10/99   PRINTED IN USA
ABBOTT LABORATORIES, NORTH CHICAGO, IL 60064, USA

A

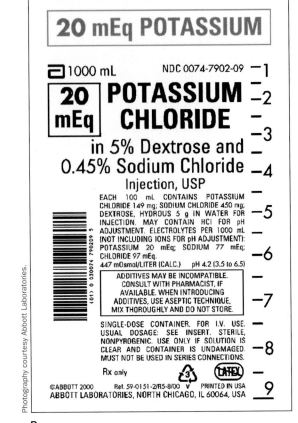

20 mEq POTASSIUM

◰ 1000 mL   NDC 0074-7902-09   —1

20   **POTASSIUM**   —2
mEq   **CHLORIDE**   —3

in 5% Dextrose and
0.45% Sodium Chloride   —4
Injection, USP

EACH 100 mL CONTAINS POTASSIUM
CHLORIDE 149 mg; SODIUM CHLORIDE 450 mg;
DEXTROSE, HYDROUS 5 g IN WATER FOR
INJECTION. MAY CONTAIN HCl FOR pH   —5
ADJUSTMENT. ELECTROLYTES PER 1000 mL
(NOT INCLUDING IONS FOR pH ADJUSTMENT):
POTASSIUM 20 mEq; SODIUM 77 mEq;
CHLORIDE 97 mEq.   —6
447 mOsmol/LITER (CALC.)   pH 4.2 (3.5 to 6.5)

ADDITIVES MAY BE INCOMPATIBLE.
CONSULT WITH PHARMACIST, IF
AVAILABLE. WHEN INTRODUCING   —7
ADDITIVES, USE ASEPTIC TECHNIQUE,
MIX THOROUGHLY AND DO NOT STORE.

SINGLE-DOSE CONTAINER. FOR I.V. USE.
USUAL DOSAGE: SEE INSERT. STERILE,
NONPYROGENIC. USE ONLY IF SOLUTION IS   —8
CLEAR AND CONTAINER IS UNDAMAGED.
MUST NOT BE USED IN SERIES CONNECTIONS.

Rx only   ♲(3)   (LATEX)
©ABBOTT 2000   Ref. 59-0151-2/R5-8/00 v   PRINTED IN USA   —9
ABBOTT LABORATORIES, NORTH CHICAGO, IL 60064, USA

B

◰ 1000 mL   NDC 0074-7983-09

0.9%
SODIUM CHLORIDE   —1
INJECTION, USP   —2

EACH 100 mL CONTAINS SODIUM   —3
CHLORIDE 900 mg IN WATER FOR
INJECTION. ELECTROLYTES PER 1000 mL:
SODIUM 154 mEq; CHLORIDE 154 mEq.
308 mOsmol/LITER (CALC).   —4
pH 5.6 (4.5 to 7.0)
ADDITIVES MAY BE INCOMPATIBLE.
CONSULT WITH PHARMACIST, IF
AVAILABLE. WHEN INTRODUCING   —5
ADDITIVES, USE ASEPTIC TECHNIQUE, MIX
THOROUGHLY AND DO NOT STORE.
SINGLE-DOSE CONTAINER. FOR
INTRAVENOUS USE. USUAL DOSAGE: SEE   —6
INSERT. STERILE, NONPYROGENIC. USE
ONLY IF SOLUTION IS CLEAR AND
CONTAINER IS UNDAMAGED. MUST NOT
BE USED IN SERIES CONNECTIONS.   —7

Rx only   ♲(3)   (LATEX)   —8

©ABBOTT 2001   Ref. 59-0016-2/R4-7/01   PRINTED IN USA   —9
ABBOTT LABORATORIES, NORTH CHICAGO, IL 60064, USA

C

◰ 1000 mL   NDC 0074-7926-09

5% DEXTROSE
and 0.45%
SODIUM CHLORIDE   —1
Injection, USP   —2

EACH 100 mL CONTAINS DEXTROSE,   —3
HYDROUS 5 g; SODIUM CHLORIDE
450 mg IN WATER FOR INJECTION.
ELECTROLYTES PER 1000 mL: SODIUM   —4
77 mEq; CHLORIDE 77 mEq.
406 mOsmol/LITER (CALC).
pH 4.3 (3.5 to 6.5).
ADDITIVES MAY BE INCOMPATIBLE.   —5
CONSULT WITH PHARMACIST, IF
AVAILABLE. WHEN INTRODUCING
ADDITIVES, USE ASEPTIC TECHNIQUE,
MIX THOROUGHLY AND DO NOT STORE.   —6
SINGLE-DOSE CONTAINER. FOR I.V. USE.
USUAL DOSAGE: SEE INSERT. STERILE,
NONPYROGENIC. USE ONLY IF
SOLUTION IS CLEAR AND CONTAINER IS   —7
UNDAMAGED. MUST NOT BE USED IN
SERIES CONNECTIONS.

Rx only   ♲(3)   (LATEX)   —8

©ABBOTT 2000   Ref. 59-0028-2/R4-10/99   PRINTED IN USA
ABBOTT LABORATORIES, NORTH CHICAGO, IL 60064, USA

—9

D

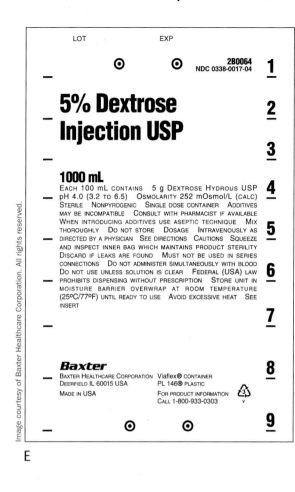

LOT   EXP

2B0064
NDC 0338-0017-04   **1**

5% Dextrose Injection USP

2

3

1000 mL   **4**

EACH 100 mL CONTAINS   5 g DEXTROSE HYDROUS USP
pH 4.0 (3.2 TO 6.5)   OSMOLARITY 252 mOsmol/L (CALC)
STERILE NONPYROGENIC SINGLE DOSE CONTAINER ADDITIVES
MAY BE INCOMPATIBLE   CONSULT WITH PHARMACIST IF AVAILABLE
WHEN INTRODUCING ADDITIVES USE ASEPTIC TECHNIQUE   MIX
THOROUGHLY   DO NOT STORE   DOSAGE   INTRAVENOUSLY AS   **5**
DIRECTED BY A PHYSICIAN   SEE DIRECTIONS   CAUTIONS   SQUEEZE
AND INSPECT INNER BAG WHICH MAINTAINS PRODUCT STERILITY
DISCARD IF LEAKS ARE FOUND   MUST NOT BE USED IN SERIES
CONNECTIONS   DO NOT ADMINISTER SIMULTANEOUSLY WITH BLOOD
DO NOT USE UNLESS SOLUTION IS CLEAR   FEDERAL (USA) LAW   **6**
PROHIBITS DISPENSING WITHOUT PRESCRIPTION   STORE UNIT IN
MOISTURE BARRIER OVERWRAP AT ROOM TEMPERATURE
(25°C/77°F) UNTIL READY TO USE   AVOID EXCESSIVE HEAT   SEE
INSERT

7

Baxter   **8**
BAXTER HEALTHCARE CORPORATION   Viaflex® CONTAINER
DEERFIELD IL 60015 USA   PL 146® PLASTIC
MADE IN USA   FOR PRODUCT INFORMATION
CALL 1-800-933-0303

9

E

LOT   EXP

2B1313
NDC 0338-0043-03   −**1**

0.45% Sodium Chloride Injection USP

−**2**

500 mL   −**3**

EACH 100 mL CONTAINS   450 mg SODIUM CHLORIDE USP
pH 5.0 (4.5 TO 7.0)   mEq/L SODIUM 77 CHLORIDE 77 HYPOTONIC
OSMOLARITY 154 mOsmol/L (CALC)   STERILE NONPYROGENIC SINGLE
DOSE CONTAINER   ADDITIVES MAY BE INCOMPATIBLE   CONSULT WITH
PHARMACIST IF AVAILABLE   WHEN INTRODUCING ADDITIVES USE ASEPTIC
TECHNIQUE   MIX THOROUGHLY   DO NOT STORE   DOSAGE   INTRAVENOUSLY
AS DIRECTED BY A PHYSICIAN   SEE DIRECTIONS   CAUTIONS   SQUEEZE AND   −**4**
INSPECT INNER BAG WHICH MAINTAINS PRODUCT STERILITY   DISCARD IF LEAKS
ARE FOUND   MUST NOT BE USED IN SERIES CONNECTIONS   DO NOT USE
UNLESS SOLUTION IS CLEAR   FEDERAL (USA) LAW PROHIBITS DISPENSING
WITHOUT PRESCRIPTION   STORE UNIT IN MOISTURE BARRIER OVERWRAP AT
ROOM TEMPERATURE (25°C/77°F) UNTIL READY TO USE   AVOID EXCESSIVE
HEAT   SEE INSERT

Baxter
BAXTER HEALTHCARE CORPORATION   Viaflex® CONTAINER
DEERFIELD IL 60015 USA   PL 146® PLASTIC
MADE IN USA   FOR PRODUCT INFORMATION
CALL 1-800-933-0303

F

⊟ 1000 mL   NDC 0074-7941-09

5% DEXTROSE and 0.9% SODIUM CHLORIDE Injection, USP

−1

−2

EACH 100 mL CONTAINS DEXTROSE,   −3
HYDROUS 5 g; SODIUM CHLORIDE
900 mg IN WATER FOR INJECTION.
ELECTROLYTES PER 1000 mL: SODIUM   −4
154 mEq; CHLORIDE 154 mEq.
560 mOsmol/LITER (CALC).
pH 4.3 (3.5 to 6.5).
ADDITIVES MAY BE INCOMPATIBLE.   −5
CONSULT WITH PHARMACIST, IF
AVAILABLE. WHEN INTRODUCING
ADDITIVES, USE ASEPTIC TECHNIQUE,
MIX THOROUGHLY AND DO NOT STORE.   −6
SINGLE-DOSE CONTAINER. FOR I.V. USE.
USUAL DOSAGE: SEE INSERT. STERILE,
NONPYROGENIC. USE ONLY IF
SOLUTION IS CLEAR AND CONTAINER IS   −7
UNDAMAGED. MUST NOT BE USED IN
SERIES CONNECTIONS.

Rx only ⟨3⟩ (LATEX)   −8

©ABBOTT 2000   Ref. 59-0035-2/R4-10/99   PRINTED IN USA
ABBOTT LABORATORIES, NORTH CHICAGO, IL 60064, USA

−9

G

⊟ 500 mL   NDC 0074-7929-03

LACTATED RINGER'S and 5% DEXTROSE Injection, USP

−1

EACH 100 mL CONTAINS DEXTROSE, HYDROUS 5 g; SODIUM
LACTATE, ANHYD. 310 mg; SODIUM CHLORIDE 600 mg;
POTASSIUM CHLORIDE 30 mg; CALCIUM CHLORIDE, DIHYDRATE
20 mg IN WATER FOR INJECTION. pH ADJUSTED WITH HCl.   −2
ELECTROLYTES PER 1000 mL (NOT INCLUDING pH ADJUSTMENT):
SODIUM 130 mEq; POTASSIUM 4 mEq; CALCIUM 3 mEq; CHLORIDE
109 mEq; LACTATE 28 mEq. 525 mOsmol/LITER (CALC). pH 4.9 (4.0
to 6.5). CAUTION: DO NOT ADMINISTER CALCIUM CONTAINING
SOLUTIONS CONCURRENTLY WITH STORED BLOOD. NOT FOR USE
IN THE TREATMENT OF LACTIC ACIDOSIS. ADDITIVES MAY BE
INCOMPATIBLE. CONSULT WITH PHARMACIST, IF AVAILABLE.
WHEN INTRODUCING ADDITIVES, USE ASEPTIC TECHNIQUE, MIX   −3
THOROUGHLY AND DO NOT STORE. SINGLE-DOSE CONTAINER.
FOR I.V. USE. USUAL DOSAGE: SEE INSERT. STERILE,
NONPYROGENIC. USE ONLY IF SOLUTION IS CLEAR AND
CONTAINER IS UNDAMAGED. MUST NOT BE USED IN SERIES
CONNECTIONS.

Rx only ⟨3⟩ (LATEX)
©ABBOTT 1999   Ref. 59-0001-2/R5-9/99   PRINTED IN USA   −4
ABBOTT LABORATORIES, NORTH CHICAGO, IL 60064, USA

H

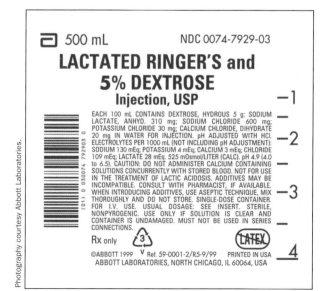

CALCULATING COMPONENTS OF IV SOLUTIONS WHEN EXPRESSED AS A PERCENT

Recall from Chapter 8 that solution strength expressed as a percent (%) indicates the number of g per 100 mL. Understanding this concept allows you to calculate the total amount of solute per IV order.

It is not necessary to perform this calculation each time you administer IV fluids, but this concept is important because it helps you understand that IV solutions provide much more than fluid. They also provide other components.

EXAMPLE 1 ■

Order: D_5W 1,000 mL IV q.8h

Calculate the amount of dextrose in 1,000 mL of D_5W.

This can be calculated using ratio-proportion.

Recall that percent indicates g per 100 mL; for example, D_5 is 5% dextrose or 5 g dextrose per 100 mL of solution.

$$\frac{5 \text{ g}}{100 \text{ mL}} \times \frac{X \text{ g}}{1,000 \text{ mL}}$$

$$100X = 5,000$$

$$\frac{100X}{100} = \frac{5,000}{100}$$

$$X = 50 \text{ g}$$

1,000 mL of D_5W contains 50 g of dextrose.

EXAMPLE 2 ■

Order: $D_5 \frac{1}{4}NS$ 500 mL IV q.6h

Calculate the amount of dextrose and sodium chloride in 500 mL of $D_5 \frac{1}{4}$ NS.

D_5 = dextrose 5% = 5 g dextrose per 100 mL

$$\frac{5 \text{ g}}{100 \text{ mL}} \times \frac{X \text{ g}}{500 \text{ mL}}$$

$$100X = 2,500$$

$$\frac{100X}{100} = \frac{2,500}{100}$$

$$X = 25 \text{ g (dextrose)}$$

$\frac{1}{4}NS$ = 0.225% NaCl = 0.225 g NaCl per 100 mL

(Recall that NS, or normal saline, is 0.9% NaCl; therefore, $\frac{1}{4}NS$ is $\frac{1}{4} \times 0.9\% = 0.225\%$ NaCl.)

$$\frac{0.225 \text{ g}}{100 \text{ mL}} \times \frac{X \text{ g}}{500 \text{ mL}}$$

$$100X = 112.5$$

$$\frac{100X}{100} = \frac{112.5}{100}$$

$$X = 1.125 \text{ g (NaCl)}$$

500 mL $D_5 \frac{1}{4}NS$ contains 25 g dextrose and 1.125 g sodium chloride.

Now you know what you are administering to your patient when IV solutions are prescribed, such as D₅W. Think, "I am hanging D₅W intravenous solution. Do I know what this fluid contains? Yes, it contains dextrose as the solute and water as the solvent in the concentration of 5 g of dextrose in every 100 mL of solution." Regular monitoring and careful understanding of intravenous infusions cannot be stressed enough.

QUICK REVIEW
- Solution concentration expressed as a percent is the number of g of solute per 100 mL solution.

Review Set 33

Calculate the amount of dextrose and/or sodium chloride in each of the following IV solutions.

1. 1,000 mL of D₅NS

   dextrose _____ g

   sodium chloride _____ g

2. 500 mL of D₅ $\frac{1}{2}$NS

   dextrose _____ g

   sodium chloride _____ g

3. 250 mL of D₁₀W

   dextrose _____ g

4. 750 mL of NS

   sodium chloride _____ g

5. 500 mL of D₅ 0.225% NaCl

   dextrose _____ g

   sodium chloride _____ g

6. 3 L of D₅NS

   dextrose _____ g

   sodium chloride _____ g

7. 0.5 L of D₁₀ $\frac{1}{4}$NS

   dextrose _____ g

   sodium chloride _____ g

8. 300 mL of D₁₂ 0.9% NaCl

   dextrose _____ g

   sodium chloride _____ g

9. 2 L of D₅ 0.225% NaCl

   dextrose _____ g

   sodium chloride _____ g

10. 0.75 L of 0.45% NaCl

   sodium chloride _____ g

After completing these problems, see page 701 to check your answers.

IV SITES

IV fluids may be ordered via a *peripheral line,* such as a vein in the arm or leg, or sometimes a scalp vein for infants, if other sites are inaccessible. Blood flowing through these veins can usually dilute the components in IV fluids. Glucose or dextrose is usually concentrated between 5% and 10% for short-term IV therapy. Peripheral veins can accommodate a maximum glucose concentration of 12%. The rate of infusion in peripheral veins should not exceed 200 mL in 1 hour.

IV fluids that are transparent flow smoothly into relatively small peripheral veins. When blood transfusion or replacement is needed, a larger vein is preferred to facilitate ease of blood flow. Whole blood or its components, especially packed cells, can be viscous and must be infused within a short period of time.

IV fluids may also be ordered via a *central line,* in which a special catheter is inserted to access a large vein, for example, in the chest. The subclavian vein may also be used for a central line. Central lines may be accessed either directly through the chest wall or indirectly via a neck vein or peripheral vein in the arm. If a peripheral vein is used to access a central vein, you may see the term *peripherally inserted central catheter* or *PICC line.* Larger veins can accommodate higher concentrations of glucose (up to 35%) and other nutrients and faster rates of IV fluids (greater than 200 mL in 1 hour). They are often utilized if the patient is expected to need IV therapy for an extended period.

 ## MONITORING IVs

The nurse is responsible for monitoring the patient regularly during an IV infusion.

 CAUTION

Generally, the IV site and infusion should be checked at least every 30 minutes to 1 hour (according to hospital policy) for the volume of remaining fluids, correct infusion rate, and signs of complications.

The major complications associated with IV therapy are phlebitis, infiltration, and infection at the IV site. *Phlebitis* occurs when the vein becomes irritated, red, or painful. (THINK: *warm and cordlike vein.*) *Infiltration* is when the IV catheter becomes dislodged from the vein and IV fluid escapes into the subcutaneous tissue. (THINK: *cool and puffy skin.*) Should phlebitis or infiltration occur, the IV is discontinued and another IV site is chosen to restart the IV. The patient should be instructed to notify the nurse of any pain or swelling.

PRIMARY AND SECONDARY IVs

Primary IV tubing packaging and set are shown in Figures 15-6, 15-7(a), and 15-7(b). This IV set is used for a typical or *primary IV.* Primary IV tubing includes a drip chamber, one or more injection ports, and a roller clamp and is long enough to be attached to the hub of the IV catheter positioned in the patient's vein. The drip chamber is squeezed until it is half full of IV fluid, and IV fluid is run through the tubing prior to attaching it to the IV catheter to ensure that no air is in the tubing. The nurse can either regulate the rate manually using the roller clamp (Figure 15-7a) or place the tubing in an electronic infusion pump (Figures 15-13 through 15-15).

Secondary IV tubing is used when giving medications. Secondary tubing is "piggybacked" into the primary line (Figure 15-8). This type of tubing generally is shorter and also contains a drip chamber and roller clamp. This gives access to the primary IV catheter without having to start another IV. You will notice that in this type of setup, the *secondary IV* set, or *piggyback,* is hung higher than the primary IV to allow the secondary set of medication to infuse first. When administering primary IV fluids, choose primary IV tubing; when hanging piggybacks, select secondary IV tubing. IV piggybacks are discussed further at the end of this chapter.

FIGURE 15-6   Primary intravenous infusion set package label

CLEARLINK System	**2C8541s**
CONTINU-FLO Solution Set with DUO-VENT Spike 105" (2.7 m) 3 Luer Activated Valves Male Luer Lock Adapter	**10** 10 drops/mL Approx.

FIGURE 15-7(a)   Standard straight gravity-flow IV system

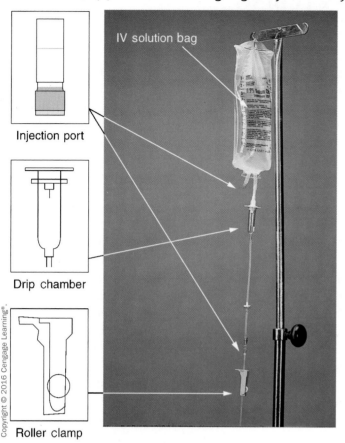

IV solution bag

Injection port

Drip chamber

Roller clamp

FIGURE 15-8   IV with piggyback (IV PB)

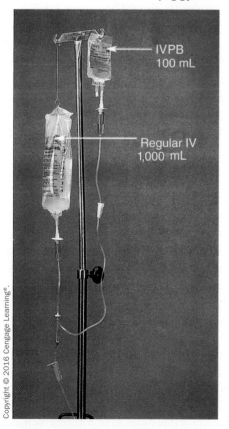

IVPB
100 mL

Regular IV
1,000 mL

FIGURE 15-7(b)   1 liter IV solution bag: The numerals 1–9 indicate 100 mL each: 1 = 100 mL, 2 = 200 mL . . . 9 = 900 mL, for a total IV solution volume of 1,000 mL

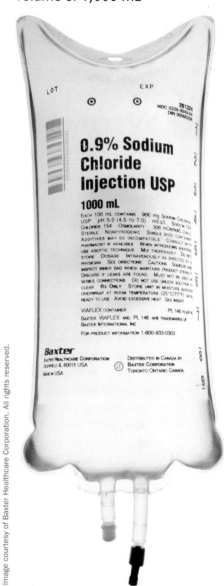

0.9% Sodium Chloride Injection USP

1000 mL

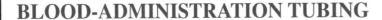

BLOOD-ADMINISTRATION TUBING

When blood is administered, a standard blood set (Figure 15-9) or a Y-type blood set (Figure 15-10) is commonly used. The "Y" refers to the two spikes that are attached above the drip chamber. One spike is attached to the blood container, and the other spike is attached to normal saline. Normal saline is used to dilute packed cells and to flush the IV tubing at the beginning and at the end of the transfusion. Blood is usually infused manually by gravity, and the roller clamp on the line is used to adjust the rate. Some electronic pumps may also be used for infusion of blood. In such cases, the nurse would program the pump in mL/h, and then the pump would regulate the blood infusion. Blood infusion is calculated the same as any other IV fluid.

IV FLOW RATE

The *flow rate* of an IV infusion is ordered by the physician. It is usually prescribed in mL/h and measured in mL/h or gtt/min. Later sections of this chapter will describe these calculations. It is the nurse's responsibility to regulate, monitor, and maintain this flow rate. Regulation of intravenous therapy is a critical skill in nursing. Because the fluids administered are infusing directly into the patient's circulatory system, careful monitoring is essential to be sure the patient does not receive too much or too little IV fluid and medication. It is also important for the nurse to accurately set and maintain the flow rate to administer the prescribed volume of the IV solution within the specified time period. The nurse records the IV fluids administered and IV flow rates on the IV administration record (IVAR) (Figure 15-11).

IV solutions are usually ordered for a certain volume to run for a stated period of time, such as *125 mL/h* or *1,000 mL q.8h.* The nurse will use electronic or manual regulating equipment to monitor the flow rate. The calculations you must perform to set the flow rate will depend on the equipment used to administer the IV solutions.

Nurses often label IV bags with a tape marking the infusion times (Figure 15-12), which provides a quick visual check if the IV is infusing on time as prescribed. These labels are attached to the IV bag and indicate the start and stop times of the infusion, as well as how the IV should be progressing. Each hour, from the start time to the stop time, the nurse should mark the label at the level where the solution should be. As a convenience, stock IV bags may be supplied with custom labels with pre-marked time intervals (Figure 15-12a). The hourly intervals are marked for liter bags infusing over 6, 8, 10, and 12 hours. Nurses may also use plain tape and mark the hourly time intervals manually (Figure 15-12b). The example in Figure 15-12 demonstrates an infusion tape adhered to a liter IV bag (1,000 mL) with a flow rate to be set at 25 gtt/min. The nurse intends to infuse the 1 L in 10 hours at 100 mL/h. Each hour is marked on the tape, beginning at 0700 (7:00 AM) when the IV started and ending at 1700 (5:00 PM) when the IV should be complete.

ELECTRONICALLY REGULATED IVs

Most often, IV solutions are regulated electronically by an infusion device—i.e., an IV pump. The use of an electronic IV pump will be determined by the need to strictly regulate the IV. Manufacturers supply special volumetric tubing that must be used with their infusion devices. This special tubing ensures accurate, consistent IV infusions. Each device can be set for a specific flow rate and will set off an alarm if this rate is interrupted. Electronic units today are powered by direct current (from a wall outlet) as well as an internal rechargeable battery. The battery takes over when the unit is unplugged to allow for portability and patient ambulation.

Infusion pumps represent significant threats to patient safety, with various performance problems leading to both over- and underinfusion, as well as delays in therapy administration. The U.S. Food and Drug Administration (FDA, 2010a) reported that from 2005 to 2009, infusion pump manufacturers recalled 87 different pumps to address safety issues. During the same period, the FDA received more than 56,000 adverse-event reports associated with IV pumps, including numerous injuries and deaths. Infusion

FIGURE 15-9 Standard blood set

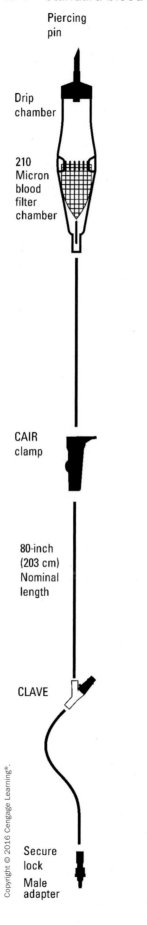

Piercing
pin

Drip
chamber

210
Micron
blood
filter
chamber

CAIR
clamp

80-inch
(203 cm)
Nominal
length

CLAVE

Secure
lock

Male
adapter

FIGURE 15-10 Y-type blood set

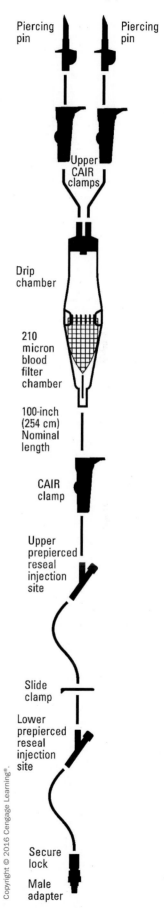

Piercing
pin

Piercing
pin

Upper
CAIR
clamps

Drip
chamber

210
micron
blood
filter
chamber

100-inch
(254 cm)
Nominal
length

CAIR
clamp

Upper
prepierced
reseal
injection
site

Slide
clamp

Lower
prepierced
reseal
injection
site

Secure
lock

Male
adapter

FIGURE 15-11 Intravenous administration record

Page: 1 of 1	I.V. Order	DATE: 11/10/xx through					
Correct		Rate	Time	Initial	Site / Infusion Port	Pump / Other	Tubing Change
✓	$D_5\frac{1}{2}NS$	100 mL/h	0900	GP	LH / PIV	☑ ✓	✓

CIRCULATORY ACCESS SITE

Time	Gauge	Length	Type	Site	# Attempts	Dressing Change	Site Condition	IV Lock	Initial	Time Catheter D/C Intact	Site Condition	Reason Code	Initial
0800	22	1½"	I	LH	1	✓	0	☐	GP				
								☐					
								☐					
								☐					

Type:
I - Insyte
B - Butterfly
C - Cathlon
CVC - CVC
T - Tunnelled
IP - Implanted Port
PICC - PICC
A - Arterial Line
SG - Swan Ganz
DL - Dual Lumen Peripheral
UAC - UAC
UVC - UVC

Site:
L - Left
R - Right
H - Hand
FA - Forearm
UA - Upper Arm
SC - Subclavian
C - Chest

A - Antecubital
F - Femoral
J - Jugular
FT - Foot
S - Scalp
U - Umbilical
RA - Radial

Dressing Change:
T - Transparent
A - Air Occlusive
B - Bandaid
PR - Pressure Dressing

Reason Code:
1 - Infiltrate
2 - Physician Order
3 - Patient Removed
4 - Clotted
5 - Phlebitis
6 - Site Rotation
7 - Leaking
8 - Positional
9 - Not Patent
10 - Family Refused
Other:
D - Dial-a-flow

Infusion Port:
PIV - Peripheral IV
CVC - CVC
SG - Swan Ganz
D - Distal
M - Middle
P - Proximal
R - Red
BL - Blue
V - Venous
S - Sideport
AN - Access Needle
A - Arterial

Site Condition:
0
1+
2+
3+
4+
5+

Tubing Change:
P - Primary
S - Secondary
E - Extension
T - 3 Way Stopcock
H - Hemodynamic

ALLERGIES: NKA

Initial / Signature - Circulatory Access Site(s) checked hourly.
GP / G. Pickar, R.N. ____ / ____
____ / ____ ____ / ____
____ / ____ ____ / ____
Reconciled by: _____

Smith, James   43y   M

Dr. Jones   Medical Service

Admitted   11-10-xx   Rm 237-1

Adm. # 6634297

IV ADMINISTRATION RECORD

FIGURE 15-12(a)   Section of
1 liter (1,000 mL) IV bag labeled
with pre-marked custom tape

FIGURE 15-12(b)   Section of
1 liter (1,000 mL) IV bag labeled
with plain tape

Follow the marking in the white
column to infuse 1 liter in 10 h.

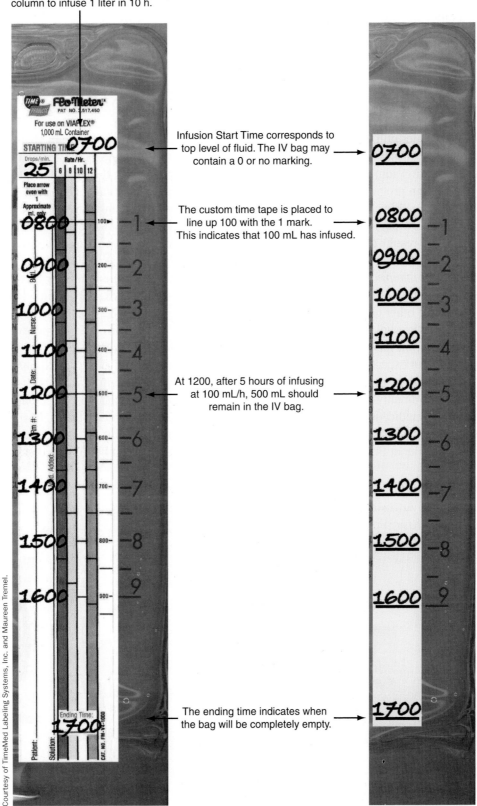

Infusion Start Time corresponds to
top level of fluid. The IV bag may
contain a 0 or no marking.

The custom time tape is placed to
line up 100 with the 1 mark.
This indicates that 100 mL has infused.

At 1200, after 5 hours of infusing
at 100 mL/h, 500 mL should
remain in the IV bag.

The ending time indicates when
the bag will be completely empty.

pump efficacy is an ongoing concern of the FDA. The organization closely monitors problems with infusion pumps and maintains an active web site for clinicians, pharmacists, product engineers, managers, and patients. The site includes examples of current pump safety issues; such as, software problems, alarm errors, inadequate user interface design, broken components, battery failures, fire, sparks, and shocks (FDA, 2014). While infusion pumps are designed to improve patient safety and provide more accurate delivery of IV therapy, they can present serious problems.

There are several strategies recommended by the FDA (2010b) to reduce patient risk when using infusion pumps: planning ahead, labeling, and frequent checking. Planning ahead includes having a backup plan to replace IV pumps with mechanical or electrical failures, such as maintaining a backup unit or temporarily switching to a manually regulated IV, and calling on another nurse to monitor a high-acuity patient while securing an alternate infusion device. Labeling the IV bag with time-strip indicators (Figure 15-12) and using intermittent volume control devices (Figure 16-3, page 538) are two other plan-ahead strategies utilized to ensure safe and accurate IV therapy. IV fluid and medication labels should be prominently displayed on the infusion pump and the tubing at the port of entry. Apply the Six Rights of safe medication administration to IV pumps: right patient is getting the right fluid and medication via the right IV pump programmed to deliver the right dosage at the right rate and volume with the right documentation. Double-check high-alert drugs such as heparin or insulin with another clinician; this is especially critical when infusing with an IV pump. Double-checks should be done alone and apart from one another, and results compared. Finally, careful patient and device monitoring for over- or underinfusion and per your facility's required time frames will reduce risk of serious patient injury.

Infusion pumps (Figure 15-13) do not rely on gravity but maintain the flow by displacing fluid at the prescribed rate. Resistance to flow within the system causes positive pressure in relation to the flow rate. The nurse or other user may preset a pressure-alarm threshold. When the pressure sensed by the device reaches this threshold, the device stops pumping and sets off an alarm. The amount of change in pressure that results from infiltration or phlebitis may be insufficient to reach the alarm threshold. Therefore, users should not expect the device to stop infusing in the presence of these conditions.

A *syringe pump* (Figure 15-14) is a type of electronic infusion pump. It is used to infuse fluids or medications directly from a syringe. It is most often used in the neonatal and pediatric areas when small volumes of medication are delivered at low rates. It is also used in anesthesia, hospice, labor and delivery, and critical care when the drug cannot be mixed with other solutions or medications or to reduce the volume of diluent fluid delivered to the patient. Syringe pumps can be regulated using up to 16 different

FIGURE 15-13 Alaris® system with large-volume infusion pumps and Auto-ID module for medication administration (primary infusion pump and two secondary pumps)

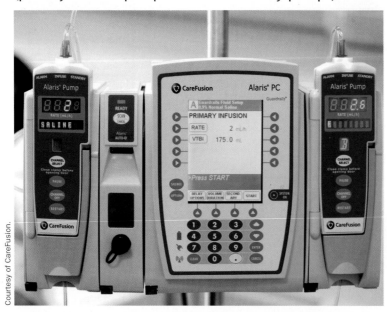

Courtesy of CareFusion.

FIGURE 15-14(a) Alaris® system with syringe
module used in neonatal unit

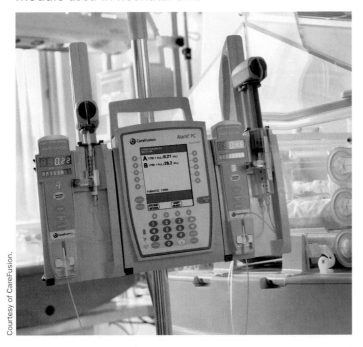

Courtesy of CareFusion.

FIGURE 15-14(b) Syringe pump

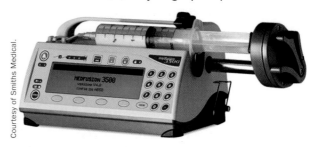

Courtesy of Smiths Medical.

modes, including mL/h, volume/time, dose or body-weight modes, mass modes such as units/h, and other specialty modes.

A *patient-controlled analgesia (PCA) pump* (Figure 15-15) is used to allow the patient to self-administer IV medication to control postoperative and other types of severe pain. The physician or other prescribing practitioner orders the pain medication, which is contained in a prefilled syringe locked securely in the IV pump. The patient presses the control button and receives the pain medication immediately rather than waiting for someone to bring it. The dose, frequency, and a safety "lock out" time are

FIGURE 15-15(a) Alaris® system with PCA (patient-controlled analgesia) module, along with pump module for use as primary and secondary infusions and physiological respiratory monitoring modules

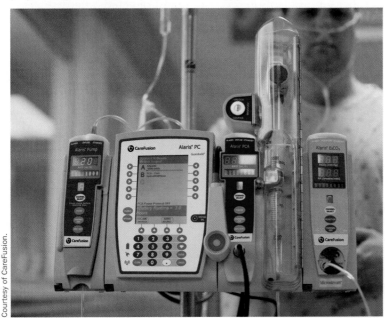

Courtesy of CareFusion.

FIGURE 15-15(b) Syndeo PCA (patient-controlled analgesia) syringe pump

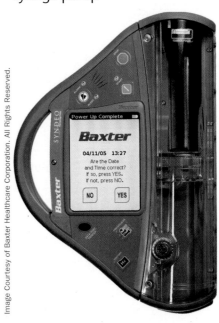

Image Courtesy of Baxter Healthcare Corporation. All Rights Reserved.

ordered and programmed into the pump, which delivers an individual therapeutic dose. The pump stores information about the frequency and dosage of the drug requested by and delivered to the patient. The nurse can display this information to document and evaluate pain-management effectiveness.

CAUTION

All electronic infusion devices must be monitored frequently (at least every 30 minutes to 1 hour) to ensure proper and safe functioning. Check the policy in your facility.

CALCULATING FLOW RATES FOR INFUSION PUMPS IN mL/h

When an electronic infusion pump is used, the IV volume is ordered by the physician and programmed into the device by the nurse. These devices are regulated in mL/h. Usually, the physician orders the IV volume to be delivered in mL/h. If not, the nurse must calculate it.

RULE

To regulate an IV volume by electronic infusion pump calibrated in mL/h, calculate:

$$\frac{\text{Total mL ordered}}{\text{Total h ordered}} = \text{mL/h}$$ (rounded to a whole number or tenths, depending on equipment)

or use ratio-proportion: $\frac{\text{Total mL}}{\text{Total h}} = \frac{\text{X mL}}{\text{1 h}}$

CAUTION

Some IV pumps are capable of delivering IV fluids in tenths of a milliliter. Check the equipment you have available before deciding to round flow rates to whole milliliters per hour (mL/h). For this text, we will assume that the equipment you have available is programmable in whole milliliters only, so you should round mL/h to a whole number for problems in this text, unless directed otherwise.

EXAMPLE ■

Order reads: D₅W 250 mL IV *over the next 2 h by infusion pump*

Step 1	**Think**	The pump is set by the rate of mL per hour. So, if 250 mL is to be infused in 2 hours, how much will be infused in 1 hour? Yes, 125 mL will be infused in 1 hour. You would set the pump at 125 mL per hour.
Step 2	**Calculate**	Use the formula:

$$\frac{\text{Total mL ordered}}{\text{Total h ordered}} = \text{mL/h}$$

$$\frac{\overset{125}{\cancel{250}} \text{ mL}}{\underset{1}{\cancel{2}} \text{ h}} = \frac{125 \text{ mL}}{1 \text{ h}} = 125 \text{ mL/h}$$

Therefore, set the pump at 125 mL per hour (125 mL/h).

This can also be solved using the ratio-proportion method. In fact, the formula *is* a ratio-proportion. Let's look at this more closely.

The ratio-proportion method used to calculate mL/h looks almost the same as the formula method.

$$\frac{\text{Total mL}}{\text{Total h}} = \frac{\text{X mL}}{1\text{ h}}$$

$$\frac{250\text{ mL}}{2\text{ h}} \diagup\!\!\!\!\diagdown \frac{\text{X mL}}{1\text{ h}}$$

$$2\text{X} = 250$$

$$\frac{2\text{X}}{250} = \frac{250}{250}$$

$$\text{X} = 125\text{ mL (per 1 hour)}$$

But, the formula to divide *total mL* by *total h* is quite simple. You can use either formula or ratio-proportion.

In most cases it is easy to calculate mL/h by dividing total mL by total h. However, an IV with medication added or an IV PB may be ordered to be administered in *less than 1 hour* by an electronic infusion device, but the pump must still be set in mL/h.

RULE

$$\frac{\text{Total mL ordered}}{\text{Total min ordered}} = \frac{\text{X mL/h}}{60\text{ min/h}}$$

X = mL/h (rounded to a whole number or tenths, depending on equipment)

EXAMPLE ▪

Order: *ampicillin 500 mg IV in 50 mL D$_5$ $\frac{1}{2}$NS in 30 min by infusion pump*

Step 1   **Think**   The infusion pump is set at the rate of mL per hour. If 50 mL is to be infused in 30 minutes, then 100 mL will be infused in 60 minutes, because 100 mL is twice as much as 50 mL and 60 minutes is twice as much as 30 minutes. Set the rate of the infusion pump at 100 mL/h to infuse 50 mL per 30 min.

Step 2   **Calculate** $\dfrac{\text{Total mL ordered}}{\text{Total min ordered}} = \dfrac{\text{X mL/h}}{60\text{ min/h}}$

$$\frac{50\text{ mL}}{30\text{ min}} \diagup\!\!\!\!\diagdown \frac{\text{X mL/h}}{60\text{ min/h}}$$

$$30\text{X} = 3{,}000$$

$$\frac{30\text{X}}{30} = \frac{3{,}000}{30}$$

$$\text{X} = 100\text{ mL/h}$$

CAUTION

Typical values of mL/h to expect in calculations are in the range of 50 to 200 mL/h. Use this guideline as part of checking for reasonable answers.

QUICK REVIEW

For electronic infusion regulators:

- $\dfrac{\text{Total mL ordered}}{\text{Total h ordered}} = \text{mL/h}$

- If the infusion time is less than 1 hour, then
  $\dfrac{\text{Total mL ordered}}{\text{Total min ordered}} = \dfrac{\text{X mL/h}}{60\text{ min/h}}$

- Round mL/h to a whole number or tenths, depending on equipment.

Review Set 34

Calculate the flow rate at which you will program the electronic infusion pump for the following IV orders.

1. D$_5$W 1 L IV to infuse in 10 h

   Flow rate: _____ mL/h

2. NS 1,800 mL IV to infuse in 15 h

   Flow rate: _____ mL/h

3. D$_5$W 2,000 mL IV in 24 h

   Flow rate: _____ mL/h

4. NS 100 mL IV PB in 30 min

   Flow rate: _____ mL/h

5. antibiotic in 30 mL D$_5$W IV in 15 min

   Flow rate: _____ mL/h

6. NS 2.5 L IV in 20 h

   Flow rate: _____ mL/h

7. D$_5$LR 500 mL IV in 4 h

   Flow rate: _____ mL/h

8. 0.45% NaCl 600 mL IV in 3 h

   Flow rate: _____ mL/h

9. antibiotic in 150 mL D$_5$W IV in 2 h

   Flow rate: _____ mL/h

10. NS 3 L IV in 24 h

    Flow rate: _____ mL/h

11. LR injection 1.5 L IV in 24 h

    Flow rate: _____ mL/h

12. D$_{10}$W 240 mL IV in 10 h

    Flow rate: _____ mL/h

13. D$_5$W 750 mL IV in 5 h

    Flow rate: _____ mL/h

14. D$_5$NS 1.5 L IV in 12 h

    Flow rate: _____ mL/h

15. D$_5$ 0.45% NaCl 380 mL IV in 9 h

    Flow rate: _____ mL/h

After completing these problems, see pages 701–702 to check your answers.

MANUALLY REGULATED IVs

As a backup to an IV pump, or when an electronic infusion pump is unavailable, the clinician can use a standard straight gravity-flow IV system to administer fluids, medications, and nutrients. In this case, the nurse must manually regulate the IV flow rate. To do this, the nurse must calculate the ordered IV rate based on a certain *number of drops per minute (gtt/min)*. This actually represents the ordered milliliters per hour, as you will shortly see in the calculation.

The number of drops falling per minute into the IV drip chamber (Figures 15-7a and 15-16) is counted and regulated by opening or closing the roller clamp. You place your digital or analog watch with a second hand at the level of the drip chamber and count the drops as they fall during a 1-minute period or fraction thereof (referred to as the *watch count*). This manual, gravity-flow rate depends on the IV tubing calibration, called the *drop factor*.

RULE
Drop factor = gtt/mL

The drop factor is the number of drops per milliliter (gtt/mL) that a particular IV tubing set will deliver. It is determined by the size of the tubing or needle releasing the drops into the drip chamber (Figure 15-16).

FIGURE 15-16   Intravenous drip chambers; comparison of (a) macrodrops and (b) microdrops

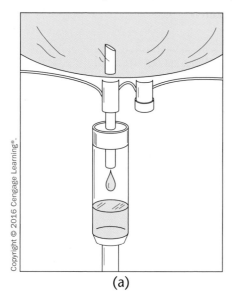
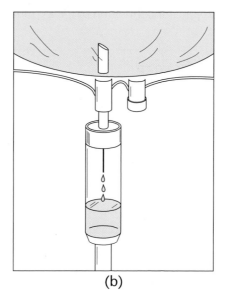

(a)   (b)

The drop factor is stated on the IV tubing package and varies according to the manufacturer of the IV equipment. For example, the tubing depicted in Figure 15-6 delivers 10 gtt/mL. The wider tubing delivers larger drops (macrodrops); therefore, there are fewer drops in 1 mL (Figure 15-16a). The small needle delivers very small drops; therefore, there are many drops in 1 mL (Figure 15-16b). The standard microdrop IV tubing is available in various sizes that deliver 10, 15, or 20 drops per mL (gtt/mL). The microdrop tubing delivers 60 gtt/mL. Hospitals typically stock one macrodrop tubing for routine adult IV administration and the microdrop tubing for situations requiring more exact measurement or to manage a very slow infusion rate.

Figure 15-16 compares macrodrops and microdrops. Figure 15-17 illustrates the size and number of drops in 1 mL for each drop factor. Notice that the fewer the number of drops per milliliter, the larger the actual drop size.

QUICK REVIEW
- Drop factor = gtt/mL
- The drop factor is stated on the IV tubing package.
- Macrodrop factors: 10, 15, or 20 gtt/mL
- Microdrop factor: 60 gtt/mL

FIGURE 15-17   Comparison of calibrated drop factors (enlarged to show detail)

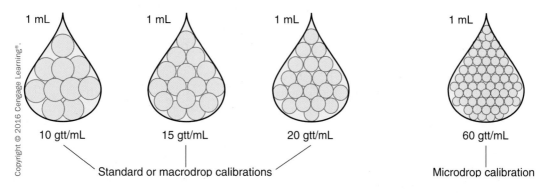

Review Set 35

Identify the drop factor calibration of the IV tubing pictured.

▣ **LATEX-FREE**   No. 4967

PRIMARY I.V. SET,
Convertible Pin, 80 Inch
with Backcheck Valve
and 2 Injection Sites
Piggyback

1. _____ gtt/mL

▣ **LifeShield®** *LATEX-FREE*   No. 11409

HEMA® II Y-TYPE BLOOD SET,
Nonvented, 100 Inch
with 2 Prepierced Injection Sites
and Secure Lock

2. _____ gtt/mL

CLEARLINK System

CONTINU-FLO Solution Set   2C6546s

105" (2.7 m)
3 Injection Sites
Male Luer Lock Adapter
with Retractable Collar

**60 drops/mL
Approx.**

3. _____ gtt/mL

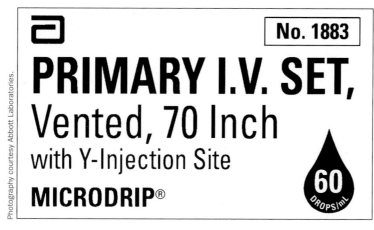

4. _____ gtt/mL

CLEARLINK System

CONTINU-FLO Solution Set 2C6541s
with DUO-VENT Spike
106" (2.7 m), 3 Injection Sites
Male Luer Lock Adapter

10
10 drops/mL
Approx.

5. _____ gtt/mL

After completing these problems, see page 702 to check your answers.

CALCULATING FLOW RATES FOR MANUALLY-REGULATED IVs IN gtt/min

In this section, you will learn two methods to calculate IV flow rate for manually-regulated IVs: the formula method and the shortcut method.

Formula Method

The formula method can be used to determine the flow rate in drops per minute (gtt/min).

RULE

The formula method to calculate IV flow rate for manually regulated IVs ordered in mL/h or for a prescribed number of minutes is:

$$\frac{V}{T} \times C = R$$

$$\frac{\text{Volume (mL)}}{\text{Time (min)}} \times \text{Calibration or drop factor (gtt/mL)} = \text{Rate (gtt/min)}$$

In this formula:

V: *volume to be infused* designated in mL; ordered by the prescriber (primary infusion) or recommended by the pharmacist or a drug reference guide (such as for an IV PB medication)

T: *time required to infuse V,* converted to minutes; ordered by the prescriber (primary infusion) or recommended by the pharmacist or a drug reference guide (such as for an IV PB medication)

C: *calibration of tubing* (drop factor) in gtt/mL; noted on package

R: *rate of flow* in gtt/min. THINK: the unknown is the watch count.

The rate of IV fluid and IV medications is expressed as a specific volume to be infused in a certain time period. Most IV fluid orders are written as X mL/h, which means X mL in 60 minutes. However, some IV medications are to be administered in less than 1 hour—for example, over 30 minutes.

MATH TIP

When using the formula method to calculate IV flow rates, carry calculations to one decimal place. Round gtt/min to the nearest whole number, because you can watch count only whole drops.

Let's look at some examples of how to calculate the flow rate or watch count in gtt/min.

EXAMPLE 1 ■

The physician orders D_5W 1 L IV at 125 mL/h. The infusion set is calibrated for a drop factor of 10 gtt/mL. Calculate the IV flow rate in gtt/min. Notice that the mL units cancel out, leaving gtt/min.

$$\frac{V}{T} \times C = \frac{125 \text{ mL}}{60 \text{ min}} \times 10 \text{ gtt/mL} = \frac{125 \text{ mL}}{\underset{6}{60} \text{ min}} \times \frac{\overset{1}{10} \text{ gtt}}{1 \text{ mL}} = \frac{125 \text{ gtt}}{6 \text{ min}} = 20.8 \text{ gtt/min} = 21 \text{ gtt/min}$$

Use your watch to count the drops, and adjust the roller clamp to deliver 21 gtt/min.

EXAMPLE 2 ■

Order: **Lactated Ringer's 500 mL IV at 150 mL/h.** The drop factor is 15 gtt/mL.

$$\frac{V}{T} \times C = \frac{150 \text{ mL}}{\underset{4}{60} \text{ min}} \times \overset{1}{15} \text{ gtt/mL} = \frac{150 \text{ gtt}}{4 \text{ min}} = 37.5 \text{ gtt/min} = 38 \text{ gtt/min}$$

EXAMPLE 3 ■

Order: **ampicillin 500 mg IV in 100 mL of NS to infuse over 45 min**

The drop factor is 20 gtt/mL. Notice that the time is less than 1 hour. Also notice that the 500 mg does not figure into the flow rate calculations, because it is the dosage of ampicillin dissolved in the IV fluid. Only the *total volume of 100 mL* is needed to complete the calculations.

$$\frac{V}{T} \times C = \frac{100 \text{ mL}}{45 \text{ min}} \times 20 \text{ gtt/mL} = \frac{2,000 \text{ gtt}}{45 \text{ min}} = 44.4 \text{ gtt/min} = 44 \text{ gtt/min}$$

MATH TIP

When the IV drop factor is 60 gtt/mL (microdrop sets), then the calculated flow rate in gtt/min will result in the same number as the volume ordered in mL/h.

EXAMPLE 4 ■

Order: D_5NS 500 mL IV at 50 mL/h. The drop factor is 60 gtt/mL.

$$\frac{V}{T} \times C = \frac{50 \text{ mL}}{\underset{1}{60} \text{ min}} \times \overset{1}{60} \text{ gtt/mL} = 50 \text{ gtt/min}$$

Notice that the order of 50 mL/h is the *same* as the flow rate of 50 gtt/min when the drop factor is 60 gtt/mL. This will always be the rule when the drop factor is 60 gtt/mL.

Sometimes the prescriber will order a total IV volume to be infused over a total number of hours. In such cases, first calculate the mL/h (rounded to tenths), then calculate gtt/min (rounded to a whole number).

RULE

The formula method to calculate IV flow rate for manually-regulated IVs ordered in total volume and total hours is:

Step 1 $\frac{\text{Total mL}}{\text{Total hours}}$ = mL/h (round result to tenths)

Step 2 $\frac{V}{T} \times C = R$ (round result to a whole number)

EXAMPLE ■

Order: NS IV 3,000 mL per 24 h. Drop factor is 15 gtt/min.

Step 1 $\frac{\text{Total mL}}{\text{Total h}} = \frac{3,000 \text{ mL}}{24 \text{ h}} = 125 \text{ mL/h}$

Step 2 $\frac{V}{T} \times C = R$

$\frac{125 \text{ mL}}{60 \text{ min}} \times 15 \text{ gtt/mL} = \frac{125 \text{ mL}}{\underset{4}{60} \text{ min}} \times \frac{\overset{1}{15} \text{ gtt}}{1 \text{ mL}} = \frac{125 \text{ gtt}}{4 \text{ min}} = 31.2 \text{ gtt/min} = 31 \text{ gtt/min}$

CAUTION

Typical values of gtt/min to expect in calculations are in the range of 20 to 100 gtt/min. Use this guideline as part of checking for reasonable answers.

QUICK REVIEW

■ The formula method to calculate the flow rate, or watch count, in gtt/min for manually-regulated IV rates ordered in mL/h or mL/min is:

$\frac{V}{T} \times C = R$: $\frac{\text{Volume (mL)}}{\text{Time (min)}} \times$ Calibration or drop factor (gtt/mL) = Rate (gtt/min)

■ When total volume and total hours are ordered, first calculate mL/h.

■ When the IV drop factor is 60 gtt/mL (microdrop sets), then the calculated flow rate in gtt/min will result in the same number as the volume ordered in mL/h.

■ Round gtt/min to a whole number. You can only count whole drops.

Review Set 36

1. State the rule for the formula method that is used to calculate IV flow rate in gtt/min when mL/h are known. _____

Calculate the flow rate or watch count in gtt/min.

2. Order: D$_5$W 3,000 mL IV at 125 mL/h

   Drop factor: 10 gtt/mL

   _____ gtt/min

3. Order: LR 250 mL IV at 50 mL/h

   Drop factor: 60 gtt/mL

   _____ gtt/min

4. Order: **NS 100 mL bolus IV to infuse in 60 min**

   Drop factor: 20 gtt/mL

   _____ gtt/min

5. Order: **$D_5\frac{1}{2}$NS IV with 20 mEq KCl per liter to run at 25 mL/h**

   Drop factor: 60 gtt/mL

   _____ gtt/min

6. Order: **two 500 mL units of whole blood IV to be infused in 4 h**

   Drop factor: 20 gtt/mL

   _____ gtt/min

7. Order: **$D_5\frac{1}{4}$NS 1 L to infuse in 6 h**

   Drop factor: 15 gtt/mL

   _____ gtt/min

8. Order: **D_5NS 1 L IV at 150 mL/h**

   Drop factor: 20 gtt/mL

   _____ gtt/min

9. Order: **NS 150 mL bolus IV to infuse in 45 min**

   Drop factor: 15 gtt/mL

   _____ gtt/min

10. Order: **D_5W antibiotic solution 80 mL IV to infuse in 60 min**

    Drop factor: 60 gtt/mL

    _____ gtt/min

11. Order: **packed red blood cells 480 mL IV to infuse in 4 h**

    Drop factor: 10 gtt/mL

    _____ gtt/min

12. Order: **D_5W IV at 120 mL/h**

    Drop factor: 15 gtt/mL

    _____ gtt/min

13. Order: **D_5 0.45% NaCl IV at 50 mL/h**

    Drop factor: 20 gtt/mL

    _____ gtt/min

14. Order: **LR 2,500 mL IV at 165 mL/h**

    Drop factor: 20 gtt/mL

    _____ gtt/min

15. Order: **D_5LR 3,500 mL IV to run at 160 mL/h**

    Drop factor: 15 gtt/mL

    _____ gtt/min

After completing these problems, see page 702 to check your answers.

Shortcut Method

By converting the volume and time in the formula method to mL per h (or mL per 60 min), you can use a shortcut to calculate flow rate. This shortcut is derived from the number in the drop factor (C), which cancels out each time and reduces the 60 min (T). You are left with the *drop factor constant*. Look at these examples.

EXAMPLE 1 ■

Administer **normal saline 1,000 mL IV at 125 mL/h** with a microdrop infusion set calibrated for 60 gtt/mL. Use the formula $\frac{V}{T} \times C = R$.

$$\frac{V}{T} \times C = \frac{125 \text{ mL}}{60 \text{ min}} \times 60 \text{ gtt/mL} = \frac{125 \text{ gtt}}{1 \text{ min}} = 125 \text{ gtt/min}$$

The drop factor constant for an infusion set with 60 gtt/mL is 1. Therefore, to administer 125 mL/h, set the flow rate at 125 gtt/min. Recall that when the drop factor is 60, then the number of gtt/min = the number of mL/h.

EXAMPLE 2 ■

Administer NS 1,000 mL IV at 125 mL/h with 20 gtt/mL infusion set.

$$\frac{V}{T} \times C = \frac{125 \text{ mL}}{\underset{3}{60} \text{ min}} \times \overset{1}{20} \text{ gtt/mL} = \frac{125 \text{ gtt}}{③ \text{ min}} = 41.6 \text{ gtt/min} = 42 \text{ gtt/min}$$

Drop factor constant = 3

Each drop factor constant is obtained by dividing 60 by the drop factor calibration from the infusion set.

REMEMBER

Drop Factor	Drop Factor Constant
10 gtt/mL	$\frac{60}{10} = 6$
15 gtt/mL	$\frac{60}{15} = 4$
20 gtt/mL	$\frac{60}{20} = 3$
60 gtt/mL	$\frac{60}{60} = 1$

Most hospitals consistently use infusion equipment manufactured by one company. Each manufacturer typically supplies one macrodrop and one microdrop system. You will become familiar with the supplier used where you work; therefore, the shortcut method is practical, quick, and simple to use.

RULE

The shortcut method to calculate IV flow rate is:

$$\frac{\text{mL/h}}{\text{Drop factor constant}} = \text{gtt/min}$$

Let's review four examples using the shortcut method.

EXAMPLE 1 ■

Order reads: D₅W 1,000 mL IV at 125 mL/h. The infusion set is calibrated for a drop factor of 10 gtt/mL. Drop factor constant: 6

$$\frac{\text{mL/h}}{\text{Drop factor constant}} = \text{gtt/min}$$

$$\frac{125 \text{ mL/h}}{6} = 20.8 \text{ gtt/min} = 21 \text{ gtt/min}$$

EXAMPLE 2 ■

Order reads: LR 1,000 mL IV at 150 mL/h. The drop factor is 15 gtt/mL. Drop factor constant: 4

$$\frac{\text{mL/h}}{\text{Drop factor constant}} = \text{gtt/min}$$

$$\frac{150 \text{ mL/h}}{4} = 37.5 \text{ gtt/min} = 38 \text{ gtt/min}$$

EXAMPLE 3 ■

Order reads: D₅ $\frac{1}{2}$NS 200 mL IV in 2 h. The drop factor is 20 gtt/mL. Drop factor constant: 3

Step 1 $\frac{\text{Total mL}}{\text{Total h}} = \text{mL/h}$

$$\frac{200}{2} = 100 \text{ mL/h}$$

Step 2 $\dfrac{\text{mL/h}}{\text{Drop factor constant}} = \text{gtt/min}$

$$\dfrac{100 \text{ mL/h}}{3} = 33.3 \text{ gtt/min} = 33 \text{ gtt/min}$$

EXAMPLE 4 ■

Order reads: D₅NS 500 mL IV at 50 mL/h. The drop factor is 60 gtt/mL. Drop factor constant: 1

$$\dfrac{\text{mL/h}}{\text{Drop factor constant}} = \text{gtt/min}$$

$$\dfrac{50 \text{ mL/h}}{1} = 50 \text{ gtt/min}$$

Remember: When the drop factor is 60 (microdrop), set the flow rate at the same number of gtt/min as the number of mL/h.

CAUTION

For the shortcut method to work, the rate has to be written in mL/h. The shortcut method will not work if the time is less than 1 hour or is calculated in minutes, such as 30 or 90 minutes.

QUICK REVIEW

■ The drop factor constant is 60 divided by the drop factor.

Drop Factor	Drop Factor Constant
10 gtt/mL	6
15 gtt/mL	4
20 gtt/mL	3
60 gtt/mL	1 → Set the flow rate at the same number of gtt/min as the number of mL/h.

■ $\dfrac{\text{mL/h}}{\text{Drop factor constant}} = \text{gtt/min}$

Review Set 37

1. The drop factor constant is derived by dividing _____ by the drop factor calibration.

Determine the drop factor constant for each of the following infusion sets.

2. 60 gtt/mL _____

3. 20 gtt/mL _____

4. 15 gtt/mL _____

5. 10 gtt/mL _____

6. State the rule for the shortcut method to calculate the IV flow rate in gtt/min. _____

_____

Calculate the IV flow rate in gtt/min using the shortcut method.

7. Order: D₅W 1,000 mL IV to infuse at 200 mL/h

   Drop factor: 15 gtt/mL

   Flow rate: _____ gtt/min

8. Order: D₅W 750 mL IV to infuse at 125 mL/h

   Drop factor: 20 gtt/mL

   Flow rate: _____ gtt/min

9. Order: D₅W 0.45% saline 500 mL IV to infuse at 165 mL/h

   Drop factor: 10 gtt/mL

   Flow rate: _____ gtt/min

10. Order: NS 2 L IV to infuse at 60 mL/h

    Drop factor: microdrop infusion set

    Flow rate: _____ gtt/min

11. Order: D₅W 400 mL IV to infuse at 50 mL/h

    Drop factor: 10 gtt/mL

    Flow rate: _____ gtt/min

12. Order: NS 3 L IV to infuse at 125 mL/h

    Drop factor: 15 gtt/mL

    Flow rate: _____ gtt/min

13. Order: D₅LR 500 mL IV to infuse in 6 h

    Drop factor: 20 gtt/mL

    Flow rate: _____ gtt/min

14. Order: 0.45% NaCl 0.5 L IV to infuse in 20 h

    Drop factor: 60 gtt/mL

    Flow rate: _____ gtt/min

15. Order: D₅ 0.9% NaCl 650 mL IV to infuse in 10 h

    Drop factor: 10 gtt/mL

    Flow rate: _____ gtt/min

After completing these problems, see page 702 to check your answers.

CALCULATING FLOW RATES FOR MANUALLY-REGULATED IVs USING A DIAL-FLOW CONTROLLER

Regulating IV flow rate by adjusting the roller clamp is simple to do, but usually requires a few readjustments until the desired flow rate is achieved. A dial-flow controller is widely used to reduce the inconvenience and time spent with the repeated estimation of the required tightness of the roller clamp. These controllers work on the same principles as the roller clamp, but the addition of a dial with numbers on it helps to take out some of the guesswork when adjusting the flow. While dial-flow controllers are widely used as a cost-saving alternative to electronic infusion devices, dial-flow controllers have not been shown to be more accurate than a general IV set alone. Inconsistencies may still result from differences in the height of the IV and level of remaining fluid in the bag.

CAUTION

Dial-flow controllers are convenient, time-saving devices for manually regulated IVs. Flow rate calibrations in mL/h on the dial are estimates and must be verified by drop count. Failure to verify drop rate may result in insufficient or excessive intravenous infusions.

There is a wide variety of dial-flow controllers available for use. Some are supplied as complete infusion sets (Figure 15-18a) and others as extension tubing (Figure 15-18b). Controller dials may be fully closed or open for free flow and are marked with a range of adjustable flow rates as slow as 5–10 mL/h to rapid rates as fast as 250 mL/h (Figure 15-18c). Flow rates may be easily set up initially without relying on the drip chamber by simply turning the dial to a gradation mark corresponding to the desired rate. The numbers on the dial provide an approximate flow rate. However, the drops still need to be counted to check if the flow rate determined by the position of the dial is accurate. Numerals on the dial should be considered estimates and be verified by drip count.

FIGURE 15-18   Examples of dial-flow controllers: **(a)** complete infusion set; **(b)** extension tubing; **(c)** controller settings

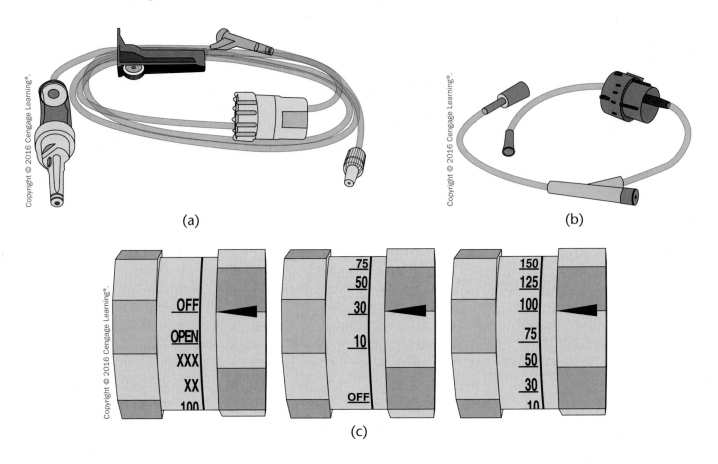

(a)   (b)

(c)

EXAMPLE 1 ■

Order: D₅W 1,000 mL IV at 75 mL/h. The infusion set is calibrated for a drop factor of 15 gtt/mL.

Turn dial of controller to 75 mL/h.

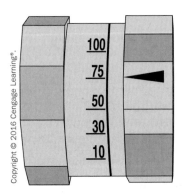

Use formula method to determine flow rate in drops per minute (gtt/min).

$$\frac{V}{T} \times C = \frac{75 \text{ mL}}{60 \text{ min}} \times 15 \text{ gtt/mL} = \frac{75 \text{ mL}}{\underset{4}{60} \text{ min}} \times \frac{\overset{1}{15} \text{ gtt}}{1 \text{ mL}} = \frac{75 \text{ gtt}}{4 \text{ min}} = 18.75 \text{ gtt/min} = 19 \text{ gtt/min}$$

Verify the accuracy of the controller using watch count. The number of drops counted in 60 seconds is 19. The controller is delivering the correct rate. Continue to monitor periodically throughout the infusion.

EXAMPLE 2 ■

Order: D₅W 1,000 mL IV at 200 mL/h. The infusion set is calibrated for a drop factor of 10 gtt/mL.

Turn dial of controller to 200 mL/h.

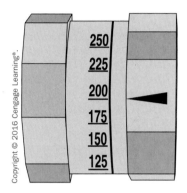

To verify accuracy this time, let's use the shortcut method to determine flow rate in drops per minute (gtt/min). Drop factor constant: 6

$$\frac{\text{mL/h}}{\text{Drop factor constant}} = \text{gtt/min} \qquad \frac{200 \text{ mL/h}}{6} = 33.3 \text{ gtt/min} = 33 \text{ gtt/min}$$

In order to count for less than one full minute (60 seconds), you can count for a portion of a minute, such as 15 or 20 seconds. Divide the number of drops per minute by 3 to determine that the drop count should be 11 drops per 20 seconds (or 33 drops per minute).

THINK: 60 sec ÷ 3 = 20 sec
33 gtt ÷ 3 = 11 gtt

Now check the accuracy of the controller using watch count for 20 seconds. You find that the actual number of drops counted in 20 seconds is 15, not 11. So you know the IV is infusing too rapidly. The dial will need to be adjusted somewhat, in the same manner as a roller clamp. A minor adjustment to slow the infusion by tightening the controller may be made by turning the dial to a position slightly less than 200 gtt/min.

Turn dial of controller between 200 mL/h and 175 mL/h but closer to 200 mL/h.

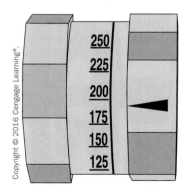

Again, verify the accuracy of the new setting on the controller using watch count. The number of drops counted in 20 seconds is now 11 (or 33 in 60 seconds). Now the controller is delivering the correct rate. Continue to monitor periodically throughout the infusion.

> **QUICK REVIEW**
>
> For dial-flow controllers:
>
> ■ Controller dials are marked in mL/h.
>
> ■ Turn the dial to the calibration mark that corresponds to the ordered hourly flow rate in mL/h.
>
> ■ Use formula $\frac{V}{T} \times C$ or shortcut $\frac{mL/h}{\text{Drop factor constant}}$ = gtt/min methods to verify accuracy of drop rate.
>
> ■ Adjust the dial to control accuracy and verify adjusted rate as needed.
>
> ■ As with all IV infusions, continue to monitor for accuracy and safety periodically throughout the infusion.

Review Set 38

Place an arrow on the dial-flow controller to mark the correct position to provide an estimated flow rate for the ordered manually regulated IV infusions.

1. Order: *0.45% NaCl 3,000 mL IV for 24 h*

   Drop factor: 15 gtt/mL

   Flow rate: _____ mL/h

   Flow rate: _____ gtt/min

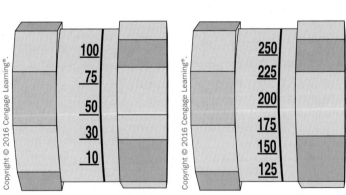

2. Order: *D₅W 200 mL IV to run at 100 mL/h*

   Drop factor: microdrop, 60 gtt/mL

   Flow rate: _____ gtt/min

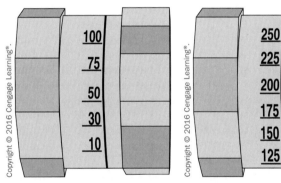

3. Order: *D₅NS 800 mL IV for 8 h*

   Drop factor: 20 gtt/mL

   Flow rate: _____ mL/h

   Flow rate: _____ gtt/min

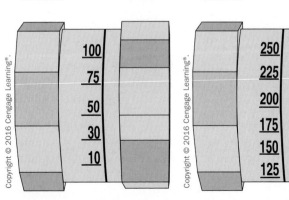

4. Order: NS 1,000 mL IV at 50 mL/h

   Drop factor: 60 gtt/mL

   Flow rate: _____ gtt/min

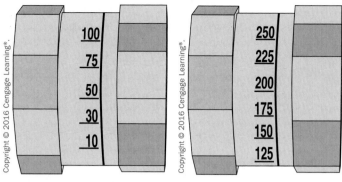

5. Order: D₅W 1,500 mL IV for 12 h

   Drop factor: 15 gtt/mL

   Flow rate: _____ mL/h

   Flow rate: _____ gtt/min

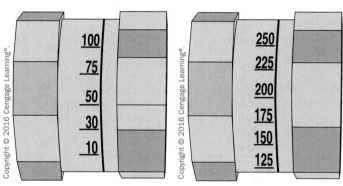

6. Order: theophylline 0.5 g IV
   in 250 mL D₅W to run for 2 h

   Drop factor: 60 gtt/mL

   Flow rate: _____ mL/h

   Flow rate: _____ gtt/min

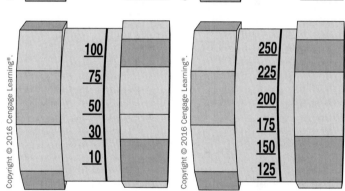

7. Order: D₅ 0.45% NaCl 2,500 mL IV
   at 105 mL/h

   Drop factor: 20 gtt/mL

   Flow rate: _____ gtt/min

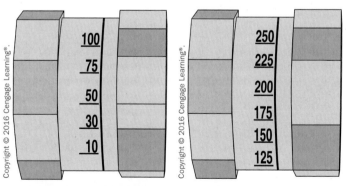

8. Order: D₅ 0.45% NaCl 500 mL IV
   at 100 mL/h

   Drop factor: 10 gtt/mL

   Flow rate: _____ gtt/min

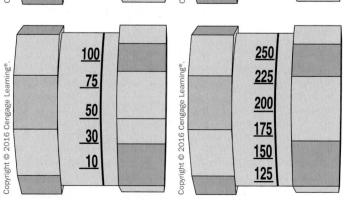

9. Order: **NS 1,200 mL IV at 150 mL/h**

   Drop factor: 10 gtt/mL

   Flow rate: _____ gtt/min

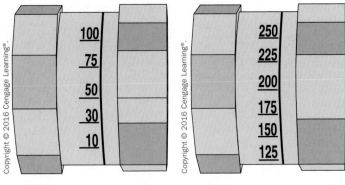

10. Order: **LR 500 mL IV to infuse over 4 h**

    Drop factor: 20 gtt/mL

    Flow rate: _____ mL/h

    Flow rate: _____ gtt/min

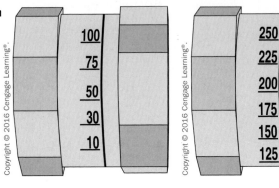

After completing these problems, see pages 703–704 to check your answers.

ADJUSTING IV FLOW RATE

IV fluids, especially those with medicines added (called *additives*), are viewed as medications with specific dosages (rates of infusion, in this case). It is the responsibility of the nurse to maintain this rate of flow through careful calculations and close observation at regular intervals. Various circumstances, such as gravity, condition, and movement of the patient, can alter the set flow rate of an IV, causing the IV to run ahead of, or behind, schedule.

CAUTION

It is not the discretion of the nurse to arbitrarily speed up or slow down the IV flow rate to get it back on schedule. This practice can result in serious conditions of over- or underhydration and electrolyte imbalance. Avoid off-schedule IV flow rates by regularly monitoring IVs at least every 30 minutes to 1 hour. Check your agency policy.

During your regular monitoring of the IV, if you find that the rate is not progressing as scheduled, or is significantly ahead of, or behind, schedule, the physician may need to be notified as warranted by the patient's condition, the hospital policy, or good nursing judgment. Some hospital policies allow the flow rate per minute to be adjusted by a certain percentage of variation. A safe rule is that the flow rate per minute may be adjusted by *up to 25% more or less* than the original prescribed rate, depending on the condition of the patient. In such cases, assess the patient. If the patient is stable, recalculate the flow rate to administer the total remaining milliliters over the number of hours remaining in the original order.

RULE

- Check for institutional policy regarding correcting off-schedule IV rates and the percentage of variation allowed. This variation should not exceed 25%.

- If adjustment is permitted, use the following formula to recalculate the mL/h and gtt/min for the time remaining and the percentage of variation.

Step 1 $\dfrac{\text{Remaining volume}}{\text{Remaining hours}}$ = **Recalculated mL/h**

Step 2 $\dfrac{V}{T} \times C = R$ **(gtt/min)**

Step 3 $\dfrac{\text{Adjusted IV flow rate } - \text{ Ordered IV flow rate}}{\text{Ordered IV flow rate}}$ = **% variation**

The percent variation will be positive (+) if the administration is slow and the rate has to be increased, and negative (−) if the administration is too fast and the rate has to be decreased.

EXAMPLE 1 ▪

The order reads D$_5$W *1,000 mL IV at 125 mL/h for 8 h.* The drop factor is 10 gtt/mL, and the IV is correctly set at 21 gtt/min. You would expect that, after 4 hours, one half of the total, or 500 mL, of the solution would be infused (125 mL/h̶ × 4 h̶ = 500 mL). However, during regular hourly IV monitoring at the fourth hour after starting the IV, you find 600 milliliters remaining. The rate of flow is *behind schedule,* and the hospital allows a 25% IV flow variation with careful patient assessment and if the patient's condition is stable. The patient is stable, so you decide to compute a new flow rate for the remaining 600 milliliters, to complete the IV fluid order in the remaining 4 hours.

Step 1 $\dfrac{\text{Remaining volume}}{\text{Remaining hours}}$ = Recalculated mL/h

$$\frac{600 \text{ mL}}{4 \text{ h}} = 150 \text{ mL/h}$$

Step 2 $\dfrac{V}{T} \times C = \dfrac{150 \text{ m̶L̶}}{\underset{6}{60} \text{ min}} \times \overset{1}{1\!0} \text{ gtt/m̶L̶} = \dfrac{150 \text{ gtt}}{6 \text{ min}} = 25 \text{ gtt/min}$ (adjusted flow rate)

You could also use the shortcut method.

$$\frac{\text{mL/h}}{\text{Drop factor constant}} = \text{gtt/min}$$

$$\frac{150 \text{ mL/h}}{6} = 25 \text{ gtt/min}$$

Step 3 $\dfrac{\text{Adjusted gtt/min } - \text{ Ordered gtt/min}}{\text{Ordered gtt/min}} = \%$ of variation

$\dfrac{25 - 21}{21} = \dfrac{4}{21} = 0.19 = 19\%$; within the acceptable 25% of variation, depending on policy and patient's condition

Compare 25 gtt/min (in the last example) with the starting flow rate of 21 gtt/min. You can see that adjusting the total remaining volume over the total remaining hours changes the flow rate by only 4 gtt/min. Most patients can tolerate this small amount of increase per minute over several hours. However, trying to catch up the lost 100 milliliters in 1 hour can be dangerous. To infuse an extra 100 milliliters in 1 hour, with a drop factor of 10 gtt/mL, you would need to speed up the IV to a much faster rate. Let's see what that additional amount to increase the rate would be.

$\dfrac{V}{T} \times C = \dfrac{100 \text{ m̶L̶}}{\underset{6}{60} \text{ min}} \times \overset{1}{1\!0} \text{ gtt/m̶L̶} = \dfrac{100 \text{ gtt}}{6 \text{ min}} = 16.6 \text{ gtt/min} = 17 \text{ gtt/min}$ more than the original rate

To catch up the IV over the next hour, the flow rate would have to be 17 drops per minute faster than the original 21 drops per minute rate. The infusion would have to be set at $17 + 21 = 38$ gtt/min for 1 hour and then slowed to the original rate. Such an increase would be $\frac{38 - 21}{21} = \frac{17}{21} = 81\%$ greater than the ordered rate. This could present a serious problem. **Do not do it! If permitted by hospital policy, the flow rate for the remainder of the order must be recalculated when the IV is off schedule and should not exceed a 25% adjustment, unless instructed otherwise by a physician.**

EXAMPLE 2 ▪

The order reads: **LR 500 mL IV to run over 10 h at 50 mL/h.** The drop factor is 60 gtt/mL, and the IV is correctly infusing at 50 gtt/min. It is $2\frac{1}{2}$ hours since the IV was started, but there has been no regular IV monitoring. You find 300 mL remaining. Almost half of the total volume has already infused in about one quarter the time. This IV infusion is *ahead of schedule*. You would compute a new flow rate of 300 mL to complete the IV fluid order in the remaining $7\frac{1}{2}$ hours. The patient would require close assessment for fluid overload.

Step 1 $\dfrac{\text{Remaining volume}}{\text{Remaining hours}} = \text{Recalculated mL/h}$

$$\frac{300 \text{ mL}}{7.5 \text{ h}} = 40 \text{ mL/h}$$

Time remaining is $7\frac{1}{2}$ h $(10 \text{ h} - 2\frac{1}{2} \text{ h})$

Step 2 $\dfrac{V}{T} \times C = \dfrac{40 \text{ mL}}{60 \text{ min}} \times \overset{1}{\cancel{60}} \text{ gtt/mL} = 40 \text{ gtt/min}$ (adjusted flow rate)

Or, you know that when the drop factor is 60, then mL/h = gtt/min.

Step 3 $\dfrac{\text{Adjusted gtt/min} - \text{Ordered gtt/min}}{\text{Ordered gtt/min}} = \%$ of variation

$$\frac{40 - 50}{50} = \frac{-10}{50} = -0.2 = -20\%, \text{ within the acceptable 25\% of variation}$$

Remember: A negative percent of variation (in this case, -20%) indicates that the adjusted flow rate will be decreased.

RULE
Shortcut for IV rate adjustment check (Step 3):
Ordered IV rate ± (Ordered IV rate ÷ 4) = Acceptable IV adjustment range

You know that you can adjust the flow rate by as much as ±25%, and you know that $25\% = \frac{1}{4}$. Therefore, after recalculating the adjusted flow rate, you can check the safety of the recalculated rate by using a shortcut that does not include percents. To do this, you divide the ordered rate by 4 and add or subtract the result from the ordered rate to determine the acceptable range of adjustment.

In Example 1, the ordered rate is 21 gtt/min, and the recalculated rate is 25 gtt/min. Is this within the safe range? Use the shortcut to calculate the acceptable range.

Ordered IV rate ± (Ordered IV rate ÷ 4) = Acceptable IV adjustment range
$21 + (21 ÷ 4) = 21 + 5.25 = 26.25 = 26$ gtt/min
$21 - (21 ÷ 4) = 21 - 5.25 = 15.75 = 16$ gtt/min

The safe range is 16 to 26 gtt/min. Yes, 25 gtt/min is within the safe ±25% range.

This may be an easier calculation for you than working with percents. Let's look again at Example 2. The ordered rate is 50 gtt/min, and the recalculated rate is 40 gtt/min. What is the acceptable range?

Ordered IV rate $\pm$ (Ordered IV rate $\div$ 4) = Acceptable IV adjustment range
$$50 + (50 \div 4) = 50 + 12.5 = 62.5 = 63 \text{ gtt/min}$$
$$50 - (50 \div 4) = 50 - 12.5 = 37.5 = 38 \text{ gtt/min}$$

The safe range is 38 to 63 gtt/min. Yes, it is safe to slow the rate to 40 gtt/min, which is within the safe $\pm25\%$ range.

A safe rule is that the recalculated flow rate should not vary from the ordered rate by more than 25%. If the recalculated rate does vary from the order by more than 25%, contact your supervisor or the doctor for further instructions. The original order may have to be revised. Regular monitoring helps to prevent or minimize this problem.

Patients who require close monitoring for IV fluids will most likely have the IV regulated by an electronic infusion device. Because of the nature of the patient conditions, speeding up or slowing down these IVs, if off schedule, is not recommended. If an IV regulated by an electronic infusion pump is off schedule or inaccurate, you should suspect that the infusion pump may need recalibration. Consult with your supervisor, as appropriate.

QUICK REVIEW

- Regular IV monitoring and patient assessment at least every 30 minutes to 1 hour is important to maintain the prescribed IV flow rate.

- Do not arbitrarily speed up or slow down IV flow rates that are off schedule.

- Check hospital policy regarding adjustment of off-schedule IV flow rates and the percentage of variation allowed. If permitted, a safe rule is a maximum 25% variation for patients in stable condition.

- Use the remaining time and the remaining IV fluid volume to recalculate the off-schedule IV flow rate:

Step 1 $\dfrac{\text{Remaining volume}}{\text{Remaining hours}} = \text{Recalculated mL/h}$

Step 2 $\dfrac{V}{T} \times C = R \text{ (gtt/min)}$

Step 3 $\dfrac{\text{Adjusted IV flow rate} - \text{Ordered IV flow rate}}{\text{Ordered IV flow rate}} = \% \text{ variation}$

- Contact the prescribing health care professional for a new IV fluid order if the recalculated IV flow rate variation exceeds the allowed variation or if the patient's condition is unstable.

Review Set 39

Compute the flow rate in drops per minute. Hospital policy permits recalculation of IVs when off schedule, with a maximum variation in rate of 25% for patients who are stable. Compute the percent of variation.

1. Order: **Lactated Ringer's 1,500 mL IV for 12 h at 125 mL/h**

   Drop factor: 20 gtt/mL

   Original flow rate: _____ gtt/min

   After 6 hours, there are 850 mL remaining; describe your action now.

Time remaining: _____ h

Recalculated flow rate: _____ mL/h

Recalculated flow rate: _____ gtt/min

Variation: _____ %

Action: _____

2. Order: **Lactated Ringer's 1,000 mL IV for 6 h at 167 mL/h**

   Drop factor: 15 gtt/mL

   Original flow rate: _____ gtt/min

   After 4 hours, there are 360 mL remaining; describe your action now.

   Time remaining: _____ h

   Recalculated flow rate: _____ mL/h

   Recalculated flow rate: _____ gtt/min

   Variation: _____ %

   Action: _____

3. Order: **D$_5$W 1,000 mL IV for 8 h at 125 mL/h**

   Drop factor: 20 gtt/mL

   Original flow rate: _____ gtt/min

   After 4 hours, there are 800 mL remaining; describe your action now.

   Time remaining: _____ h

   Recalculated flow rate: _____ mL/h

   Recalculated flow rate: _____ gtt/min

   Variation: _____ %

   Action: _____

4. Order: **NS 2,000 mL IV for 12 h at 167 mL/h**

   Drop factor: 10 gtt/mL

   Original flow rate: _____ gtt/min

   After 8 hours, there are 750 mL remaining; describe your action now.

   Time remaining: _____ h

   Recalculated flow rate: _____ mL/h

   Recalculated flow rate: _____ gtt/min

   Variation: _____ %

   Action: _____

5. Order: **NS 1,000 mL IV for 8 h at 125 mL/h**

   Drop factor: 10 gtt/mL

   Original flow rate: _____ gtt/min

   After 4 hours, there are 750 mL remaining; describe your action now.

   Time remaining: _____ h

Recalculated flow rate: _____ mL/h

Recalculated flow rate: _____ gtt/min

Variation: _____ %

Action: _____

6. Order: **NS 2,000 mL IV for 16 h at 125 mL/h**

   Drop factor: 15 gtt/mL

   Original flow rate: _____ gtt/min

   After 6 hours, 650 mL of fluid have infused; describe your action now.

   Solution remaining: _____ mL

   Time remaining: _____ h

   Recalculated flow rate: _____ mL/h

   Recalculated flow rate: _____ gtt/min

   Variation: _____ %

   Action: _____

7. Order: **NS 900 mL IV for 6 h at 150 mL/h**

   Drop factor: 20 gtt/mL

   Original flow rate: _____ gtt/min

   After 3 hours, there are 700 mL remaining; describe your action now.

   Time remaining: _____ h

   Recalculated flow rate: _____ mL/h

   Recalculated flow rate: _____ gtt/min

   Variation: _____ %

   Action: _____

8. Order: **D₅NS 500 mL IV for 5 h at 100 mL/h**

   Drop factor: 20 gtt/mL

   Original flow rate: _____ gtt/min

   After 2 hours, there are 250 mL remaining; describe your action now.

   Time remaining: _____ h

   Recalculated flow rate: _____ mL/h

   Recalculated flow rate: _____ gtt/min

   Variation: _____ %

   Action: _____

9. Order: **NS 1 L IV for 20 h at 50 mL/h**

   Drop factor: 15 gtt/mL

   Original flow rate: _____ gtt/min

   After 10 hours, there are 600 mL remaining; describe your action now.

   Time remaining: _____ h

Recalculated flow rate: _____ mL/h

Recalculated flow rate: _____ gtt/min

Variation: _____ %

Action: _____

10. Order: D₅W 1,000 mL IV for 10 h at 100 mL/h

Drop factor: 60 gtt/mL

Original flow rate: _____ gtt/min

After 5 hours, there are 500 mL remaining; describe your action now.

Time remaining: _____ h

Recalculated flow rate: _____ mL/h

Recalculated flow rate: _____ gtt/min

Variation: _____ %

Action: _____

After completing these problems, see pages 704–705 to check your answers.

INTERMITTENT IV INFUSIONS

Sometimes the patient needs to receive supplemental fluid therapy and/or IV medications but does not need continuous replacement or maintenance IV fluids. Several intermittent IV infusion systems are available to administer IV drugs. These include IV PB, IV locks for IV push drugs, the ADD-Vantage system, and volume control sets (such as Buretrol). Volume control sets are discussed in Chapter 16.

IV Piggybacks

A medication may be ordered to be dissolved in a small amount of IV fluid (usually 50 to 100 mL) and run piggyback to the regular IV fluids (Figure 15-8). Recall that the IV PB (or secondary IV) requires a secondary IV set.

The IV PB medication may come premixed by the manufacturer or pharmacy, or the nurse may need to prepare it. Whichever the case, it is always the responsibility of the nurse to accurately and safely administer the medication. The infusion time may be less than 60 minutes, so it is important to carefully read the order and recommended infusion time.

Sometimes the physician's order for the IV PB medication will not include an infusion time or rate. It is understood, when this is the case, that the nurse will follow the manufacturer's guidelines for infusion rates, keeping in mind the amount of fluid accompanying the medication and any standing orders that limit fluid amounts or rates. Appropriate infusion times are readily available in many drug reference books. Reference books are usually available on most nursing units, or you can consult with a hospital pharmacist.

EXAMPLE 1 ■

Order: *cefazolin 0.5 g in 100 mL D₅W IV PB to run over 30 min*

Drop factor: 20 gtt/mL

What is the flow rate in gtt/min?

$$\frac{V}{T} \times C = \frac{100 \text{ mL}}{\underset{3}{30 \text{ min}}} \times \overset{2}{20} \text{ gtt/mL} = \frac{200 \text{ gtt}}{3 \text{ min}} = 66.6 \text{ gtt/min} = 67 \text{ gtt/min}$$

EXAMPLE 2 ■

If an electronic infusion pump is used to administer the same order as in Example 1, remember that you would need to program the device in mL/h.

| Step 1 | **Think** | If 100 mL will be administered in 30 minutes, or one-half hour, then 200 mL will be administered in twice this time, or 60 minutes. |

| Step 2 | **Calculate** | Use ratio-proportion to calculate mL/h. |

$$\frac{100 \text{ mL}}{30 \text{ min}} \times \frac{X \text{ mL/h}}{60 \text{ min/h}}$$

$$30X = 6{,}000$$

$$\frac{30X}{30} = \frac{6{,}000}{30}$$

$$X = 200 \text{ mL/h}$$

Set the electronic IV PB regulator to 200 mL/h. Remember, though, that the actual volume of 100 mL will be infused in 30 minutes.

Saline and Heparin IV Locks for IV Push Drugs

IV locks can be attached to the hub of the IV catheter that is positioned in the vein. The lock may be referred to as a *saline lock,* meaning that saline is used to flush or maintain the IV catheter patency, or a *heparin lock* if heparin is used to maintain the IV catheter patency. Sometimes a more general term, such as *intermittent peripheral infusion device,* may be used. Medications can be given *IV push,* meaning that a syringe is attached to the lock and medication is pushed in. An *IV bolus,* usually a quantity of IV fluid, can be run in over a specified period of time through an IV setup that is attached to the lock. Using either a saline or a heparin lock allows for intermittent medication and fluid infusion. Heparin and saline locks are also being used for outpatient and home care medication therapy.

CAUTION

Remember: As you learned in Chapter 11, heparin is a high-alert drug and comes in many dosage strengths, or concentrations. A heparin lock flush is usually concentrated to 10 units/mL or 100 units/mL. Much higher concentrations of heparin are given IV or subcut, so carefully check the concentration. Refer to the policy at your hospital or health care agency regarding the frequency, volume, and concentration of heparin to be used to maintain an IV lock.

Dosage calculations for IV push injections are the same as calculations for intramuscular (IM) injections. The IV push route of administration is often preferred when immediate onset of action is desired for persons with small or wasted muscle mass or poor circulation, or for drugs that have limited absorption when injected into body tissues. The IV route of administration is also generally preferred over IM when IV access is available, because repeated IM injections can be painful. Therefore, when a peripheral IV is in place, an IM route is avoided.

Drug literature and institutional guidelines recommend an acceptable rate (per minute or per incremental amount of time) for IV push drug administration. Most timed IV push administration recommendations are for 1 to 5 minutes or more. For smooth manual administration of IV push drugs, calculate the incremental volume to administer over 15-second intervals. You should time the administration with a digital or sweep second-hand watch or clock.

CAUTION

IV drugs are rapidly distributed in the blood stream. Never infuse IV push drugs more rapidly than recommended by agency policy or pharmacology literature. Some drugs require further dilution after reconstitution for IV push administration. Carefully read package inserts and reputable drug resources for minimum dilution and minimum time for IV administration.

EXAMPLE 1 ▪

Order: Ativan 3 mg IV push 20 min preoperatively

Supply: Ativan 4 mg/mL with drug literature guidelines of *IV infusion not to exceed 2 mg/min*

How much Ativan should you prepare?

Step 1   **Convert**   No conversion is necessary.

Step 2   **Think**   You want to give less than 1 mL.

Step 3   **Calculate** $\dfrac{\text{Dosage on hand}}{\text{Amount on hand}} = \dfrac{\text{Dosage desired}}{\text{X Amount desired}}$

$$\frac{4\ mg}{1\ mL} \diagdown\!\!\!\!\diagup \frac{3\ mg}{X\ mL}$$

$$4X = 3$$

$$\frac{4X}{4} = \frac{3}{4}$$

$$X = 0.75\ mL$$

What is a safe infusion time?

In this example, 2 mg/min is the recommended infusion rate to deliver the supply dosage.

Use ratio-proportion method to calculate the time required to administer the drug dosage as ordered.

$$\frac{\text{Dosage recommended}}{\text{Time recommended}} = \frac{\text{Dosage desired}}{\text{X Time desired}}$$

$$\frac{2\ mg}{1\ min} \diagdown\!\!\!\!\diagup \frac{3\ mg}{X\ min}$$

$$2X = 3$$

$$\frac{2X}{2} = \frac{3}{2}$$

$$X = 1.5\ min$$

Administer 0.75 mL over 1.5 min.

How much should you infuse every 15 seconds?

Convert: 1 min = 60 sec; 1.5 m̶i̶n̶ × 60 sec/m̶i̶n̶ = 90 sec

$$\frac{0.75\ mL}{90\ sec} \diagdown\!\!\!\!\diagup \frac{X\ mL}{15\ sec}$$

$$90X = 11.25$$

$$\frac{90X}{90} = \frac{11.25}{90}$$

X = 0.125 mL = 0.13 mL of Ativan 4 mg/mL, infused IV push every 15 seconds, delivers 3 mg of Ativan at the recommended rate of 2 mg/min

This is a small amount. Use a 1 mL syringe to prepare 0.75 mL, and slowly administer 0.13 mL every 15 seconds.

EXAMPLE 2 ▪

Order: Cefizox 1,500 mg bolus stat

Supply: Cefizox 2 g powder with directions, *For direct IV administration, reconstitute each 1 g in 10 mL sterile water and give slowly over 3 to 5 minutes.*

How much Cefizox should you prepare?

Step 1   **Convert**   1 g = 1,000 mg

2 g = 2.000. = 2,000 mg

Step 2   **Think**   If 1 g (or 1,000 mg) requires 10 mL for dilution, then 2 g (or 2,000 mg) requires twice this amount, or 20 mL, for dilution. Therefore, to administer 1,500 mg, you will prepare more than 10 mL and less than 20 mL.

Step 3   **Calculate** $\dfrac{\text{Dosage on hand}}{\text{Amount on hand}} = \dfrac{\text{Dosage desired}}{\text{X Amount desired}}$

$$\frac{2{,}000\ \text{mg}}{20\ \text{mL}} \diagdown\!\!\!\!\diagup \frac{1{,}500\ \text{mg}}{\text{X mL}}$$

$$2{,}000\text{X} = 30{,}000$$

$$\frac{2{,}000\text{X}}{2{,}000} = \frac{30{,}000}{2{,}000}$$

$$\text{X} = 15\ \text{mL}$$

What is a safe infusion time?

This amount is larger than the Ativan dosage from Example 1, so you should use the longer infusion time recommendation (1 g per 5 min). Remember the unknown X is the amount of time to infuse the dosage desired.

$$\frac{\text{Dosage recommended}}{\text{Time recommended}} = \frac{\text{Dosage desired}}{\text{X Time desired}}$$

$$\frac{1{,}000\ \text{mg}}{5\ \text{min}} \diagdown\!\!\!\!\diagup \frac{1{,}500\ \text{mg}}{\text{X min}}$$

$$\frac{1{,}000\text{X}}{1{,}000} = \frac{7{,}500}{1{,}000}$$

$$\text{X} = 7.5\ \text{min}$$

Administer 15 mL over 7.5 min.

How much should you infuse every 15 seconds?

Convert: 1 min = 60 sec

7.5 m̶i̶n̶ × 60 sec/m̶i̶n̶ = 450 sec

$$\frac{15\ \text{mL}}{450\ \text{sec}} \diagdown\!\!\!\!\diagup \frac{\text{X mL}}{15\ \text{sec}}$$

$$450\text{X} = 225$$

$$\frac{450\text{X}}{450} = \frac{225}{450}$$

X = 0.5 mL of Cefizox 2 g per 20 mL, infused IV push every 15 seconds, delivers 1,500 mg of Cefizox at the rate of 1 g per 5 min

Use a 20 mL syringe to prepare 15 mL, and slowly infuse 0.5 mL every 15 seconds.

ADD-Vantage System

Another type of IV medication setup commonly used in hospitals is the ADD-Vantage system by Abbott Laboratories (Figure 15-19). This system uses a specially designed IV bag with a medication vial port. The medication vial comes with the ordered dosage and medication prepared in a powder form. The medication vial is attached to the special IV bag, and together they become the IV PB container. The powder is dissolved by the IV fluid and used within a specified time. This system maintains asepsis and eliminates the extra time and equipment (syringe and diluent vials) associated with reconstitution of powdered medications. Several drug manufacturers market many common IV antibiotics that use products similar to the ADD-Vantage system.

FIGURE 15-19   ADD-Vantage system: Medications can be added to another solution being infused

1 ASSEMBLE **USE ASEPTIC TECHNIQUE**

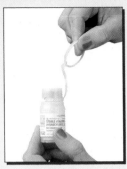 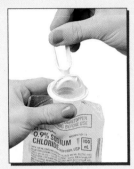 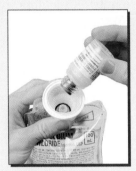

Swing the pull ring over the top of the vial and pull down far enough to start the opening. Then pull straight up to remove the cap. Avoid touching the rubber stopper and vial threads.

Hold diluent container and gently grasp the tab on the pull ring. Pull up to break the tie membrane. Pull back to remove the cover. Avoid touching the inside of the vial port.

Screw the vial into the vial port until it will go no further. **Recheck the vial to ensure that it is tight.** Label appropriately.

2 ACTIVATE **PULL PLUG/STOPPER TO MIX DRUG WITH DILUENT**

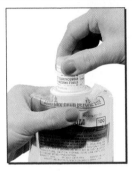 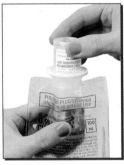 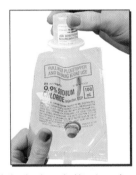

Hold the vial as shown. Push the drug vial down into container and grasp the inner cap of the vial through the walls of the container.

Pull the inner cap from the drug vial: allow drug to fall into diluent container for fast mixing. Do not force stopper by pushing on one side of inner cap at a time.

Verify that the plug and rubber stopper have been removed from the vial. The floating stopper is an indication that the system has been activated.

3 MIX AND ADMINISTER **WITHIN THE SPECIFIED TIME**

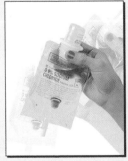 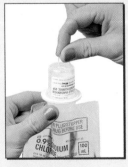 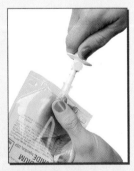

Mix container contents thoroughly to ensure complete dissolution. Look through bottom of vial to verify complete mixing. Check for leaks by squeezing container firmly. If leaks are found, discard unit.

Pull up hanger on the vial.

Remove the white administration port cover and spike (pierce) the container with the piercing pin. Administer within the specified time.

Photography courtesy Abbott Laboratories.

QUICK REVIEW

- Intermittent IV infusions usually require more or less than 60 minutes of infusion time.
- Calculate IV PB flow rate in gtt/min: $\frac{V}{T} \times C = R$.
- Use a proportion to calculate IV PB flow rate in mL/h for an electronic infusion device.
- Use the three-step dosage calculation method to calculate the amount to give for IV push medications: convert, think, calculate.
- Use the ratio-proportion method to calculate safe IV push time in minutes and seconds as recommended by a reputable drug reference.

Review Set 40

Calculate the IV PB or IV push flow rate.

1. Order: Ancef 1 g in 100 mL D$_5$W IV PB to be infused over 45 min

    Drop factor: 60 gtt/mL

    Flow rate: _____ gtt/min

2. Order: Ancef 1 g in 100 mL D$_5$W IV PB to be administered by electronic infusion pump to infuse in 45 min

    Flow rate: _____ mL/h

3. Order: cefazolin 500 mg IV PB diluted in 50 mL D$_5$W to infuse in 15 min

    Drop factor: 15 gtt/mL

    Flow rate: _____ gtt/min

4. Order: cefazolin 500 mg IV PB diluted in 50 mL D$_5$W to infuse in 15 min by an electronic infusion pump

    Flow rate: _____ mL/h

5. Order: 50 mL IV PB antibiotic solution to infuse in 30 min

    Drop factor: 60 gtt/mL

    Flow rate: _____ gtt/min

6. Order: Zosyn 3 g in 100 mL D$_5$W IV PB to be infused over 40 min

    Drop factor: 10 gtt/mL

    Flow rate: _____ gtt/min

7. Order: Unasyn 1.5 g in 50 mL D$_5$W IV PB to be infused over 15 min

    Drop factor: 15 gtt/mL

    Flow rate: _____ gtt/min

8. Order: Merrem 1 g in 100 mL D$_5$W IV PB to be infused over 30 min

    Use electronic infusion pump.

    Flow rate: _____ mL/h

9. Order: cefoxitin 750 mg in 50 mL NS IV PB to be infused over 20 min

    Use electronic infusion pump.

    Flow rate: _____ mL/h

10. Order: oxacillin sodium 900 mg in 125 mL D$_5$W IV PB to be infused over 45 min

    Use electronic infusion pump.

    Flow rate: _____ mL/h

11. Order: Unasyn 0.5 g in 100 mL D$_5$W IV PB to be infused over 15 min

    Drop factor: 20 gtt/mL

    Flow rate: _____ gtt/min

12. Order: cefotetan 500 mg in 50 mL NS IV PB to be infused over 20 min

    Drop factor: 10 gtt/mL

    Flow rate: _____ gtt/min

13. Order: Merrem 1 g in 100 mL D$_5$W IV PB to be infused over 50 min

    Use electronic infusion pump.

    Flow rate: _____ mL/h

14. Order: oxacillin sodium 900 mg in 125 mL D$_5$W IV PB to be infused over 45 min

    Drop factor: 20 gtt/mL

    Flow rate: _____ gtt/min

15. Order: Zosyn 1.3 g in 100 mL D$_5$W IV PB to be infused over 30 min

    Drop factor: 60 gtt/mL

    Flow rate: _____ gtt/min

16. Order: Lasix 120 mg IV push stat

    Supply: Lasix 10 mg/mL with drug insert, which states, *IV injection not to exceed 40 mg/min.*

    Give: _____ mL per _____ min

    or _____ mL per 15 sec

17. Order: phenytoin 150 mg IV push stat

    Supply: phenytoin 250 mg per 5 mL with drug insert, which states, *IV infusion not to exceed 50 mg/min.*

    Give: _____ mL per _____ min

    or _____ mL per 15 sec

18. Order: morphine sulfate 6 mg IV push q.3h p.r.n., pain

    Supply: morphine sulfate 10 mg/mL with drug reference recommendation, which states, *IV infusion not to exceed 2.5 mg/min.*

    Give: _____ mL per _____ min

    or _____ mL per 15 sec

19. Order: cimetidine 300 mg IV push stat

    Supply: cimetidine 300 mg per 2 mL

    Package insert instructions: *For direct IV injection, dilute 300 mg in 0.9% NaCl to a total volume of 20 mL. Inject over at least 2 minutes.*

    Prepare _____ mL cimetidine

    Dilute with _____ mL 0.9% NaCl for a total of 20 mL of solution.

    Administer _____ mL/min or _____ mL per 15 sec

20. Order: midazolam hydrochloride 1.5 mg IV push stat

    Supply: midazolam hydrochloride 1 mg/mL

    Instructions: *Slowly titrate to the desired effect, using no more than 1.5 mg initially, given over 2-minute period.*

    Prepare _____ mL midazolam hydrochloride

    Give _____ mL/min or _____ mL per 15 sec

After completing these problems, see page 705 to check your answers.

CALCULATING IV INFUSION TIME AND VOLUME

Intravenous solutions are usually ordered to be administered at a prescribed number of milliliters per hour, such as **Lactated Ringer's 1,000 mL IV to run at 125 mL/h.** You may need to calculate the total infusion time so that you can anticipate when to add a new bag or bottle, or when to discontinue the IV.

RULE
To calculate IV infusion time:

$$\frac{\text{Total volume}}{\text{mL/h}} = \textbf{Total hours}$$

Or use ratio-proportion: Ratio for prescribed flow rate in mL/h = Ratio for total mL per X total hours

$$\frac{\text{mL}}{\text{h}} = \frac{\text{Total mL}}{\text{X Total h}}$$

EXAMPLE 1 ▪

LR 1,000 mL IV to run at 125 mL/h. How long will this IV last?

$$\frac{\overset{8}{\cancel{1,000\text{ mL}}}}{\underset{1}{\cancel{125\text{ mL/h}}}} = 8\text{ h}$$

Or, use ratio-proportion.

$$\frac{125 \text{ mL}}{1 \text{ h}} \diagdown\!\!\!\!\diagup \frac{1,000 \text{ mL}}{X \text{ h}}$$

$$125X = 1,000$$

$$\frac{125X}{125} = \frac{1,000}{125}$$

$$X = 8 \text{ h}$$

MATH TIP

When calculating IV infusion time, use fractions for hours that are not whole numbers. They are more exact than rounded decimal numbers. For calculations involving time, rounded decimals are harder to use.

EXAMPLE 2 ■

D$_5$W 1,000 mL IV to infuse at 60 mL/h to begin at 0600. At what time will this IV be complete?

$$\frac{1,000 \text{ mL}}{60 \text{ mL/h}} = 16\frac{2}{3} \text{ h}; \frac{2}{3} \text{ h} \times 60 \text{ min/h} = 40 \text{ min}; \text{ Total time: 16 h and 40 min}$$

Or, use ratio-proportion.

$$\frac{60 \text{ mL}}{1 \text{ h}} \diagdown\!\!\!\!\diagup \frac{1,000 \text{ mL}}{X \text{ h}}$$

$$60X = 1,000$$

$$\frac{60X}{60} = \frac{1,000}{60}$$

$$X = 16\frac{2}{3} \text{ h} = 16 \text{ h and 40 min}$$

The IV will be complete at 0600 + 1640 = 2240 (or 10:40 PM).

If the IV is regulated in mL/h, you can also calculate the total volume that will infuse over a specific time.

RULE

To calculate IV volume:

Total hours × mL/h = Total mL

Or use ratio-proportion: Ratio for ordered mL/h = Ratio for X total mL per total hours

$$\frac{\text{mL}}{\text{h}} = \frac{\text{X Total mL}}{\text{Total h}}$$

EXAMPLE ■

Your patient's IV is running on an infusion pump set at the rate of 100 mL/h. How much will be infused during the next 8 hours?

$$8 \text{ h} \times 100 \text{ mL/h} = 800 \text{ mL}$$

Or, use ratio-proportion:

$$\frac{100 \text{ mL}}{1 \text{ h}} \diagdown\!\!\!\!\diagup \frac{X \text{ mL}}{8 \text{ h}}$$

$$X = 800 \text{ mL}$$

QUICK REVIEW

- The formula to calculate IV infusion time, when mL is known:

$$\frac{\text{Total volume}}{\text{mL/h}} = \text{Total hours}$$

or use ratio-proportion: $\frac{\text{mL}}{\text{h}} = \frac{\text{Total mL}}{\text{X total h}}$

- The formula to calculate total infusion volume, when mL/h are known:

Total hours × mL/h = Total mL

Or, use ratio-proportion: $\frac{\text{mL}}{\text{h}} = \frac{\text{X total mL}}{\text{Total h}}$

Review Set 41

Calculate the infusion time for the following IV orders:

1. Order: D$_5$W 500 mL IV at 90 mL/h

   Time: _____ h and _____ min

2. Order: Lactated Ringer's 1,000 mL IV at 100 mL/h

   Time: _____ h and _____ min

3. Order: D$_5$ Lactated Ringer's 800 mL IV at 125 mL/h

   Time: _____ h and _____ min

Calculate the infusion time and completion time for the following IVs.

4. At 1600 hours, the nurse started D$_5$W 1,200 mL IV at 100 mL/h.

   Infusion time: _____ h _____ min

   Completion time: _____

5. At 1530 hours, the nurse starts D$_5$W 2,000 mL IV to run at 125 mL/h.

   Infusion time: _____ h _____ min

   Completion time: _____

Calculate the total volume (mL) to be infused per 24 hours.

6. An IV of D$_5$ Lactated Ringer's is infusing on an electronic infusion pump at 125 mL/h.

   Total volume: _____ mL per 24 h

Calculate total volume and completion time (if requested) for the following IV orders.

7. Order: 0.9% sodium chloride IV infusing at 65 mL/h for 4 h

   Volume: _____ mL

8. Order: D$_5$W IV infusing at 150 mL/h for 2 h

   Volume: _____ mL

9. Order: D$_5$LR IV at 75 mL/h for 8 h

   Volume: _____ mL

10. Order: **At 2000 hours start 0.45% NaCl IV at 90 mL/h for 4 h**

    Volume: _____ mL

    Completion time: _____

After completing these problems, see page 706 to check your answers.

CLINICAL REASONING SKILLS

Drug reference guides provide recommendations for the rate at which IV push medications should be administered. Nurses should calculate the volume to be administered over short intervals of time to prevent the medication from being administered too quickly. If the volume of medication is very small, it may need to be diluted further to give the nurse more control over the rate.

ERROR

Not being able to push the plunger of a syringe slowly enough and administering an IV push medication too rapidly

Possible Scenario

A patient who had recently undergone abdominal surgery was complaining of severe incisional pain. The postoperative orders included *hydromorphone 1 mg IV slow push q.2h for moderate to severe* pain. The supply of hydromorphone available on the surgical unit was 2 mg/mL. According to a drug reference guide, it is recommended that the solution be diluted with at least 5 mL of sterile water or 0.9% NaCl for injection and administered slowly at a rate not to exceed 2 mg over 3 to 5 minutes, which for the ordered amount of 1 mg would be 1.5 to 2.5 minutes. The nurse did not review the administration guidelines but did intend to give the medication as slowly as possible. The nurse correctly calculated the amount to give and drew up the correct dose of 0.5 mL into a 3 mL syringe, but did not dilute the dose further. Unfortunately, when administering the medication, the plunger moved too quickly, infusing the entire 0.5 mL dose immediately. The nurse was very concerned and remained with the patient for 10 minutes to assess for any adverse effects. The patient felt relief of pain, fell asleep, and did not display any notable adverse consequences.

Potential Outcome

Hydromorphone is an opioid analgesic and is considered a high-alert drug. Two potentially serious adverse effects include respiratory depression and confusion. Infusing an IV push medication too rapidly places the patient at greater risk for these and other serious adverse effects.

Prevention

The nurse would have had more control if the volume of solution in the syringe was larger. The 3 mL syringe will not hold a volume of 5 mL, and most larger syringes do not have a marking to accurately measure 0.5 mL. The medication should be diluted by first drawing up 0.5 mL of hydromorphone into a 1 mL or 3 mL syringe, as the nurse did. Then, using a 10 mL syringe, the 5 mL of the recommended diluent should be drawn up. The needle should be removed and the plunger pulled back to leave at least 0.5 mL of air. The nurse should then add the small volume of hydromorphone into the larger syringe by inserting the needle of the smaller syringe directly into the barrel. The excess air should be removed, leaving the resulting 5.5 mL volume of diluted solution. A new sterile needle or protective cap should then be placed on the 10 mL syringe until it is inserted into the IV tubing. There will now be 5.5 mL to infuse over the recommended 3 to 5 minutes. In order to determine the minimum rate of the IV push injection, divide the total volume (5.5 mL) by time (3 min) to calculate mL/min.

$$5.5 \text{ mL} \div 3 \text{ min} = 1.83 \text{ mL/min} = 1.8 \text{ mL/min}$$

The nurse may also push a slightly smaller amount per minute for the slower rate of 5 minutes.

$$5.5 \text{ mL} \div 5 \text{ min} = 1.1 \text{ mL/min}$$

Therefore, the nurse may safely administer the IV push dose of hydromorphone by using a watch and slowly injecting a diluted volume of 1.1 to 1.8 mL (approximately 1 to 2 mL) per min or 0.275 to 0.45 mL (approximately 0.3 to 0.5 mL) per 15 sec.

CLINICAL REASONING SKILLS   It is important to understand backup methods for managing intravenous infusions when electronic infusion pumps malfunction or are unavailable.

ERROR

Failing to verify accuracy of a dial-flow controller or use time tape to manage a manually regulated IV infusion

Possible Scenario

Upon admission to the medical unit of a community hospital, a patient is ordered to receive an intravenous infusion of D$_5$½ NS at 200 mL/h and the anti-infective ampicillin 1 g IV PB q.6h. The nurse is unable to obtain an electronic infusion pump due to an unusually high patient census. The nurse decides to set up the IV tubing using a dial-flow controller until a pump becomes available. At 2000, the nurse attaches the extension tubing to the liter of IV fluid, connects the tubing to the patient, and turns the controller dial to the 200 mL/h marking. At 2400, the nurse prepares the first dose of ampicillin, as prescribed. The nurse added the reconstituted powdered medication to a 100 mL IV PB, attached another dial-flow controller extension tubing connected to the patient, and turned the second controller dial to the 100 mL/h marking. The nurse returns to the patient's bedside at 0100 expecting the medication infusion to be complete and the liter of IV fluid to need replacement. The nurse is surprised to find that the IV PB still has approximately 25 mL remaining and the liter bag has 100 mL remaining. The nurse verifies the dials are still set at 200 mL/h and 100 mL/h, waits until the infusions are complete, removes the IV PB, and replaces the liter of fluid.

Potential Outcome

The nurse, who was more experienced with electronic infusion pumps than manually regulated IV infusions, was apparently unaware that the mL/h calibrations on the dial-flow controller are only estimated rates. Inconsistency in the flow rate may have resulted from the height of the IV, the level of remaining fluid in the bag, or the condition of the IV site. In this case, both infusions were running slower than the settings indicated. The patient who was in need of hydration received less than the ordered amount of replacement fluid. The ampicillin should have infused within 1 hour of reconstitution to retain potency. There was a risk that the patient did not receive the ordered dosage of ampicillin. While the consequences in this situation were not life threatening, the potential outcomes would be more serious for a severely ill patient or one receiving a high-alert medication.

Prevention

Electronic infusion pumps are an added safety and convenience for administering intravenous therapy; however, they may not always be available due to malfunction or limited supply. Nurses must be knowledgeable in techniques for manually regulated IVs in the event that a backup method is needed. Calibrations for mL/h on dial-flow controllers should be considered approximate rates and always checked for accuracy with a watch count at the outset of the infusion and then again periodically. In this case, if the nurse calculated the correct infusion rates in gtt/min and counted the actual drops, the infusions would have immediately been found to be running slower and the dial could have been adjusted to the correct rate. An additional backup method to improve surveillance of manually regulated IV infusions is the time tape. If the nurse had placed a simple time tape on the liter bag when it was started at 2000, it would have become evident sooner that the infusion was falling behind schedule. Dial-flow controller package instructions and nursing drug guides generally provide handy references for these less frequently used skills.

PRACTICE PROBLEMS—CHAPTER 15

Compute the flow rate in drops per minute or milliliters per hour as requested. For these situations, hospital policy permits recalculating IVs, when off schedule, with a maximum variation in rate of 25%.

1. Order: *ampicillin 500 mg dissolved in 100 mL D$_5$W IV to run for 1 h*

   Drop factor: 10 gtt/mL

   Flow rate: _____ gtt/min

2. Order: *D$_5$W 1,000 mL IV per 24 h*

   Drop factor: 60 gtt/mL

   Flow rate: _____ gtt/min

3. Order: *D$_5$LR 1,500 mL IV to run for 12 h*

   Drop factor: 20 gtt/mL

   Flow rate: _____ gtt/min

4. Order: *D$_5$RL 200 mL IV for 24 h*

   Drop factor: 60 gtt/mL

   Flow rate: _____ gtt/min

5. Order: *D$_{10}$W 1 L IV to run from 1000 to 1800*

   Drop factor: On electronic infusion pump

   Flow rate: _____ mL/h

6. See question 5. At 1100, there are 800 mL remaining. Describe your nursing action now. _____

   _____

7. Order: *NS 1,000 mL followed by D$_5$W 2,000 mL IV to run for 24 h*

   Drop factor: 15 gtt/mL

   Flow rate: _____ gtt/min

8. Order: *NS 2.5 L IV to infuse at 125 mL/h*

   Drop factor: 20 gtt/mL

   Flow rate: _____ gtt/min

9. Order: *D$_5$W 1,000 mL IV for 6 h*

   Drop factor: 15 gtt/mL

   After 2 hours, 800 mL remain. Describe your nursing action now. _____

   _____

The IV tubing package in the accompanying figure is the IV system available in your hospital for manually regulated, straight gravity-flow IV administration with macrodrop. The patient has an order for *D$_5$W 500 mL IV q.4h* written at 1515, and you start the IV at 1530. Questions 10 through 20 refer to this situation.

◰ LATEX-FREE   **No. 4967**

PRIMARY I.V. SET,
Convertible Pin, 80 Inch
with Backcheck Valve
and 2 Injection Sites
Piggyback

Abbott Laboratories, Inc.

15 DROPS/mL

10. How much IV fluid will the patient receive in 24 hours? _____ mL

11. Who is the manufacturer of the IV infusion-set tubing? _____

12. What is the drop factor calibration for the IV infusion-set tubing? _____

13. What is the drop factor constant for the IV infusion-set tubing? _____

14. Using the shortcut (drop factor constant) method, calculate the flow rate of the IV as ordered. Show your work.

    Shortcut-method calculation: _____

    Flow rate: _____ gtt/min

15. Using the formula method, calculate the flow rate of the IV as ordered. Show your work.

    Formula-method calculation: _____

    Flow rate: _____ gtt/min

16. At what time should you anticipate that the first IV bag of 500 mL D_5W will be completely infused? _____

17. How much IV fluid should be infused by 1730? _____ mL

18. At 1730, you notice that the IV has 210 mL remaining. After assessing your patient and confirming that his or her condition is stable, what should you do? _____

    _____

19. After consulting the physician, you decide to use an electronic infusion pump to better regulate the flow rate. The physician orders that the pump be set to infuse 500 mL every 4 hours. You should set the pump for _____ mL/h.

20. The next day, the physician adds the order **amoxicillin 250 mg in 50 mL D_5W IV PB to infuse in 30 min q.6h.** The patient is still on the IV pump. To infuse the IV PB, set the pump for _____ mL/h.

21. List the components and concentration strengths of the IV fluid $D_{2.5} \frac{1}{2}NS$.

    _____

22. Calculate the amount of dextrose and sodium chloride in D_5NS 500 mL.

    dextrose _____ g

    NaCl _____ g

23. Labetalol may be safely infused by IV push at a rate of 2 mg/min. What is a safe infusion time to administer 10 mg? _____ min

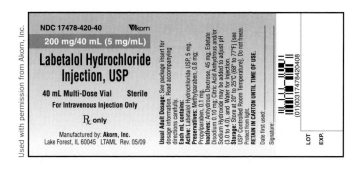

Labetalol is available in the supply pictured. To administer 10 mg IV push, prepare _____ mL and slowly inject IV at the rate of _____ mL/min or _____ mL per 30 sec.

24. Diltiazem may be safely infused by IV push at a rate of 10 mg/min. What is a safe infusion time to administer 35 mg? _____ min

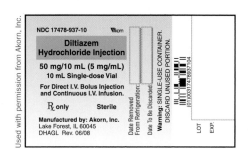

Diltiazem is available in the supply pictured. To administer 35 mg IV push, prepare _____ mL and slowly inject IV at the rate of _____ mL/min or _____ mL per 15 sec.

25. Midazolam may be safely infused by IV push at a rate of 0.5 mg/min. What is a safe infusion time to administer 3 mg? _____ min

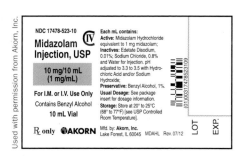

Midazolam is available in the supply pictured. To administer 3 mg IV push, prepare _____ mL and slowly inject IV at the rate of _____ mL/min or _____ mL per 30 sec.

26. Protamine sulfate may be safely infused by IV push at a rate of 5 mg/min. What is a safe infusion time to administer 50 mg? _____ min

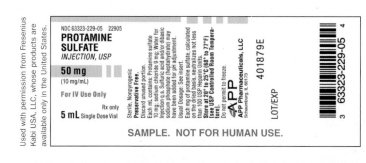

Protamine sulfate is available in the supply pictured. To administer 50 mg IV push, prepare _____ mL and slowly inject IV at the rate of _____ mL/min or _____ mL per 15 sec.

For questions 27–31, observe the setting on the dial-flow controller. First, identify the intended rate of flow, then calculate the expected flow rate in gtt/min using the specified extension tubing.

27. 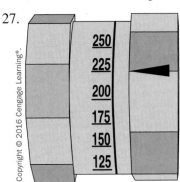 _____ mL/h   Tubing: 10 gtt/mL   _____ gtt/min

28. 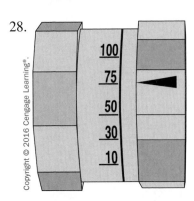 _____ mL/h   Tubing: 60 gtt/mL   _____ gtt/min

29. 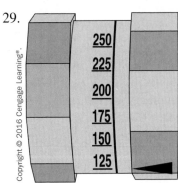 _____ mL/h   Tubing: 20 gtt/mL   _____ gtt/min

30. 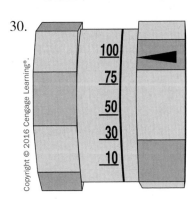 _____ mL/h   Tubing: 15 gtt/mL   _____ gtt/min

31. 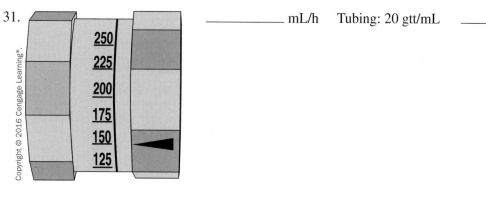 _____ mL/h   Tubing: 20 gtt/mL   _____ gtt/min

For each IV order in questions 32 through 47, use the drop factor to calculate the flow rate in gtt/min.

Order: D₅W 1 L IV *to infuse in 12 h*

32. Drop factor 10 gtt/mL   Flow rate: _____ gtt/min

33. Drop factor 15 gtt/mL   Flow rate: _____ gtt/min

34. Drop factor 20 gtt/mL   Flow rate: _____ gtt/min

35. Drop factor 60 gtt/mL   Flow rate: _____ gtt/min

Order: D₅NS 2 L IV *to infuse in 20 h*

36. Drop factor 10 gtt/mL   Flow rate: _____ gtt/min

37. Drop factor 15 gtt/mL   Flow rate: _____ gtt/min

38. Drop factor 20 gtt/mL   Flow rate: _____ gtt/min

39. Drop factor 60 gtt/mL   Flow rate: _____ gtt/min

Order: 0.45% NaCl 1,000 mL IV *at 200 mL/h*

40. Drop factor 10 gtt/mL   Flow rate: _____ gtt/min

41. Drop factor 15 gtt/mL   Flow rate: _____ gtt/min

42. Drop factor 20 gtt/mL   Flow rate: _____ gtt/min

43. Drop factor 60 gtt/mL   Flow rate: _____ gtt/min

Order: D₅ 0.9% NaCl 500 mL IV *at 45 mL/h*

44. Drop factor 10 gtt/mL   Flow rate: _____ gtt/min

45. Drop factor 15 gtt/mL   Flow rate: _____ gtt/min

46. Drop factor 20 gtt/mL   Flow rate: _____ gtt/min

47. Drop factor 60 gtt/mL   Flow rate: _____ gtt/min

48. You make rounds before your lunch break and find that a patient has 60 mL of IV fluid remaining of an intermittent IV ordered at 125 mL/h on an IV pump and with a saline lock. What volume will be infused during the 30 minutes you will be at lunch? _____ mL

    What should you alert your relief nurse to watch for and do while you are off the unit? _____

    _____

49. Your shift is 0700 to 1500. You make rounds at 0730 and find 400 mL remaining on an IV of D₅ 0.45% NaCl that is regulated on an electronic infusion pump at the ordered rate of 75 mL/h. The order specifies a continuous infusion. At what time should you anticipate hanging the next IV bag? _____

50. Describe the clinical reasoning you would use to prevent this medication error.

Possible Scenario

Suppose the physician ordered D₅LR 1,000 mL IV at 125 mL/h for an elderly patient just returning from the OR following abdominal surgery. The nurse gathered the IV solution and IV tubing, which had a drop factor of 20 gtt/mL. The nurse did not check the package for the drop factor and assumed it was 60 gtt/mL. The manual rate was calculated this way:

$$\frac{125 \text{ mL}}{60 \text{ min}} \times 60 \text{ gtt/mL} = 125 \text{ gtt/min} \qquad \textbf{INCORRECT}$$

The nurse infused the D₅LR at 125 gtt/min for 8 hours. During shift report, the patient called for the nurse, complaining of shortness of breath. On further assessment, the nurse heard crackles in the patient's lungs and noticed that the patient's third 1,000 mL bottle of D₅LR this shift was nearly empty already. At this point, the nurse realized that the IV rate was in error. The nurse was accustomed to using the 60 gtt/mL IV setup and therefore calculated the drip rate using the 60 gtt/mL (microdrop) drop factor. However, the tubing used delivered a 20 gtt/mL (macrodrop) drop factor. The nurse never looked at the drop factor on the IV set package and assumed it was a 60 gtt/mL set.

Potential Outcome

This situation represents very serious errors. The patient developed signs of fluid overload and could have developed congestive heart failure due to the excessive IV rate. The physician would have been notified and likely ordered Lasix (a diuretic) to help eliminate the excess fluid. The patient likely would have been transferred to the ICU for closer monitoring.

Prevention

_____

_____

After completing these problems, see pages 706–708 to check your answers.

🖰 Be sure to use the online software for additional practice!

REFERENCES

U.S. Food and Drug Administration (FDA). (2010a). White paper: Infusion pump improvement initiative. Retrieved from http://www.fda.gov/medicaldevices/productsandmedicalprocedures/GeneralHospitalDevicesandSupplies/InfusionPumps/ucm205424.htm

U.S. Food and Drug Administration (FDA). (2010b). Infusion pump risk reduction strategies for clinicians. Retrieved from http://www.fda.gov/MedicalDevices/ProductsandMedicalProcedures/GeneralHospitalDevicesandSupplies/InfusionPumps/ucm205406.htm

U.S. Food and Drug Administration (FDA). (2014). Examples of reported infusion pump problems. Retrieved from http://www.fda.gov/MedicalDevices/ProductsandMedicalProcedures/GeneralHospitalDevicesandSupplies/InfusionPumps/ucm202496.htm

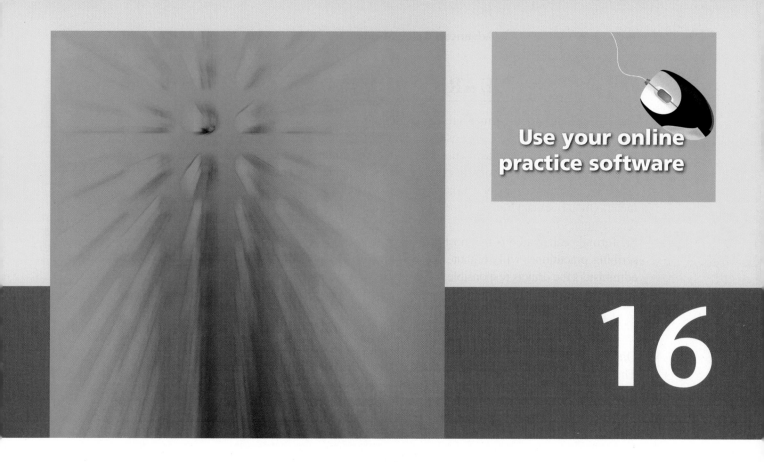

16

Body Surface Area and Advanced Pediatric Calculations

OBJECTIVES

Upon mastery of Chapter 16, you will be able to perform advanced calculations for children and apply these advanced concepts across the life span. To accomplish this, you will also be able to:

- Determine the body surface area (BSA) using a calculation formula or a nomogram scale.
- Compute the safe amount of drug to be administered when ordered according to the BSA.
- Calculate intermittent intravenous (IV) medications administered with IV infusion-control sets.
- Calculate the minimal and maximal dilution with which an IV medication can be safely prepared and delivered via modes such as a syringe pump.
- Calculate pediatric IV maintenance fluids.

This chapter will focus on additional and more advanced calculations used frequently by pediatric nurses. It will help you understand the unique drug and fluid management required by a growing child. Further, these concepts, which are most commonly related to children, are also applied to adults in special situations. Let's start by looking at the BSA method of calculating a dosage, and then we'll discuss checking for the accuracy and safety of a particular drug order.

BODY SURFACE AREA METHOD

The BSA is an important measure in calculating dosages for infants and children. BSA is also used for selected adult populations, such as those undergoing open-heart surgery or radiation therapy, severe burn victims, and those with renal disease. Regardless of patient age, antineoplastic agents (chemotherapy drugs) and an increasing number of other highly potent drug classifications are being prescribed based on BSA.

BSA is a mathematical estimate using the patient's *height* and *weight*. BSA is expressed in square meters (**m²**). BSA can be determined by formula calculation or by using a chart, referred to as a *nomogram*, that estimates the BSA. Because drug dosages recommended by BSA measurement are potent, and because the formula calculation is the most accurate, we will begin with the formulas. In most situations, the prescribing practitioner will compute the BSA for drugs ordered by this method. However, the nurse who administers the drug is responsible for verifying safe dosage, which may require calculating the BSA.

BSA Formula

One BSA formula is based on metric measurement of height in centimeters and weight in kilograms. The other is based on household measurement of height in inches and weight in pounds. Either is easy to compute using the square root function on a calculator. BSA calculators are also readily available on the Internet.

RULE

To calculate BSA in m² based on metric measurement of height and weight:

- $$\text{BSA (m}^2) = \sqrt{\frac{\text{ht (cm)} \times \text{wt (kg)}}{3,600}}$$

To calculate BSA in m² based on household measurement of height and weight:

- $$\text{BSA (m}^2) = \sqrt{\frac{\text{ht (in)} \times \text{wt (lb)}}{3,131}}$$

Let's apply both formulas and see how the BSA measurements compare.

MATH TIP

Notice that in addition to metric versus household measurement, the other difference between the two BSA formulas is in the denominators of the fraction within the square root sign.

EXAMPLE 1 ■

Use the metric formula to calculate the BSA of an infant whose length is 50 cm (20 in) and weight is 3.2 kg (7 lb).

$$\text{BSA (m}^2) = \sqrt{\frac{\text{ht (cm)} \times \text{wt (kg)}}{3,600}} = \sqrt{\frac{50 \times 3.2}{3,600}} = \sqrt{\frac{160}{3,600}} = \sqrt{0.044444} = 0.210 \text{ m}^2 = 0.21 \text{ m}^2$$

MATH TIP

To perform BSA calculations using the metric formula on most calculators, follow this sequence: multiply height in cm by weight in kg; divide by 3,600; press =; then press √ to arrive at m². Round m² to hundredths (two decimal places). For Example 1 above, enter 50 × 3.2 ÷ 3,600 = 0.044444 and press √ to arrive at 0.210, rounded to 0.21 m².

Or use the BSA formula based on household measurement.

$$\text{BSA (m}^2) = \sqrt{\frac{\text{ht (in)} \times \text{wt (lb)}}{3{,}131}} = \sqrt{\frac{20 \times 7}{3{,}131}} = \sqrt{\frac{140}{3{,}131}} = \sqrt{0.044714} = 0.211 \text{ m}^2 = 0.21 \text{ m}^2$$

MATH TIP

To use the calculator for the household formula, follow this sequence: multiply height in inches by weight in pounds; divide by 3,131; press =; then press √ to arrive at the m². Round m² to hundredths (two decimal places). For Example 1, enter 20 × 7 ÷ 3,131 = 0.044714 and press √ to arrive at 0.211, rounded to 0.21 m².

EXAMPLE 2 ■

Calculate the BSA of a child whose height is 105 cm (42 inches) and weight is 31.8 kg (70 lb).

Metric:

$$\text{BSA (m}^2) = \sqrt{\frac{\text{ht (cm)} \times \text{wt (kg)}}{3{,}600}} = \sqrt{\frac{105 \times 31.8}{3{,}600}} = \sqrt{\frac{3{,}339}{3{,}600}} = \sqrt{0.9275} = 0.963 \text{ m}^2 = 0.96 \text{ m}^2$$

Household:

$$\text{BSA (m}^2) = \sqrt{\frac{\text{ht (in)} \times \text{wt (lb)}}{3{,}131}} = \sqrt{\frac{42 \times 70}{3{,}131}} = \sqrt{\frac{2{,}940}{3{,}131}} = \sqrt{0.938997} = 0.969 \text{ m}^2 = 0.97 \text{ m}^2$$

MATH TIP

There is a slight variation in m² calculated by the metric and household methods because of the rounding used to convert centimeters and inches; 1 in = 2.54 cm, which is rounded to 2.5 cm. The results of the two methods, however, are practically equivalent.

EXAMPLE 3 ■

Calculate the BSA of an adult whose height is 173 cm (69 inches) and weight is 88.6 kg (195 lb).

Metric:

$$\text{BSA (m}^2) = \sqrt{\frac{\text{ht (cm)} \times \text{wt (kg)}}{3{,}600}} = \sqrt{\frac{173 \times 88.6}{3{,}600}} = \sqrt{\frac{15{,}327.8}{3{,}600}} = \sqrt{4.257722} = 2.063 \text{ m}^2 = 2.06 \text{ m}^2$$

Household:

$$\text{BSA (m}^2) = \sqrt{\frac{\text{ht (in)} \times \text{wt (lb)}}{3{,}131}} = \sqrt{\frac{69 \times 195}{3{,}131}} = \sqrt{\frac{13{,}455}{3{,}131}} = \sqrt{4.297349} = 2.073 \text{ m}^2 = 2.07 \text{ m}^2$$

These examples show that either metric or household measurement of height and weight results in essentially the same calculated BSA value.

BSA Nomogram

Some practitioners use a chart called a *nomogram* that *estimates* the BSA by plotting the height and weight and simply connecting the dots with a straight line. Figure 16-1 shows the most well-known BSA chart, the West Nomogram (Kliegman, Stanton, St. Geme, Schor, & Behrman, 2011). It is used for both children and adults for heights up to 240 cm or 90 inches, and weights up to 80 kg or 180 lb.

CAUTION

Notice that the increments of measurement and the spaces on the BSA nomogram are not consistent. Be sure you correctly read the numbers and the calibration values between them.

FIGURE 16-1   Body surface area (BSA) is determined by drawing a straight line from the patient's height (1) in the far left column to his or her weight (2) in the far right column. The intersection of the line with surface area (SA) column (3) is the estimated BSA (m²). For infants and children of normal height and weight, BSA may be estimated from weight alone by referring to the enclosed area.

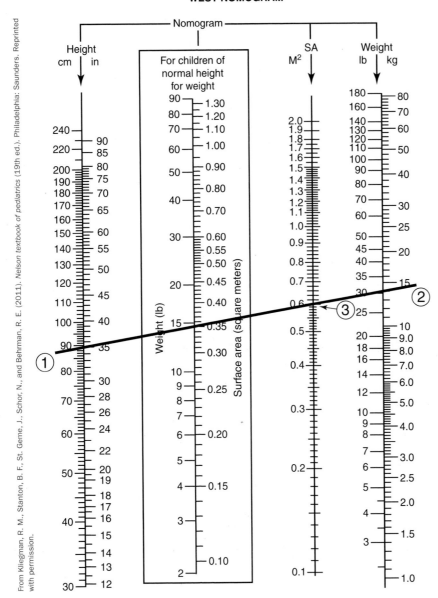

From Kliegman, R. M., Stanton, B. F., St. Geme, J., Schor, N., and Behrman, R. E. (2011). *Nelson textbook of pediatrics* (19th ed.). Philadelphia: Saunders. Reprinted with permission.

For a child of normal height for weight, the BSA can be determined on the West Nomogram, using the weight alone. (Notice the enclosed column to the center left.) Normal height and weight standards can be found on pediatric growth and development charts.

CAUTION

To use the normal column on the West Nomogram, you must be familiar with normal height and weight standards for children. If you are unsure, use both height and weight to estimate BSA. Do not guess.

QUICK REVIEW

- BSA is used to calculate select dosages across the life span, most often for children.
- BSA is calculated by height and weight and expressed in m^2.
- The following metric and household formulas are the preferred methods of calculating BSA:

Metric: $BSA\ (m^2) = \sqrt{\dfrac{ht\ (cm) \times wt\ (kg)}{3,600}}$

Household: $BSA\ (m^2) = \sqrt{\dfrac{ht\ (in) \times wt\ (lb)}{3,131}}$

- Nomograms can be used to estimate BSA, by correlating height and weight measures to m^2.

Review Set 42

Use the formula method to determine the BSA. Round to two decimal places.

1. A child measures 36 inches tall and weighs 40 lb. _____ m^2

2. An adult measures 190 cm tall and weighs 105 kg. _____ m^2

3. A child measures 94 cm tall and weighs 18 kg. _____ m^2

4. A teenager measures 153 cm tall and weighs 46 kg. _____ m^2

5. An adult measures 175 cm tall and weighs 85 kg. _____ m^2

6. A child measures 41 inches tall and weighs 76 lb. _____ m^2

7. An adult measures 62 inches tall and weighs 140 lb. _____ m^2

8. A child measures 28 inches tall and weighs 18 lb. _____ m^2

9. A teenager measures 160 cm tall and weighs 64 kg. _____ m^2

10. A child measures 65 cm tall and weighs 15 kg. _____ m^2

11. A child measures 55 inches tall and weighs 70 lb. _____ m^2

12. A child measures 92 cm tall and weighs 24 kg. _____ m^2

Find the BSA on the West Nomogram (Figure 16-1) for a child of normal height and weight.

13. 4 lb _____ m^2 14. 42 lb _____ m^2 15. 17 lb _____ m^2

Find the BSA on the West Nomogram (Figure 16-1) for children with the following heights and weights.

16. 41 inches and 32 lb _____ m^2

17. 21 inches and 8 lb _____ m^2

18. 140 cm and 30 kg _____ m^2

19. 80 cm and 11 kg _____ m^2

20. 106 cm and 25 kg _____ m^2

After completing these problems, see page 708 to check your answers.

BSA DOSAGE CALCULATIONS

Once the BSA is obtained, the drug dosage can be verified by consulting a reputable drug resource for the recommended dosage. Package inserts, the American Hospital Formulary Service *AHFS Drug Information*, *Delmar Nurse's Drug Handbook*, or other drug references contain pediatric and adult dosages. Remember to carefully read the reference to verify if the drug dosage is calculated in *m² per dose* or *m² per day*.

Use the following rule to calculate dosage based on body mass measured in m². Notice that the calculation is similar to that used for determining dosage based on body weight (such as mg/kg) learned in Chapter 14.

RULE

To verify safe pediatric dosage based on BSA:

1. Determine BSA in m².

2. Calculate the safe dosage based on **BSA: mg/m² × m² = X mg**

3. Compare the ordered dosage to the recommended dosage, and decide if the dosage is safe.

4. If the dosage is safe, calculate the amount to give and administer the dose. If the dosage seems unsafe, consult with the ordering practitioner before administering the drug.

Note: Recommended dosage may specify mg/m², mcg/m², g/m², units/m², milliunits/m², or mEq/m².

EXAMPLE 1 ■

A child is 126 cm tall and weighs 23 kg. The drug order reads: Vincasar 1.8 mg IV at 10 AM. Is this dosage safe for this child? The recommended dosage as noted on the package insert is 2 mg/m² (with the dosage further diluted for IV administration). Supply: see label, Figure 16-2.

1. **Determine BSA.** The child's BSA is 0.9 m² (using the metric BSA formula).

$$\text{BSA (m}^2) = \sqrt{\frac{\text{ht (cm)} \times \text{wt (kg)}}{3{,}600}} = \sqrt{\frac{126 \times 23}{3{,}600}} = \sqrt{\frac{2{,}898}{3{,}600}} = \sqrt{0.805} = 0.897 \text{ m}^2 = 0.9 \text{ m}^2$$

2. **Calculate recommended dosage.** mg/m² × m² = 2 mg/m² × 0.9 m² = 1.8 mg

3. **Decide if the dosage is safe.** The dosage ordered is 1.8 mg, and 1.8 mg is the amount recommended by BSA. The dosage is safe. How much should you give?

FIGURE 16-2 Vincasar 1 mg/mL label

4. **Calculate 1 dose.**

Step 1   **Convert**   No conversion is necessary.

Step 2   **Think**   You want to give more than 1 mL and less than 2 mL. At 1 mg per mL, it is obvious that you want to give 1.8 mL.

Step 3   **Calculate** $\dfrac{\text{Dosage on hand}}{\text{Amount on hand}} = \dfrac{\text{Dosage desired}}{\text{X Amount desired}}$

$$\frac{1 \text{ mg}}{1 \text{ mL}} \diagdown\!\!\!\!\diagup \frac{1.8 \text{ mg}}{\text{X mL}}$$

$$\text{X} = 1.8 \text{ mL}$$

NDC 0703-4402-11

VINCASAR PFS®
(vincristine sulfate injection, USP)

PRESERVATIVE FREE SOLUTION
1 mg/mL

FATAL IF GIVEN INTRATHECALLY
FOR INTRAVENOUS USE ONLY
Single Dose Vial
REFRIGERATE
Protect From Light

sicor™
SICOR Pharmaceuticals, Inc.,
Irvine, CA 92618

(01)00307034402115

440202

EXAMPLE 2 ▪

A 2-year-old child with herpes simplex is 35 inches tall and weighs 30 lb. The drug order reads *acyclovir 100 mg IV b.i.d.* Is this order safe? The drug reference recommends 250 mg/m² q.8h for children younger than 12 years and older than 6 months. Acyclovir is supplied as Zovirax 500 mg injection, with directions to reconstitute with 10 mL sterile water for injection for a concentration of 50 mg/mL (with the dosage further diluted for IV administration).

1. **Determine BSA.** The child's BSA is 0.6 m² (using the West Nomogram, Figure 16-1).

2. **Calculate recommended dosage.** mg/m² × m² = 250 mg/m̶² × 0.6 m̶² = 150 mg

3. **Decide if the dosage is safe.** The dosage of 100 mg b.i.d. is not safe—the single dosage is too low. Further, the drug should be administered 3 times per day q.8h, not b.i.d. or 2 times per day.

4. **Confer with the prescriber.**

QUICK REVIEW

Safe dosage based on BSA: mg/m² × m², compared to recommended dosage.

Review Set 43

1. What is the dosage of 1 dose of interferon alpha-2b required for a child with a BSA of 0.82 m² if the recommended dosage is 2 million units/m²? _____ units

2. What is the total daily dosage range of mitomycin required for a child with a BSA of 0.59 m² if the recommended dosage range is 10 to 20 mg/m²/day? _____ mg/day to _____ mg/day

3. What is the dosage of calcium EDTA required for an adult with a BSA of 1.47 m² if the recommended dosage is 500 mg/m²? _____ mg

4. What is the total daily dosage of thiotepa required for an adult with a BSA of 2.64 m² if the recommended dosage is 6 mg/m²/day? _____ mg. After 4 full days of therapy, this patient will have received a total of _____ mg of thiotepa.

5. What is the dosage of acyclovir required for a child with a BSA of 1 m² if the recommended dosage is 250 mg/m²? _____ mg

6. A child is 30 inches tall and weighs 25 pounds.

   Order: *Zovirax 122.5 mg IV q.8h*

   Supply: Zovirax 500 mg with directions to reconstitute with 10 mL sterile water for injection for a final concentration of 50 mg/mL.

   Recommended dosage from drug insert: 250 mg/m²

   BSA = _____ m²

   Recommended dosage for this child: _____ mg

   Is the ordered dosage safe? _____

   If safe, give _____ mL.

   If not safe, what should you do? _____

7. A child is 45 inches tall and weighs 55 pounds.

   Order: *methotrexate 2.9 mg IV daily*

   Supply: methotrexate 2.5 mg/mL

Recommended dosage from drug insert: 3.3 mg/m²

BSA = _____ m²

Recommended dosage for this child: _____ mg

Is the ordered dosage safe? _____

If safe, give _____ mL.

If not safe, what should you do? _____

8. Order: **Benoject 22 mg IV q.8h.** Child has BSA of 0.44 m². The recommended safe dosage of Benoject is 150 mg/m²/day in divided dosages every 6 to 8 hours.

   Recommended daily dosage for this child: _____ mg/day

   Recommended single dosage for this child: _____ mg/dose

   Is the ordered dosage safe? _____

   If not safe, what should you do? _____

9. Order: **quinidine 198 mg p.o. daily for 5 days.** Child has BSA of 0.22 m². The recommended safe dosage of quinidine is 900 mg/m²/day given for 5 days.

   Recommended dosage for this child: _____ mg/dose

   Is the dosage ordered safe? _____

   If not safe, what should you do? _____

   How much quinidine would this child receive over 5 days of therapy? _____ mg

10. Order: **deferoxamine mesylate IV per protocol.** Child has BSA of 1.02 m².

    Protocol: 600 mg/m² initially followed by 300 mg/m² at 4-hour intervals for 2 doses; then give 300 mg/m² q.12h for 2 days. Calculate the total dosage received.

    Initial dosage: _____ mg

    Total for 2 q.4h dosages: _____ mg

    Total for 2 days of q.12h dosages: _____ mg

    Total dosage child would receive: _____ mg

11. Order: **Fludara 10 mg/m² bolus over 15 minutes followed by a continuous IV infusion of 30.5 mg/m²/day.** Child has BSA of 0.81 m². The bolus dosage is _____ mg, and the continuous 24-hour IV infusion will contain _____ mg of Fludara.

12. Order: **isotretinoin 83.75 mg IV q.12h** for a child with a BSA of 0.67 m². The recommended dosage range is 100 to 250 mg/m²/day in 2 divided doses.

    Recommended daily dosage range for this child: _____ mg/day to _____ mg/day

    Recommended single dosage range for this child: _____ mg/dose to _____ mg/dose

    Is the ordered dosage safe? _____

    If not, what should you do? _____

13. Order: **Cerubidine 9.6 mg IV on day 1 and day 8 of cycle**

    Protocol: 25 to 45 mg/m² on days 1 and 8 of cycle. Child has BSA of 0.32 m².

    Recommended dosage range for this child: _____ mg/dose to _____ mg/dose

    Is the ordered dosage safe? _____

    If not safe, what should you do? _____

Answer questions 14 and 15 based on the following information.

The recommended dosage of Oncaspar is 2,500 units/m²/dose IV daily × 14 days for adults and children with a BSA greater than 0.6 m².

Supply: Oncaspar 750 units/mL with directions to dilute in 100 mL D_5W and give over 2 hours. You will administer the drug via infusion pump.

14. Order: *Give Oncaspar 2,050 units IV today at 1600.* Child is 100 cm tall and weighs 24 kg. The child's BSA is _____ m².

    The recommended dosage for this child is _____ units. Is the ordered dosage of Oncaspar safe? _____

    If yes, add _____ mL of Oncaspar for a total IV fluid volume of _____ mL. Set the IV infusion pump at _____ mL/h.

    If the order is not safe, what should you do? _____

15. Order: *Oncaspar 4,050 units IV stat* for an adult patient who is 162 cm tall and weighs 58.2 kg. The patient's BSA is _____ m². The recommended dosage of Oncaspar for this adult is _____ units.

    Is the ordered dosage of Oncaspar safe? _____

    If safe, you would add _____ mL of Oncaspar for a total IV fluid volume of _____ mL. Set the infusion pump at _____ mL/h.

    If the order is not safe, what should you do? _____

After completing these problems, see pages 708–709 to check your answers.

PEDIATRIC VOLUME-CONTROL SETS

Volume-control sets (Figure 16-3) are most frequently used to administer hourly fluids and intermittent IV medications to children. The fluid chamber will hold 100 to 150 milliliters of fluid to be infused in a specified time period as ordered, usually 60 minutes or less. The medication is added to the IV fluid in the chamber for a prescribed dilution volume.

The volume of fluid in the chamber is filled by the nurse every 1 to 2 hours or as needed. Only small, prescribed quantities of fluid are added, and the clamp above the chamber is fully closed. The IV bag acts only as a reservoir to hold future fluid infusions. The patient is protected from receiving more volume than intended. This is especially important for children, because they can tolerate only a narrow range of fluid volume. This differs from standard IV infusions that run directly from the IV bag through the drip chamber and IV tubing into the patient's vein.

Volume-control sets may also be used to administer intermittent IV medications to adults with fluid restrictions, such as for heart or kidney disease. An electronic pump may also be used to regulate the flow rate. When used, the electronic device will sound an alarm when the chamber empties.

With the expanded use of IV pumps, volume-control devices (such as Buretrol) are less common in practice. However, as a safety device for controlling the volume of fluid administered to children and critically ill patients of any age, they are still available. Nurses should be familiar with how to use them and be able to calculate the IV flow rate.

Intermittent IV Medication Infusion via Volume-Control Set

Children receiving IV medications may have a saline or heparin lock in place of a continuous IV infusion. The nurse will inject the medication into the volume-control set chamber, add an appropriate volume of IV fluid to dilute the drug, and attach the IV tubing to the child's IV lock to infuse over a specified period of time. Realize that when the chamber empties, some medication still remains in the

FIGURE 16-3   Volume-control set

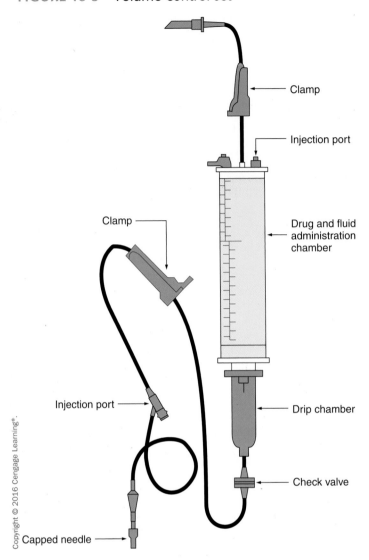

drip chamber, the IV tubing, and the IV lock above the child's vein. After the chamber has emptied and the medication has infused, a flush of IV fluid is given to be sure all the medication has cleared the tubing. There is no standard amount of fluid used to flush peripheral or central IV lines. Because tubing varies by manufacturer, the flush can vary from 15 mL to as much as 50 mL, according to the overall length of the tubing and extra extensions added. Verify your hospital policy on the correct volume for flushing peripheral and central IV lines in children. For the purpose of sample calculations, this text uses a 15 mL volume to flush a peripheral IV line, unless specified otherwise.

To calculate the IV flow rate for the volume-control set, you must consider the total fluid volume of the medication, the IV fluid used for dilution, and the volume of IV flush fluid. Volume-control sets are microdrip sets with a drop factor of 60 gtt/mL.

EXAMPLE ▪

Order: *Claforan 250 mg IV q.6h in 50 mL* $D_5\frac{1}{4}NS$ *to infuse in 30 min followed by a 15 mL flush.* Child has a saline lock.

Supply: see label (Figure 16-4)

Instructions from package insert for IV use:
Add 10 mL diluent for a total volume of 11 mL with a concentration of 180 mg/mL.

FIGURE 16-4   Claforan 2 g label

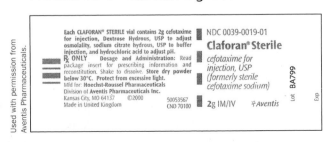

Step 1　Calculate the total volume of the intermittent IV medication and the IV flush.

$$50 \text{ mL} + 15 \text{ mL} = 65 \text{ mL}$$

Step 2　Calculate the flow rate of the IV medication and the IV flush. Remember: The drop factor is 60 gtt/mL.

$$\frac{V}{T} \times C = \frac{\overset{}{65 \text{ mL}}}{\underset{1}{\cancel{30} \text{ min}}} \times \overset{2}{\cancel{60}} \text{ gtt/mL} = 130 \text{ gtt/min}$$

Step 3　Calculate the volume of the medication to be administered.

$$\frac{\text{Dosage on hand}}{\text{Amount on hand}} = \frac{\text{Dosage desired}}{\text{X Amount desired}}$$

$$\frac{180 \text{ mg}}{1 \text{ mL}} \overset{\diagup}{\diagdown} \frac{250 \text{ mg}}{\text{X mL}}$$

$$180\text{X} = 250$$

$$\frac{180\text{X}}{180} = \frac{250}{180}$$

$$\text{X} = 1.38 = 1.4 \text{ mL}$$

Step 4　Add 1.4 mL reconstituted Claforan to the chamber and fill with IV fluid to a volume of 50 mL. This provides the prescribed total volume of 50 mL in the chamber.

Step 5　Set the flow rate of the 50 mL of intermittent IV medication for 130 gtt/min. Follow with the 15 mL flush, also set at 130 gtt/min. When complete, detach IV tubing and follow saline lock policy.

The patient may also have an intermittent medication ordered as part of a continuous infusion at a prescribed IV volume per hour. In such cases, the patient is to receive the same fluid volume each hour, regardless of the addition of intermittent medications. This means that the total prescribed fluid volume must include the intermittent IV medication volume.

EXAMPLE ■

Order: D₅NS IV at 30 mL/h for continuous infusion and gentamicin 30 mg IV q.8h over 30 min

Supply: see label (Figure 16-5)

An electronic infusion pump is in use with the volume-control set.

FIGURE 16-5　Gentamicin 80 mg per 2 mL label

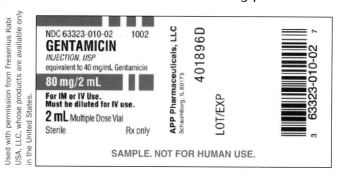

Step 1　Calculate the dilution volume required to administer the gentamicin at the prescribed continuous flow rate of 30 mL/h.

　　Think　If 30 mL infuses in 1 h, then $\frac{1}{2}$ of 30 mL, or 15 mL, will infuse in $\frac{1}{2}$ h, or 30 min.

　　Calculate　Use ratio-proportion to verify your estimate.

$$\frac{30 \text{ mL}}{60 \text{ min}} \overset{\diagup}{\diagdown} \frac{\text{X mL}}{30 \text{ min}}$$

$$60\text{X} = 900$$

$$\frac{60\text{X}}{60} = \frac{900}{60}$$

$$\text{X} = 15 \text{ mL (in 30 min)}$$

Therefore, the IV fluid dilution volume required to administer 30 mg of gentamicin in 30 minutes is 15 mL to maintain the prescribed, continuous infusion rate of 30 mL/h.

Step 2   Determine the volume of gentamicin and IV fluid to add to the volume-control chamber.

$$\frac{\text{Dosage on hand}}{\text{Amount on hand}} = \frac{\text{Dosage desired}}{\text{X Amount desired}}$$

$$\frac{40 \text{ mg}}{1 \text{ mL}} \diagdown\!\!\!\diagup \frac{30 \text{ mg}}{\text{X mL}}$$

$$40X = 30$$

$$\frac{40X}{40} = \frac{30}{40}$$

$$X = 0.75 \text{ mL}$$

Add 0.75 mL gentamicin and fill the chamber with D_5NS to the total volume of 15 mL.

Step 3   Set the infusion pump to 30 mL/h to deliver 15 mL of intermittent IV gentamicin solution in 30 minutes. Resume the regular IV, which will also flush out the tubing. The continuous flow rate will remain at 30 mL/h.

QUICK REVIEW

- Volume-control sets have a drop factor of 60 gtt/mL.

- The total volume of the medication, the IV dilution fluid, and the IV flush fluid must be considered to calculate flow rates when using volume-control sets.

- Use ratio-proportion to calculate flow rates for intermittent medications when a continuous IV rate in mL/h is prescribed.

Review Set 44

Calculate the IV flow rate to administer the following IV medications by using a volume-control set, and determine the amount of IV fluid and medication to be added to the chamber. The ordered time includes the flush volume.

1. Order: **Antibiotic X 60 mg IV q.8h in 50 mL D_5NS over 45 min. Flush with 15 mL.**

   Supply: Antibiotic X 60 mg per 2 mL

   Flow rate: _____ gtt/min

   Add _____ mL medication and _____ mL IV fluid to the chamber.

2. Order: **Medication Y 75 mg IV q.6h in 60 mL $D_5\frac{1}{4}NS$ over 60 min. Flush with 15 mL.**

   Supply: Medication Y 75 mg per 3 mL

   Flow rate: _____ gtt/min

   Add _____ mL medication and _____ mL IV fluid to the chamber.

3. Order: **Antibiotic Z 15 mg IV b.i.d. in 25 mL 0.9% NaCl over 20 min. Flush with 15 mL.**

   Supply: Antibiotic Z 15 mg per 3 mL

   Flow rate: _____ gtt/min

   Add _____ mL medication and _____ mL IV fluid to the chamber.

4. Order: **Ancef 0.6 g IV q.12h in 50 mL D_5NS over 60 min on an infusion pump. Flush with 30 mL.**

   Supply: Ancef 1 g per 10 mL

   Flow rate: _____ mL/h

   Add _____ mL medication and _____ mL IV fluid to the chamber.

5. Order: *Cleocin 150 mg IV q.8h in 32 mL D₅NS over 60 min on an infusion pump. Flush with 28 mL.*

   Supply: Cleocin 150 mg/mL

   Flow rate: _____ mL/h

   Add _____ mL medication and _____ mL IV fluid to the chamber.

   Total IV volume after 3 doses are given is _____ mL.

Calculate the amount of IV fluid to be added to the volume-control chamber for questions 6 through 10.

6. Order: *0.9% NaCl at 50 mL/h for continuous infusion with Ancef 250 mg IV q.8h to be infused over 30 min by volume-control set*

   Supply: Ancef 125 mg/mL

   Add _____ mL medication and _____ mL IV fluid to the chamber.

7. Order: *D₅W at 30 mL/h for continuous infusion with Medication X 60 mg q.6h to be infused over 20 min by volume-control set*

   Supply: Medication X 60 mg per 2 mL

   Add _____ mL medication and _____ mL IV fluid to the chamber.

8. Order: *D₅ 0.225% NaCl IV at 85 mL/h with erythromycin 600 mg IV q.6h to be infused over 40 min by volume-control set*

   Supply: erythromycin 50 mg/mL

   Add _____ mL medication and _____ mL IV fluid to the chamber.

9. Order: *D₅NS IV at 66 mL/h with Fortaz 720 mg IV q.8h to be infused over 40 min by volume-control set*

   Supply: Fortaz 1 g per 10 mL

   Add _____ mL medication and _____ mL IV fluid to the chamber.

10. Order: *D₅ 0.45% NaCl IV at 48 mL/h with doxycycline 75 mg IV q.12h to be infused over 2 h by volume-control set*

    Supply: doxycycline 100 mg per 10 mL

    Add _____ mL medication and _____ mL IV fluid to the chamber.

After completing these problems, see pages 709–710 to check your answers.

MINIMAL DILUTIONS FOR IV MEDICATIONS

IV medications in infants and young children (or adults on limited fluids) are often prescribed to be given in the smallest volume or *maximal safe concentration* to prevent fluid overload. Consult a pediatric reference, *Hospital Formulary,* or drug insert to assist you in problem solving. These types of medications are usually given via an electronic infusion pump.

Many pediatric IV medications allow a dilution *range* or a minimum and maximum allowable concentration. A solution of *lower* concentration may be given if the patient can tolerate the added volume (called *minimal safe concentration, maximal dilution,* or *largest volume*). A solution of *higher* concentration (called *maximal safe concentration, minimal dilution,* or *smallest volume*) must not exceed the recommended dilution instructions. Recall that the greater the volume of diluent or solvent, the less concentrated the resulting solution. Likewise, less volume of diluent or solvent results in a more concentrated solution.

CAUTION

An excessively high concentration of an IV drug can cause vein irritation and potentially life-threatening toxic effects. Accurate dilution calculation is a critical skill.

Let's examine how to follow the drug reference recommendations for a minimal IV drug dilution, when a minimal and maximal range is given for an IV drug dilution.

RULE

Ratio for recommended drug dilution equals ratio for desired drug dilution.

EXAMPLE 1 ▪

The physician orders *vancomycin 40 mg IV q.12h* for an infant who weighs 4,000 g. What is the minimal amount of IV fluid in which the vancomycin can be safely diluted? Look at the package insert provided for your reference (Figure 16-6) and find the *recommended maximal safe concentration* (10 mg/mL).

$$\frac{10 \text{ mg}}{1 \text{ mL}} \times \frac{40 \text{ mg}}{X \text{ mL}}$$

$$10X = 40$$

$$\frac{10X}{10} = \frac{40}{10}$$

$$X = 4 \text{ mL (This is the minimal amount of IV fluid.)}$$

FIGURE 16-6 Portion of simulated vancomycin package insert

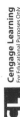

STERILE VANCOMYCIN HYDROCHLORIDE, USP
INTRAVENOUS

DOSAGE AND ADMINISTRATION

Infusion-related events are related to both the concentration and the rate of administration of vancomycin. Concentrations of no more than 5 mg/mL and rates of no more than 10 mg/min are recommended in adults (see also age-specific recommendations). In selected patients in need of fluid restriction, <u>a concentration up to 10 mg/mL may be used</u>; use of such higher concentrations may increase the risk of infusion-related events. An infusion rate of 10 mg/min or less is associated with fewer infusion-related events. Infusion-related events may occur, however, at any rate or concentration.

Copyright © 2016 Cengage Learning®.

Cengage Learning
For Educational Purposes Only

EXAMPLE 2 ▪

The physician orders *Claforan 1.2 g IV q.8h* for a child who weighs 36 kg. The recommended safe administration of Claforan for intermittent IV administration is a final concentration of 20 to 60 mg/mL to infuse over 15 to 30 minutes. What is the minimal amount of IV fluid to safely dilute this dosage? (Remember that this represents the **maximal safe concentration**.)

Step 1	**Convert**	1.2 g = 1.200. = 1,200 mg

Step 2   **Think**   1,200 is more than 10 times 60; in fact, it is 20 times 60. So you need at least 20 mL to dilute the drug.

Step 3   **Calculate** $\dfrac{60 \text{ mg}}{1 \text{ mL}} \underset{\times}{\times} \dfrac{1,200 \text{ mg}}{X \text{ mL}}$

$$60X = 1,200$$

$$\frac{60X}{60} = \frac{1,200}{60}$$

$$X = 20 \text{ mL (minimal dilution for maximal safe concentration)}$$

What is the maximal amount of IV fluid recommended to safely dilute this drug to the minimal safe concentration?

Step 1   **Convert**   1.2 g = 1,200 mg

Step 2   **Think**   1,200 is more than 50 times 20; in fact, it is 60 times 20. So you can use up to 60 mL to dilute the drug.

Step 3   **Calculate** $\dfrac{20 \text{ mg}}{1 \text{ mL}} \underset{\times}{\times} \dfrac{1,200 \text{ mg}}{X \text{ mL}}$

$$20X = 1,200$$

$$\frac{20X}{20} = \frac{1,200}{20}$$

$$X = 60 \text{ mL (maximal dilution for minimal safe concentration)}$$

CALCULATION OF DAILY VOLUME FOR MAINTENANCE FLUIDS

Another common pediatric IV formula involves the calculation of 24-hour maintenance IV fluids for children.

RULE

Use this formula to calculate the daily rate of pediatric maintenance IV fluids:

- 100 mL/kg/day for first 10 kg of body weight
- 50 mL/kg/day for next 10 kg of body weight
- 20 mL/kg/day for each kg above 20 kg of body weight

This formula uses the child's weight in kilograms to estimate the 24-hour total fluid need, including oral intake. It does not include replacement for losses such as those due to diarrhea, vomiting, or fever. This accounts only for fluid needed to maintain normal cellular metabolism and fluid turnover.

Pediatric IV solutions that run over 24 hours usually include a combination of glucose, saline, and potassium chloride and are *hypertonic* solutions (see Figure 15-5). Dextrose (glucose) for energy is usually concentrated between 5% and 12% for peripheral infusions. Sodium chloride is usually concentrated between 0.225% and 0.9% ($\frac{1}{4}$NS up to NS). Further, 20 mEq per liter of potassium chloride (20 mEq KCl/L) are usually added to continuous pediatric infusions. Any dextrose and saline combination without potassium should be used only as an intermittent or short-term IV fluid in children. Be wary of isotonic solutions such as 5% dextrose in water and 0.9% sodium chloride. They do not contribute enough electrolytes and can quickly lead to water intoxication.

> ⚠ **CAUTION**
> A red flag should go up in your mind if either plain 5% dextrose in water or 0.9% sodium chloride (normal saline) is running continuously for an infant or child. Consult the ordering practitioner immediately!

Let's examine the daily rate of maintenance fluids and the hourly flow rate for the children in the following examples. Assume for these examples that the IV pump is programmable in whole numbers, not tenths of a milliliter.

EXAMPLE 1 ■
Child who weighs 6 kg

100 mL/kg/day × 6 kg = 600 mL/day or per 24 h

$$\frac{600 \text{ mL}}{24 \text{ h}} = 25 \text{ mL/h}$$

EXAMPLE 2 ■
Child who weighs 12 kg

100 mL/kg/day × 10 kg = 1,000 mL/day (for first 10 kg)

50 mL/kg/day × 2 kg = 100 mL/day (for the remaining 2 kg)

Total: 1,000 mL/day + 100 mL/day = 1,100 mL/day or per 24 h

$$\frac{1,100 \text{ mL}}{24 \text{ h}} = 45.8 \text{ mL/h} = 46 \text{ mL/h}$$

EXAMPLE 3 ■
Child who weighs 24 kg

100 mL/kg/day × 10 kg = 1,000 mL/day (for first 10 kg)

50 mL/kg/day × 10 kg = 500 mL/day (for next 10 kg)

20 mL/kg/day × 4 kg = 80 mL/day (for the remaining 4 kg)

Total: 1,000 mL/day + 500 mL/day + 80 mL/day = 1,580 mL/day or per 24 h

$$\frac{1,580 \text{ mL}}{24 \text{ h}} = 65.8 \text{ mL/h} = 66 \text{ mL/h}$$

QUICK REVIEW

- Minimal and maximal dilution volumes for some IV drugs are recommended to prevent fluid overload and to minimize vein irritation and toxic effects.

- The ratio for recommended dilution equals the ratio for desired drug dilution.

- When mixing IV drug solutions,

  - the *smaller* the added volume, the *stronger* or *higher* the resulting *concentration* (minimal dilution).

  - the *larger* the added volume, the *weaker* (more dilute) or *lower* the resulting *concentration* (maximal dilution).

- Daily volume of pediatric maintenance IV fluids based on body weight is:

  - 100 mL/kg/day for first 10 kg

  - 50 mL/kg/day for next 10 kg

  - 20 mL/kg/day for each kg above 20

Review Set 45

Calculate the following. Assume IV pumps measure whole milliliters.

1. If a child is receiving **chloramphenicol 400 mg IV q.6h** and the maximum concentration is 100 mg/mL, what is the minimum volume of fluid in which the medication can be safely diluted? _____ mL

2. If a child is receiving **gentamicin 25 mg IV q.8h** and the minimal concentration is 1 mg/mL, what is the maximum volume of fluid in which the medication can be safely diluted? _____ mL

3. Calculate the total volume and hourly IV flow rate for a 25 kg child receiving maintenance IV fluids. Infuse _____ mL at _____ mL/h.

4. Calculate the total volume and hourly IV flow rate for a 13 kg child receiving maintenance IV fluids. Infuse _____ mL at _____ mL/h.

5. Calculate the total volume and hourly IV flow rate for a 77 lb child receiving maintenance IV fluids. Infuse _____ mL at _____ mL/h.

6. Calculate the total volume and hourly IV flow rate for a 3,500 g infant receiving maintenance IV fluids. Infuse _____ mL at _____ mL/h.

7. A child is receiving 350 mg of a certain medication IV, and the minimal and maximal dilution range is 30 to 100 mg/mL. What is the minimum volume (maximal concentration) and the maximum volume (minimal concentration) for safe dilution? _____ mL (minimum volume); _____ mL (maximum volume). (Hint: The equipment measures whole mL; round up to the next whole mL.)

8. A child is receiving 52 mg of a certain medication IV, and the minimal and maximal dilution range is 0.8 to 20 mg/mL. What is the minimum volume and the maximum volume of fluid for safe dilution? _____ mL (minimum volume); _____ mL (maximum volume)

9. A child is receiving 175 mg of a certain medication IV, and the minimal and maximal dilution range is 5 to 75 mg/mL. What is the minimum volume and the maximum volume of fluid for safe dilution? _____ mL (minimum volume); _____ mL (maximum volume)

10. You are making rounds on your pediatric patients and you notice that a 2-year-old child who weighs 14 kg has 1,000 mL of normal saline infusing at the rate of 50 mL/h. You decide to question this order. What is your rationale? _____

_____

After completing these problems, see page 710 to check your answers.

CLINICAL REASONING SKILLS

Let's look at an example in which the nurse *prevents* a medication error by calculating the safe dosage of a medication before administering the drug to an infant.

ERROR

Dosage that is too high for an infant

Possible Scenario

Suppose a physician ordered KCl (*potassium chloride*) 25 mEq IV per 500 mL of $D_5\frac{1}{2}NS$ to infuse at the rate of 20 mL/h.

The infant weighs $10\frac{1}{2}$ lb and is 24 in long. KCl (potassium chloride) for IV injection is supplied as 2 mEq/mL. The nurse looked up potassium chloride in a drug reference and noted that the safe dosage of potassium chloride is up to 3 mEq/kg or 40 mEq/m²/day. The nurse calculated the infant's dosage as 14.4 mEq/day based on body weight and 11.2 mEq/day based on BSA.

First the nurse converted lb to kg.

$10\frac{1}{2}$ lb = 10.5 lb, 1 kg = 2.2 lb

$$\frac{1 \text{ kg}}{2.2 \text{ lb}} \diagdown\diagup \frac{X \text{ kg}}{10.5 \text{ lb}}$$

$$\frac{2.2X}{2.2} = \frac{10.5}{2.2}$$

$$X = 4.8 \text{ kg}$$

3 mEq/kg/day × 4.8 kg = 14.4 mEq/day

$$\text{BSA (m}^2) = \sqrt{\frac{\text{ht (in)} \times \text{wt (lb)}}{3{,}131}} = \sqrt{\frac{24 \times 10.5}{3{,}131}} = \sqrt{\frac{252}{3{,}131}} = \sqrt{0.080485} = 0.283 \text{ m}^2 = 0.28 \text{ m}^2$$

40 mEq/m²/day × 0.28 m² = 11.2 mEq/day

The nurse further calculated that, at the rate ordered, the infant would receive 480 mL of IV fluid per day, which is a reasonable daily rate of pediatric maintenance IV fluids.

20 mL/h × 24 h/day = 480 mL/day

Maintenance pediatric IV fluids:

100 mL/kg/day for first 10 kg: 100 mL/kg/day × 4.8 kg = 480 mL/day

But then the nurse calculated that the infant would receive 1 mEq KCl (potassium chloride) per hour.

$$\frac{25 \text{ mEq}}{500 \text{ mL}} \diagdown\diagup \frac{X \text{ mEq}}{20 \text{ mL}}$$

$$500X = 500$$

$$X = 1 \text{ mEq}$$

Finally, the nurse calculated that, at this rate, the infant would receive 24 mEq/day, which is approximately twice the safe dosage. Therefore, the order is unsafe.

1 mEq/h × 24 h/day = 24 mEq/day

The nurse notified the physician and questioned the order. The physician responded, "Thank you. You are correct. I intended to order one half that amount of potassium chloride, or 25 mEq per L, which should have been 12.5 mEq per 500 mL. This was my error, and I am glad that you caught it."

Potential Outcome

If the nurse had not questioned the order, the infant would have received twice the safe dosage. The infant likely would have developed signs of hyperkalemia that could lead to ventricular fibrillation, muscle weakness progressing to flaccid quadriplegia, respiratory failure, and possibly death.

Prevention

In this instance, the nurse prevented a medication error by checking the safe dosage and notifying the physician before administering the infusion. Let this be you!

PRACTICE PROBLEMS—CHAPTER 16

Calculate the volume for one safe dosage. Refer to the BSA formulas or the West Nomogram below (Figure 16-7) as needed to answer questions 1 through 20.

FIGURE 16-7 West Nomogram for estimation of body surface area

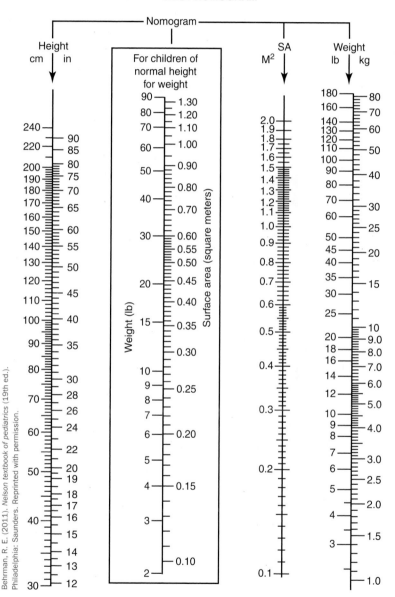

WEST NOMOGRAM

Metric:

$$BSA\ (m^2) = \sqrt{\frac{ht\ (cm) \times wt\ (kg)}{3,600}}$$

Household:

$$BSA\ (m^2) = \sqrt{\frac{ht\ (in) \times wt\ (lb)}{3,131}}$$

From Kliegman, R. M., Stanton, B. F., St. Geme, J., Schor, N., and Behrman, R. E. (2011). *Nelson textbook of pediatrics* (19th ed.). Philadelphia: Saunders. Reprinted with permission.

1. Order: **vincristine 2 mg direct IV stat** for a child who weighs 85 pounds and is 50 inches tall

   Recommended dosage of vincristine for children: 1.5 to 2 mg/m² 1 time/week; inject slowly over a period of 1 minute.

   Supply: vincristine 1 mg/mL

   BSA (per formula) of this child: _____ m²

   Recommended dosage range for this child: _____ mg to _____ mg

Is the ordered dosage safe? _____

If safe, give _____ mL/min or _____ mL per 15 sec.

If not, what should you do? _____

2. Use the BSA nomogram to calculate the safe oral dosage and amount to give of mercaptopurine for a child of normal proportions who weighs 25 pounds.

   Recommended dosage: 80 mg/m^2/day once daily p.o.

   Supply: mercaptopurine 50 mg/mL

   BSA: _____ m^2

   Safe dosage: _____ mg

   Give: _____ mL

3. Use the BSA nomogram to calculate the safe IV dosage of sargramostim for a 1-year-old child who is 25 inches tall and weighs 20 pounds.

   Recommended dosage: 250 mcg/m^2/day once daily IV

   BSA: _____ m^2

   Safe dosage: _____ mcg

4. Sargramostim is available in a solution strength of 500 mcg per 10 mL. Calculate 1 dose for the child in question 3.

   Give: _____ mL

5. Use the BSA nomogram to determine the BSA for a child who is 35 inches tall and weighs 40 pounds.

   BSA: _____ m^2

6. The child in question 5 will receive levodopa. The recommended oral dosage of levodopa is 0.5 g/m^2. What is the safe dosage for this child?

   Safe dosage: _____ mg

7. Levodopa is supplied in 100 mg and 250 mg capsules. Calculate 1 dose for the child in question 6.

   Give: _____ of the _____ mg capsule(s)

8. Use the BSA nomogram to determine the safe IM dosage of Oncaspar for a child who is 42 inches tall and weighs 45 pounds. The recommended IM dosage is 2,500 units/m^2/dose.

   BSA: _____ m^2

   Safe dosage: _____ units

9. Oncaspar is reconstituted to 750 units/mL. Calculate 1 dose for the child in question 8.

   Give: _____ mL

10. Should the Oncaspar in question 9 be given in one injection? _____

11. A child is 140 cm tall and weighs 43.5 kg. The recommended IV dosage of Adriamycin is 20 mg/m^2. Use the BSA formula to calculate the safe IV dosage of Adriamycin for this child.

    BSA: _____ m^2

    Safe dosage: _____ mg

12. Calculate the dose amount of Adriamycin for the child in question 11.

    Supply: Adriamycin 2 mg/mL

    Give: _____ mL

For questions 13 through 20, use the BSA formulas to calculate the BSA value.

13. Height: 5 ft 6 in   Weight: 136 lb   BSA: _____ m^2

14. Height: 4 ft   Weight: 80 lb   BSA: _____ m^2

15. Height: 60 cm   Weight: 6 kg   BSA: _____ m^2

16. Height: 68 in   Weight: 170 lb   BSA: _____ m^2

17. Height: 164 cm   Weight: 58 kg   BSA: _____ m^2

18. Height: 100 cm   Weight: 17 kg   BSA: _____ m^2

19. Height: 64 in   Weight: 63 kg   BSA: _____ m^2

20. Height: 85 cm   Weight: 11.5 kg   BSA: _____ m^2

21. What is the safe dosage of 1 dose of interferon alpha-2b required for a child with a BSA of 0.28 m^2 if the recommended dosage is 2 million units/m^2? _____ units

22. What is the safe dosage of calcium EDTA required for an adult with a BSA of 2.17 m^2 if the recommended dosage is 500 mg/m^2? _____ mg or _____ g

23. What is the total daily dosage range of mitomycin required for a child with a BSA of 0.19 m^2 if the recommended dosage range is 10 to 20 mg/m^2/day? _____ mg/day to _____ mg/day

24. What is the total safe daily dosage of thiotepa required for an adult with a BSA of 1.34 m^2 if the recommended dosage is 6 mg/m^2/day? _____ mg/day

25. After 5 full days of therapy receiving the recommended dosage, the patient in question 24 will have received a total of _____ mg of thiotepa.

For questions 26 through 38, the IV pump measures whole milliliters.

26. Order: **Ancef 0.42 g IV q.12h in 30 mL D$_5$NS over 30 min by volume-control set on an electronic infusion pump. Flush with 15 mL.**

    Supply: Ancef 500 mg per 5 mL

    Total IV fluid volume: _____ mL

    Flow rate: _____ mL/h

    Add _____ mL Ancef and _____ mL D$_5$NS to the chamber.

27. After 7 days of IV therapy, the patient referred to in question 26 will have received a total of _____ mL of Ancef.

28. Order: **clindamycin 285 mg IV q.8h in 45 mL D$_5$NS over 60 min by volume-control set on an electronic infusion pump. Flush with 15 mL.**

    Supply: clindamycin 75 mg per 0.5 mL

    Total IV fluid volume: _____ mL

    Flow rate: _____ mL/h

    Add _____ mL clindamycin and _____ mL D$_5$NS to the chamber.

29. When the patient in question 28 has received 4 days of therapy with clindamycin, she will have received a total clindamycin volume of _____ mL.

30. Order: **D$_5$ 0.225% NaCl IV at 65 mL/h $\bar{c}$ erythromycin 500 mg IV q.6h to be infused over 40 min**

    You will use a volume-control set and flush with 15 mL.

    Supply: erythromycin 50 mg/mL

    Add _____ mL of erythromycin and _____ mL D$_5$ 0.225% NaCl to the chamber.

31. When the patient in question 30 has received 5 days of therapy with erythromycin, he will have received a total erythromycin volume of _____ mL.

32. Order: D₅ 0.45% NaCl IV at 66 mL/h with Fortaz 620 mg IV q.8h to be infused over 40 min

    You will use a volume-control set and flush with 15 mL.

    Supply: Fortaz 0.5 g per 5 mL

    Add _____ mL Fortaz and _____ mL D₅ 0.45% NaCl to the chamber.

33. When the patient in question 32 has received 7 days of therapy with Fortaz, she will have received a total Fortaz volume of _____ mL.

For questions 34 through 38, calculate the daily volume of pediatric maintenance IV fluids using:

    100 mL/kg/day for first 10 kg of body weight

    50 mL/kg/day for next 10 kg of body weight

    20 mL/kg/day for each kg of body weight above 20 kg

34. Calculate the total volume and hourly IV flow rate for a child who weighs 10 kg and who is receiving maintenance fluids.

    Infuse _____ mL at _____ mL/h.

35. Calculate the total volume and hourly IV flow rate for a 21 kg child receiving maintenance fluids.

    Infuse _____ mL at _____ mL/h.

36. Calculate the total volume and hourly IV flow rate for a 78 lb child receiving maintenance fluids.

    Infuse _____ mL at _____ mL/h.

37. Calculate the total volume and hourly IV flow rate for a 33 lb child receiving maintenance fluids.

    Infuse _____ mL at _____ mL/h.

38. Calculate the total volume and hourly IV flow rate for a 2,400 g infant receiving maintenance fluids.

    Infuse _____ mL at _____ mL/h.

For questions 39 through 49, verify the safety of the following pediatric dosages ordered. If the dosage is safe, calculate 1 dose and the IV volume to infuse 1 dose.

Order for a child weighing 15 kg:

D₅ 0.45% NaCl IV at 53 mL/h c̄ ampicillin 275 mg IV q.4h infused over 40 min by volume-control set

Recommended dosage: ampicillin 100 to 125 mg/kg/day in 6 divided doses

Supply: ampicillin 1 g per 10 mL

39. Safe daily dosage range for this child: _____ mg/day to _____ mg/day

    Safe single dosage range for this child: _____ mg/dose to _____ mg/dose

    Is the ordered dosage safe? _____ If safe, give _____ mL/dose.

    If not safe, describe your action. _____

40. IV fluid volume to be infused in 40 min: _____ mL

    Add _____ mL ampicillin and _____ mL D₅ 0.45% NaCl to the chamber.

For questions 41 and 42, order for a child who weighs 27 lb:

D₅NS IV at 46 mL/h c̄ oxacillin 308 mg IV q.6h to be infused over 30 min by volume-control set

Recommended dosage: oxacillin 100 mg/kg/day in 4 divided doses

Supply: oxacillin 500 mg per 10 mL

41. Child's weight: _____ kg

    Safe daily dosage for this child: _____ mg/day

    Safe single dosage for this child: _____ mg/dose

    Is the ordered dosage safe? _____ If safe, give _____ mL/dose.

    If not safe, describe your action. _____

42. IV fluid volume to be infused in 30 min: _____ mL

    Add _____ mL oxacillin and _____ mL D$_5$ NS to the chamber.

For questions 43 and 44, order for a child who weighs 22 kg:

D$_5$ 0.225% NaCl IV at 50 mL/h c̄ Amikin 165 mg IV q.8h to be infused over 30 min by volume-control set

Recommended dosage: Amikin 15 to 22.5 mg/kg/day in 3 divided doses q.8h

Supply: Amikin 100 mg per 2 mL

43. Safe daily dosage range for this child: _____ mg/day to _____ mg/day

    Safe single dosage range for this child: _____ mg/dose to _____ mg/dose

    Is the ordered dosage safe? _____ If safe, give _____ mL/dose.

    If not safe, describe your action. _____

44. IV fluid volume to be infused in 30 min: _____ mL

    Add _____ mL Amikin and _____ mL D$_5$ 0.225% NaCl to the chamber.

For questions 45 and 46, order for a child who weighs 9 kg:

D$_5$NS IV at 38 mL/h c̄ Timentin 800 mg IV q.4h to be infused over 40 min by volume-control set

Recommended dosage: Timentin 200 to 300 mg/kg/day in 6 divided doses every 4 hours

Supply: Timentin 200 mg/mL

45. Safe daily dosage range for this child: _____ mg/day to _____ mg/day

    Safe single dosage range for this child: _____ mg/dose to _____ mg/dose

    Is the ordered dosage safe? _____ If safe, give _____ mL/dose.

    If not safe, describe your action. _____

46. IV fluid volume to be infused in 40 min: _____ mL

    Add _____ mL Timentin and _____ mL D$_5$ NS to the chamber.

For questions 47 through 49, order for a child who weighs 55 lb:

D$_5$NS IV at 60 mL/h c̄ penicillin G potassium 525,000 units q.4h to be infused over 20 min by volume-control set

Recommended dosage: penicillin G potassium 100,000 to 250,000 units/kg/day in 6 divided doses q.4h

Supply: penicillin G potassium 200,000 units/mL

47. Child's weight: _____ kg

    Safe daily dosage range for this child: _____ units/day to _____ units/day

    Safe single dosage range for this child: _____ units/dose to _____ units/dose

48. Is the ordered dosage safe? _____ If safe, give _____ mL/dose.

    If not safe, describe your action. _____

49. IV fluid volume to be infused in 20 min: _____ mL

    Add _____ mL penicillin G potassium and _____ mL D$_5$ NS to the chamber.

50. Describe the clinical reasoning you would use to prevent the following medication error.

    Possible Scenario

    Suppose the physician came to the pediatric oncology unit to administer chemotherapy to a critically ill child whose cancer symptoms had recurred suddenly. The nurse assigned to care for the child was floated from the adult oncology unit and was experienced in administering chemotherapy to adults. The physician, recognizing the nurse, said, "Oh good, you know how to calculate and prepare chemo. Go draw up 2 mg/m^2 of vincristine for this child so I can get his chemotherapy started quickly." The nurse consulted the child's chart and saw the following weights written on his assessment sheet: 20/.45. No height was recorded.

    On the adult unit, that designation means __X__ kg or __Y__ lb. The nurse took the West Nomogram and estimated the child's BSA based on his weight of 45 lb to be 0.82 m^2. The nurse calculated 2 mg/m^2 × 0.82 m^2 = 1.64 mg. Vincristine is supplied as 1 mg/1 mL, so the nurse further calculated that 1.6 mL was the dose and drew it up in a 3 mL syringe. As the nurse handed the syringe to the physician, the amount looked wrong. The physician asked the nurse how that amount was obtained. When the nurse told the physician that the estimated BSA from the child's weight (45 pounds) was 0.82 m^2 and that the dosage was 2 mg/m^2 × 0.82 m^2 = 1.64 mg, or 1.6 mL, the physician said, "No! This child's *BSA is 0.45 m^2*. I wrote it myself next to his weight—20 pounds." The physician, despite the need to give the medication as soon as possible, took the necessary extra step and examined the amount of medication in the syringe. Though the physician knew and trusted the nurse, the amount of medication in the syringe did not seem right. Perhaps the physician had figured a ballpark amount of about 1 mL and the volume the nurse brought in made the physician question what was calculated. The correct dosage calculations are:

    2 mg/m^2 × 0.45 m^2 = 0.9 mg

    $$\frac{\text{Dosage on hand}}{\text{Amount on hand}} = \frac{\text{Dosage desired}}{\text{X Amount desired}}$$

    $$\frac{1 \text{ mg}}{1 \text{ mL}} \diagdown\!\!\!\!\diagup \frac{0.9 \text{ mg}}{\text{X mL}}$$

    X = 0.9 mL

    Potential Outcome

    The child, already critically ill, could have received almost double the amount of medication had the physician rushed to give the dose calculated and prepared by someone else. This excessive amount of medication probably could have caused a fatal overdose. What should have been done to prevent this error?

    Prevention

    _____

    _____

After completing these problems, see pages 711–713 to check your answers.

◢ Be sure to use the online software for additional practice!

REFERENCE

Kliegman, R. M., Stanton, B. F., St. Geme, J., Schor, N., & Behrman, R.E. (2011). *Nelson textbook of pediatrics* (19th ed.). Philadelphia, PA: Saunders.

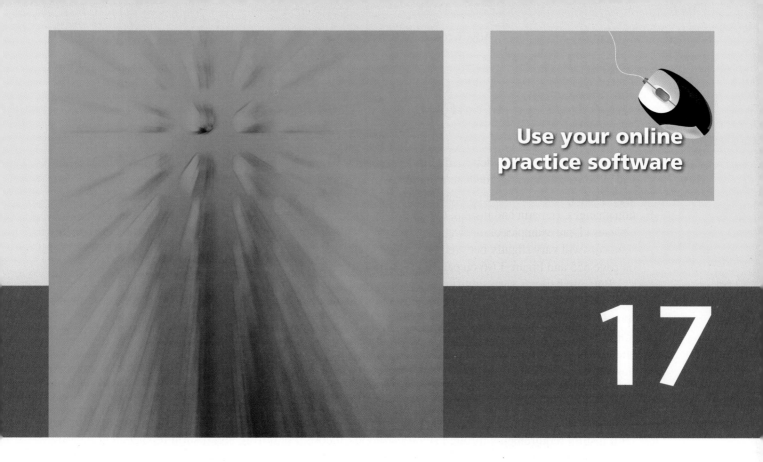

17

Advanced Adult Intravenous Calculations

OBJECTIVES

Upon mastery of Chapter 17, you will be able to perform advanced adult intravenous (IV) calculations and apply these skills to patients across the life span. To accomplish this, you will also be able to:

- Initiate and manage continuous infusions of critical medications (such as heparin and insulin) using protocol to:
  - Calculate a bolus dosage and volume.
  - Calculate a continuous infusion dosage (units/h) and rate (mL/h).
  - Monitor and make necessary adjustments to continuous intravenous therapy.
  - Observe patients for serious adverse reactions and administer antidote as needed.
- Calculate the flow rate and assess safe dosages for critical care IV medications administered over a specified time period.
- Calculate the flow rate for primary IV and IV piggyback (IV PB) solutions for patients with restricted fluid intake requirements.

Nurses are becoming increasingly more responsible for the administration of high-alert IV medications in the critical care areas as well as on general nursing units. Patients in life-threatening situations require thorough and timely interventions that frequently involve specialized, potent drugs. This chapter focuses on advanced adult IV calculations with special requirements that can be applied to patients across the life span.

CALCULATING IV DOSAGES AND FLOW RATES USING CLINICAL PROTOCOLS

Clinical protocols are preapproved orders for routine therapies, monitoring guidelines, and diagnostic procedures for patients with identified clinical problems. These orders are common in practice settings where patients' needs require immediate attention. Clinical protocols give the nurse legal protection to intervene appropriately and administer medication without contacting the prescriber each time the patient's condition changes. Heparin and insulin, two high-alert medications for which you learned to calculate dosages in Chapter 11, are examples of medications given intravenously that are ordered using standard protocols. Specific protocols will vary slightly between practitioners and agencies; however, two typical protocols (Figure 17-1 on page 555 and Figure 17-6 on page 566) are provided in this chapter as samples for study purposes.

Because patients vary significantly in weight, the intravenous heparin dosage is individualized based on the patient's weight. The heparin protocol orders depicted in Figure 17-1 are based on patient weight rounded to the nearest 10 kg (line 1). Some facilities use the patient's exact weight in kilograms. It is important to know the protocol for your clinical setting. When the patient's response to heparin therapy changes, as measured by the aPTT blood clotting value (activated partial thromboplastin time measured in seconds), the heparin dosage is adjusted as indicated in lines 11 to 15 of Figure 17-1.

Insulin dosage must be closely matched with insulin needs. For hospitalized patients, the dosage must be monitored and adjusted to meet special conditions such as infection, surgery, pregnancy, and drug-to-drug interactions. Nurses follow standard protocols to ensure that insulin dosage is coordinated with insulin requirements through rigorous blood glucose monitoring and insulin replacement therapy. The insulin protocol orders in Figure 17-6 provide instructions to use specific dosage grids for three levels of therapy based on potential resistance to insulin. If the patient is nondiabetic, the insulin infusion is started on the lowest level—i.e., Level 1. Diabetic patients begin insulin replacement on Level 2 and may need to move to the Level 3 insulin dosage grid if the therapy has proven ineffective.

For both the heparin and insulin protocols, as well as other protocols for critical medications, the administration process is the same and includes three sequential actions: 1) bolus, 2) continuous infusion, and 3) rebolus and/or adjust infusion rate.

RULE

To administer critical intravenous medications according to protocol, follow three sequential actions:

Action 1 **Bolus:** Determine the need for a bolus dose (a large dose to rapidly achieve a therapeutic effect) according to patient condition specified in the protocol. Select the right supplied drug, calculate, and administer the right amount by IV push or direct IV infusion.

Action 2 **Continuous infusion:** Acquire the right concentration of the continuous solution from the pharmacy (or mix the IV PB bag by selecting the right supplied drug), calculate to determine the amount required to provide the ordered dosage, and calculate and set the flow rate as determined by protocol.

Action 3 **Rebolus and/or adjust infusion rate:** Based on patient monitoring, determine if additional bolus is needed or if the continuous infusion rate needs to be increased, decreased, or discontinued.

CAUTION

Remember that high-alert drugs require independent double verification (of the order, test results, calculations, and drug preparation) by two clinicians who are alone and apart from each other, and who later compare results.

Let's apply all three actions beginning with the heparin protocol, and then we will work through the same process with the insulin protocol.

IV Heparin Protocol

Heparin protocols will vary slightly between facilities. For problems in this text, we will use a sample Standard Weight-Based Heparin Protocol (Figure 17-1), but you will use the protocol that has been adopted by the specific agency where you practice. In order to have consistent monitoring from shift to shift, the nurse must document the initiation of the protocol, serial aPTT values, and any resulting boluses and infusion rate changes. Figure 17-3 (page 561) is an example of a handwritten heparin protocol worksheet.

FIGURE 17-1   Sample heparin therapy protocol

SAMPLE STANDARD WEIGHT-BASED HEPARIN PROTOCOL		
For all patients on heparin drips:		
1. Weight in KILOGRAMS. Required for order to be processed: _____ kg (round to nearest 10 kg).		
2. Heparin 25,000 units in 250 mL of $\frac{1}{2}$NS; boluses to be given as 1,000 units/mL.		
3. aPTT q.6h or 6 hours after rate change; daily after two consecutive therapeutic aPTTs.		
4. CBC initially and repeat every _____ day(s).		
5. Obtain aPTT and PT/INR on day 1 prior to initiation of therapy.		
6. Guaiac stool initially, then every _____ day(s) until heparin discontinued. Notify if positive.		
7. Neuro checks every _____ hours while on heparin. Notify physician of any changes.		
8. Discontinue aPTT and CBC once heparin drip is discontinued unless otherwise ordered.		
9. Notify physician of any bleeding problems.		
10. Bolus with 80 units/kg. Start drip at 18 units/kg/h.		
11. If aPTT is less than 35 secs:	Rebolus with 80 units/kg and increase rate by 4 units/kg/h.	
12. If aPTT is 36 to 44 secs:	Rebolus with 40 units/kg and increase rate by 2 units/kg/h.	
13. If aPTT is 45 to 75 secs:	Continue current rate.	
14. If aPTT is 76 to 90 secs:	Decrease rate by 2 units/kg/h.	
15. If aPTT is greater than 90 secs:	Hold heparin for 1 hour and decrease rate by 3 units/kg/h.	
ONLY USE 1,000 unit/mL HEPARIN FOR BOLUSES		
WEIGHT	**INITIAL BOLUS** (VOL.)	**INITIAL INFUSION** (RATE)
40 kg	3,200 units (3.2 mL)	700 units/h (7 mL/h)
50 kg	4,000 units (4 mL)	900 units/h (9 mL/h)
60 kg	4,800 units (4.8 mL)	1,100 units/h (11 mL/h)
70 kg	5,600 units (5.6 mL)	1,300 units/h (13 mL/h)
80 kg	6,400 units (6.4 mL)	1,400 units/h (14 mL/h)
90 kg	7,200 units (7.2 mL)	1,600 units/h (16 mL/h)
100 kg	8,000 units (8 mL)	1,800 units/h (18 mL/h)
110 kg	8,800 units (8.8 mL)	2,000 units/h (20 mL/h)
120 kg	9,600 units (9.6 mL)	2,200 units/h (22 mL/h)
130 kg	10,400 units (10.4 mL)	2,300 units/h (23 mL/h)
140 kg	11,200 units (11.2 mL)	2,500 units/h (25 mL/h)
150 kg	12,000 units (12 mL)	2,700 units/h (27 mL/h)

Action 1: Bolus

A bolus dosage is a large dose of a medication given to rapidly achieve the needed therapeutic concentration in the bloodstream. Notice that the heparin protocol defines the bolus dosage that should be given based on the patient's weight and the results of the patient's blood tests. Let's first consider the initial bolus dosage ordered.

EXAMPLE 1 ▪

Your patient, who weighs 110 lb, has orders to start on Standard Weight-Based Heparin Protocol at 0900. The result of the baseline aPTT is 29 seconds. Refer to Figure 17-1, lines 1, 2, and 10 as we work through this example.

Protocol order: Bolus with 80 units/kg (line 10, Figure 17-1)

Supply: Automated dispensing cabinet (ADC) matrix drawer with vials of heparin in various concentrations (Figure 17-2)

FIGURE 17-2 · **(a)** Heparin 1,000 units/mL; **(b)** 10,000 units/mL

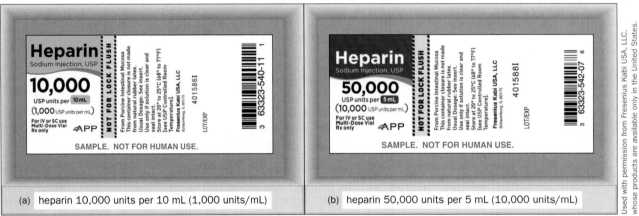

(a) heparin 10,000 units per 10 mL (1,000 units/mL)   (b) heparin 50,000 units per 5 mL (10,000 units/mL)

RULE

To calculate the heparin bolus:

1. Calculate the dosage (units) of the heparin bolus based on patient's weight (kg):

   units/kg × kg = units

2. Calculate the volume (mL) of the bolus to prepare using the ratio-proportion approach:

   $$\frac{\text{Dosage on hand}}{\text{Amount on hand}} = \frac{\text{Dosage desired}}{\text{X Amount desired}}$$

Note: This rule also applies to other bolus drugs ordered in units/kg, milliunits/kg, mg/kg, mcg/kg, g/kg, or mEq/kg.

Let's prepare the initial IV bolus, using the Three-Step Approach to dosage calculations that you have used throughout the book.

Step 1   **Convert**   No conversion is necessary for the medications, but the patient's weight needs to be converted to kilograms to calculate the correct bolus dosage by weight.

Equivalent: 1 kg = 2.2 lb

$$\frac{1\ kg}{2.2\ lb} \diagup\!\!\!\!\diagdown \frac{X\ kg}{110\ lb}$$

$$2.2X = 110$$

$$\frac{2.2X}{2.2} = \frac{110}{2.2}$$

$$X = 50\ kg$$

Step 2   **Think**   The patient is ordered to receive an initial bolus of 80 units/kg. According to the grid provided, the initial bolus dosage for a patient weighing 50 kg is 4,000 units or 4 mL. But because heparin is supplied in various concentrations, you must know which concentration to use. You must not draw up 4 mL of just any vial of heparin. The protocol specifically requires the use of the 1,000 units/mL concentration of heparin (line 2). The grid only provides the initial bolus, so the nurse will have to calculate any additional boluses needed throughout the therapy. We will calculate the bolus now to verify the grid and then use this same calculation process for additional boluses. Carefully compare the two supplied concentrations. At first glance, you might think the supply you need is unavailable in the ADC. However, on closer inspection you will see that the strength per total volume (10,000 units per 10 mL; 50,000 units per 5 mL) is printed on both heparin labels as the primary expression of strength. The strength per milliliter is located in the parentheses (1,000 units/mL; 10,000 units/mL) directly below the strength per total volume. Select one vial from the ADC compartment labeled 1,000 units/mL (Figure 17-2a, page 556), and check the label again to be certain it is of the desired concentration.

Step 3   **Calculate**   the dosage (units) of the heparin bolus based on the patient's weight (kg).

units/kg $\times$ kg = 80 units/kg $\times$ 50 kg = 4,000 units

The patient should receive 4,000 units heparin as a bolus (verifies grid).

Calculate   the volume (mL) of the bolus to prepare.

$$\frac{\text{Dosage on hand}}{\text{Amount on hand}} = \frac{\text{Dosage desired}}{\text{X Amount desired}}$$

$$\frac{1,000 \text{ units}}{1 \text{ mL}} \diagdown\!\!\!\!\diagup \frac{4,000 \text{ units}}{\text{X mL}}$$

$$\frac{1,000\text{X}}{1,000} = \frac{4,000}{1,000}$$

$$1,000\text{X} = 4,000$$

$$\text{X} = 4 \text{ mL (verifies grid)}$$

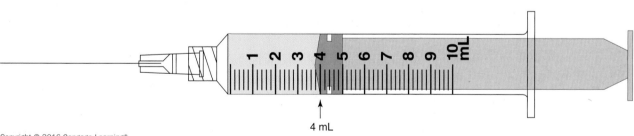

4 mL

Measure 4 mL of heparin from the 1,000 units/mL supply in a 10 mL syringe. Because 6 mL remain in the vial, label the vial with date and time opened and store safely for next use. Provide order, vial, and syringe to another nurse for independent verification and documentation. Document the patient's weight, the initial bolus, and the initial infusion rate in the designated spaces at the top of the heparin protocol worksheet (Figure 17-3, page 561).

CAUTION

Heparin is a high-alert medication. Read heparin labels very carefully. Health care agencies are transitioning from old to new regulations for label content and design in response to a recent announcement by the U.S. Pharmacopeial Convention (USP). Heparin labels must now print the strength per total volume as the primary expression of strength, followed in close proximity by the strength per milliliter (mL) (Institute for Safe Medication Practices, 2013). Be aware that both the old and new labels may be available until current supplies are depleted. To avoid serious medication errors, always identify the concentration of the supply as well as the total volume in the container.

Action 2: Continuous Infusion

A continuous infusion is a controlled method of drug administration in which the rate and quality of drug administration can be precisely adjusted over time. Often, IV solutions with heparin, insulin, or other added high-alert drugs come premixed from the hospital pharmacy. There will be times when nurses will need to mix the IV solution for the continuous infusion. Let's continue with your patient in the previous example by following the protocol to prepare the IV heparin solution and calculate the initial infusion rate.

EXAMPLE 2 ■

In addition to receiving the bolus dose, your patient from Example 1 will need to have the continuous infusion started according to protocol.

Protocol order for heparin solution: heparin 25,000 units in 250 mL $\frac{1}{2}$NS (line 2, Figure 17-1, page 555)

Supply: ADC matrix drawer with vials of heparin in various concentrations (Figure 17-2, page 556)

Let's prepare the IV solution using the Three-Step Approach to dosage calculations.

Step 1	**Convert**	Remember: You already know that 110 lb = 50 kg. The order and the supplied dosages are in the same unit of measurement: units. No conversion is necessary.
Step 2	**Think**	It is clear to see that the 50,000 units per 5 mL supply dosage (Figure 17-2b, page 556) is the vial that will provide 25,000 units. If there are 50,000 units in the 5 mL vial, then there are 10,000 units in 1 mL, which is stated on the label in the parentheses. This order for 25,000 units is supplied by half of the total volume in the vial, or 2.5 mL. Select one vial from the ADC compartment labeled 50,000 units per 5 mL (Figure 17-2b), and check the label again to be certain it is of the desired concentration.

Step 3 **Calculate**

$$\frac{\text{Dosage on hand}}{\text{Amount on hand}} = \frac{\text{Dosage desired}}{\text{X Amount desired}}$$

$$\frac{10,000 \text{ units}}{1 \text{ mL}} \diagdown \frac{25,000 \text{ units}}{\text{X mL}}$$

$$10,000\text{X} = 25,000$$

$$\frac{10,000\text{X}}{10,000} = \frac{25,000}{10,000}$$

$$\text{X} = 2.5 \text{ mL (verifies estimate)}$$

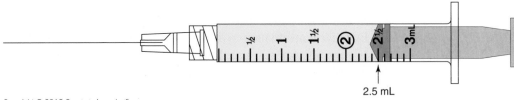

2.5 mL

Measure 2.5 mL of heparin from the 10,000 units/mL supply in a 3 mL syringe. Provide order, vial, and syringe to another nurse for independent verification and documentation. Add to the 250 mL IV PB bag of 0.45% sodium chloride $\left(\frac{1}{2}NS\right)$ through the injection port. There will be 2.5 mL of this highly concentrated, high-alert drug remaining in the vial. Either discard the vial immediately or label with date and time opened, and store safely. Prepare a label with the patient's name, drug name and concentration, dosage and amount added, date and time prepared, and your signature, and place the label on the IV PB bag.

Protocol order for initial infusion rate: Start drip at 18 units/kg/h (line 10, Figure 17-1, page 555)

Supply: heparin 25,000 units in 250 mL

RULE

To calculate the continuous flow rate of the IV heparin solution in mL/h:

1. Calculate the dosage (units/h) of the initial continuous infusion based on patient's weight (kg):

   units/kg/h × kg = units/h

2. Calculate the continuous infusion rate (mL/h) using ratio and proportion:

   Ratio of supply dosage on hand is equivalent to ratio of desired dosage rate

   $$\frac{\text{Dosage on hand}}{\text{Amount on hand}} = \frac{\text{Dosage desired/h}}{\text{X Amount desired/h}}$$

Note: This rule applies to drugs ordered in units/kg/h, milliunits/kg/h, mg/kg/h, mcg/kg/h, g/kg/h, or mEq/kg/h.

Now let's calculate the initial infusion rate using the Three-Step Approach to dosage calculations.

Step 1 Convert   The order and the supplied dosages are in the same unit of measurement: units. No conversion is necessary. Remember: You already know that the patient's weight of 110 lb = 50 kg.

Step 2 Think   According to the grid provided, the initial continuous infusion rate for a patient weighing 50 kg is 900 units/h (9 mL/h). Remember that the grid only provides the initial infusion rate, so the nurse will have to calculate any necessary infusion rate increases or decreases throughout the therapy. We will calculate the infusion rate now to verify the grid and then use this same calculation process for any needed adjustments in the rate. The solution prepared is 25,000 units per 250 mL. You need 900 units for the dose; 900 units is less than $\frac{1}{2}$ but more than $\frac{1}{3}$ of 25,000 units. So you will need less than 125 mL but more than 80 mL. You can also use ratio and proportion to determine how many units are in 1 mL. If there are 25,000 units per 250 mL, how many units are there in 1 mL? Set up the ratio and proportion like this:

$$\frac{25,000 \text{ units}}{250 \text{ mL}} \diagtimes \frac{\text{X units}}{1 \text{ mL}}$$

$$250X = 25,000$$

$$\frac{250X}{250} = \frac{25,000}{250}$$

$$X = 100 \text{ units}\qquad \text{There are 100 units of heparin per 1 mL.}$$

Now you know that with the concentration of heparin solution used for this protocol, each mL infused will contain 100 units of heparin. So if you want to administer 900 units of heparin, you want 9 times 1 mL, or 9 mL.

Step 3   **Calculate**   the dosage (units/h) of the continuous infusion increase based on the patient's weight (kg).

units/kg/h × kg = 18 units/kg/h × 50 kg = 900 units/h (verifies grid)

Calculate   the new hourly infusion rate (mL/h) using a ratio-proportion approach:

$$\frac{\text{Dosage on hand}}{\text{Amount on hand}} = \frac{\text{Dosage desired/h}}{\text{X Amount desired/h}}$$

$$\frac{100 \text{ units}}{1 \text{ mL}} \diagdown \frac{900 \text{ units/h}}{\text{X mL/h}}$$

$$100\text{X} = 900$$

$$\frac{100\text{X}}{100} = \frac{900}{100}$$

$$\text{X} = 9 \text{ mL/h (verifies grid and estimate)}$$

As you can see, knowing the units per mL simplifies the calculation. In fact, for many protocols, the concentrations for the solutions are specifically chosen to help make the calculations easier, thereby reducing the risk of error. The rate on the chart included with the protocol is verified by our calculations. Remember that, while the chart is convenient to refer to when setting up the initial infusion, it is not to be used for any needed adjustment to the infusion rate throughout the therapy. This high-alert medication will be infused using an electronic IV infusion pump. For this example, we will assume that the infusion pump available is designed to infuse at the mL/h rate using whole numbers only. It is important to verify the calibration of the IV pump in your clinical setting. Some IV pumps are programmable in tenths of a milliliter. Set the rate on the pump for the initial infusion at 9 mL/h. Ask another nurse for independent verification of the initial infusion rate.

Action 3: Rebolus and/or Adjust Infusion Rate

The anticoagulant heparin is used to prevent formation of thrombi (intravenous blood clots) by suppressing clotting factors, such as thrombin. The most significant complication of treatment is life-threatening hemorrhage. The goal of heparin therapy is to reduce the body's ability to clot to a level that is low enough to prevent thrombosis but not so low that it causes spontaneous bleeding. Response to heparin therapy is highly variable from one individual patient to another. The activated partial thromboplastin time (aPTT) is a blood test that measures the time it takes blood to clot. The aPTT is used during anticoagulation therapy to determine the right dosage of the drug. It is the nurse's responsibility to monitor the patient for bleeding and adjust the dosage of heparin based on periodic measurements of aPTT and the heparin protocol.

EXAMPLE 3 ■

At 1500, 6 hours after the initiation of the heparin infusion, your patient on the heparin protocol has an aPTT test done (line 3, Figure 17-1, page 555). One hour later, at 1600, the result is reported to be 43 seconds. This result is documented on the heparin protocol worksheet (Figure 17-3, page 561). The clotting time measured has lengthened from 26 seconds to 43 seconds but has not reached the target time. According to the protocol, you will rebolus with 40 units/kg and increase the amount of IV heparin by 2 units/kg/h (line 12, Figure 17-1) and then recheck the aPTT in 6 hours. You will use the same calculation skills you learned in the previous examples for the initial bolus and to set the initial infusion rate. (Note: Example 3 continues on page 562.)

FIGURE 17-3   Sample heparin protocol worksheet

STANDARD WEIGHT-BASED HEPARIN PROTOCOL WORKSHEET

Round patient's total body weight to nearest 10 kg: __50__ kg.

DO NOT change the weight based on daily measurements.

FOUND ON THE ORDER FORM
Initial Bolus (80 units/kg): __4,000__ units __4__ mL
Initial Infusion Rate (18 units/kg/h): __900__ units/h __9__ mL/h

Make adjustments to the heparin drip rate as directed by the order form.

ALL DOSES ARE ROUNDED TO THE NEAREST 100 UNITS.

Date	Time	aPTT sec	Bolus units	Rate Change units/h	Rate Change mL/h	New Rate mL/h	RN 1 initial	RN 2 initial
1/22/14	1500	43	-----------	-----------	-----------	-----------	MT	-----------
1/22/14	1600	-----------	2,000	100	1	10	MT	GP

If aPTT is	Then
Less than 35 secs:	Rebolus with 80 units/kg and increase rate by 4 units/kg/h.
36 to 44 secs:	Rebolus with 40 units/kg and increase rate by 2 units/kg/h.
45 to 75 secs:	Continue current rate.
76 to 90 secs:	Decrease rate by 2 units/kg/h.
Greater than 90 secs:	Hold heparin for 1 hour and decrease rate by 3 units/kg/h.

Signatures	Initials
M. Tremel, RN	MT
G. Pickar, RN	GP

RULE

To calculate the heparin rebolus and adjust the continuous infusion rate:

1. Calculate the dose (units) of the heparin bolus based on aPTT results and patient's weight (kg):

units/kg × kg = units

2. Calculate the volume (mL) of the bolus to prepare using the ratio-proportion approach:

$$\frac{\text{Dosage on hand}}{\text{Amount on hand}} = \frac{\text{Dosage desired/h}}{\text{X Amount desired/h}}$$

3. Calculate the dosage (units/h) of the continuous infusion adjustment based on aPTT results and patient's weight (kg):

units/kg/h × kg = units/h

4. Calculate the adjustment to the hourly infusion rate (mL/h) using ratio and proportion:

$$\frac{\text{Dosage on hand}}{\text{Amount on hand}} = \frac{\text{Dosage desired/h}}{\text{X Amount desired/h}}$$

5. Calculate the new hourly infusion rate (mL/h):

current rate (mL/h) ± adjustment (mL/h) = new rate (mL/h)

Note: This rule also applies to other rebolus or continuous infusion drugs ordered in units/kg/h, milliunits/kg/h, mg/kg/h, mcg/kg/h, g/h, or mEq/kg/h.

Protocol order: Rebolus with 40 units/kg and increase rate by 2 units/kg/h (line 12, Figure 17-1, page 555)

Supply: Vial of heparin 1,000 units/mL with 6 mL remaining from Example 1; IV PB of heparin 25,000 units in 250 mL currently infusing

Calculate the adjusted infusion rate using the Three-Step Approach to dosage calculations.

Step 1	**Convert**	Remember that you already know that the patient's weight of 110 lb = 50 kg and that no unit conversion is necessary.
Step 2	**Think**	The patient now needs to receive a bolus of 40 units/kg. You cannot use the grid provided, because it lists the dosage for the initial bolus of 80 units/kg. You will need to calculate the dose, so think: if the patient now needs half of the initial bolus order, the dose should be half of the bolus dose, which was 4 mL. The bolus should now be 2 mL. Additionally, the continuous infusion is set at a rate of 18 units/kg/h, or 9 mL per hour. The rate will need to be increased by 2 units/kg/h, which should provide an hourly rate of slightly more than 9 mL.
Step 3	**Calculate**	the dosage (units) of the heparin rebolus based on patient's weight (kg).

units/kg × kg = 40 units/k̶g̶ × 50 k̶g̶ = 2,000 units

The patient should receive 2,000 units heparin as a rebolus.

Calculate the volume (mL) of the rebolus to prepare. Remember that you will use the 1,000 units/mL supply to measure the amount of heparin for the rebolus.

$$\frac{\text{Dosage on hand}}{\text{Amount on hand}} = \frac{\text{Dosage desired}}{\text{X Amount desired}}$$

$$\frac{1,000 \text{ units}}{1 \text{ mL}} \diagdown\diagup \frac{2,000 \text{ units}}{\text{X mL}}$$

$$1,000X = 2,000$$

$$\frac{1,000X}{1,000} = \frac{2,000}{1,000}$$

$$X = 2 \text{ mL (verifies estimate)}$$

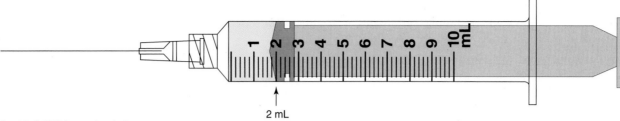

2 mL

Measure 2 mL of heparin from the 1,000 units/mL supply in a 10 mL syringe. You may use the vial with 6 mL remaining from the initial bolus if it was safely labeled and stored. There will now be 4 mL remaining, which you may store safely for the next use. Provide order, vial, and syringe to another nurse for independent verification and documentation.

Calculate   the dosage (units/h) of the continuous infusion increase based on patient's weight (kg).

units/kg/h × kg = 2 units/k̶g̶/h × 50 k̶g̶ = 100 units/h

The infusion rate should be increased by 100 units per hour.

Calculate   the adjustment to the hourly infusion rate (mL/h).

$$\frac{\text{Dosage on hand}}{\text{Amount on hand}} = \frac{\text{Dosage desired/h}}{\text{X Amount desired/h}}$$

$$\frac{100 \text{ units}}{1 \text{ mL}} \diagdown \frac{100 \text{ units/h}}{\text{X mL/h}}$$

$$100X = 100$$

$$\frac{100X}{100} = \frac{100}{100}$$

$$X = 1 \text{ mL/h}$$

Calculate   the new hourly infusion rate (mL/h).

9 mL/h + 1 mL/h = 10 mL/h (verifies estimate)

Increase the rate on the pump to 10 mL/h. Ask another nurse for independent verification of the infusion rate adjustment. Document the time and dose of the bolus and the infusion rate changes on the heparin protocol worksheet (Figure 17-3, page 561). Plan to recheck the aPTT at 2200, which is 6 hours after the rebolus and infusion rate change, not 6 hours since the last lab work.

You have now worked through the three sequential actions needed to safely initiate, monitor, and maintain continuous intravenous infusions of high-alert medications. The principles learned with the heparin examples may be applied to calculations of boluses and continuous infusions for other critical medications.

Heparin Overdose

Intravenous infusions of high-alert medications require vigilance to ensure that the patient receives the correct dosage and that serious side effects are recognized and treated promptly. In addition to safely preparing the medication according to protocol, the nurse must be prepared to administer an antidote in the case of life-threatening adverse reactions. Adverse reactions may be the result of expected risks due to individual patient variation, but may also occur due to calculation error or intravenous pump malfunction. Protamine sulfate is the antidote to severe heparin overdose. Let's consider a potential situation when protamine sulfate might be indicated.

EXAMPLE 4 ■

Your patient on the heparin protocol has been receiving intravenous heparin according to protocol for 21 hours. After periodic adjustments, the infusion rate is currently set for 12 mL/h, which is equal to 12,000 units/h. The most recent aPTT result was 94 seconds, which according to protocol required the infusion to be stopped for 1 hour and then decreased by 3 units/kg/h (line 15, Figure 17-1, page 555). While waiting to resume the heparin infusion, the patient care technician reports to the nurse that the patient's blood pressure has dropped, pulse has increased, and that urine is very dark. Recognizing that these are all signs of possible hemorrhage, the nurse contacts the physician, who orders **protamine sulfate 12 mg slow IV push**. The recommended infusion rate is no faster than 20 mg per minute. Calculate this emergency dose using the Three-Step Approach to dosage calculations.

Order: **protamine sulfate 12 mg slow IV push**

Supply: See Figure 17-4

FIGURE 17-4   Protamine sulfate 50 mg (10 mg/mL)

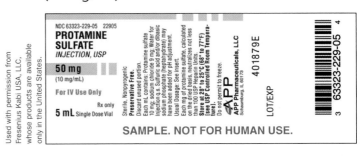

Step 1	**Convert**	The order and the supplied dosages are in the same unit of measurement: mg. No conversion is necessary.
Step 2	**Think**	There are 50 mg in the entire 5 mL vial, but the concentration is also stated as 10 mg/mL. Because 12 mg is slightly larger than 10 mg, you will need slightly more than 1 mL. The rate should be no faster than 20 mg per minute. Because 12 mg is slightly larger than $\frac{1}{2}$ of 20 mg, the dose should be injected in slightly more than $\frac{1}{2}$ minute.
Step 3	**Calculate**	$\dfrac{\text{Dosage on hand}}{\text{Amount on hand}} = \dfrac{\text{Dosage desired}}{\text{X Amount desired}}$

$$\frac{10 \text{ mg}}{1 \text{ mL}} \diagdown \frac{12 \text{ mg}}{\text{X mL}}$$

$$10\text{X} = 12$$

$$\frac{10\text{X}}{10} = \frac{12}{10}$$

$$\text{X} = 1.2 \text{ mL (verifies estimate)}$$

Draw up 1.2 mL in a 3 mL syringe and inject as an IV push.

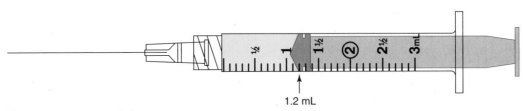

1.2 mL

Recall from Chapter 15 that ratio-proportion can be used to calculate the time required to administer IV push medications.

Rate: 20 mg/min or 20 mg per 60 sec

$$\frac{\text{Dosage on hand}}{\text{Amount on hand}} = \frac{\text{Dosage desired}}{\text{X Amount desired}}$$

$$\frac{20 \text{ mg}}{60 \text{ sec}} \diagdown\!\!\!\diagup \frac{12 \text{ mg}}{\text{X sec}}$$

$$20X = 720$$

$$\frac{20X}{20} = \frac{720}{20}$$

$$X = 36 \text{ sec (verifies estimate)}$$

Infuse 1.2 mL of protamine sulfate over at least 36 seconds.

Use ratio and proportion to calculate how much to push each 15 seconds, to slowly titrate the infusion.

$$\frac{1.2 \text{ mL}}{36 \text{ sec}} \diagdown\!\!\!\diagup \frac{\text{X mL}}{15 \text{ sec}}$$

$$36X = 18 \text{ sec}$$

$$\frac{36X}{36} = \frac{18}{36}$$

$$X = 0.5 \text{ mL (every 15 sec)}$$

IV Insulin Protocol

It has been shown that critically ill diabetic patients who have tight management of blood glucose levels have reduced morbidity and mortality. There is increased use of intravenous insulin protocols in the intensive care units and on some medical-surgical units to maintain tight control over hyperglycemia. While there is no universal protocol for intravenous insulin infusions, most are similar in approach. In this text, we will use the sample critical care intravenous insulin protocol (Figure 17-6, page 566) to calculate insulin dosage, but in your clinical practice, you will use the protocol that has been adopted by your health care agency. According to the sample protocol, the target level for blood glucose control is 70 to 110 mg/dL. As with the heparin protocol, we will use the same three sequential actions: 1) bolus, 2) continuous infusion, and 3) rebolus and/or adjust infusion rate.

EXAMPLE 1 ■

Individual patients' insulin needs vary and are regulated based on the measurement of blood glucose. The sample insulin protocol provides three levels of insulin dosage, depending on expected individual response to insulin therapy. Rapid- or short-acting insulin may be used for intravenous infusions. The sample protocol uses regular U-100 insulin (line 1, Figure 17-6). The insulin available is pictured in Figure 17-5.

FIGURE 17-5 Humulin R regular U-100 insulin

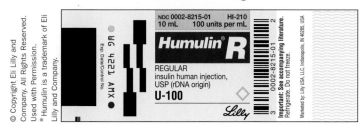

FIGURE 17-6   Sample intravenous insulin therapy protocol

	Sample Critical Care Intravenous Insulin Protocol Orders
TARGET	**BLOOD GLUCOSE LEVEL 70 to 110 mg/dL**
Insulin Solution	1. 100 units **regular U-100 insulin** in 100 mL of 0.9% NaCl, to be titrated based on grid for Levels 1, 2, or 3.
Initial Infusion	2. Start nondiabetic patients at Level 1. Advance to Level 2 if TARGET range not reached after 2 hours on Level 1. 3. Start diabetic patients at Level 2. Advance to Level 3 if TARGET range not reached after 2 hours on Level 2. 4. Do not initiate insulin infusion unless blood glucose greater than 110 mg/dL.
Monitoring	5. Check blood glucose prior to start of insulin infusion. 6. Check blood glucose every hour thereafter. 7. When glucose is 80 to 110 mg/dL for 3 hours, check glucose every 2 hours. 8. Resume monitoring every hour if blood glucose greater than 120 mg/dL for 2 hours.

Blood Glucose Less than 80 mg/dL	9. If patient has blood glucose less than 80 mg/dL:
	   a. Refer to regular insulin infusion rate column in grid tables for management instructions.
	   b. If necessary to reinitiate insulin infusion, start one level below previous level.
	   c. Call physician for symptomatic hypoglycemia or blood glucose less than 50 mg/dL, even if treated.

Sample Grid for Titration of Intravenous Insulin—Level 2

LEVEL 2: DO NOT INITIATE insulin drip unless blood glucose is greater than 110 mg/dL.

Blood Glucose (mg/dL)	Regular U-100 Insulin Bolus	Regular Insulin Infusion Rate: 100 Units of Regular U-100 Insulin in 100 mL NaCl
Less than 70	Give $\frac{1}{2}$ of 50 mL amp of 50% dextrose	HOLD insulin infusion $\times$ 60 minutes and check blood glucose every 15 minutes until equal to or greater than 80.
70 to 79	0	HOLD insulin infusion $\times$ 60 minutes and check blood glucose every 15 minutes until equal to or greater than 80.
80 to 110	0	2 units/h
111 to 125	0	3 units/h
126 to 149	0	4 units/h
150 to 165	0	5 units/h
166 to 179	0	6 units/h
180 to 209	0	8 units/h
210 to 239	10 units IV push	12 units/h
240 to 269	10 units IV push	16 units/h
270 to 299	10 units IV push	20 units/h
300 to 350	10 units IV push	25 units/h
Greater than 350	Notify physician	

For this example, we will provide insulin coverage for an insulin-dependent diabetic who is recovering in the intensive care unit from extensive surgery. According to protocol (line 3, Figure 17-6, page 566), the sample Level 2 grid for titration of insulin will be used for this patient. (For simplicity, the Level 1 and Level 3 grids, used for less critical or more critical situations respectively, have been omitted.) The point-of-care blood glucose measurement of this patient is 226 mg/dL, as tested upon admission to the intensive care unit.

Action 1   **Bolus:** Unlike the heparin protocol, the initial insulin bolus dose is not based on patient weight, but glucose level alone. A bolus dose is not always required. In this instance, the patient's blood glucose level of 226 mg/dL falls between 210 and 239 mg/dL, which requires a bolus of 10 units U-100 regular insulin. Draw up 10 units in a 30-unit Lo-Dose insulin syringe.

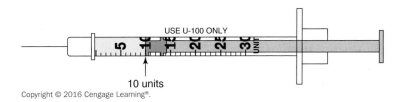

Provide the order, point-of-care glucose measurement, insulin vial, and syringe to another nurse for independent verification and documentation.

Action 2   **Continuous infusion:** Often, insulin or other high-alert drugs come premixed from the hospital pharmacy. But there will be times when nurses will need to mix the IV solution for the continuous infusion. Let's continue with our patient example by following the protocol to prepare the IV insulin solution (line 1, Figure 17-6) and then by calculating the initial infusion rate for the blood glucose level of this patient (226 mg/dL, which is in the range on the Level 2 grid of 210 to 239 mg/dL).

Protocol order insulin solution: 100 units regular insulin in 100 mL of 0.9% NaCl

Draw up 100 units of regular U-100 insulin in a standard U-100 insulin syringe.

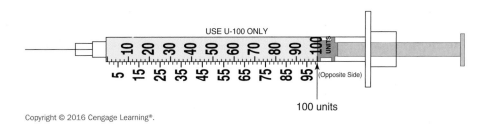

Provide the order, point-of-care glucose measurement, insulin vial, and syringe to another nurse for independent verification and documentation. Inject the 100 units into the 100 mL IV PB bag of 0.9% NaCl (NS or normal saline). Prepare a label with the patient's name, drug name and concentration, dosage and amount added, date and time prepared, and your signature. Secure the label on the IV PB bag.

Protocol order insulin infusion rate: Now we will calculate the hourly infusion rate with the same formula we used to calculate the heparin infusion.

RULE

To calculate the continuous flow rate of IV solutions mL/h using the ratio-proportion approach:

$$\frac{\text{Dosage on hand}}{\text{Amount on hand}} = \frac{\text{Dosage desired/h}}{\text{X Amount desired/h}}$$

Note: This rule also applies to other continuous infusion drugs ordered in units/h, milliunits/h, mg/h, mcg/h, g/h, or mEq/h.

The patient's blood glucose level of 226 mg/dL falls between 210 and 239 mg/dL, which requires an infusion rate of 12 units/h.

$$\frac{\text{Dosage on hand}}{\text{Amount on hand}} = \frac{\text{Dosage desired/h}}{\text{X Amount desired/h}}$$

$$\frac{100 \text{ units}}{100 \text{ mL}} \diagdown \frac{12 \text{ units/h}}{\text{X mL/h}}$$

$$100X = 1{,}200$$

$$\frac{100X}{100} = \frac{1{,}200}{100}$$

$$X = 12 \text{ mL/h}$$

For this problem, we will assume that the infusion pump available is designed to infuse at a mL/h rate using whole numbers only. Set the rate on the pump for the initial infusion at 12 mL/h. Ask another nurse for independent verification of the initial infusion rate.

Action 3   **Rebolus and/or adjust infusion rate:** The insulin protocol requires hourly blood glucose monitoring until the glucose level is 80 to 110 mg/dL for 3 hours (lines 6 and 7, Figure 17-6, page 566). For the patient in this example, 1 hour after the infusion is started, the point-of-care blood glucose measurement is 206 mg/dL. What will you do?

Rebolus: Is a bolus necessary now? 206 mg/dL falls between 180 and 209 mg/dL. According to the grid, no bolus is needed at this time.

Adjust infusion rate: According to the grid, for a glucose measurement of 206 mg/dL, the rate should be set for 8 units per hour. Now that we know there is 1 unit/mL, we will give 8 times as much, or 8 mL/h. While this seems obvious, let's use ratio and proportion one more time to verify our estimate.

$$\frac{\text{Dosage on hand}}{\text{Amount on hand}} = \frac{\text{Dosage desired/h}}{\text{X Amount desired/h}}$$

$$\frac{1 \text{ unit}}{1 \text{ mL}} \diagdown \frac{8 \text{ units/h}}{\text{X mL/h}}$$

$$1X = 8$$

$$\frac{1X}{1} = \frac{8}{1}$$

$$X = 8 \text{ mL/h}$$

Reduce the rate on the infusion pump from 12 mL/h to 8 mL/h. Ask another nurse for independent verification of the change in infusion rate. Remember: In order to have consistent monitoring from shift to shift, the nurse must document the time and dose of the bolus and infusion rate changes on a standard worksheet.

Insulin Overdose

Hypoglycemia (blood glucose below 50 mg/dL) occurs when insulin levels exceed insulin needs. This may result from an overdose of insulin during intravenous infusion due to expected risks because of individual patient variation, but may also occur because of calculation error or intravenous pump malfunction. Rapid treatment of hypoglycemia is required to prevent irreversible brain damage or even death. For this reason, protocols for insulin and other high-alert drugs frequently include standard orders for severe adverse reactions. The sample protocol for intravenous insulin infusion provides an order for 50% dextrose in the case of hypoglycemia. It is supplied for emergency use in a prefilled ampule of 25 g per 50 mL.

EXAMPLE 2 ▪

After periodic adjustments in the insulin infusion rate, the patient care technician reports that your patient in the previous example was acting confused during the point-of-care glucose monitoring, which was 65 mg/dL. According to the protocol, the nurse should give $\frac{1}{2}$ amp (ampule) of 50% dextrose, hold the insulin infusion for 60 minutes, and check blood glucose every 15 minutes until it is greater than or equal to 80 mg/dL.

Protocol order: *Give $\frac{1}{2}$ amp of 50% dextrose*

Supply: 50 mL ampule of 50% dextrose

Calculate: $\frac{1}{2} \times 50 \text{ mL} = \frac{\overset{25}{\cancel{50}}}{\underset{1}{\cancel{2}}} \text{ mL} = 25 \text{ mL}$

To administer $\frac{1}{2}$ amp of 50% dextrose, you will need to give 25 mL by IV push. You should discard 25 mL, leaving 25 mL in the ampule, and then push the entire amount remaining through an infusion port near the IV insertion site. It is not safe to insert the ampule with the entire amount into the port and then try to push only 25 mL. It is very difficult to push a 50% dextrose solution, and you could push forcefully and inject more than the ordered amount.

According to protocol, increase glucose monitoring to every 15 minutes until greater than 80 mg/dL. The physician must be notified for symptomatic hypoglycemia or blood glucose that is less than 50 mg/dL, even if treated (line 9c, Figure 17-6, page 566). Your patient showed the hypoglycemic symptom of confusion. Notify the physician.

QUICK REVIEW

- Many hospitals use standard protocols to initiate and maintain continuous infusion therapy for critical medications such as heparin and insulin.

- Protocols may be based on weight in kilograms, and dose adjustments are made based on blood tests or other patient data such as physical assessment findings.

- To calculate mL/h when you know units/h and units/mL:

$$\frac{\textbf{Dosage on hand}}{\textbf{Amount on hand}} = \frac{\textbf{Dosage desired/h}}{\textbf{X Amount desired/h}}$$

- Document boluses and changes to infusion rate on the flowsheet for consistent monitoring and maintenance of infusions.

- Be prepared to administer an antidote, if severe adverse reactions occur.

Review Set 46

Calculate the flow rate. The infusion pumps are calibrated to deliver whole mL.

1. Order: *0.45% NS 1,000 mL IV $\bar{c}$ heparin 25,000 units to infuse at 1,000 units/h*

    Flow rate: _____ mL/h

2. Order: *D$_5$W 500 mL IV $\bar{c}$ heparin 40,000 units to infuse at 1,100 units/h*

    Flow rate: _____ mL/h

3. Order: *0.45% NS 500 mL IV $\bar{c}$ heparin 25,000 units to infuse at 500 units/h*

    Flow rate: _____ mL/h

4. Order: D₅W 500 mL IV c̄ heparin 40,000 units to infuse at 1,500 units/h

   Flow rate: _____ mL/h

5. Order: D₅W 1 L IV c̄ heparin 25,000 units to infuse at 1,200 units/h. On rounds, you assess the patient and observe that the infusion pump is set at 120 mL/h.

   At what rate should the pump be set? _____ mL/h

   What should your action be? _____

6. Order: D₅W 500 mL IV with heparin 25,000 units to infuse at 800 units/h

   Flow rate: _____ mL/h

Questions 7 through 10 refer to a patient who weighs 165 lb and has IV heparin ordered per the following Weight-Based Heparin Protocol. With this variation of the heparin protocol, you will not round the patient's weight, and instead you will use the patient's actual weight. The infusion pumps are calibrated to deliver whole mL.

Weight-Based Heparin Protocol:

Heparin IV infusion: Heparin 25,000 units in 250 mL of $\frac{1}{2}$NS

IV boluses: Use heparin 1,000 units/mL.

Calculate the patient's weight in kg. Weight: _____ kg

Bolus with heparin 80 units/kg. Then initiate heparin drip at 18 units/kg/h. Obtain aPTT every 6 hours, and adjust dosage and rate as follows:

If aPTT is less than 35 seconds: Rebolus with 80 units/kg and increase rate by 4 units/kg/h.

If aPTT is 36 to 44 seconds: Rebolus with 40 units/kg and increase rate by 2 units/kg/h.

If aPTT is 45 to 75 seconds: Continue current rate.

If aPTT is 76 to 90 seconds: Decrease rate by 2 units/kg/h.

If aPTT is greater than 90 seconds: Hold heparin for 1 hour and then decrease rate by 3 units/kg/h.

---

7. Convert the patient's weight to kg: _____ kg

   Calculate the initial heparin bolus dosage: _____ units

   Calculate the bolus dose: _____ mL

   Calculate the initial heparin infusion rate: _____ units/h, or _____ mL/h

8. Six hours later at 0900, the patient's aPTT is 33 seconds. According to the protocol, what will your action be?

   Rebolus with _____ units, or _____ mL.

   Increase infusion rate by _____ units/h, or _____ mL/h, for a new rate of _____ mL/h.

9. At 1500, the patient's aPTT is 40 seconds. According to the protocol, what will your action be?

   Rebolus with _____ units or _____ mL.

   Increase infusion rate by _____ units/h, or _____ mL/h, for a new rate of _____ mL/h.

10. At 2100, the patient's aPTT is 60 seconds. What will your action be according to the protocol?

    _____

Questions 11 through 15 refer to a seriously ill patient in the critical care unit who has insulin-dependent diabetes. Use the following grid for titration of intravenous insulin. An IV pump is used, and it is calibrated to deliver whole milliliters.

Sample Grid for Titration of Intravenous Insulin—Level 2		
LEVEL 2: DO NOT INITIATE insulin drip unless blood glucose is greater than 110 mg/dL.		
Blood Glucose (mg/dL)	**Regular U-100 Insulin Bolus**	**Regular Insulin Infusion Rate: 100 Units of Regular U-100 Insulin in 100 mL NaCl**
Less than 70	Give $\frac{1}{2}$ of 50 mL amp of 50% dextrose	HOLD insulin infusion × 60 minutes and check blood glucose every 15 minutes until equal to or greater than 80.
70 to 79	0	HOLD insulin infusion × 60 minutes and check blood glucose every 15 minutes until equal to or greater than 80.
80 to 110	0	2 units/h
111 to 125	0	3 units/h
126 to 149	0	4 units/h
150 to 165	0	5 units/h
166 to 179	0	6 units/h
180 to 209	0	8 units/h
210 to 239	10 units IV push	12 units/h
240 to 269	10 units IV push	16 units/h
270 to 299	10 units IV push	20 units/h
300 to 350	10 units IV push	25 units/h
Greater than 350	Notify physician	

11. The blood glucose level at the start of the infusion is 320 mg/dL. Is a bolus dose of insulin required? _____ If so, what is the required bolus dosage? _____ units

12. The insulin solution prepared for the continuous infusion is 100 units U-100 regular insulin in 100 mL of 0.9% NaCl. What should be the rate at the start of the infusion? _____ mL/h

13. One hour later, the blood glucose level is 198 mg/dL. Is a bolus dose of insulin required? _____ If so, what is the required dosage? _____ units

14. What should be the new rate for the continuous infusion? _____ mL/h

15. After monitoring and adjusting insulin doses over 4 hours, the blood glucose level is 72 mg/dL. What should your action be at this time? _____

After completing these problems, see pages 713–714 to check your answers.

CRITICAL CARE IV CALCULATIONS: CALCULATING FLOW RATE OF AN IV MEDICATION TO BE GIVEN OVER A SPECIFIED TIME PERIOD

With increasing frequency, medications are ordered for patients in critical care situations as a prescribed amount to be administered in a specified time period, such as *X mg per minute*. Such medications are usually administered by electronic infusion devices programmed in mL/h. Unless stated otherwise, for calculations you can assume that the IV pump is calibrated to deliver whole milliliters. Careful monitoring of patients receiving life-threatening therapies is a critical nursing skill.

IV Medication Ordered per Minute

RULE

To determine the flow rate (mL/h) for IV medications ordered per minute (such as mg/min):

Step 1   Calculate the dosage flow rate in mL/min:

Ratio for supply dosage on hand is equivalent to the desired dosage flow rate. In this case it is *per minute.*

$$\frac{\text{Dosage on hand}}{\text{Amount of solution on hand}} = \frac{\text{Dosage desired/min}}{\text{X Amount desired/min}}$$

Step 2   Calculate the flow rate in mL/h of the volume to administer per minute:

$$\frac{\text{Volume on hand}}{\text{Min to be infused}} = \frac{\text{X volume to be infused/h}}{\text{60 min/h}}$$

Or,

mL/min × 60 min/h = mL/h

Note: The order may specify mg/min, mcg/min, g/min, units/min, milliunits/min, or mEq/min.

EXAMPLE 1 ■

Order: **lidocaine 2 g IV in 500 mL D₅W at 2 mg/min via infusion pump.** You must prepare and hang 500 mL of D₅W IV solution that has 2 g of lidocaine added to it. Then, you must regulate the flow rate so the patient receives 2 mg of the lidocaine every minute. Determine the flow rate for the IV pump calibrated to deliver tenths of a mL/h.

Step 1   Calculate mL/min (change mg/min to mL/min).

$$\frac{\text{Dosage on hand}}{\text{Amount of solution on hand}} = \frac{\text{Dosage desired/min}}{\text{X Amount desired/min}}$$

Dosage on hand: 2 g = 2,000 mg

Amount of solution on hand: 500 mL

Dosage desired/min: 2 mg/min

Amount desired/min: X mL/min

$$\frac{2,000 \text{ mg}}{500 \text{ mL}} \diagdown \frac{2 \text{ mg/min}}{\text{X mL/min}}$$

$$2,000\text{X} = 1,000$$

$$\frac{2,000\text{X}}{2,000} = \frac{1,000}{2,000}$$

$$\text{X} = 0.5 \text{ mL/min}$$

Step 2   Determine the flow rate in mL/h (change mL/min to mL/h).

$$\frac{\text{Volume on hand}}{\text{Min to be infused}} = \frac{\text{X volume to be infused/h}}{\text{60 min/h}}$$

Now you know the following information:

Volume on hand: 0.5 mL

Minutes to infuse 0.5 mL: 1 min

Minutes per hour: 60 min/h

Flow rate: X mL/h

$$\frac{0.5 \text{ mL}}{1 \text{ min}} \diagdown \frac{\text{X mL/h}}{60 \text{ min/h}}$$

$$X = 30 \text{ mL/h}$$

Or, you know that there are 60 minutes per hour, so you can just multiply mL/min by 60 min/h. Notice that *min* cancel out so you have *mL/h* remaining.

mL/min × 60 min/h = mL/h

0.5 mL/m̶i̶n̶ × 60 m̶i̶n̶/h = 30 mL/h

Regulate the flow rate to 30 mL/h to deliver 2 mg/min of lidocaine that is prepared at the concentration of 2 g per 500 mL of D_5W IV solution.

EXAMPLE 2 ■

Order: **nitroglycerin 125 mg IV in 500 mL D_5W to infuse at 42 mcg/min**

Calculate the flow rate in mL/h to program the infusion pump.

Step 1　Calculate mL/min (change mcg/min to mL/min).

First, convert mg to mcg: 1 mg = 1,000 mcg

$$\frac{1 \text{ mg}}{1,000 \text{ mcg}} \diagdown \frac{125 \text{ mg}}{\text{X mcg}}$$

$$X = 125,000 \text{ mcg}$$

Then, calculate mL/min:

$$\frac{\text{Dosage on hand}}{\text{Amount of solution on hand}} = \frac{\text{Dosage desired/min}}{\text{X Amount desired/min}}$$

$$\frac{125,000 \text{ mcg}}{500 \text{ mL}} \diagdown \frac{42 \text{ mcg/min}}{\text{X mL/min}}$$

$$125,000\text{X} = 21,000$$

$$\frac{125,000\text{X}}{125,000} = \frac{21,000}{125,000}$$

$$X = 0.168 \text{ mL/min} = 0.17 \text{ mL/min}$$

Step 2　Determine the flow rate in mL/h (change mL/min to mL/h).

$$\frac{\text{Volume on hand}}{\text{Min to be infused}} = \frac{\text{X Volume to be infused/h}}{60 \text{ min/h}}$$

$$\frac{0.17 \text{ mL}}{1 \text{ min}} \diagdown \frac{\text{X mL/h}}{60 \text{ min/h}}$$

$$X = 10.2 \text{ mL/h} = 10 \text{ mL/h}$$

Or, you can just multiply mL/min by 60 min/h.

mL/min × 60 min/h = mL/h

0.17 mL/m̶i̶n̶ × 60 m̶i̶n̶/h = 10.2 mL/h = 10 mL/h

Regulate the flow rate to 10 mL/h to deliver 42 mcg/min of nitroglycerin that is prepared at the concentration of 125 mg per 500 mL of D_5W IV solution.

IV MEDICATION ORDERED PER KILOGRAM PER MINUTE

The physician may also order the amount of medication in an IV solution that a patient should receive in a specified time period per kilogram of body weight. An electronic infusion device is usually used to administer these orders.

RULE

To determine the flow rate (mL/h) for IV medications ordered per minute (such as mg/min):

Step 1   Convert to like units, such as mg to mcg or lb to kg.

Step 2   Calculate desired dosage per minute: mg/kg/min × kg = mg/min.

Step 3   Calculate the dosage flow rate in mL/min:

$$\frac{\text{Dosage on hand}}{\text{Amount of solution on hand}} = \frac{\text{Dosage desired/min}}{\text{X Amount desired/min}}$$

Step 4   Calculate the flow rate in mL/h of the volume to administer per minute:

$$\frac{\text{Volume on hand}}{\text{Min to be infused}} = \frac{\text{X volume to be infused/h}}{\text{60 min/h}}$$

Or,

mL/min × 60 min/h = mL/h

Note: The order may specify mg/min, mcg/min, g/min, units/min, milliunits/min, or mEq/min; or mg/h, mcg/h, g/h, units/h, milliunits/h, or mEq/h.

EXAMPLE 1 ▪

Order: *250 mL of IV solution with 225 mg of a medication to infuse at 3 mcg/kg/min via infusion pump* for a person who weighs 110 lb.

Determine the flow rate in mL/h.

Step 1   Convert mg to mcg: 1 mg = 1,000 mcg.

$$\frac{1 \text{ mg}}{1,000 \text{ mcg}} \diagdown \frac{225 \text{ mg}}{\text{X mcg}}$$

$$X = 225,000 \text{ mcg}$$

Convert lb to kg: 1 kg = 2.2 lb

$$\frac{1 \text{ kg}}{2.2 \text{ lb}} \diagup \frac{\text{X kg}}{110 \text{ lb}}$$

$$2.2X = 110$$

$$\frac{2.2X}{2.2} = \frac{110}{2.2}$$

$$X = 50 \text{ kg}$$

Step 2   Calculate desired mcg/min.

3 mcg/k̶g̶/min × 50 k̶g̶ = 150 mcg/min

Step 3   Calculate mL/min.

$$\frac{\text{Dosage on hand}}{\text{Amount of solution on hand}} = \frac{\text{Dosage desired/min}}{\text{X Amount desired/min}}$$

$$\frac{225,000 \text{ mcg}}{250 \text{ mL}} \diagdown\diagup \frac{150 \text{ mcg/min}}{\text{X mL/min}}$$

$$225,000\text{X} = 37,500$$

$$\frac{225,000\text{X}}{225,000} = \frac{37,500}{225,000}$$

$$\text{X} = 0.166 \text{ mL/min} = 0.17 \text{ mL/min}$$

Step 4   Calculate mL/h.

$$\frac{\text{Volume on hand}}{\text{Min to be infused}} = \frac{\text{X Volume to be infused/h}}{60 \text{ min/h}}$$

$$\frac{0.17 \text{ mL}}{1 \text{ min}} \diagdown\diagup \frac{\text{X mL/h}}{60 \text{ min/h}}$$

$$\text{X} = 10.2 \text{ mL/h} = 10 \text{ mL/h}$$

Or, you can just multiply mL/min by 60 min/h.

mL/min × 60 min/h = mL/h

0.17 mL/~~min~~ × 60 ~~min~~/h = 10.2 mL/h = 10 mL/h

For a person who weighs 110 lb, or 50 kg, regulate the IV flow rate to 10 mL/h to deliver 150 mcg/min (3 mcg/kg/min) of the drug, which is prepared at the concentration of 225 mg per 250 mL of IV solution.

Titrating IV Drugs

Sometimes IV medications may be prescribed to be administered at an initial dosage over a specified time period and then continued at a different dosage and time period. These situations are common in obstetrics and critical care. Medications such as magnesium sulfate, dopamine, Isuprel, and Pitocin are ordered to be *titrated,* or *regulated,* to obtain measurable physiologic responses. Dosages will be adjusted until the desired effect is achieved. In some cases, a loading or bolus dose is infused and monitored closely. Most IV medications that require titration usually start at the lowest dosage and are increased or decreased as needed. An upper titration limit is usually set and is not exceeded unless the desired response is not obtained. A new drug order is then required.

Let's look at some of these situations.

RULE

To calculate flow rate (mL/h) for IV medications ordered over a specific time period (such as mg/min):

Step 1   Calculate mg/mL.

Step 2   Calculate mL/h.

Note: The order may specify mg/min, mcg/min, g/min, units/min, milliunits/min, or mEq/min; or it may specify mg/h, mcg/h, g/h, units/h, milliunits/h, or mEq/h.

EXAMPLE 1 ■

Order: RL 1,000 mL IV c̄ magnesium sulfate 20 g. Start with bolus of 4 g for 30 min, then maintain a continuous infusion at 2 g/h

1. What is the flow rate in whole mL/h for the bolus order?

Step 1   Calculate the bolus dosage in g/mL.

There are 20 g in 1,000 mL. How many mL are necessary to infuse 4 g?

$$\frac{\text{Dosage on hand}}{\text{Amount of solution on hand}} = \frac{\text{Dosage desired}}{\text{X Amount desired}}$$

$$\frac{20\ \text{g}}{1{,}000\ \text{mL}} \times \frac{4\ \text{g}}{\text{X mL}}$$

$$20\text{X} = 4{,}000$$

$$\frac{20\text{X}}{20} = \frac{4{,}000}{20}$$

$$\text{X} = 200\ \text{mL}$$

Therefore, 200 mL contain 4 g, to be administered over 30 min.

Step 2   Calculate the bolus rate in mL/h.

What is the flow rate in mL/h to infuse 200 mL (which contain 4 g of magnesium sulfate)? Remember 1 h = 60 min.

$$\frac{\text{Volume on hand}}{\text{Min to be infused}} = \frac{\text{X volume to be infused/h}}{60\ \text{min/h}}$$

$$\frac{200\ \text{mL}}{30\ \text{min}} \times \frac{\text{X mL/h}}{60\ \text{min/h}}$$

$$30\text{X} = 12{,}000$$

$$\frac{30\text{X}}{30} = \frac{12{,}000}{30}$$

$$\text{X} = 400\ \text{mL/h}$$

Set the infusion pump at 400 mL/h to deliver the bolus of 4 g for 30 min as ordered.

Now calculate the continuous IV rate in mL/h.

2. What is the flow rate in mL/h for the continuous infusion of magnesium sulfate of 2 g/h? You know from the bolus dosage calculation that 200 mL contain 4 g.

$$\frac{\text{Dosage on hand}}{\text{Amount of solution on hand}} = \frac{\text{Dosage desired/h}}{\text{X Amount desired/h}}$$

$$\frac{4\ \text{g}}{200\ \text{mL}} \times \frac{2\ \text{g/h}}{\text{X mL/h}}$$

$$4\text{X} = 400$$

$$\frac{4\text{X}}{4} = \frac{400}{4}$$

$$\text{X} = 100\ \text{mL/h}$$

After the bolus has infused in the first 30 min, reset the infusion pump to 100 mL/h to deliver the continuous infusion of 2 g/h of magnesium sulfate.

EXAMPLE 2 ■

Let's look at an example using Pitocin (a drug used to induce or augment labor) measured in units and milliunits. The physician wrote an order to induce labor: LR 1,000 mL IV c̄ Pitocin 20 units. Begin a continuous infusion IV at 1 milliunit/min, increase by 1 milliunit/min q.15 min to a maximum of 20 milliunits/min

1. What is the flow rate in whole mL/h to deliver 1 milliunit/min?

   In this example, the medication is measured in units (instead of g or mg).

Step 1 Calculate milliunits/mL.

Convert: 1 unit = 1,000 milliunits; 20 units = 20,000 milliunits

$$\frac{\text{Dosage on hand}}{\text{Amount of solution on hand}} = \frac{\text{Dosage desired}}{\text{X Amount desired}}$$

Dosage on hand: 20,000 milliunits

Amount of solution on hand: 1,000 mL

Dosage desired: 1 milliunit

$$\frac{20,000 \text{ milliunits}}{1,000 \text{ mL}} \diagdown\diagup \frac{1 \text{ milliunit}}{\text{X mL}}$$

$$20,000X = 1,000$$

$$\frac{20,000X}{20,000} = \frac{1,000}{20,000}$$

$$X = 0.05 \text{ mL}$$

Therefore, 0.05 mL contains 1 milliunit of Pitocin, or there is 1 milliunit per 0.05 mL.

Step 2 Calculate mL/h.

What is the flow rate in mL/h to infuse 0.05 mL/min (which is 1 milliunit Pitocin/min)?

$$\frac{\text{Volume on hand}}{\text{Min to be infused}} = \frac{\text{X Volume to be infused/h}}{60 \text{ min/h}}$$

$$\frac{0.05 \text{ mL}}{1 \text{ min}} \diagdown\diagup \frac{\text{X mL/h}}{60 \text{ min/h}}$$

$$X = 3 \text{ mL/h}$$

Set the infusion pump at 3 mL/h to infuse Pitocin 1 milliunit/min as ordered.

2. What is the maximum flow rate in mL/h that the Pitocin infusion can be set for the titration as ordered? Notice that the order allows a maximum of 20 milliunits/min. You know from the bolus dosage calculation that there is 1 milliunit per 0.05 mL.

$$\frac{\text{Dosage on hand}}{\text{Amount of solution on hand}} = \frac{\text{Dosage desired/min}}{\text{X Amount desired/min}}$$

Dosage on hand: 1 milliunit

Amount of solution: 0.05 mL

Dosage desired: 20 milliunits/min

$$\frac{1 \text{ milliunit}}{0.05 \text{ mL}} \diagdown\diagup \frac{20 \text{ milliunits/min}}{\text{X mL/min}}$$

$$X = 0.05 \times 20$$

$$X = 1 \text{ mL/min}$$

Now convert mL/min to mL/h, so you can program the electronic infusion device.

$$\frac{\text{Volume on hand}}{\text{Min to be infused}} = \frac{\text{X volume to be infused/h}}{60 \text{ min/h}}$$

$$\frac{1 \text{ mL}}{1 \text{ min}} \diagup\hspace{-0.8em}\diagdown \frac{\text{X mL/h}}{60 \text{ min/h}}$$

$$X = 60 \text{ mL/h}$$

Or, you can just multiply mL/min by 60 min/h.

mL/min $\times$ 60 min/h = mL/h

1 mL/~~min~~ $\times$ 60 ~~min~~/h = 60 mL/h

You know that 1 milliunit/min is infused at 3 mL/h.

$$\frac{3 \text{ mL/h}}{1 \text{ milliunit/min}} \diagup\hspace{-0.8em}\diagdown \frac{\text{X mL/h}}{20 \text{ milliunits/min}}$$

$$X = 60 \text{ mL/h}$$

Rate of 60 mL/h will deliver 20 milliunits/min.

Verifying Safe IV Medication Dosage Recommended per Minute

It is also a critical nursing skill to be sure that patients are receiving safe dosages of medications. Therefore, you must also be able to convert critical care IVs with additive medications to **mg/h** or **mg/min** to check safe or normal dosage ranges.

RULE

To check safe dosage of IV medications ordered in mL/h:

Step 1   Calculate mg/h.

Step 2   Calculate mg/min.

Step 3   Compare recommended dosage and ordered dosage to decide if the dosage is safe.

Note: The ordered and recommended dosages may specify mg/min, mcg/min, g/min, units/min, milliunits/min, or mEq/min.

EXAMPLE ■

The drug reference states that the recommended dosage of lidocaine is 1 to 4 mg/min. The patient has an order for D₅W 500 mL IV c̄ lidocaine 1 g to infuse at 30 mL/h. Is the lidocaine dosage within the safe range?

Step 1   Calculate mg/h.

Convert: 1 g = 1,000 mg

Remember, the unknown X is mg/h. Notice that X is in the numerator of the second ratio in this proportion.

$$\frac{\text{Dosage on hand}}{\text{Amount of solution on hand}} = \frac{\text{X Dosage desired/h}}{\text{Amount desired/h}}$$

$$\frac{1{,}000 \text{ mg}}{500 \text{ mL}} \diagup\hspace{-0.8em}\diagdown \frac{\text{X mg/h}}{30 \text{ mL/h}}$$

$$500\text{X} = 30{,}000$$

$$\frac{500\text{X}}{500} = \frac{30{,}000}{500}$$

$$X = 60 \text{ mg/h} \qquad \text{60 mg are administered in 1 hour when the flow rate is 30 mL/h.}$$

Step 2   Calculate mg/min. THINK: It is obvious that 60 mg/h is the same as 60 mg per 60 min or 1 mg/min.

$$\frac{60 \text{ mg}}{60 \text{ min}} \underset{\diagup}{\overset{\diagdown}{\times}} \frac{X \text{ mg}}{1 \text{ min}}$$

$$60X = 60$$

$$\frac{60X}{60} = \frac{60}{60}$$

$$X = 1 \text{ mg}$$

Rate is 1 mg/min.

Step 3   Compare ordered and recommended dosages.

1 mg/min of lidocaine is within the safe range of 1 to 4 mg/min. The dosage is safe.

Likewise, IV medications ordered as mL/h and recommended in mg/kg/min require verification of their safety or normal dosage range.

RULE

To check safe dosage of IV medications recommended in mg/kg/min and ordered in mL/h:

Step 1   Convert to like units, such as mg to mcg or lb to kg.

Step 2   Calculate recommended mg/min.

Step 3   Calculate ordered mg/h.

Step 4   Calculate ordered mg/min.

Step 5   Compare ordered and recommended dosages. Decide if the dosage is safe.

Note: The ordered and recommended dosages may specify mg/kg/min, mcg/kg/min, g/kg/min, units/kg/min, milliunits/kg/min, or mEq/kg/min.

EXAMPLE ▪

The recommended dosage range of sodium nitroprusside for adults is 0.3 to 10 mcg/kg/min. The patient has an order for D$_5$W 100 mL IV with nitroprusside 420 mg to infuse at 1 mL/h. The patient weighs 154 lb. Is the nitroprusside dosage within the normal range?

Step 1   Convert lb to kg.

$$\frac{1 \text{ kg}}{2.2 \text{ lb}} \underset{\diagup}{\overset{\diagdown}{\times}} \frac{X \text{ kg}}{154 \text{ lb}}$$

$$2.2X = 154$$

$$\frac{2.2X}{2.2} = \frac{154}{2.2}$$

$$X = 70 \text{ kg}$$

Convert mg to mcg: 420 mg = 420.000. = 420,000 mcg

Step 2   Calculate recommended mcg/min range.

minimum: 0.3 mcg/kg/min × 70 kg = 21 mcg/min

maximum: 10 mcg/kg/min × 70 kg = 700 mcg/min

Step 3   Calculate ordered mcg/h.

$$\frac{\text{Dosage on hand}}{\text{Amount on hand}} = \frac{\text{Dosage desired/h}}{\text{X Amount desired/h}}$$

$$\frac{420,000 \text{ mcg}}{100 \text{ mL}} \times \frac{\text{X mcg/h}}{1 \text{ mL/h}}$$

$$100\text{X} = 420,000$$

$$\frac{100\text{X}}{100} = \frac{420,000}{100}$$

$$\text{X} = 4,200 \text{ mcg/h}$$

Step 4   Calculate ordered mcg/min.

You know 1 h = 60 min; therefore, 4,200 mcg/h = 4,200 mcg per 60 min. How many mcg can be infused in 1 min?

$$\frac{4,200 \text{ mcg}}{60 \text{ min}} \times \frac{\text{X mcg}}{1 \text{ min}}$$

$$60\text{X} = 4,200$$

$$\frac{60\text{X}}{60} = \frac{4,200}{60}$$

$$\text{X} = 70 \text{ mcg (per minute)}$$

This is also a simple division problem.

$$\frac{4,200 \text{ mcg}}{60 \text{ min}} = 70 \text{ mcg/min}$$

Step 5   Compare ordered and recommended dosages. Decide if the dosage is safe. Because 70 mcg/min is within the allowable range of 21 to 700 mcg/min, the ordered dosage is safe.

QUICK REVIEW

- For IV medications ordered in mg/min:

  Step 1   Calculate mL/min.

  Step 2   Calculate mL/h.

- To check safe dosages of IV medications recommended in mg/min and ordered in mL/h:

  Step 1   Calculate mg/h.

  Step 2   Calculate mg/min.

  Step 3   Compare recommended and ordered dosages. Decide if the dosage is safe.

- To check safe dosage of IV medications recommended in mg/kg/min and ordered in mL/h:

  Step 1   Convert to like units, such as mg to mcg or lb to kg.

  Step 2   Calculate recommended mg/min.

  Step 3   Calculate ordered mg/h.

  Step 4   Calculate ordered mg/min.

  Step 5   Compare ordered and recommended dosages. Decide if the dosage is safe.

Review Set 47

For questions 1 to 5, compute the flow rate for the medications to be administered by IV pump calibrated in tenths of a mL/h.

1. Order: lidocaine 2 g IV per 1,000 mL D$_5$W at 4 mg/min

   Rate: _____ mL/min and _____ mL/h

2. Order: procainamide 0.5 g IV per 250 mL D$_5$W at 2 mg/min

   Rate: _____ mL/min and _____ mL/h

3. Order: isoproterenol 2 mg IV per 500 mL D$_5$W at 6 mcg/min

   Rate: _____ mL/min and _____ mL/h

4. Order: medication X 450 mg IV per 500 mL NS at 4 mcg/kg/min

   Weight: 198 lb

   Weight: _____ kg   Give: _____ mcg/min

   Rate: _____ mL/min and _____ mL/h

5. Order: dopamine 800 mg in 500 mL NS IV at 15 mcg/kg/min

   Weight: 70 kg

   Give: _____ mcg/min

   Rate: _____ mL/min and _____ mL/h

Refer to this order for questions 6 through 8.

Order: D$_5$W 500 mL IV c̄ dobutamine hydrochloride 500 mg to infuse at 15 mL/h. The patient weighs 125 lb. Recommended range: 2.5 to 10 mcg/kg/min

6. What mcg/min range of dobutamine should this patient receive? _____ to _____ mcg/min

7. What mg/min range of dobutamine should this patient receive? _____ to _____ mg/min

8. Is the dobutamine as ordered within the safe range? _____

Refer to this order for questions 9 and 10.

Order: D$_5$W 500 mL IV c̄ procainamide 2 g to infuse at 60 mL/h. Normal range: 2 to 6 mg/min

9. How many mg/min of procainamide is the patient receiving? _____ mg/min

10. Is the dosage of procainamide within the normal range? _____

11. Order: magnesium sulfate 20 g IV in LR 500 mL. Start with a bolus of 2 g to infuse over 30 min. Then maintain a continuous infusion at 1 g/h. IV pump delivers whole mL/h.

    Rate: _____ mL/h for bolus

    _____ mL/h for continuous infusion

12. The following order is to induce labor. The IV pump delivers whole mL/h.

    Pitocin 15 units IV in 250 mL LR. Begin a continuous infusion at the rate of 1 milliunit/min.

    Rate: _____ mL/h

Refer to this order for questions 13 through 15.

Order: D$_5$W 1,000 mL IV with terbutaline sulfate 10 mg to infuse at 150 mL/h

Normal dosage range: 10 to 80 mcg/min

13. How many mg/min of terbutaline is the patient receiving? _____ mg/min

14. How many mcg/min of terbutaline is the patient receiving? _____ mcg/min

15. Is the dosage of terbutaline within the normal range? _____

After completing these problems, see pages 715–716 to check your answers.

LIMITING INFUSION VOLUMES

Calculating IV rates to include the IV piggyback (IV PB) volume may be necessary to limit the total volume of IV fluid a patient receives. To do this, you must calculate the flow rate for both the regular IV and the piggyback IV. In such instances of restricted fluids, the piggyback IVs are to be included as part of the total prescribed IV volume and time.

RULE

Follow these six steps to calculate the flow rate of an IV, which includes IV PB.

Step 1	IV PB flow rate:	$\frac{V}{T} \times C = R$
		or use $\dfrac{mL/h}{\text{Drop factor constant}} = R$
Step 2	Total IV PB time:	**Time for 1 dose × # of doses in 24 h**
Step 3	Total IV PB volume:	**Volume of 1 dose × # of doses in 24 h**
Step 4	Total regular IV volume:	**Total volume − IV PB volume = Regular IV volume**
Step 5	Total regular IV time:	**Total time − IV PB time = Regular IV time**
Step 6	Regular IV flow rate:	$\frac{V}{T} \times C = R$
		or use $\dfrac{mL/h}{\text{Drop factor constant}} = R$

EXAMPLE 1 ■

Order: D₅LR 3,000 mL IV for 24 h with cefazolin 1 g IV PB per 100 mL D₅W q.6h to run 1 hour. Limit total fluids to 3,000 mL daily.

The drop factor is 10 gtt/mL.

Note: The order intends that the patient receive a maximum of 3,000 mL in 24 hours. Remember: When fluids are restricted, the piggybacks are to be *included* in the total 24-hour intake, not added to it.

Step 1   Calculate the flow rate of the IV PB.

$$\frac{V}{T} \times C = \frac{100 \text{ mL}}{60 \text{ min}} \times \overset{1}{10} \text{ gtt/mL} = \frac{100 \text{ gtt}}{6 \text{ min}} = 16.6 \text{ gtt/min} = 17 \text{ gtt/min}$$

or $\dfrac{mL/h}{\text{Drop factor constant}}$ = gtt/min (drop factor constant is 6)

$$\frac{100 \text{ mL/h}}{6} = 16.6 \text{ gtt/min} = 17 \text{ gtt/min}$$

Set the flow rate for the IV PB at 17 gtt/min to infuse 1 g cefazolin in 100 mL over 1 hour, or 60 min.

Step 2   Calculate the total time the IV PB will be administered.

q.6h = 4 times per 24 h; 4 × 1 h = 4 h

Step 3 Calculate the total volume of the IV PB.

100 mL × 4 = 400 mL IV PB per 24 hours

Step 4 Calculate the volume of the regular IV fluids to be administered between IV PB doses. Total volume of regular IV minus total volume of IV PB: 3,000 mL − 400 mL = 2,600 mL

Step 5 Calculate the total regular IV fluid time or the time between IV PB doses. Total IV time minus total IV PB time: 24 h − 4 h = 20 h

Step 6 Calculate the flow rate of the regular IV.

$$\text{mL/h} = \frac{2,600 \text{ mL}}{20 \text{ h}} = 130 \text{ mL/h}$$

$$\frac{V}{T} \times C = \frac{130 \text{ mL}}{\underset{6}{60} \text{ min}} \times \overset{1}{10} \text{ gtt/mL} = \frac{130 \text{ gtt}}{6 \text{ min}} = 21.6 \text{ gtt/min} = 22 \text{ gtt/min}$$

or $\dfrac{\text{mL/h}}{\text{Drop factor constant}} = \text{gtt/min}$ (drop factor constant is 6)

$$\frac{130 \text{ mL/h}}{6} = 21.6 \text{ gtt/min} = 22 \text{ gtt/min}$$

Set the regular IV of D_5LR at the flow rate of 22 gtt/min. Then after 5 hours, switch to the cefazolin IV PB at the flow rate of 17 gtt/min for 1 hour. Repeat this process 4 times in 24 hours.

EXAMPLE 2 ▪

Order: NS 2,000 mL IV for 24 h with 80 mg gentamicin in 80 mL IV PB q.8h to run for 30 min. Limit fluid intake to 2,000 mL daily.

Drop factor: 15 gtt/mL

Calculate the flow rate for the regular IV and for the IV PB. IV pump is calibrated in whole mL/h.

Step 1 IV PB flow rate:

$$\frac{V}{T} \times C = \frac{80 \text{ mL}}{\underset{2}{30} \text{ min}} \times \overset{1}{15} \text{ gtt/mL} = \frac{80 \text{ gtt}}{2 \text{ min}} = 40 \text{ gtt/min}$$

Step 2 Total IV PB time: q.8h = 3 times per 24 h; 3 × 30 min = 90 min

$$90 \text{ min} \div 60 \text{ min/h} = 90 \text{ min} \times 1 \text{ h/60 min} = 1\frac{1}{2} \text{ h}$$

Step 3 Total IV PB volume: 80 mL × 3 = 240 mL

Step 4 Total regular IV volume: 2,000 mL − 240 mL = 1,760 mL

Step 5 Total regular IV time: $24 \text{ h} - 1\frac{1}{2} \text{ h} = 22\frac{1}{2} \text{ h} = 22.5 \text{ h}$

Step 6 Regular IV flow rate:

$$\text{mL/h} = \frac{1,760 \text{ mL}}{22.5 \text{ h}} = 78.2 \text{ mL/h} = 78 \text{ mL/h}$$

$$\frac{V}{T} \times C = \frac{78 \text{ mL}}{\underset{4}{60} \text{ min}} \times \overset{1}{15} \text{ gtt/mL} = \frac{78 \text{ gtt}}{4 \text{ min}} = 19.5 \text{ gtt/min} = 20 \text{ gtt/min}$$

or $\dfrac{\text{mL/h}}{\text{Drop factor constant}} = R$ (drop factor constant is 4)

$$\frac{78 \text{ mL/h}}{4} = 19.5 \text{ gtt/min} = 20 \text{ gtt/min}$$

Set the regular IV of NS at the flow rate of 20 gtt/min. After $7\frac{1}{2}$ hours, switch to the gentamicin IV PB at the flow rate of 40 gtt/min for 30 minutes. Repeat this process 3 times in 24 hours.

Patients receiving a primary IV at a specific rate via an electronic infusion pump may require that the infusion rate be altered when a secondary (piggyback) medication is being administered. To do this, calculate the flow rate of the secondary medication in mL/h as you would the primary IV, and reset the infusion device.

Some infusion pumps allow you to set the flow rate for the secondary IV independent of the primary IV. Upon completion of the secondary infusion, the infusion device automatically returns to the original flow rate. If this is not the case, be sure to manually readjust the primary flow rate after the completion of the secondary set.

QUICK REVIEW

■ To calculate the flow rate of a regular IV with an IV PB and restricted fluids, calculate:

Step 1   IV PB flow rate

Step 2   Total IV PB time

Step 3   Total IV PB volume

Step 4   Total regular IV volume

Step 5   Total regular IV time

Step 6   Regular IV flow rate

Review Set 48

Calculate the flow rates for the IV and IV PB orders. These patients are on limited fluid volume (restricted fluids). IV pumps are calibrated in whole mL.

1. Orders: NS 3,000 mL IV for 24 h

    Limit total IV fluids to 3,000 mL daily.

    penicillin G potassium 1,000,000 units IV PB q.4h in 100 mL NS to run for 30 min

    Drop factor: 10 gtt/mL

    IV PB flow rate: _____ gtt/min

    IV flow rate: _____ gtt/min

2. Orders: D$_5$W 1,000 mL IV for 24 h

    Limit total IV fluids to 1,000 mL daily.

    gentamicin 40 mg q.i.d. in 40 mL IV PB to run 1 h

    Drop factor: 60 gtt/mL

    IV PB flow rate: _____ gtt/min

    IV flow rate: _____ gtt/min

3. Orders: D$_5$LR 3,000 mL IV for 24 h

    Limit total IV fluids to 3,000 mL daily.

    ampicillin 0.5 g q.6h IV PB in 50 mL D$_5$W to run 30 min

    Drop factor: 15 gtt/mL

    IV PB flow rate: _____ gtt/min

    IV flow rate: _____ gtt/min

4. Orders: $\frac{1}{2}$NS 2,000 mL IV for 24 h

   Limit total IV fluids to 2,000 mL daily.

   chloramphenicol 500 mg per 50 mL NS IV PB q.6h to run 1 h

   Drop factor: 60 gtt/mL

   IV PB flow rate: _____ gtt/min

   IV flow rate: _____ gtt/min

5. Orders: LR 1,000 mL IV for 24 h

   Limit total IV fluids to 1,000 mL daily.

   cefazolin 250 mg IV PB per 50 mL D$_5$W q.8h to run 1 h

   Drop factor: 60 gtt/mL

   IV PB flow rate: _____ gtt/min

   IV flow rate: _____ gtt/min

6. Orders: D$_5$LR 2,400 mL IV for 24 h

   Limit total IV fluids to 2,400 mL daily.

   cefazolin 1 g IV PB q.6h in 50 mL D$_5$W to run 30 min

   Drop factor: On electronic infusion pump

   IV PB flow rate: _____ mL/h

   IV flow rate: _____ mL/h

7. Orders: NS 2,000 mL IV for 24 h

   Limit total IV fluids to 2,000 mL daily.

   gentamicin 100 mg IV PB q.8h in 100 mL D$_5$W to run in over 30 min

   Drop factor: On electronic infusion pump

   IV PB flow rate: _____ mL/h

   IV flow rate: _____ mL/h

8. Orders: D$_5$ 0.45% NS 3,000 mL IV to run 24 h

   Limit total IV fluids to 3,000 mL daily.

   ranitidine 50 mg q.6h in 50 mL D$_5$W to infuse 15 min

   Drop factor: On electronic infusion pump

   IV PB flow rate: _____ mL/h

   IV flow rate: _____ mL/h

9. Orders: D$_5$NS 1,500 mL IV to run 24 h

   Limit total IV fluids to 1,500 mL daily.

   cefazolin 500 mg IV PB per 50 mL D$_5$W q.8h to run 1 h

   Drop factor: 20 gtt/mL

   IV PB flow rate: _____ gtt/min

   IV flow rate: _____ gtt/min

10. Orders: NS 2,700 mL IV for 24 h

      Limit total IV fluids to 2,700 mL per day.

      gentamicin 60 mg in 60 mL D₅W IV PB q.8h to run for 30 min

Drop factor: On electronic infusion pump

IV PB flow rate: _____ mL/h

IV flow rate: _____ mL/h

After completing these problems, see pages 716–718 to check your answers.

CLINICAL REASONING SKILLS

Knowing the therapeutic dosage of a given medication is a critical nursing skill. Let's look at an example in which the order was unclear and the nurse did not verify the order with the appropriate person.

ERROR

Failing to clarify an order

Possible Scenario

Suppose the physician ordered a heparin infusion for a patient with thrombophlebitis who weighs 100 kg. The facility uses the Standard Weight-Based Heparin Protocol as seen in Figure 17-1 (page 555). The order was written this way:

heparin 25,000 units in 250 mL ½NS IV at 18000/h

The order was difficult to read, and the nurse asked a coworker to help her decipher it. They both agreed that it read 18,000 units per hour. The nurse calculated mL/h to be:

$$\frac{\text{Dosage on hand}}{\text{Amount of solution on hand}} = \frac{\text{Dosage desired/h}}{\text{X Amount desired/h}}$$

$$\frac{25,000 \text{ units}}{250 \text{ mL}} \diagdown \frac{18,000 \text{ units/h}}{\text{X mL/h}} \qquad \textbf{INCORRECT}$$

$$25,000\text{X} = 4,500,000$$

$$\frac{25,000\text{X}}{25,000} = \frac{4,500,000}{25,000}$$

$$\text{X} = 180 \text{ mL/h}$$

The nurse proceeded to start the heparin drip at 180 mL/h. The patient's aPTT prior to initiation of the infusion was 37 seconds. Six hours into the infusion, an aPTT was drawn according to protocol. The nurse was shocked when the results returned and were 95 seconds, which is abnormally high. The nurse called the physician, who asked, "What is the rate of the heparin drip?" The nurse replied, "I have the infusion set at 180 mL/h so that the patient receives the prescribed amount of 18,000 units per hour." The physician was astonished and replied, "I ordered the drip at 1,800 units per hour, not 18,000 units per hour."

Potential Outcome

The physician would likely have discontinued the heparin; ordered protamine sulfate, the antidote for heparin overdosage; and obtained another aPTT. The patient may have started to show signs of abnormal bleeding, such as blood in the urine, bloody nose, and increased tendency to bruise.

Prevention

The physician intended to order 1,800 units/h, but wrote 1800 U/h, which appeared to the nurse to read 18000/h. She had misinterpreted the U to be a 0. The order as written is unclear, unsafe, and incomplete. Contacting the physician and requesting a clarification of the order would be the appropriate preventative action. Instead the nurse missed three opportunities to prevent this error.

First, the order as written is unclear. The prescriber should use commas for emphasis to write amounts of 1,000 and greater. More important, it does not follow The Joint Commission's *Official "Do Not Use" List* of abbreviations acronyms, and symbols. The physician should have written out *units* instead of using the outdated abbreviation *U*. This policy error alone regarding acceptable notation should automatically signal to the nurse to contact the physician to clarify the order. Guessing about the exact meaning of an order is dangerous, as this scenario demonstrates.

The second missed opportunity is that the order interpreted by the nurse was unsafe. The Standard Weight-Based Heparin Protocol recommends a safe heparin infusion rate of 1,800 units/h, or 18 mL/h (with a supply dosage of 25,000 units per 250 mL or 100 units/mL), for an individual weighing 100 kg. It is the responsibility of the individual administering a medication to be sure the Six Rights of medication administration are observed. The first three rights state that the *"right patient must receive the right drug in the right amount."* The order of 18,000 units as understood by the nurse resulted in an overdose that was 10 times the recommended amount of heparin.

Third, the order as interpreted by the nurse was incomplete. If the nurse correctly interpreted the order as 18000/h, then no unit of measure was specified, which is a medication error that requires contact with the physician for correction. An incomplete order must not be filled.

You may ask, "Could an error such as this really happen?" The answer is, "Definitely yes," which is why the Joint Commission has written their policy and why nurses must verify every order and take care to calculate accurately.

PRACTICE PROBLEMS—CHAPTER 17

Unless stated otherwise, IV pumps are calibrated in whole mL/h.

1. Order: **heparin 25,000 units in 250 mL 0.45% NS to infuse at 1,200 units/h**

   Drop factor: On electronic infusion pump

   Flow rate: _____ mL/h

2. Order: **thiamine 100 mg per L D₅W IV to infuse at 5 mg/h**

   Drop factor: On electronic infusion pump

   Flow rate: _____ mL/h

3. Order: **magnesium sulfate 4 g in 500 mL D₅W at 500 mg/h**

   Drop factor: On electronic infusion pump

   Flow rate: _____ mL/h

4. A patient is to receive **D₅W 500 mL c̄ heparin 20,000 units at 1,400 units/h.**

   Set the infusion pump at _____ mL/h.

5. At the rate of 4 mL/min, how long will it take to administer 1.5 L of IV fluid?
   _____ h and _____ min

6. Order: **lidocaine 2 g in 500 mL D₅W IV to run at 4 mg/min**

   Drop factor: On electronic infusion pump calibrated in tenths of a mL/h

   Flow rate: _____ mL/h

7. Order: lidocaine 1 g IV in 250 mL D₅W at 3 mg/min

   Drop factor: On electronic infusion pump calibrated in tenths of a mL/h

   Flow rate: _____ mL/h

8. Order: procainamide 1 g IV in 500 mL D₅W to infuse at 2 mg/min

   Drop factor: On electronic infusion pump calibrated in tenths of a mL/h

   Flow rate: _____ mL/h

9. Order: dobutamine 250 mg IV in 250 mL D₅W to infuse at 5 mcg/kg/min

   Weight: 80 kg

   Drop factor: On electronic infusion pump calibrated in tenths of a mL/h

   Flow rate: _____ mL/h

10. Your patient has an order for D₅W 1 L IV with 2 g lidocaine added infusing at 75 mL/h. The recommended continuous IV dosage of lidocaine is 1 to 4 mg/min. Is this dosage safe? _____

11. Orders: Restricted fluids: 3,000 mL D₅NS IV for 24 h

    chloramphenicol 1 g IV PB in 100 mL NS q.6h to run 1 h

    Drop factor: 10 gtt/mL

    Flow rate: _____ gtt/min IV PB and _____ gtt/min primary IV

12. Order: Restricted fluids: 3,000 mL D₅W IV for 24 h

    ampicillin 500 mg in 50 mL D₅W IV PB q.i.d. for 30 min

    Drop factor: On electronic infusion pump

    Flow rate: _____ mL/h IV PB and _____ mL/h primary IV

13. Order: 50 mg nitroprusside IV in 500 mL D₅W to infuse at 3 mcg/kg/min

    Weight: 125 lb

    Drop factor: On electronic infusion pump calibrated in tenths of a mL/h

    Flow rate: _____ mL/h

14. Order: potassium chloride 40 mEq to each liter IV fluid

    Situation: IV discontinued with 800 mL remaining

    How much potassium chloride infused? _____

15. A patient's infusion rate is 125 mL/h. The rate is equivalent to _____ mL/min.

16. Order: ½NS 1,500 mL IV to run at 100 mL/h. Calculate the infusion time. _____ h

17. Order: potassium chloride 40 mEq/L D₅W IV to infuse at 2 mEq/h

    Rate: _____ mL/h

18. Order: heparin 50,000 units/L D₅W IV to infuse at 1,250 units/h

    Rate: _____ mL/h

19. If the minimal dilution for tobramycin is 5 mg/mL and you are giving 37 mg, what is the least amount of fluid in which you could safely dilute the dosage? _____ mL

20. Order: oxytocin 10 units IV in 500 mL NS. Infuse 4 milliunits/min for 20 min, followed by 6 milliunits/min for 20 min. Use electronic infusion pump.

    Rate: _____ mL/h for first 20 min

    Rate: _____ mL/h for next 20 min

21. Order: magnesium sulfate 20 g IV in 500 mL of LR solution. Start with a bolus of 3 g to infuse over 30 min. Then maintain a continuous infusion at 2 g/h.

    You will use an electronic infusion pump.

    Rate: _____ mL/h for bolus

    Rate: _____ mL/h for continuous infusion

22. Order: Pitocin 15 units IV in 500 mL of LR solution. Infuse at 1 milliunit/min.

    You will use an electronic infusion pump.

    Rate: _____ mL/h

23. Order: heparin drip 40,000 units/L D_5W IV to infuse at 1,400 units/h

    Drop factor: On infusion pump

    Flow rate: _____ mL/h

Refer to this order for questions 24 and 25.

Order: magnesium sulfate 4 g IV in 500 mL D_5W at 500 mg/h on an infusion pump

24. What is the solution concentration? _____ mg/mL

25. What is the hourly flow rate? _____ mL/h

Calculate the drug concentration of the following IV solutions as requested.

26. A solution containing 80 units of oxytocin in 1,000 mL of D_5W: _____ milliunits/mL

27. A solution containing 200 mg of nitroglycerin in 500 mL of D_5W: _____ mg/mL

28. A solution containing 4 mg of isoproterenol in 1,000 mL of D_5W: _____ mcg/mL

29. A solution containing 2 g of lidocaine in 500 mL of D_5W: _____ mg/mL

Refer to this order for questions 30 through 32.

Order: venuronium bromide IV 1 mg/kg/min to control respirations for a patient who is ventilated

30. The patient weighs 220 pounds, which is equal to _____ kg.

31. The available venuronium bromide 20 mg is dissolved in 100 mL NS. This available solution concentration is _____ mg/mL, which is equivalent to _____ mcg/mL.

32. The IV is infusing at the rate of 1 mcg/kg/min on an infusion pump calibrated in tenths of a mL/h. The hourly rate is _____ mL/h.

Refer to these orders for questions 33 through 38.

Orders: Restricted fluids: 3,000 mL per 24 h. Primary IV of D_5LR running via infusion pump. ampicillin 3 g IV PB q.6h in 100 mL of D_5W over 30 min gentamicin 170 mg IV PB q.8h in 50 mL of D_5W to infuse in 1 h

33. Calculate the IV PB flow rates. ampicillin: _____ mL/h; gentamicin: _____ mL/h

34. Calculate the total IV PB time. _____ h

35. Calculate the total IV PB volume. _____ mL

36. Calculate the total regular IV volume. _____ mL

37. Calculate the total regular IV time. _____ h

38. Calculate the regular IV flow rate. _____ mL/h

39. A patient who weighs 190 lb receives *dopamine 800 mg in 500 mL of* D$_5$W *IV at 4 mcg/kg/min.* As the patient's blood pressure drops, the nurse titrates the drip to 12 mcg/kg/min as ordered.

What is the initial flow rate for the IV pump calibrated in tenths of a mL/h? _____ mL/h

After titration, what is the flow rate? _____ mL/h

Questions 40 through 44 refer to a seriously ill patient in the critical care unit who has insulin-dependent diabetes. Use the following grid for titration of intravenous insulin. An IV pump, calibrated to deliver whole milliliters, will be used.

Sample Grid for Titration of Intravenous Insulin—Level 2		
LEVEL 2: DO NOT INITIATE insulin drip unless blood glucose is greater than 110 mg/dL.		
Blood Glucose (mg/dL)	**Regular U-100 Insulin Bolus**	**Regular Insulin Infusion Rate: 100 Units of Regular U-100 Insulin in 100 mL NaCl**
Less than 70	Give $\frac{1}{2}$ of 50 mL amp of 50% dextrose	HOLD insulin infusion × 60 minutes and check blood glucose every 15 minutes until equal to or greater than 80.
70 to 79	0	HOLD insulin infusion × 60 minutes and check blood glucose every 15 minutes until equal to or greater than 80.
80 to 110	0	2 units/h
111 to 125	0	3 units/h
126 to 149	0	4 units/h
150 to 165	0	5 units/h
166 to 179	0	6 units/h
180 to 209	0	8 units/h
210 to 239	10 units IV push	12 units/h
240 to 269	10 units IV push	16 units/h
270 to 299	10 units IV push	20 units/h
300 to 350	10 units IV push	25 units/h
Greater than 350	Notify physician	

40. The blood glucose level at the start of the infusion is 215 mg/dL. Is a bolus dose of insulin required? _____ If so, what is the required bolus dosage? _____ units

41. The insulin solution prepared for the continuous infusion is 100 units U-100 regular insulin in 100 mL of 0.9% NaCl. What should be the rate at the start of the infusion? _____ mL/h

42. One hour later, the blood glucose level is 129 mg/dL. Is a bolus dose of insulin required? _____ If so, what is the required dosage? _____ units

43. What should be the new rate for the continuous infusion? _____ mL/h

44. After monitoring and adjusting insulin doses over 4 hours, the blood glucose level is 68 mg/dL. What should your action be at this time? _____

Questions 45 through 49 refer to your patient who has left-leg deep vein thrombosis. He has orders for IV heparin therapy. He weighs 225 lb. On admission, his aPTT is 25 seconds. You initiate therapy at 1130 on 5/10/xx. Follow the Standard Weight-Based Heparin Protocol (Figure 17-7), and record your answers on the Standard Weight-Based Heparin Protocol Worksheet (Figure 17-8).

45. What is the patient's weight in kilograms? Calculate the weight as instructed in the protocol and record weight on the worksheet. _____ kg.

   What does the protocol indicate for the standard bolus dosage of heparin? _____ units/kg

46. Calculate the dosage of heparin that should be administered for the bolus for this patient, and record your answer on the worksheet. _____ units

   What does the protocol indicate as the required solution concentration (supply dosage) of heparin to use for the bolus? _____ units/mL

   Calculate the dose volume of heparin that should be administered for the bolus for this patient, and record your answer on the worksheet. _____ mL

47. What does the protocol indicate for the initial infusion rate? _____ units/kg/h

   Calculate the dosage of heparin this patient should receive each hour, and record your answer on the worksheet. _____ units/h

   What does the protocol indicate as the required solution concentration (supply dosage) of heparin to use for the initial infusion? _____ units/mL

   Calculate the heparin solution volume this patient should receive each hour to provide the correct infusion for his weight, and record your answer on the worksheet. _____ mL/h

48. According to the protocol, how often should the patient's aPTT be checked? q. _____ h

   At 1730, the patient's aPTT is 37 seconds. Calculate the new heparin bolus and record your answer on the worksheet. Give _____ units/kg or _____ units measured as _____ mL.

   Calculate the change in heparin infusion rate (increase or decrease) and record on the worksheet. How much should you change the infusion rate? _____ by _____ units/kg/h or _____ units/h for a rate of _____ mL/h

   Calculate the new infusion rate and record on the worksheet. _____ mL/h

49. At 2330, the patient's aPTT is 77 seconds. What should you do now?

   _____

   Calculate the new infusion rate and record your answer on the worksheet. _____ mL/h

FIGURE 17-7 Heparin Protocol

Standard Weight-Based Heparin Protocol

For all patients on heparin drips:
   1. Weight in kilograms (round to nearest 10 kg). Required for order to be processed: _____ kg
   2. Heparin 25,000 units in 250 mL of $\frac{1}{2}$NS. Boluses to be given as 1,000 units/mL.
   3. aPTT q.6h or 6 hours after rate change; daily after two consecutive therapeutic aPTTs.
   4. CBC initially and repeat every _____ days(s).
   5. Obtain aPTT and PT/INR on day 1 prior to initiation of therapy.
   6. Guaiac stool initially, then every _____ day(s) until heparin discontinued. Notify if positive.
   7. Neuro checks every _____ hours while on heparin. Notify physician of any changes.
   8. Discontinue aPTT and CBC once heparin drip is discontinued, unless otherwise ordered.
   9. Notify physician of any bleeding problems.
   10. Bolus with 80 units/kg. Start drip at 18 units/kg/h.
   11. If aPTT is less than 35 secs: Rebolus with 80 units/kg and increase rate by 4 units/kg/h.
   12. If aPTT is 36 to 44 secs: Rebolus with 40 units/kg and increase rate by 2 units/kg/h.
   13. If aPTT is 45 to 75 secs: Continue current rate.
   14. If aPTT is 76 to 90 secs: Decrease rate by 2 units/kg/h.
   15. If aPTT is greater than 90 secs: Hold heparin for 1 hour and decrease rate by 3 units/kg/h.

FIGURE 17-8 Heparin Protocol Worksheet

STANDARD WEIGHT-BASED HEPARIN PROTOCOL WORKSHEET

Round patient's total body weight to nearest 10 kg: _____ kg.

DO NOT change the weight based on daily measurements.

FOUND ON THE ORDER FORM

Initial Bolus (80 units/kg): _____ units _____ mL

Initial Infusion Rate (18 units/kg/h): _____ units/h _____ mL/h

---

Make adjustments to the heparin drip rate as directed by the order form.

ALL DOSES ARE ROUNDED TO THE NEAREST 100 UNITS.

Date	Time	aPTT	Bolus	Rate Change units/h	Rate Change mL/h	New Rate	RN 1	RN 2

If aPTT is	Then
Less than 35 secs:	Rebolus with 80 units/kg and increase rate by 4 units/kg/h.
36 to 44 secs:	Rebolus with 40 units/kg and increase rate by 2 units/kg/h.
45 to 75 secs:	Continue current rate.
76 to 90 secs:	Decrease rate by 2 units/kg/h.
Greater than 90 secs:	Hold heparin for 1 hour and decrease rate by 3 units/kg/h.

Signatures _____ Initials _____

_____

_____

_____

_____

50. Describe the strategy you would implement to prevent this medication error.

Possible Scenario

Suppose the physician writes an order to induce labor, as follows: **Pitocin 20 U IV added to 1 liter of LR beginning at 1 mU/min, then increase by 1 mU/min q 15 min to a maximum of 20 mU/min until adequate labor is reached.** The labor and delivery unit stocks Pitocin ampules 10 units per mL in boxes of 50 ampules. The nurse preparing the IV solution misread the order as "20 mL of Pitocin added to 1 liter of Lactated Ringer's . . ." and pulled 20 ampules of Pitocin from the supply shelf. Another nurse, seeing this nurse drawing up medication from several ampules, asked what the nurse was preparing. When the nurse described the IV solution being prepared, he suddenly realized he had misinterpreted the order.

Potential Outcome

The amount of Pitocin that was being drawn up (20 mL) to be added to the IV solution would have been 10 units/mL × 20 mL = 200 units of Pitocin, 10 times the ordered amount of 20 units. Starting this Pitocin solution, even at the usual slow rate, would have delivered an excessively high amount of Pitocin that could have led to fatal consequences for both the fetus and laboring mother. What should the nurse have done to avoid this type of error?

Prevention

_____

_____

After completing these problems, see pages 718–722 to check your answers.

Be sure to use the online software for additional practice!

REFERENCE

Institute for Safe Medication Practices. (2013). Medication safety alert. Important change with heparin labels. Retrieved from http://www.ismp.org/NAN/files/NAN-20130610.pdf

SECTION 4 SELF-EVALUATION

Chapter 15—Intravenous Solutions, Equipment, and Calculations

1. Which of the following IV solutions is normal saline?

   _____ 0.45% NaCl   _____ 0.9% NaCl   _____ D₅W

2. What is the solute and concentration of 0.9% NaCl? _____

3. What is the solute and concentration of 0.45% NaCl? _____

Use the following information to answer questions 4 and 5.

Order: D_5 0.45% NaCl 1,000 mL IV q.8h

4. The IV solution contains _____ g dextrose.

5. The IV solution contains _____ g sodium chloride.

6. Order: 0.45% NaCl 500 mL IV q.6h. The IV solution contains _____ g sodium chloride.

Refer to this order for questions 7 and 8.

Order: D_{10} 0.9% NaCl 750 mL IV q.8h

7. The IV solution contains _____ g dextrose.

8. The IV solution contains _____ g sodium chloride.

9. Are most electronic infusion devices calibrated in gtt/min, mL/h, mL/min, or gtt/mL? _____

Use the following information to answer questions 10 through 13.

Mrs. Wilson has an order to receive 2,000 mL of D_5NS IV fluids over 24 h. An electronic infusion pump is not available. The nurse sets up IV tubing calibrated for a drop factor of 15 gtt/mL and attaches a dial-flow controller.

10. What rate should be set on the dial-flow controller? _____ mL/h
    Mark the spot where you would position the dial mark on the image of the dial-flow controller.

11. Verify the rate of the dial-flow controller with a watch count using the IV flow rate formula for manual IVs. What should the drop rate be? _____ gtt/min

12. What constant would you use if you wanted to calculate the flow rate using the shortcut method? _____

13. A liter bag was hung at 0800, when would you expect to hang a new liter of fluid? Answer using both the 24-hour clock and traditional time. 24-hour clock: _____ traditional time: _____

Copyright © 2016 Cengage Learning®

100
75
50
30
10

Use the following information to answer questions 14 through 16.

As you continue on your rounds, you find Mr. Boyd with an infiltrated IV and decide to restart it and regulate it on an electronic infusion pump calibrated in whole mL/h. The orders specify:

NS 1,000 mL IV c̄ 20 mEq KCl q.8h

cefazolin 250 mg IV PB per 100 mL NS q.8h over 30 min

Limit IV total fluids to 3,000 mL daily.

14. Interpret Mr. Boyd's IV and medication orders. _____

_____

15. Regulate the electronic infusion pump for Mr. Boyd's standard IV at _____ mL/h.

16. Regulate the electronic infusion pump for Mr. Boyd's IV PB at _____ mL/h.

17. Order: **D₅LR 1,200 mL IV at 100 mL/h.** You start this IV at 1530 and, during your nursing
    assessment at 2200, you find 650 mL remaining. The flow rate is 100 gtt/min using a microdrip
    infusion set. Describe your action now. _____

_____

Chapter 16—Body Surface Area and Advanced Pediatric Calculations

Calculate the hourly maintenance IV rate for the children described in questions 18 through 21. Use the
following recommendations:

    First 10 kg of body weight: 100 mL/kg/day

    Next 10 kg of body weight: 50 mL/kg/day

    Each additional kg over 20 kg of body weight: 20 mL/kg/day

18. A child who weighs 40 lb requires _____ mL/day for maintenance IV fluids.

19. The infusion rate for the same child who weighs 40 lb is _____ mL/h.

20. An infant who weighs 1,185 g requires _____ mL/day for maintenance IV fluids.

21. The infusion rate for the same infant who weighs 1,185 g is _____ mL/h.

Use the BSA formula method on the following page to answer questions 22 through 24.

22. Height: 30 in   Weight: 24 lb   BSA: _____ m²

23. Height: 155 cm   Weight: 39 kg   BSA: _____ m²

24. Height: 52 in   Weight: 65 lb   BSA: _____ m²

Questions 25 through 31 refer to the following situation.

A child who is 28 in tall and weighs 25 lb will receive 1 dosage of cisplatin IV. The recommended dosage is 37 to 75 mg/m² once every 2 to 3 weeks. The order reads **cisplatin 18.5 mg IV at 1 mg/min today
at 1500 hours.** You have available a 50 mg vial of cisplatin. Reconstitution directions state to *add
50 mL of sterile water to yield 1 mg/mL.* Minimal dilution instructions require 2 mL of IV solution for
every 1 mg of cisplatin.

25. According to the West nomogram on the following page, the child's BSA is _____ m².

26. The safe dosage range for this child is _____ mg to _____ mg.

27. Is this dosage safe? _____.

28. If safe, you will prepare _____ mL. If not, describe your action. _____

_____

29. How many mL of IV fluid are required for safe dilution of the cisplatin? _____ mL

30. Given the ordered rate of 1 mg/min, set the infusion pump at _____ mL/h.

31. How long will this infusion take? _____ min

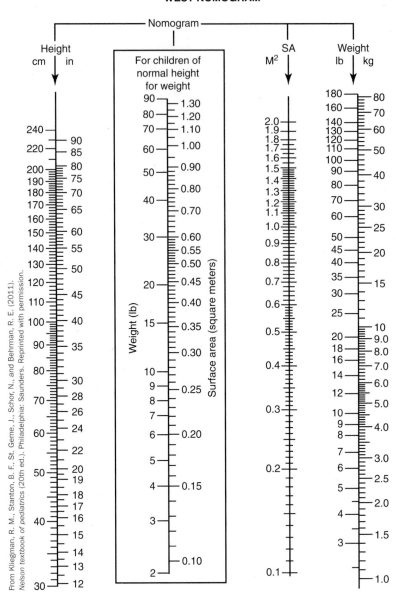

WEST NOMOGRAM

Metric:
$$BSA\ (m^2) = \sqrt{\frac{ht\ (cm) \times wt\ (kg)}{3{,}600}}$$

Household:
$$BSA\ (m^2) = \sqrt{\frac{ht\ (in) \times wt\ (lg)}{3{,}131}}$$

From Kliegman, R. M., Stanton, B. F., St. Geme, J., Schor, N., and Behrman, R. E. (2011). *Nelson textbook of pediatrics* (20th ed.). Philadelphia: Saunders. Reprinted with permission.

Questions 32 through 35 refer to the following situation.

Order: **Vincasar 1.6 mg IV stat**. The child is 50 inches tall and weighs 40 lb. The label represents the Vincasar solution you have available. The recommended dosage of Vincasar is 2 mg/m² daily.

32. According to the West nomogram, the child's BSA is _____ m².

33. The recommended safe dosage for this child is _____ mg.

34. Is the dosage ordered safe? _____

35. If safe, you will prepare _____ mL Vincasar to add to the IV. If not safe, describe your action.

_____

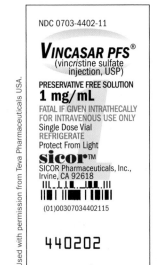

NDC 0703-4402-11

VINCASAR PFS®
(vin*cri*stine sulfate
injection, USP)

PRESERVATIVE FREE SOLUTION
1 mg/mL
FATAL IF GIVEN INTRATHECALLY
FOR INTRAVENOUS USE ONLY
Single Dose Vial
REFRIGERATE
Protect From Light
sicor™
SICOR Pharmaceuticals, Inc.,
Irvine, CA 92618

(01)00307034402115

440202

36. Order: NS IV for continuous infusion at 40 mL/h c̄ Ancef 250 mg IV q.8h over 30 min by volume control set

    Available: Ancef 125 mg/mL

    Add _____ mL NS and _____ mL Ancef to the chamber to infuse at 40 mL/h.

37. Order: Timentin 750 mg IV q.6h. Recommended minimal dilution (maximal concentration) is 100 mg/mL. Calculate the number of mL to be used for minimal dilution of the Timentin as ordered. _____ mL

Chapter 17—Advanced Adult Intravenous Calculations

Unless stated otherwise, IV pumps are calibrated to deliver whole mL/h.

Use the following information to answer questions 38 through 41.

Mr. Smith is on restricted fluids. His IV order is: NS 1,500 mL IV q.24h c̄ 300,000 units penicillin G potassium IV PB in 100 mL NS q.4h over 30 min. The infusion set is calibrated at 60 gtt/mL.

38. Set Mr. Smith's regular IV at _____ gtt/min.

39. Set Mr. Smith's IV PB at _____ gtt/min.

Later during your shift, an electronic infusion pump becomes available. You decide to use it to regulate Mr. Smith's IVs.

40. Regulate Mr. Smith's regular IV at _____ mL/h.

41. Regulate Mr. Smith's IV PB at _____ mL/h.

42. Order: potassium chloride 40 mEq/L D_5W IV at 2 mEq/h

    Regulate the infusion pump at _____ mL/h.

43. Order: nitroglycerin 25 mg/L D_5W IV at 5 mcg/min

    Regulate the infusion pump calibrated in tenths of a mL/h at _____ mL/h.

Refer to this order for questions 44 through 47.

Order: Induce labor c̄ Pitocin 15 units/L LR IV continuous infusion at 2 milliunits/min; increase by 1 milliunit/min q.30 min to a maximum of 20 milliunits/min.

44. The initial concentration of Pitocin is _____ milliunits/mL.

45. The initial Pitocin order will infuse at the rate of _____ mL/min.

46. Regulate the electronic infusion pump at _____ mL/h to initiate the order.

47. The infusion pump will be regulated at a maximum of _____ mL/h to infuse the maximum of 20 milliunits/min.

Use the following information to answer questions 48 and 49.

Order for Ms. Hill, who weighs 150 lb, to stabilize her blood pressure: dopamine 400 mg per 0.5 L D_5W at 4 mcg/kg/min titrated to 12 mcg/kg/min.

48. Regulate the electronic infusion pump calibrated in tenths of a mL/h for Ms. Hill's IV at _____ mL/h to initiate the order.

49. Anticipate that the maximum flow rate for Ms. Hill's IV to achieve the maximum safe titration would be _____ mL/h.

50. Mr. Black has an order for heparin 10,000 units in 500 mL NS IV at 750 units/h. Regulate the infusion pump at _____ mL/h.

Section 4 Board Examination Practice

To obtain licensure, you will be required to pass a board examination. The following problems represent the various types of items on the NCLEX-RN® (National Council Licensure Examination for Registered Nurses) and NCLEX-PN® (National Council Licensure Examination for Practical Nurses) exams. Whether you will be taking one of these board examinations or one from another licensure board, alternate test items such as these are good practice. For additional practice, go to the online practice software that accompanies this text to respond to more interactive test items, including those using the calculator tool.

51. NCLEX *Fill-in-the-Blank* Item

The antidote drug for heparin overdosage is _____.

Answer: _____

52. NCLEX *Multiple-Response* Item

Before administering high-alert medications, the nurse should perform independent double verification. What does this process require? (Place a check mark beside all that apply.)

Answer:

a. Two clinicians checking volume in syringe separately from each other.   _____

b. One nurse isolated, away from distractions, reviewing calculations twice.   _____

c. Independent review of order, lab tests, calculations, and amount prepared.   _____

d. Comparison of previous dose and current dose.   _____

53. NCLEX *Exhibit* Item

Patient scenario: Diabetic patient with blood glucose level of 310 mg/dL. According to the IV insulin protocol on page 599, the nurse should administer a bolus of (place a check mark beside the correct answer):

Answer:

a. $\frac{1}{2}$ amp of 50% dextrose   _____

b. 10 units IV push   _____

c. 100 units regular insulin in 100 mL of 0.9% NaCl   _____

d. 25 units/hour   _____

54. NCLEX *Drag-and-Drop / Ordered-Response* Item

Copy the tasks from the box onto the list in the proper sequence to *administer high-alert intravenous heparin by a standard weight-based protocol.*

Answer:

Check aPTT test results.
Start continuous infusion, if required.
Record weight in kilograms.
Administer bolus, if required.
Adjust infusion rate, if required.
Check aPTT test results.
Administer rebolus, if required.

_____

_____

_____

_____

_____

_____

_____

	Critical Care Intravenous Insulin Protocol Orders
TARGET	**BLOOD GLUCOSE LEVEL 70 to 110 mg/dL**
Insulin Solution	1. 100 units regular insulin in 100 mL of 0.9% NaCl, to be titrated based on grid for Levels 1, 2, or 3.
Initial Infusion	2. Start nondiabetic patients at Level 1. Advance to Level 2 if TARGET range not reached after 2 hours on Level 1.
	3. Start diabetic patients at Level 2. Advance to Level 3 if TARGET range not reached after 2 hours on Level 2.
	4. Do not initiate insulin infusion unless blood glucose greater than 110 mg/dL.
Monitoring	5. Check blood glucose prior to start of insulin infusion.
	6. Check blood glucose every hour thereafter.
	7. When glucose is 80 to 110 mg/dL for 3 hours, check glucose every 2 hours.
	8. Resume monitoring every hour if blood glucose greater than 120 mg/dL for 2 hours.
Blood Glucose Less than 80 mg/dL	9. If patient has blood glucose less than 80 mg/dL:
	a. Refer to regular insulin infusion rate column in grid tables for management instructions.
	b. If necessary to reinitiate insulin infusion, start one level below previous level.
	c. Call physician for symptomatic hypoglycemia or blood glucose less than 50 mg/dL, even if treated.

	Grid for Titration of Intravenous Insulin—Level 2

LEVEL 2: DO NOT INITIATE insulin drip unless blood glucose is greater than 110 mg/dL.

Blood Glucose (mg/dL)	Regular U-100 Insulin Bolus	Regular Insulin Infusion Rate: 100 Units of Regular U-100 Insulin in 100 mL NaCl
Less than 70	Give $\frac{1}{2}$ of 50 mL amp of 50% dextrose	HOLD insulin infusion × 60 minutes and check blood glucose every 15 minutes until equal to or greater than 80.
70 to 79	0	HOLD insulin infusion × 60 minutes and check blood glucose every 15 minutes until equal to or greater than 80.
80 to 110	0	2 units/h
111 to 125	0	3 units/h
126 to 149	0	4 units/h
150 to 165	0	5 units/h
166 to 179	0	6 units/h
180 to 209	0	8 units/h
210 to 239	10 units IV push	12 units/h
240 to 269	10 units IV push	16 units/h
270 to 299	10 units IV push	20 units/h
300 to 350	10 units IV push	25 units/h
Greater than 350	Notify physician	

55. NCLEX *Hot Box* Item

Place an X on the label(s) that the nurse could reasonably select from the ADC matrix drawer to prepare the following order.

Order: D₅W 500 mL with heparin 25,000 units IV at 1,000 units/h

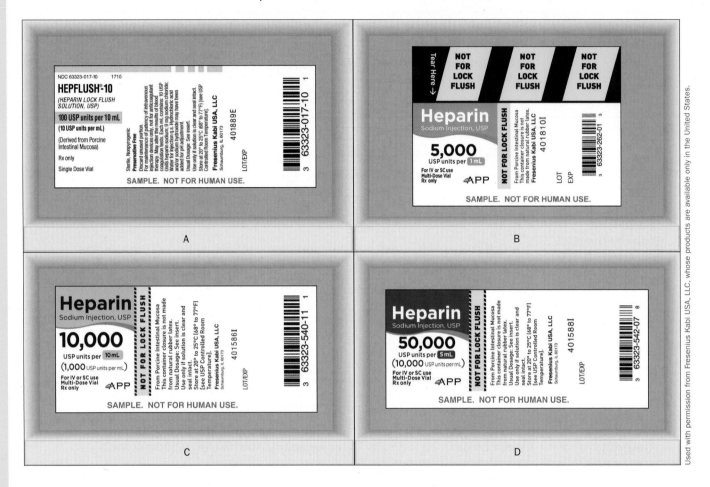

After completing these problems, refer to pages 723–726 to check your answers. Give yourself 1.8 points for each correct answer or 100 points for answering all questions correctly.

Perfect score = 100   My score = _____

Minimum mastery score = 86 (48 correct)

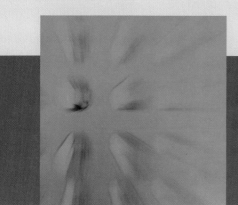

Essential Skills Evaluation: Posttest

Go back to the **Essential Skills Evaluation: Pretest** on pages 3–20 and rework the questions as a Posttest to evaluate your mastery of the essential skills of dosage calculations. Record your answers here and compare with the results of your pretest.

ESSENTIAL SKILLS EVALUATION: POSTTEST ANSWER SHEET

1. Give: _____ tablet(s)   Frequency: _____

2. Give: _____ tablet(s)   Frequency: _____

3. Choose: _____ mg capsules   Give: _____ capsule(s)   Frequency: _____

4. Give: _____ tablet(s)   Frequency: _____

5. Give: _____ tablet(s)   Frequency: _____

6. Give: _____ mL   Frequency: _____

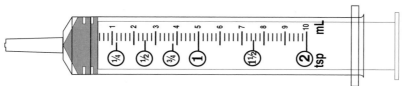

Copyright © 2016 Cengage Learning®.

7. Give: _____ mL   Frequency: _____

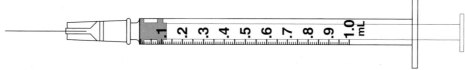

Copyright © 2016 Cengage Learning®.

8. Give: _____ mL   Frequency: _____

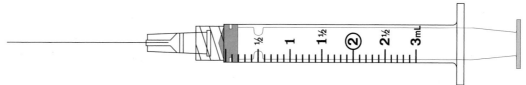

Copyright © 2016 Cengage Learning®.

9. Give: _____ mL   Frequency: _____

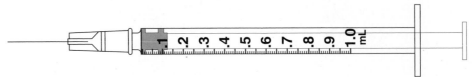

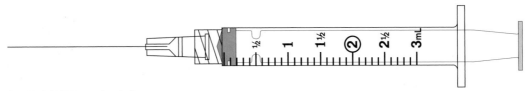

10. Give: _____ mL   Frequency: _____

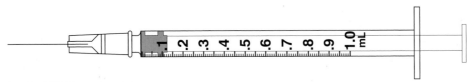

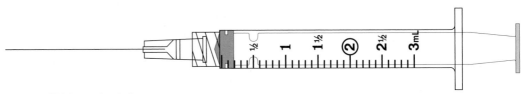

11. Give: _____ mL   Frequency: _____

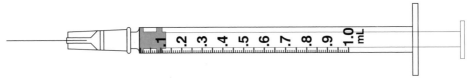

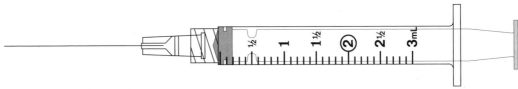

12. Give: _____ mL   Frequency: _____

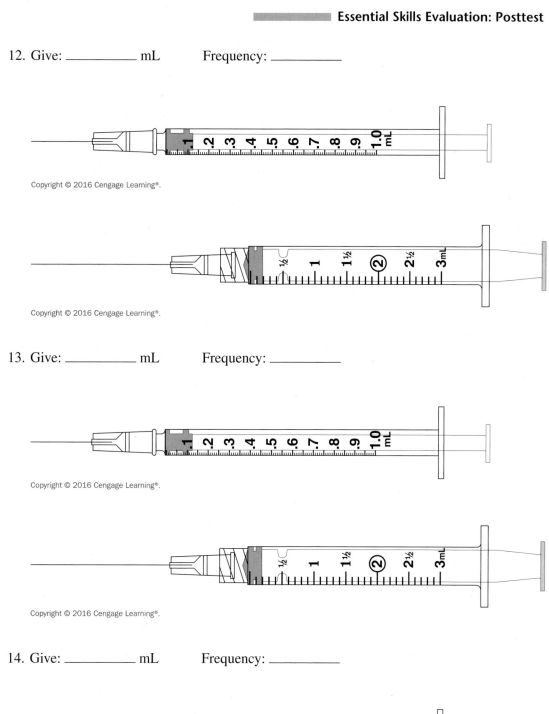

13. Give: _____ mL   Frequency: _____

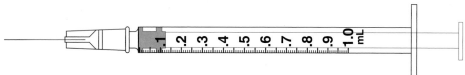

14. Give: _____ mL   Frequency: _____

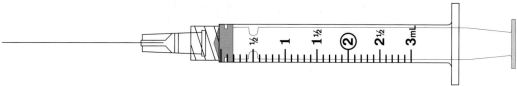

15. Give: _____ mL   Frequency: _____

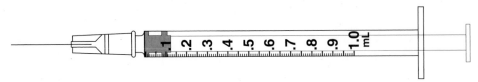

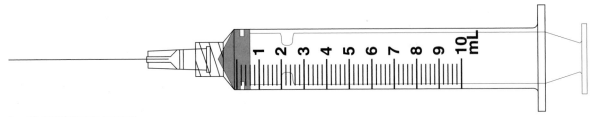

16. Give: _____ mL   Frequency: _____

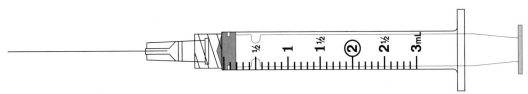

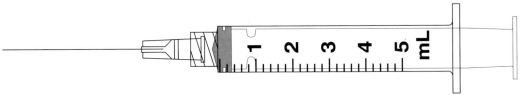

17. Give: _____ mL at _____ mL/min, which equals _____ mL per 15 sec

     Frequency: _____

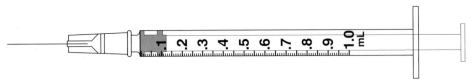

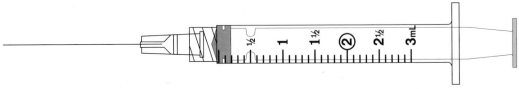

18. Add: _____ mL to the IV PB bag, and set the drip rate on the tubing to _____ gtt/min

    Frequency: _____

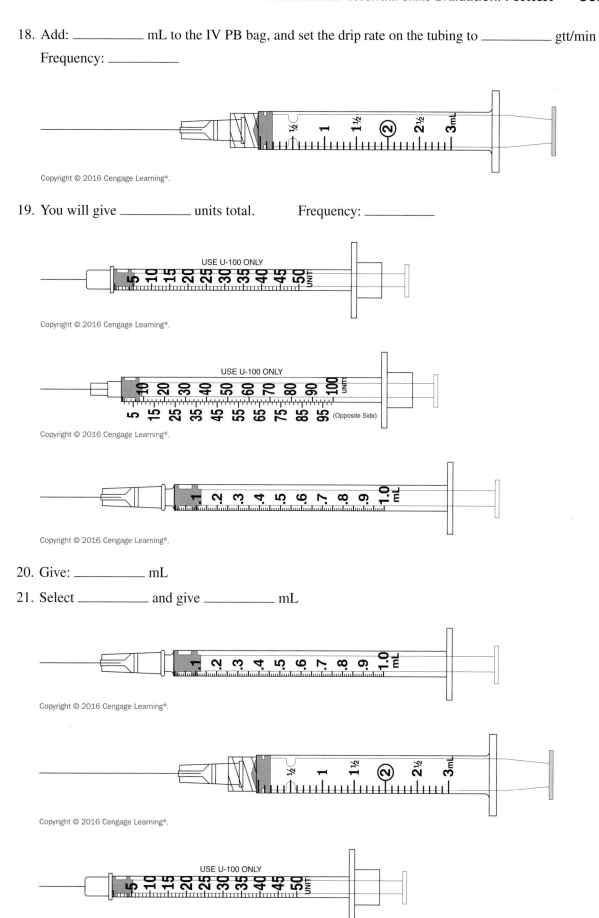

Copyright © 2016 Cengage Learning®.

19. You will give _____ units total.   Frequency: _____

Copyright © 2016 Cengage Learning®.

USE U-100 ONLY

Copyright © 2016 Cengage Learning®.

Copyright © 2016 Cengage Learning®.

20. Give: _____ mL

21. Select _____ and give _____ mL

Copyright © 2016 Cengage Learning®.

Copyright © 2016 Cengage Learning®.

USE U-100 ONLY

Copyright © 2016 Cengage Learning®.

22. Medication: _____   Give _____ mL

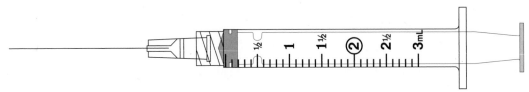

23. Yes or No: _____   Explain: _____

    _____

24. _____ tablet(s)

25. _____ mL; _____ gtt/min

26. _____ mL/h

27. _____ mL diluent; give _____ mL

28. _____ tablet(s); _____, _____, and _____ hours

29. _____ units; _____ route

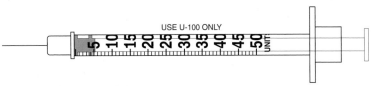

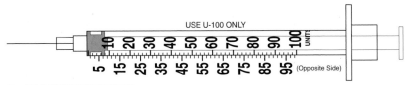

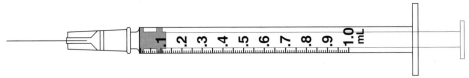

30. _____ mL

31. Yes or No: _____   Explain: _____

    _____

32. _____ mL

33. Yes or No: _____   Explain: _____

    _____

34. _____ mL   Next action: _____

35. _____ °F

36. _____ mg/dose to _____ mg/dose

37. _____ mL

38. _____ mg/dose to _____ mg/dose; Yes or No: _____

39. _____ mL; _____ gtt/min

40. _____ mL

41. _____ gtt/min

42. _____ mL

43. _____ mg; _____ mL

44. _____ dose(s)

45. _____ hours; _____ (AM/PM)

46. _____ mL

47. _____ mg per _____ mL

48. _____ mL

49.

50. **Prevention:** _____

_____

After completing these problems, see the same Answers from the Pretest on pages 627–634 to check your answers. Give yourself 2 points for each correct answer.

Perfect score = 100   My score = _____

Minimum mastery score = 90 (45 correct)

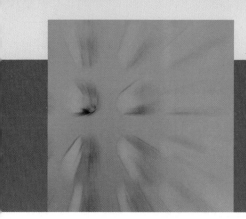

Comprehensive Skills Evaluation

T his evaluation is a comprehensive assessment of your mastery of the concepts presented in all 17 chapters of *Dosage Calculations.*

Donna Smith, a 46-year-old patient of Dr. J. Physician, has been admitted to the Progressive Care Unit (PCU) with complaints of an irregular heartbeat, shortness of breath, and chest pain (relieved by nitroglycerin). Questions 1 through 14 refer to the admitting orders on page 611 for Mrs. Smith. The following labels represent the available medications and infusion set.

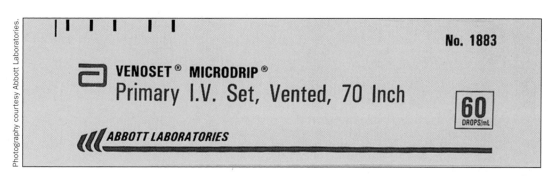

No. 1883

VENOSET® MICRODRIP®
Primary I.V. Set, Vented, 70 Inch

ABBOTT LABORATORIES

60 DROPS/mL

Photography courtesy Abbott Laboratories.

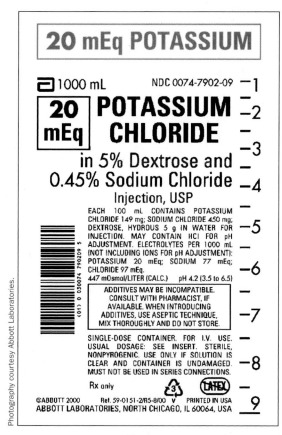

20 mEq POTASSIUM

1000 mL   NDC 0074-7902-09

20 mEq **POTASSIUM CHLORIDE**
in 5% Dextrose and
0.45% Sodium Chloride
Injection, USP

EACH 100 mL CONTAINS POTASSIUM CHLORIDE 149 mg; SODIUM CHLORIDE 450 mg; DEXTROSE, HYDROUS 5 g IN WATER FOR INJECTION. MAY CONTAIN HCl FOR pH ADJUSTMENT. ELECTROLYTES PER 1000 mL (NOT INCLUDING IONS FOR pH ADJUSTMENT): POTASSIUM 20 mEq; SODIUM 77 mEq; CHLORIDE 97 mEq.
447 mOsmol/LITER (CALC.)   pH 4.2 (3.5 to 6.5)

ADDITIVES MAY BE INCOMPATIBLE. CONSULT WITH PHARMACIST, IF AVAILABLE. WHEN INTRODUCING ADDITIVES, USE ASEPTIC TECHNIQUE, MIX THOROUGHLY AND DO NOT STORE.

SINGLE-DOSE CONTAINER. FOR I.V. USE. USUAL DOSAGE: SEE INSERT. STERILE, NONPYROGENIC. USE ONLY IF SOLUTION IS CLEAR AND CONTAINER IS UNDAMAGED. MUST NOT BE USED IN SERIES CONNECTIONS.

Rx only

©ABBOTT 2000   Ref. 59-0151-2/R5-8/00 V   PRINTED IN USA
ABBOTT LABORATORIES, NORTH CHICAGO, IL 60064, USA

Photography courtesy Abbott Laboratories.

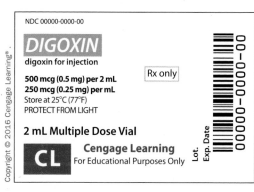

NDC 00000-0000-00

DIGOXIN
digoxin for injection

Rx only

500 mcg (0.5 mg) per 2 mL
250 mcg (0.25 mg) per mL
Store at 25°C (77°F)
PROTECT FROM LIGHT

2 mL Multiple Dose Vial

CL **Cengage Learning**
For Educational Purposes Only

Copyright © 2016 Cengage Learning®.

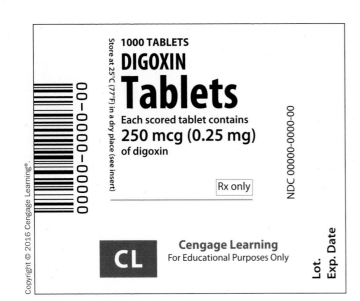

1000 TABLETS
DIGOXIN
Tablets
Each scored tablet contains
250 mcg (0.25 mg)
of digoxin

Rx only

Store at 25°C (77°F) in a dry place (see insert)

NDC 00000-0000-00

CL **Cengage Learning**
For Educational Purposes Only

Copyright © 2016 Cengage Learning®.

Lot.
Exp. Date

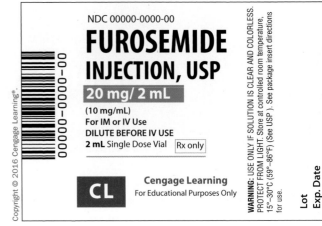

NDC 00000-0000-00
FUROSEMIDE
INJECTION, USP
20 mg / 2 mL

(10 mg/mL)
For IM or IV Use
DILUTE BEFORE IV USE
2 mL Single Dose Vial   Rx only

CL **Cengage Learning**
For Educational Purposes Only

WARNING: USE ONLY IF SOLUTION IS CLEAR AND COLORLESS. PROTECT FROM LIGHT. Store at controlled room temperature, 15°–30°C (59°–86°F). (See USP). See package insert directions for use.

Lot
Exp. Date

Copyright © 2016 Cengage Learning®.

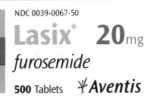

Used with permission from Aventis Pharmaceuticals.

NDC 0039-0067-50

Lasix® **20**mg
furosemide
500 Tablets   ✦*Aventis*

3 0039-0067-50 9

℞ ONLY
Each LASIX® Tablet contains 20mg furosemide. **Dosage and Administration:** See package insert for dosage information. **WARNING:** Keep out of reach of children. Do not use if bottle closure seal is broken. **Pharmacist:** Dispense in well-closed, light-resistant container with child-resistant closure. **Store at room temperature.**
Hoechst-Roussel Pharmaceuticals
Division of **Aventis Pharmaceuticals Inc.**
Kansas City, MO 64137 USA   ©2000
www.aventispharma-us.com
50058803 50058803 **50058803**

Used with permission from McNeil Consumer and Specialty Pharmaceuticals.

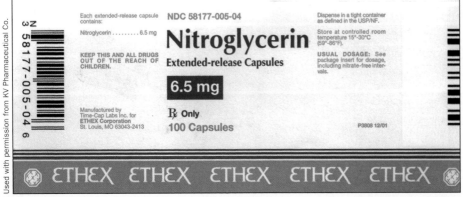

Used with permission from KV Pharmaceutical Co.

N 3 58177-005-04 6

Each extended-release capsule contains:

Nitroglycerin . . . . 6.5 mg

KEEP THIS AND ALL DRUGS OUT OF THE REACH OF CHILDREN.

NDC 58177-005-04
Nitroglycerin
Extended-release Capsules

6.5 mg

℞ Only
100 Capsules

Dispense in a tight container as defined in the USP/NF.

Store at controlled room temperature 15°-30°C (59°-86°F).

USUAL DOSAGE: See package insert for dosage, including nitrate-free intervals.

Manufactured by Time-Cap Labs Inc. for ETHEX Corporation St. Louis, MO 63043-2413

P3808 12/01

✸ ETHEX ETHEX ETHEX ETHEX ETHEX ✸

Physician's Order Form

	ENTERED	FILLED	CHECKED	VERIFIED

DATE	TIME WRITTEN	PLEASE USE BALL POINT - PRESS FIRMLY	✓	TIME NOTED	NURSE'S SIGNATURE
9/3/xx	1600	Admit to PCU, monitored bed			
		Bedrest c̄ bathroom privileges			
		nitroglycerin ER 13 mg p.o. q.8h			
		furosemide 20 mg IV Push stat, then 20 mg p.o. b.i.d.			
		digoxin 0.25 mg IV Push stat, repeat in 4 hours,		1610 GP	
		then 0.125 mg p.o. daily			
		potassium chloride 20 mEq per L D$_5$ $\frac{1}{2}$ NS IV at 80 mL/h			
		Tylenol 1 g p.o. q.4h p.r.n., headache	✓		
		Labwork: Electrolytes and CBC in am			
		Soft diet, advance as tolerated			
		J. Physician, M.D.			

AUTO STOP ORDERS: UNLESS REORDERED, FOLLOWING WILL BE D/C'D AT 0800 ON:

DATE	ORDER		PHYSICIAN SIGNATURE
		☐ CONT ☐ D/C	PHYSICIAN SIGNATURE
		☐ CONT ☐ D/C	PHYSICIAN SIGNATURE
		☐ CONT ☐ D/C	PHYSICIAN SIGNATURE

CHECK WHEN ANTIBIOTICS ORDERED   ☐ Prophylactic   ☐ Empiric   ☐ Therapeutic

ALLERGIES:
   None Known

   Chest Pain
PATIENT DIAGNOSIS

PATIENT HEIGHT   5' 6"   PATIENT WEIGHT   110 lb

Smith, Donna
ID #257-226-3

1. The progressive care unit (PCU) is short on IV pumps because of unscheduled repairs. The nurse implements a backup plan and starts a straight gravity flow IV on Mrs. Smith at 1630 hours. Calculate the watch-count flow rate for the IV fluid ordered. _____ gtt/min

2. Estimate the time and date when the nurse should plan to hang the next liter of $D_5 \frac{1}{2}$ NS.

    _____ hours on _____ (date)

3. At the present infusion rate, how much $D_5 \frac{1}{2}$ NS will Mrs. Smith receive in a 24-hour period? _____ mL/day

4. How many mEq of KCl will Mrs. Smith receive per hour and per day? _____ mEq/h; _____ mEq/day

5. Both digoxin and furosemide are ordered "stat."

    a. What does this mean? _____

    b. How frequently should the nurse administer these two stat orders? _____

6. Prior to administering the IV digoxin, the nurse consults the drug guide, which states that the recommended rate for direct IV administration of digoxin is 0.25 mg in 4 mL NS administered at the rate of 0.25 mg per 5 min.

    a. How much digoxin should the nurse administer for the stat IV order? At what rate?

    Prepare: _____ mL digoxin and add _____ mL NS for a total of _____ mL. Administer at the rate of _____ mL/min or _____ mL per 15 sec.

    b. Draw an arrow on the appropriate syringe to indicate how much digoxin to prepare.

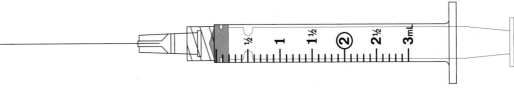

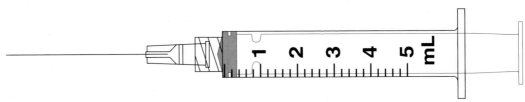

7. In addition to manual IV push administration, what other method(s) could the nurse choose for administering the direct IV digoxin order, if available?

    a. IV PB on an IV infusion pump

    b. Syringe pump

    c. Volume-control device, such as Buretrol

    d. a, b, and c

    e. b and c

8. The nurse consults the drug guide for more information about the furosemide ordered. The recommended rate for direct IV administration is 40 mg per 2 min.

   a. How much furosemide should the nurse administer for Mrs. Smith's stat dose? At what rate?

   Give: _____ mL at the rate of _____ mL/min or _____ mL per 15 sec

   b. Draw an arrow on the appropriate syringe to indicate how much furosemide to prepare.

Copyright © 2016 Cengage Learning®.

Copyright © 2016 Cengage Learning®.

9. How many digoxin tablets will Mrs. Smith need for a 24-hour period for the p.o. digoxin order? _____ tablet(s)

10. After the initial dose of furosemide, how many tablets should the nurse give Mrs. Smith for each subsequent dose? _____ tablet(s)

11. How much nitroglycerin should the nurse give Mrs. Smith for 1 dose? _____ capsule(s)

12. Mrs. Smith has a headache.

    a. How much Tylenol should the nurse give her for 1 dose? _____ tablet(s)

    b. When should the nurse give her the next dose? _____

13. Compare the drug labels for Mrs. Smith, and identify the drug(s) that is (are) supplied as generic(s).

    _____

14. An IV infusion pump that is programmable in whole milliliters becomes available for Mrs. Smith. At what rate should the nurse now set the IV pump for the continuous infusion? _____ mL/h

    Despite excellent care, Mrs. Smith's condition worsens and she is transferred into the coronary care unit (CCU) with the medical orders on page 614. CCU IV infusion pumps are programmable in tenths of a milliliter. Questions 15 through 20 refer to these orders.

		ENTERED	FILLED	CHECKED	VERIFIED

Physician's Order Form

DATE	TIME WRITTEN	PLEASE USE BALL POINT - PRESS FIRMLY	✓	TIME NOTED	NURSE'S SIGNATURE
9/4/xx	2230	Transfer to CCU			
		NPO			
		Discontinue nitroglycerin			
		lidocaine bolus 50 mg IV stat, then begin			
		lidocaine drip 2 g IV in 500 mL D_5W			
		at 2 mg/min by infusion pump			
		Increase lidocaine to 4 mg/min IV if PVCs persist			
				2235 MS	
		dopamine 400 mg IV PB in 250 mL D_5W			
		at 500 mcg/min by infusion pump			
		Increase KCl to 20 mEq per L $D_5W\frac{1}{2}NS$ IV at 50 mL/h			
		Increase furosemide to 40 mg IV q.12h			
		O_2 at 30% p̄ ABGs [arterial blood gases]			
		Labwork: Electrolytes stat and in AM and			
		ABGs stat and p.r.n.			
		J. Physician, M.D.			

AUTO STOP ORDERS: UNLESS REORDERED, FOLLOWING WILL BE D/C^D AT 0800 ON:

DATE	ORDER		PHYSICIAN SIGNATURE
		☐ CONT ☐ D/C	
		☐ CONT ☐ D/C	PHYSICIAN SIGNATURE
		☐ CONT ☐ D/C	PHYSICIAN SIGNATURE

CHECK WHEN ANTIBIOTICS ORDERED   ☐ Prophylactic   ☐ Empiric   ☐ Therapeutic

ALLERGIES:
None Known

Chest Pain
PATIENT DIAGNOSIS

PATIENT HEIGHT 5' 6"   PATIENT WEIGHT 110 lb

Smith, Donna
ID #257-226-3

15. Lidocaine is supplied in the 10 mg/mL dosage strength for Mrs. Smith. The nurse is familiar with lidocaine and knows the order is safe.

    a. How much lidocaine should the nurse administer to Mrs. Smith for the bolus? _____ mL

    b. Draw an arrow on the appropriate syringe to indicate the amount to prepare.

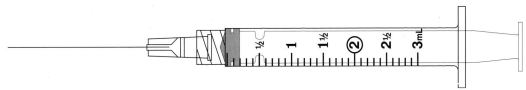

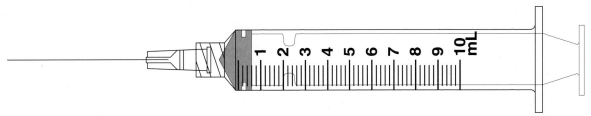

16. The CCU IV pumps are programmed in tenths of a milliliter. At what rate should the nurse initially set the IV infusion pump for the lidocaine drip? _____ mL/h

17. Dopamine is supplied for Mrs. Smith in the dosage strength of 80 mg/mL. The nurse checks the drug guide and finds that the recommended dosage of dopamine is 5 to 10 mcg/kg/min.

    a. Is the dosage ordered for Mrs. Smith safe? _____ Explain: _____

    _____

    b. If it is safe, how much dopamine should the nurse add to mix the IV PB dopamine drip?
    _____ mL

    c. If the dosage ordered is safe, draw an arrow on the appropriate syringe to indicate the amount to add to the IV PB.

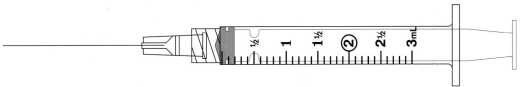

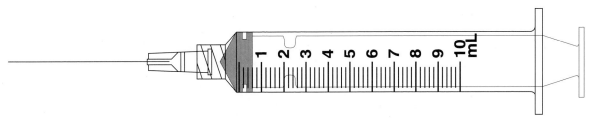

18. Calculate the rate for the IV infusion pump for the dopamine drip. _____ mL/h

19. How much dopamine will Mrs. Smith receive per hour? _____ mcg/h or _____ mg/h

20. Mrs. Smith is having increasing amounts of premature ventricular contractions (PVCs). To increase her lidocaine drip to 4 mg/min, the nurse should reprogram the IV infusion pump to _____ mL/h.

21. Julie Thomas is a 6-year-old pediatric patient who weighs 33 lb. She is in the hospital for fever of unknown origin. Julie complains of burning on urination, and her urinalysis shows *E. coli* bacterial infection. The doctor prescribes *Kantrex 75 mg IV q.8h to be administered by volume-control set on an infusion pump in 25 mL D$_5$ $\frac{1}{2}$ NS followed by 15 mL flush over 1 hour.*

The drug guide indicates that the maximum recommended dosage of Kantrex is 15 mg/kg/day IV in 3 divided doses.

a. Is the order safe? _____

    Explain: _____

b. If safe, add _____ mL Kantrex and _____ mL D$_5$ $\frac{1}{2}$ NS to the chamber, and set the flow rate for _____ mL/h.

Jamie Smith is hospitalized with a staphylococcal bone infection. He weighs 66 lb. The nurse intends to use a volume control set on an IV pump for Jamie. The pump is programmable in tenths of a milliliter. Questions 22 through 24 refer to Jamie.

Orders: D$_5$ $\frac{1}{2}$ NS IV at 50 mL/h.

        vancomycin 300 mg IV q.6h

Supply in the ADC cubby: vancomycin 500 mg per 10 mL with package insert instructions that state, "dilute further and infuse over 60 min."

Recommended dosage from drug guide: vancomycin 40 mg/kg/day IV in 4 divided doses.

22. Is this drug order safe? _____. Explain: _____

23. a. If safe, how much vancomycin should the nurse add to the chamber? _____ mL

    b. How much IV fluid should the nurse add to the chamber with the vancomycin? _____ mL

    c. How much IV fluid will Jamie receive in 24 hours? _____ mL

24. Use the following recommendations to calculate the hourly maintenance IV rate for Jamie.

First 10 kg of body weight: 100 mL/kg/day

Second 10 kg of body weight: 50 mL/kg/day

Each additional kg over 20 kg of body weight: 20 mL/kg/day

a. Jamie requires _____ mL/day for maintenance IV fluids.

b. The infusion rate should be set at _____ mL/h.

c. Does the recommended rate match the ordered rate? _____

Use the following related orders and labels to answer questions 25 through 29. Select the appropriate syringe, and mark it with the dose volume as indicated.

25. Order: Unasyn 500 mg IV q.6h in 50 mL D₅W IV PB over 30 min

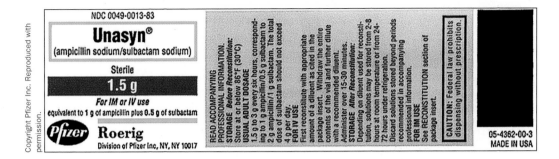

Package insert directions state:

Unasyn Vial Size	Volume Diluent to Be Added	Withdrawal Volume
1.5 g	3.2 mL	4.0 mL
3.0 g	6.4 mL	8.0 mL

To reconstitute the Unasyn, the nurse should add _____ mL diluent.

26. Prepare a reconstitution label for the Unasyn.

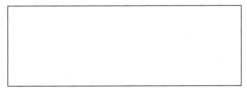

Reconstitution label

27. To prepare the IV PB for administration, the nurse should add _____ mL Unasyn to the 50 mL D₅W IV PB. Choose and mark the appropriate syringe.

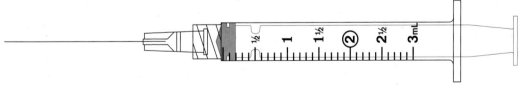

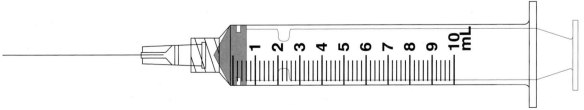

28. The IV PB Unasyn is regulated on an IV infusion pump. The nurse should set the flow rate at _____ mL/h.

29. Order: **heparin 10,000 units IV in 500 mL D₅W to infuse at 1,200 units/h**

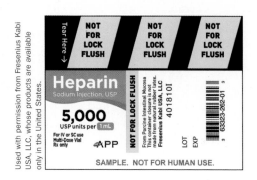

a. Add _____ mL heparin to the IV solution. Mark the dose amount on the syringe.

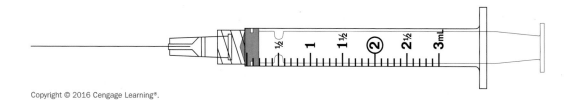

Copyright © 2016 Cengage Learning®.

b. Set the flow rate to _____ mL/h on an IV infusion pump.

Questions 30 and 31 refer to a patient who weighs 125 lb and is receiving IV heparin therapy.

30. Use the Weight-Based Heparin Protocol to calculate bolus dosage and infusion rate. The IV pump delivers tenths of a milliliter.

Weight-Based Heparin Protocol:

Heparin IV infusion: **heparin 25,000 units IV in 250 mL of $\frac{1}{2}$ NS**

IV boluses: Use heparin 1,000 units/mL

Bolus with heparin 80 units/kg. Then initiate heparin drip at 18 units/kg/h. Obtain aPTT every 6 hours, and adjust dosage and rate as follows:

If aPTT is less than 35 seconds: Rebolus with 80 units/kg and increase rate by 4 units/kg/h.

If aPTT is 36 to 44 seconds: Rebolus with 40 units/kg and increase rate by 2 units/kg/h.

If aPTT is 45 to 75 seconds: Continue current rate.

If aPTT is 76 to 90 seconds: Decrease rate by 2 units/kg/h.

If aPTT is greater than 90 seconds: Hold heparin for 1 hour and then decrease rate by 3 units/kg/h.

---

a. Convert the patient's weight to kg (rounded to tenths): _____ kg

b. Calculate the initial heparin bolus dosage: _____ units

c. Calculate the bolus dose: _____ mL

d. Calculate the initial heparin infusion rate: _____ units/h or _____ mL/h

31. At 0930, the patient's aPTT is 77 seconds.

    a. According to the protocol, what action should the nurse implement?

    _____

    _____

    b. The nurse should decrease infusion rate by _____ units/h or _____ mL/h.

    c. The nurse should reset infusion rate to _____ mL/h.

32. Order: **Humalog lispro U-100 insulin subcut ac per sliding scale**
    The patient's blood sugar at 1730 hours is 238.

Blood Glucose mg/dL	Insulin Dosage
0 to 150	0 units
151 to 250	8 units
251 to 350	13 units
351 to 400	18 units
Greater than 400	Hold insulin; call MD

Give: _____ units, which equals _____ mL (Mark dose on appropriate syringe.)

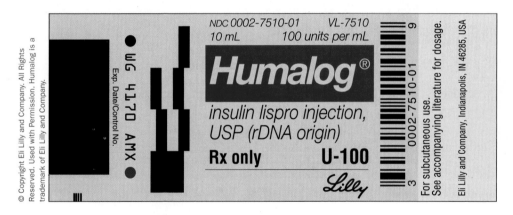

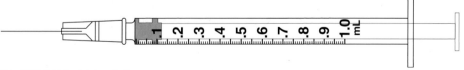

Copyright © 2016 Cengage Learning®.

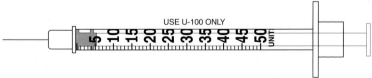

Copyright © 2016 Cengage Learning®.

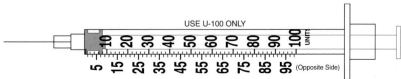

Copyright © 2016 Cengage Learning®.

33. Order: Humulin R regular U-100 insulin 15 units c̄ Humulin N NPH U-100 insulin 45 units subcut at 0730

   a. The nurse should give a total of _____ units insulin. (Remember, the nurse will get independent verification after drawing up each insulin.)

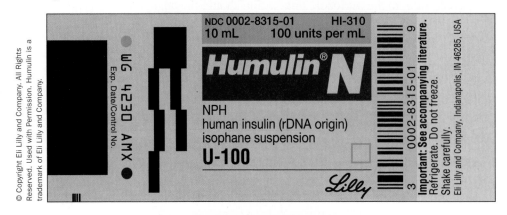

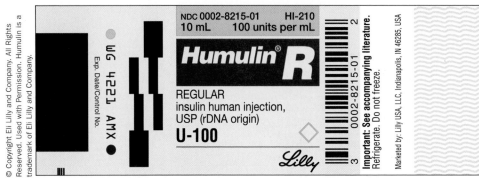

   b. Mark dose on appropriate syringe, designating measurement of both regular and NPH insulins.

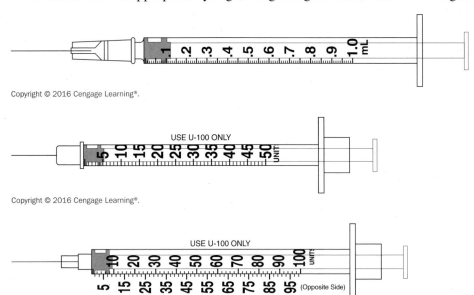

34. A patient is receiving an insulin drip of Humulin R regular U-100 insulin 300 units added to 150 mL NS IV infusing at 10 mL/h. How many units/h of insulin is this patient receiving? _____ units/h

Questions 35 and 36 refer to a child who weighs 16 lb and is admitted to the pediatric unit with vomiting and diarrhea of 3 days' duration.

Order: $\frac{1}{4}$ strength Isomil 80 mL q.3h for 4 feedings; if tolerated, increase Isomil to $\frac{1}{2}$ strength 80 mL q.3h for 4 feedings

Supply: Isomil ready-to-feed formula in 8-fl-oz cans

35. To reconstitute a full 8-fl-oz can of Isomil ready-to-feed to $\frac{1}{4}$ strength, the nurse should add _____ mL water to mix a total of _____ mL of $\frac{1}{4}$ strength reconstituted Isomil.

36. The child is not tolerating the oral feedings. Calculate this child's allowable daily and hourly IV maintenance fluids using the following recommendation.

   Daily rate of pediatric maintenance IV fluids:

   100 mL/kg for first 10 kg of body weight

   50 mL/kg for next 10 kg of body weight

   20 mL/kg for each kg above 20 kg of body weight

   Allowance: _____ mL/day or _____ mL/h

Use the following information and order to answer questions 37 through 39.

   Metric: BSA (m^2) = $\sqrt{\dfrac{\text{ht (cm)} \times \text{wt (kg)}}{3{,}600}}$ Household: BSA (m^2) = $\sqrt{\dfrac{\text{ht (in)} \times \text{wt (lb)}}{3{,}131}}$

   Order: mitomycin 28 mg IV push stat

Recommended dosage is 10 to 20 mg/m^2/single IV dose.

Patient is 5 ft 2 in tall and weighs 103 lb.

Mitomycin is available in a 40 mg vial with directions to reconstitute with 80 mL sterile water for injection and inject slowly over 10 minutes.

37. The patient's BSA is _____ m^2.

38. a. What is the recommended dosage range of mitomycin for this patient?

   _____ mg to _____ mg

   b. Is the ordered dosage safe? _____ Explain: _____

   _____

39. a. What is the concentration of mitomycin after reconstitution? _____ mg/mL

   b. If the order is safe, administer _____ mL mitomycin at the rate of _____ mL/min or _____ mL per 15 sec.

40. Calculate the amount of solutes in 1 L D$_5$ 0.45% NaCl.

   _____ g dextrose and _____ g NaCl

Use the following order and ceftriaxone label for the available drug to answer questions 41 and 42.

   Order: ceftriaxone 600 mg IV q.12h for total volume of 50 mL to infuse over 1 h via volume-control set

   The package insert states, "For IV administration, reconstitute with 9.6 mL of the specified IV diluent and each 1 mL of solution contains 100 mg of ceftriaxone."

Ceftriaxone for Injection, USP label

NDC 0703-0335-01 Rx only
Ceftriaxone for Injection, USP
1 gram
For I.M. or I.V. Use
Single Use Vial

Each vial contains: ceftriaxone sodium powder equivalent to 1 gram ceftriaxone.
For I.M. Administration : Reconstitute with 2.1 mL 1% Lidocaine Hydrochloride Injection (USP) or Sterile Water for Injection (USP). Each 1 mL of solution contains approximately 350 mg equivalent of ceftriaxone.
For I.V. Administration : See Package Insert
Usual Dosage: See Package Insert
Iss. 9/2007
39C1701450907

Storage Prior to Reconstitution: Store powder at 20° to 25°C (68° to 77°F) [See USP Controlled Room Temperature].
Protect from Light.
Storage After Reconstitution: See Package Insert
Mfd for: Teva Parenteral Medicines Irvine, CA 92618

41. The nurse should add _____ mL ceftriaxone and _____ mL IV fluid to the chamber.

42. The package insert states, ". . . recommended dilution concentration is 10 mg/mL to 40 mg/mL . . ." Is the ordered amount of IV fluid sufficient to safely dilute the ceftriaxone? _____

    Explain: _____

    _____

Use the following order and Pfizerpen label to answer questions 43 and 44.

    Order: **penicillin G potassium 400,000 units IV PB q.6h** for a child who weighs 10 kg. Recommended dosage for children: Give penicillin G potassium 150,000 to 250,000 units/kg/day in divided doses q.6h; dilute with 100 mL NS and infuse over 60 minutes.

Pfizerpen penicillin G potassium label

NDC 0049-0510-83
Buffered
Pfizerpen®
penicillin G potassium
For Injection
ONE MILLION UNITS
CAUTION: Federal law prohibits dispensing without prescription.
ROERIG *Pfizer*
A division of Pfizer Inc., N.Y., N.Y. 10017

43. a. How many units per day of penicillin G potassium will this child receive with this order? _____ units/day

    b. Is the ordered dosage safe? _____ Explain: _____

    _____

    c. If safe, reconstitute with _____ mL diluent for a concentration of _____ units/mL and prepare a reconstitution label.

    Reconstitution label

    d. Prepare to give _____ mL.

    e. If the order is not safe, what should the nurse do? _____

44. The child's IV is infusing on an IV pump programmable in whole milliliters. If the dosage is safe, set the IV flow rate at _____ mL/h.

Use the following patient information, orders, labels, and package insert to answer questions 45 through 48.

A patient has been admitted to the hospital with fever and chills, productive cough with yellow-green sputum, shortness of breath, malaise, and anorexia. Laboratory tests and X-rays confirm a diagnosis of pneumonia. The patient is complaining of nausea. The physician writes the following orders. The labels represent the drugs you have available.

Orders: NS 1,000 mL IV at 125 mL/h

ceftriaxone 1,500 mg IV PB q.8h in 100 mL NS over 30 min

promethazine 12.5 mg IV push q.4h p.r.n., nausea and vomiting

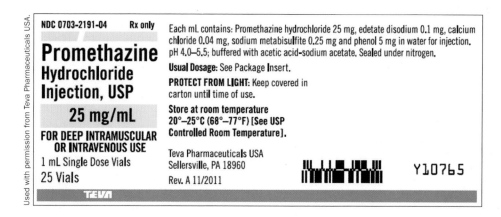

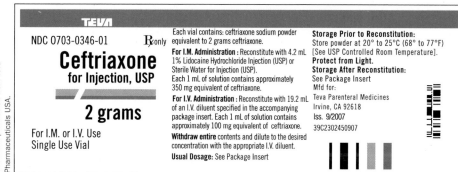

Intravenous Administration

Ceftriaxone for injection, USP should be administered intravenously by infusion over a period of 30 minutes. Concentrations between 10 mg/mL and 40 mg/mL are recommended; however, lower concentrations may be used if desired. Reconstitute vials with an appropriate IV diluent (see COMPATIBILITY AND STABILITY).

Vial Dosage Size	Amount of Diluent to be Added
250 mg	2.4 mL
500 mg	4.8 mL
1 g	9.6 mL
2 g	19.2 mL

After reconstitution, each 1 mL of solution contains approximately 100 mg equivalent of ceftriaxone. Withdraw entire contents and dilute to the desired concentration with the appropriate IV diluent.

45. The nurse starts the primary IV at 1:15 PM on an IV infusion pump. When do you estimate (using international time) that the primary IV and one IV PB administration will be completely infused and the primary IV will have to be replaced? _____ hours

46. For the direct IV administration of promethazine, the drug guide states, "not to exceed 25 mg/min." The nurse should give _____ mL of promethazine per min or _____ mL per 15 sec.

47. Calculate 1 dose of ceftriaxone: _____ mL

48. Calculate the IV PB flow rate for each dose of ceftriaxone: _____ mL/h

49. Describe the clinical reasoning that you would use to prevent this medication error.

Possible Scenario

A student nurse was preparing for medication administration. One of the orders on the medication administration record (MAR) was written as *digoxin 0.125 mg od*. The student nurse crushed the digoxin tablet. Prior to giving the medication, the nursing instructor checked the medications that the student had prepared. The instructor asked the student to explain the rationale for crushing the digoxin tablet. The student explained to the instructor that the digoxin order was for the right eye ("O.D." is an outdated abbreviation for right eye). The student planned to add a small amount of sterile water to the crushed tablet and put it in the patient's eye.

Potential Outcome

What is wrong with the digoxin order? _____

_____

What could be the result? _____

Prevention

_____

_____

50. Describe the clinical reasoning you would use to prevent this medication error.

Possible Scenario

Order: *quinapril 30 mg p.o. daily*

Supply: quinidine 300 mg tablets

A student nurse administering medications noted the difference between the order and the supply drug and questioned the staff nurse about the order and what had been administered. The nurse realized that the student was exactly right to question the order and the drug supplied, and the nurse admitted to the student that the patient had been receiving the wrong drug all week. Not only was the wrong drug supplied, the nurse also did not notice the supply was not the correct dosage. The nurse congratulated the student on these important observations and for questioning the order and drug supplied.

Potential Outcome

The student referred to a drug reference book and compared the therapeutic and side effects of both drugs. The quinapril was correctly ordered for hypertension. Quinidine is an antiarrhythmic heart medication. The staff nurse notified the physician of the medication error and the physician ordered a stat electrocardiogram. Indeed, on the electrocardiogram, the patient had a long QT interval, putting the patient at grave risk for a fatal arrythmia. The nurse and the student together completed an incident report and discussed the cause and effect of the errors, and how to prevent them.

This student nurse recognized a pair of grave errors. The student acted responsibly and courageously, putting patient safety first. Let this be you! How could these errors have been prevented initially?

Prevention

_____

_____

After completing these problems, see pages 726–732 to check your answers. Give yourself 2 points for each correct answer.

Perfect score = 100   My score = _____

Minimum mastery score = 90 (45 correct)

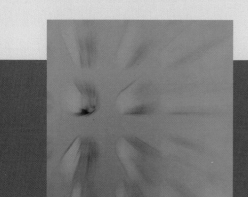

Answers

Essential Skills Evaluation: Pretest and Posttest from pages 3–20

1) $\frac{1}{2}$; 3 times a day **2)** 3; 2 times a day **3)** 10; 2; once a day **4)** $\frac{1}{2}$; every 3 hours as needed for moderate pain

5) 2; once every morning **6)** 2.5; every 8 hours

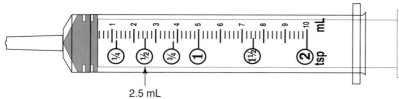

2.5 mL

7)   0.5; every 4 hours as needed for nausea

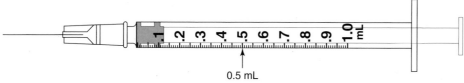

0.5 mL

8)   0.8; once, immediately

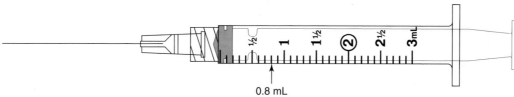

0.8 mL

9)   0.4; every 4 hours as needed for severe pain

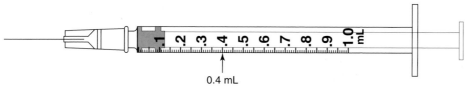

0.4 mL

10)   1.5; once, immediately

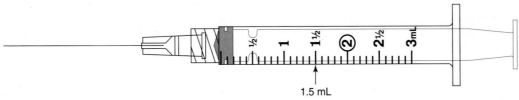

1.5 mL

11)   1.4; every 8 hours

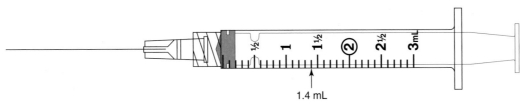

1.4 mL

12)   0.88; once, immediately

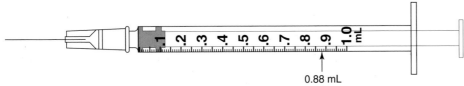

0.88 mL

13)   1; once, immediately; either syringe is appropriate

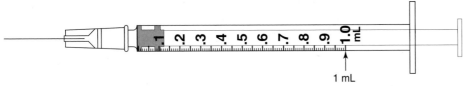

1 mL

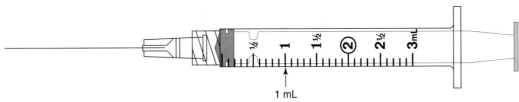

1 mL

14)   0.5; once, every morning; either syringe is appropriate

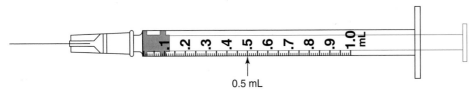

0.5 mL

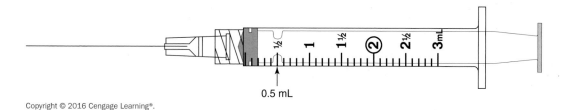

0.5 mL

15) 8; every 12 hours

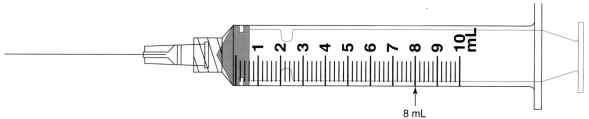

8 mL

16) 4; every 12 hours

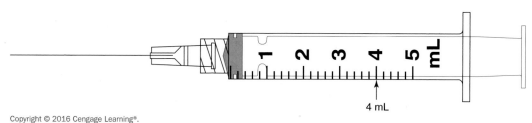

4 mL

17) 1; 1; 0.25; every 8 hours

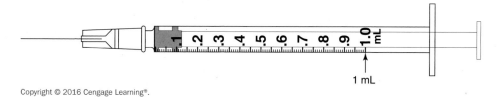

1 mL

18) 1.4; 75; every 6 hours

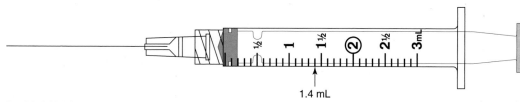

1.4 mL

19) 68; once a day before breakfast

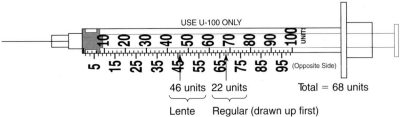

46 units   22 units   Total = 68 units

Lente   Regular (drawn up first)

20) 1

21) Benadryl; 0.7; either syringe is appropriate

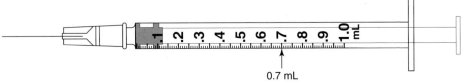

0.7 mL

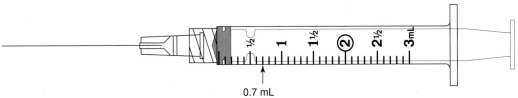

0.7 mL

22) Narcan; 1

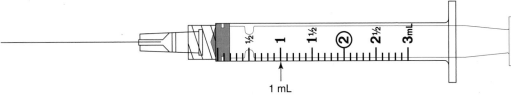

1 mL

23) Yes. Her temperature is 102.2°F. Tylenol every 4 hours as needed is indicated for fever greater than 101°F. It has been 5 hours and 5 minutes since her last dose. **24)** 2 **25)** 4; 108 **26)** 108 **27)** 8; 2 **28)** 1; 0700; 1200; 1700

29) 18; subcutaneous

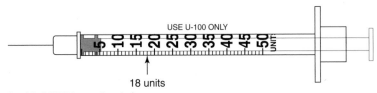

18 units

30) 77

31) Yes; the usual dosage is 20–40 mg/kg/day divided into 3 doses q.8h, which is equivalent to 67–133 mg per dose for a 22 lb (10 kg) child.

32) 4

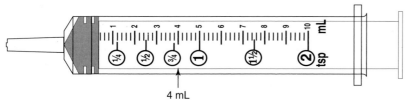

4 mL

Copyright © 2016 Cengage Learning®.

33) Yes; the usual dosage is 40 mg/kg/day divided into 3 doses q.8h, which is equivalent to 240 mg per dose for a 40 lb (approx. 18 kg) child.

34) 3; dosage is safe **35)** 103.3 **36)** 282; 423 **37)** 9.4 **38)** 250–375; Yes **39)** 1.7; 26 **40)** 880 **41)** 25 **42)** 1 **43)** 5; 5

44) 50 **45)** 0030; 12:30 AM the next day **46)** 10 **47)** 100; 1 **48)** 5

49)

> 1/30/XX, 1500, reconstituted
> as 100 mg/mL. Expires
> 1/31/XX, 1500. G.D.P.

50) Prevention: The importance of checking a medication label at least three times to verify supply dosage cannot be overemphasized. It is also important NEVER to assume that the supply dosage is the same as a supply dosage used to calculate previously. Always read the label carefully. Writing the calculation down will also help improve accuracy.

Solutions—Essential Skills Evaluation: Pretest and Posttest

1)
$$\frac{80 \text{ mg}}{1 \text{ tab}} \times \frac{40 \text{ mg}}{X \text{ tab}}$$
$$80X = 40$$
$$\frac{80X}{80} = \frac{40}{80}$$
$$X = \tfrac{1}{2} \text{ tablet}$$

2)
$$\frac{0.5 \text{ mg}}{1 \text{ tab}} \times \frac{1.5 \text{ mg}}{X \text{ tab}}$$
$$0.5X = 1.5$$
$$\frac{0.5X}{0.5} = \frac{1.5}{0.5}$$
$$X = 3 \text{ tablets}$$

3) Use 10 mg capsules; a 40 mg capsule cannot be split to provide the 20 mg dose.
$$\frac{10 \text{ mg}}{1 \text{ cap}} \times \frac{20 \text{ mg}}{X \text{ cap}}$$
$$10X = 20$$
$$\frac{10X}{10} = \frac{20}{10}$$
$$X = 2 \text{ capsules}$$

4)
$$\frac{5 \text{ mg}}{1 \text{ tab}} \times \frac{2.5 \text{ mg}}{X \text{ tab}}$$
$$5X = 2.5$$
$$\frac{5X}{5} = \frac{2.5}{5}$$
$$X = 0.5 \text{ tablet} = \tfrac{1}{2} \text{ tablet}$$

5)
$$\frac{0.15 \text{ mg}}{1 \text{ tab}} \times \frac{0.3 \text{ mg}}{X \text{ tab}}$$
$$0.15X = 0.3$$
$$\frac{0.15X}{0.15} = \frac{0.3}{0.15}$$
$$X = 2 \text{ tablets}$$

6)
$$\frac{200 \text{ mg}}{5 \text{ mL}} \times \frac{100 \text{ mg}}{X \text{ mL}}$$
$$200X = 500$$
$$\frac{200X}{200} = \frac{500}{200}$$
$$X = 2.5 \text{ mL}$$

7)
$$\frac{25 \text{ mg}}{1 \text{ mL}} \times \frac{12.5 \text{ mg}}{X \text{ mL}}$$
$$25X = 12.5$$
$$\frac{25X}{25} = \frac{12.5}{25}$$
$$X = 0.5 \text{ mL}$$

8)
$$\frac{50 \text{ mg}}{1 \text{ mL}} \times \frac{40 \text{ mg}}{X \text{ mL}}$$
$$50X = 40$$
$$\frac{50X}{50} = \frac{40}{50}$$
$$X = 0.8 \text{ mL}$$

9) $\dfrac{10 \text{ mg}}{1 \text{ mL}} \diagdown\diagup \dfrac{4 \text{ mg}}{X \text{ mL}}$

$10X = 4$

$\dfrac{10X}{10} = \dfrac{4}{10}$

$X = 0.4 \text{ mL}$

10) $\dfrac{2 \text{ mg}}{1 \text{ mL}} \diagdown\diagup \dfrac{3 \text{ mg}}{X \text{ mL}}$

$2X = 3$

$\dfrac{2X}{2} = \dfrac{3}{2}$

$X = 1.5 \text{ mL}$

11) $\dfrac{500 \text{ mg}}{2 \text{ mL}} \diagup\diagdown \dfrac{350 \text{ mg}}{X \text{ mL}}$

$500X = 700$

$\dfrac{500X}{500} = \dfrac{700}{500}$

$X = 1.4 \text{ mL}$

12) $\dfrac{80 \text{ mg}}{2 \text{ mL}} \diagdown\diagup \dfrac{35 \text{ mg}}{X \text{ mL}}$

$80X = 70$

$\dfrac{80X}{80} = \dfrac{70}{80}$

$X = 0.875 \text{ mL} = 0.88 \text{ mL}$

13) 1 mg = 1,000 mcg (known equivalent)

$\dfrac{1 \text{ mg}}{1,000 \text{ mcg}} \diagdown\diagup \dfrac{0.2 \text{ mg}}{X \text{ mcg}}$

$X = 200 \text{ mcg}$

$\dfrac{200 \text{ mcg}}{1 \text{ mL}} \diagdown\diagup \dfrac{200 \text{ mcg}}{X \text{ mL}}$

$200X = 200$

$\dfrac{200X}{200} = \dfrac{200}{200}$

$X = 1 \text{ mL}$

14) 1 mg = 1,000 mcg (known equivalent)

$\dfrac{1 \text{ mg}}{1,000 \text{ mcg}} \diagdown\diagup \dfrac{0.125 \text{ mg}}{X \text{ mcg}}$

$X = 125 \text{ mcg}$

$\dfrac{500 \text{ mcg}}{2 \text{ mL}} \diagdown\diagup \dfrac{125 \text{ mcg}}{X \text{ mL}}$

$500X = 250$

$\dfrac{500X}{500} = \dfrac{250}{500}$

$X = 0.5 \text{ mL}$

15) $\dfrac{100 \text{ mg}}{10 \text{ mL}} \diagdown\diagup \dfrac{80 \text{ mg}}{X \text{ mL}}$

$100X = 800$

$\dfrac{100X}{100} = \dfrac{800}{100}$

$X = 8 \text{ mL}$

16) 1 g = 1,000 mg (known equivalent)

$\dfrac{1 \text{ g}}{1,000 \text{ mg}} \diagdown\diagup \dfrac{0.4 \text{ g}}{X \text{ mg}}$

$X = 400 \text{ mg}$

$\dfrac{100 \text{ mg}}{1 \text{ mL}} \diagdown\diagup \dfrac{400 \text{ mg}}{X \text{ mL}}$

$100X = 400$

$\dfrac{100X}{100} = \dfrac{400}{100}$

$X = 4 \text{ mL}$

17) $\dfrac{250 \text{ mg}}{5 \text{ mL}} \diagup\diagdown \dfrac{50 \text{ mg}}{X \text{ mL}}$

$250X = 250$

$\dfrac{250X}{250} = \dfrac{250}{250}$

$X = 1 \text{ mL}$

250 mg/5 mL = 50 mg/1 mL

Do not exceed 50 mg/1 min. The 1 mL dose = 50 mg. Administer at 1 mL/1 min or 0.25 mL/15 seconds.

$\dfrac{1 \text{ mL}}{60 \text{ sec}} \diagdown\diagup \dfrac{X \text{ mL}}{15 \text{ sec}}$

$60X = 15$

$\dfrac{60X}{60} = \dfrac{15}{60}$

$X = \dfrac{1}{4} \text{ mL} = 0.25 \text{ mL}$

Either syringe could measure the amount, but the 1 mL syringe will provide greater control for pushing medication at the rate recommended.

18) $\dfrac{25 \text{ mg}}{1 \text{ mL}} \diagdown\diagup \dfrac{35 \text{ mg}}{X \text{ mL}}$

$25X = 35$

$\dfrac{25X}{25} = \dfrac{35}{25}$

$X = 1.4 \text{ mL}$

$\dfrac{V \text{ (mL)}}{T \text{ (min)}} \times C \text{ (gtt/mL)} = \dfrac{100 \text{ mL}}{20 \text{ min}} \times 15 \text{ gtt/mL}$

$= \dfrac{1,500}{20} \text{ gtt/min} = 75 \text{ gtt/min}$

19) 46 units + 22 units = 68 units (total)

20) $\dfrac{60 \text{ mg}}{2 \text{ mL}} \diagdown\diagup \dfrac{30 \text{ mg}}{X \text{ mL}}$

$60X = 60$

$\dfrac{60X}{60} = \dfrac{60}{60}$

$X = 1 \text{ mL}$

21) $\dfrac{50 \text{ mg}}{1 \text{ mL}} \diagdown\diagup \dfrac{35 \text{ mg}}{X \text{ mL}}$

$50X = 35$

$\dfrac{50X}{50} = \dfrac{35}{50}$

$X = 0.7 \text{ mL}$

22) $\dfrac{0.4 \text{ mg}}{1 \text{ mL}} \diagdown \dfrac{0.4 \text{ mg}}{X \text{ mL}}$

$\qquad 0.4X = 0.4$

$\qquad \dfrac{0.4X}{0.4} = \dfrac{0.4}{0.4}$

$\qquad X = 1 \text{ mL}$

23) $°F = 1.8°C + 32 = (1.8 \times 39) + 32 = 70.2 + 32 = 102.2°F;$

102.2°F is greater than 101°F;

$2400 - 2110 = 0250$ or 2 h 50 min before 2400;

$0215 = 2$ h 15 min after 2400;

2 h 50 min + 2 h 15 min = 5 h 5 min

24) $\dfrac{325 \text{ mg}}{1 \text{ tab}} \diagdown \dfrac{650 \text{ mg}}{X \text{ tab}}$

$\qquad 325X = 650$

$\qquad \dfrac{325X}{325} = \dfrac{650}{325}$

$\qquad X = 2 \text{ tablets}$

25) $\dfrac{25 \text{ mg}}{1 \text{ mL}} \diagdown \dfrac{100 \text{ mg}}{X \text{ mL}}$

$\qquad 25X = 100$

$\qquad \dfrac{25X}{25} = \dfrac{100}{25}$

$\qquad X = 4 \text{ mL}$

50 mL + 4 mL = 54 mL

$\dfrac{V \text{ (mL)}}{T \text{ (min)}} \times C \text{ (gtt/mL)} = \dfrac{54 \text{ mL}}{30 \text{ min}} \times 60 \text{ gtt/mL} = 108 \text{ gtt/min}$

26) Pump measured in mL/h. 54 mL in 30 min is equal to 108 mL in 60 min.

$\dfrac{54 \text{ mL}}{30 \text{ min}} \diagdown \dfrac{X \text{ mL}}{60 \text{ min}}$

$\qquad 30X = 3{,}240$

$\qquad \dfrac{30X}{30} = \dfrac{3{,}240}{30}$

$\qquad X = 108 \text{ mL}$

27) $\dfrac{500 \text{ mg}}{8 \text{ mL}} \diagdown \dfrac{125 \text{ mg}}{X \text{ mL}}$

$\qquad 500X = 1{,}000$

$\qquad \dfrac{500X}{500} = \dfrac{1{,}000}{500}$

$\qquad X = 2 \text{ mL}$

28) $\dfrac{1 \text{ g}}{1 \text{ tablet}} \diagdown \dfrac{1 \text{ g}}{X \text{ tablet}}$

$\qquad X = 1 \text{ tablet}$

31) $\dfrac{1 \text{ kg}}{2.2 \text{ lb}} \diagdown \dfrac{X \text{ kg}}{22 \text{ lb}}$

$\qquad 2.2X = 22$

$\qquad \dfrac{2.2X}{2.2} = \dfrac{22}{2.2}$

$\qquad X = 10 \text{ kg}$

Minimum dosage: 20 mg/kg/day $\times$ 10 kg = 200 mg/day

$\dfrac{200 \text{ mg}}{3 \text{ doses}} \diagdown \dfrac{X \text{ mg}}{1 \text{ dose}}$

$\qquad 3X = 200$

$\qquad \dfrac{3X}{3} = \dfrac{200}{3}$

$\qquad X = 66.6 \text{ mg/dose} = 67 \text{ mg/dose}$

Maximum dosage: 40 mg/kg/day $\times$ 10 kg = 400 mg/day

$\dfrac{400 \text{ mg}}{3 \text{ doses}} \diagdown \dfrac{X \text{ mg}}{1 \text{ dose}}$

$\qquad 3X = 400$

$\qquad \dfrac{3X}{3} = \dfrac{400}{3}$

$\qquad X = 133.3 \text{ mg/dose} = 133 \text{ mg/dose}$

32) $\dfrac{125 \text{ mg}}{5 \text{ mL}} \diagdown \dfrac{100 \text{ mg}}{X \text{ mL}}$

$\qquad 125X = 500$

$\qquad \dfrac{125X}{125} = \dfrac{500}{125}$

$\qquad X = 4 \text{ mL}$

33) $\dfrac{1 \text{ kg}}{2.2 \text{ lb}} \diagdown \dfrac{X \text{ kg}}{40 \text{ lb}}$

$\qquad 2.2X = 40$

$\qquad \dfrac{2.2X}{2.2} = \dfrac{40}{2.2}$

$\qquad X = 18.18 \text{ kg} = 18.2 \text{ kg}$

40 mg/kg/day $\times$ 18.2 kg = 728 mg/day

$\dfrac{728 \text{ mg}}{3 \text{ doses}} \diagdown \dfrac{X \text{ mg}}{1 \text{ dose}}$

$\qquad 3X = 728$

$\qquad \dfrac{3X}{3} = \dfrac{728}{3}$

$\qquad X = 242.6 \text{ mg/dose} = 243 \text{ mg/dose};$ close approximation to ordered dosage of 240 mg/dose; dosage is safe.

34) $\dfrac{400 \text{ mg}}{5 \text{ mL}} \diagdown \dfrac{240 \text{ mg}}{X \text{ mL}}$

$\qquad 400X = 1{,}200$

$\qquad \dfrac{400X}{400} = \dfrac{1{,}200}{400}$

$\qquad X = 3 \text{ mL}$

35) $°F = 1.8 °C + 32 = (1.8 \times 39.6) + 32 = 71.28 + 32$

$\qquad = 103.28°F = 103.3°F$

36) 1 kg = 2.2 lb (known equivalent)

$\dfrac{1 \text{ kg}}{2.2 \text{ lb}} \diagdown \dfrac{X \text{ kg}}{62 \text{ lb}}$

$\qquad 2.2X = 62$

$\qquad \dfrac{2.2X}{2.2} = \dfrac{62}{2.2}$

$\qquad X = 28.18 \text{ kg} = 28.2 \text{ kg}$

Minimum dosage:

$\dfrac{10 \text{ mg}}{1 \text{ kg}} \diagdown \dfrac{X \text{ mg}}{28.2 \text{ kg}}$

$\qquad X = 282 \text{ mg}$

Maximum dosage:

$\dfrac{15 \text{ mg}}{1 \text{ kg}} \diagdown \dfrac{X \text{ mg}}{28.2 \text{ kg}}$

$\qquad X = 423 \text{ mg}$

37) $\dfrac{80 \text{ mg}}{2.5 \text{ mL}} \diagdown \diagup \dfrac{300 \text{ mg}}{X \text{ mL}}$

$80X = 750$

$\dfrac{80X}{80} = \dfrac{750}{80}$

$X = 9.37 \text{ mL} = 9.4 \text{ mL}$

38) 1 kg = 2.2 lb (known equivalent)

$\dfrac{1 \text{ kg}}{2.2 \text{ lb}} \diagdown \diagup \dfrac{X \text{ kg}}{110 \text{ lb}}$

$2.2X = 110$

$\dfrac{2.2X}{2.2} = \dfrac{110}{2.2}$

$X = 50 \text{ kg}$

Minimum dosage: 20 mg/kg/day × 50 kg = 1,000 mg/day

$\dfrac{1{,}000 \text{ mg}}{4 \text{ doses}} \diagdown \diagup \dfrac{X \text{ mg}}{1 \text{ dose}}$

$4X = 1{,}000$

$\dfrac{4X}{4} = \dfrac{1{,}000}{4}$

$X = 250 \text{ mg/dose}$

Maximum dosage: 30 mg/kg/day × 50 kg = 1,500 mg/day

$\dfrac{1{,}500 \text{ mg}}{4 \text{ doses}} \diagdown \diagup \dfrac{X \text{ mg}}{1 \text{ dose}}$

$4X = 1{,}500$

$\dfrac{4X}{4} = \dfrac{1{,}500}{4}$

$X = 375 \text{ mg/dose}$

39) $\dfrac{300 \text{ mg}}{2 \text{ mL}} \diagdown \diagup \dfrac{250 \text{ mg}}{X \text{ mL}}$

$300X = 500$

$\dfrac{300X}{300} = \dfrac{500}{300}$

$X = 1.66 \text{ mL} = 1.7 \text{ mL}$

1.7 mL (medication) + 50 mL (IV fluid) = 51.7 mL = 52 mL
(to be infused)

$\dfrac{V \text{ (mL)}}{T \text{ (min)}} \times C \text{ (gtt/mL)} = \dfrac{52 \text{ mL}}{\underset{2}{20 \text{ min}}} \times \overset{1}{10} \text{ gtt/mL}$

$= \dfrac{52}{2} \text{ gtt/min} = 26 \text{ gtt/min}$

40) IV fluid: 50 mL + 50 mL = 100 mL
Oral fluid:
Gelatin: 4 fl oz
Water: 6 fl oz (3 fl oz × 2)
Apple juice: 16 fl oz
_____
                        26 fl oz

1 fl oz = 30 mL (known equivalent)

$\dfrac{30 \text{ mL}}{1 \text{ fl oz}} \diagdown \diagup \dfrac{X \text{ mL}}{26 \text{ fl oz}}$

$X = 780 \text{ mL}$

IV fluid + oral fluid = 100 mL + 780 mL = 880 mL
(total fluid intake during the 8-hour shift)

41) $\dfrac{V \text{ (mL)}}{T \text{ (min)}} \times C \text{ (gtt/mL)} = \dfrac{600 \text{ mL}}{\underset{24}{240 \text{ min}}} \times \overset{1}{10} \text{ gtt/mL}$

$= \dfrac{600}{24} \text{ gtt/min} = 25 \text{ gtt/min}$

42) $\dfrac{50 \text{ mg}}{50 \text{ mL}} \diagdown \diagup \dfrac{1 \text{ mg}}{X \text{ mL}}$

$50X = 50$

$\dfrac{50X}{50} = \dfrac{50}{50}$

$X = 1 \text{ mL}$

43) $\dfrac{1 \text{ mg}}{1 \text{ dose}} \diagdown \diagup \dfrac{X \text{ mg}}{5 \text{ doses}}$

$X = 5 \text{ mg}$

$\dfrac{1 \text{ mL}}{1 \text{ dose}} \diagdown \diagup \dfrac{X \text{ mL}}{5 \text{ doses}}$

$X = 5 \text{ mL}$

5 doses in 1 hour = 5 mg per 5 mL

44) $\dfrac{1 \text{ mg}}{1 \text{ dose}} \diagdown \diagup \dfrac{50 \text{ mg}}{X \text{ doses}}$

$X = 50 \text{ doses}$

45) $\dfrac{5 \text{ doses}}{1 \text{h}} \diagdown \diagup \dfrac{50 \text{ doses}}{X \text{ h}}$

$5X = 50$

$\dfrac{5X}{5} = \dfrac{50}{5}$

$X = 10 \text{ h}$

$\begin{array}{r} 1430 \text{ h} \\ +1000 \text{ h} \\ \hline 2430 \text{ h (0030 hours)} \end{array}$

46) 1 g = 1,000 mg (known equivalent)

After reconsitiution, the supply dosage is 100 mg/mL

$\dfrac{100 \text{ mg}}{1 \text{ mL}} \diagdown \diagup \dfrac{1{,}000 \text{ mg}}{X \text{ mL}}$

$100X = 1{,}000$

$\dfrac{100X}{100} = \dfrac{1{,}000 \text{ mg}}{X \text{ mL}}$

$X = 10 \text{ mL}$

47) 100; 1

48) 0.5 g = 0.500. = 500 mg

$\dfrac{100 \text{ mg}}{1 \text{ mL}} \diagdown \diagup \dfrac{500 \text{ mg}}{X \text{ mL}}$

$100X = 500$

$\dfrac{100X}{100} = \dfrac{500}{100}$

$X = 5 \text{ mL}$

49) Clinical reasoning indicates that the full reconstituted solution will be used up within 2 doses, so storage unrefrigerated for 24 hours is satisfactory.

Mathematics Diagnostic Evaluation from pages 28–30

1) 1,517.63 **2)** 20.74 **3)** 100.66 **4)** $323.72 **5)** 46.11 **6)** 754.5 **7)** 16.91 **8)** 19,494.7 **9)** $173.04 **10)** 403.26 **11)** 36 **12)** 2,500 **13)** $\frac{2}{3}$

14) 6.25 **15)** $\frac{4}{5}$ **16)** 40% **17)** 0.4% **18)** 0.05 **19)** 1:3 **20)** 0.02 **21)** $1\frac{1}{4}$ **22)** $6\frac{13}{24}$ **23)** $1\frac{11}{18}$ **24)** $\frac{3}{5}$ **25)** $14\frac{7}{8}$ **26)** $\frac{1}{100}$ **27)** 0.009 **28)** 320 **29)** 3

30) 0.05 **31)** 4 **32)** 0.09 **33)** 0.22 **34)** 25 **35)** 4 **36)** 0.75 **37)** 3 **38)** 500 **39)** 18.24 **40)** 2.4 **41)** $\frac{1}{5}$ **42)** 1:50 **43)** 5 tablets **44)** 2 milligrams

45) 30 kilograms **46)** 3.3 pounds **47)** 6.67 centimeters **48)** 7.5 centimeters **49)** 90% **50)** 5:1

Solutions—Mathematics Diagnostic Evaluation

3)
```
    9.50
   17.06
   32.00
   41.11
 +  0.99
 -------
  100.66
```

6)
```
 1,005.0
 - 250.5
 -------
   754.5
```

10)
```
   17.16
 × 23.5
 -------
   8580
  5148
 3432
 --------
 403.260 = 403.26
```

12)
$$0.001\overline{)2.500} = 2,500$$

19) $33\frac{1}{3}\% = \dfrac{33\frac{1}{3}}{100} = \dfrac{\frac{100}{3}}{100} = \dfrac{100}{3} \div \dfrac{100}{1} = \dfrac{100}{3} \times \dfrac{1}{100} = \dfrac{1}{3} = 1{:}3$

23)
$$1\frac{5}{6} = 1\frac{15}{18}$$
$$-\frac{2}{9} = -\frac{4}{18}$$
$$\overline{\qquad\quad 1\frac{11}{18}}$$

25) $4\frac{1}{4} \times 3\frac{1}{2} = \dfrac{17}{4} \times \dfrac{7}{2} = \dfrac{119}{8} = 14\frac{7}{8}$

29) $\dfrac{0.02 + 0.16}{0.4 - 0.34}$
```
   0.02      0.40
 + 0.16    - 0.34
 ------    ------
   0.18      0.06
```
$$\frac{0.18}{0.06} = 0.06\overline{)0.18} = 3$$

32) $\frac{1}{2}\% = 0.5\% = 0.005$
```
      18
 × 0.005
 -------
 0.090 = 0.09
```

34) $\dfrac{1{:}1,000}{1{:}100} \times 250 =$

$$\dfrac{\frac{1}{1,000}}{\frac{1}{100}} \times 250 = \dfrac{1}{1,000} \times \dfrac{100}{1} \times \dfrac{250}{1} = \dfrac{250}{10} = 25$$

45) 66 pounds $= \dfrac{66}{2.2} = 30$ kilograms or

$$\dfrac{2.2 \text{ pounds}}{1 \text{ kilogram}} \bowtie \dfrac{66 \text{ pounds}}{\text{X kilograms}}$$
$$2.2\text{X} = 66$$
$$\dfrac{2.2\text{X}}{2.2} = \dfrac{66}{2.2}$$
$$\text{X} = 30 \text{ kilograms}$$

49)
```
   50 items
 -  5 incorrect
 -------------
   45 correct
```
$\dfrac{45}{50} = \dfrac{9}{10} = 90\%$ (correct)

Review Set 1 from pages 37–38

1) $\frac{6}{6}, \frac{7}{5}$ **2)** $\dfrac{\frac{1}{100}}{\frac{1}{150}}$ **3)** $\frac{1}{4}, \frac{1}{14}$ **4)** $1\frac{2}{9}, 1\frac{1}{4}, 5\frac{7}{8}$ **5)** $\frac{3}{4} = \frac{6}{8}, \frac{1}{5} = \frac{2}{10}, \frac{3}{9} = \frac{1}{3}$ **6)** $\frac{13}{2}$ **7)** $\frac{6}{5}$ **8)** $\frac{32}{3}$ **9)** $\frac{47}{6}$ **10)** $\frac{411}{4}$ **11)** 2 **12)** 1 **13)** $3\frac{1}{3}$ **14)** $1\frac{1}{3}$ **15)** $2\frac{3}{4}$ **16)** $\frac{6}{8}$

17) $\frac{4}{16}$ **18)** $\frac{8}{12}$ **19)** $\frac{4}{10}$ **20)** $\frac{6}{9}$ **21)** $\frac{1}{100}$ **22)** $\frac{1}{10,000}$ **23)** $\frac{5}{9}$ **24)** $\frac{3}{10}$ **25)** $\frac{2}{5}$ bottle **26)** $1\frac{1}{2}$ bottles **27)** $\frac{2}{5}$ of the students are men **28)** $\frac{9}{10}$ of the questions were answered correctly **29)** $\frac{1}{2}$ dose **30)** $\frac{1}{2}$ teaspoon

Solutions—Review Set 1

8) $10\frac{2}{3} = \dfrac{(10 \times 3) + 2}{3} = \dfrac{32}{3}$

14) $\dfrac{100}{75} = 1\frac{25}{75} = 1\frac{1}{3}$

18) $\dfrac{2}{3} = \dfrac{2 \times 4}{3 \times 4} = \dfrac{8}{12}$

25) 10 ounces − 6 ounces = 4 ounces remaining

$\dfrac{4}{10} = \dfrac{4 \div 2}{10 \div 2} = \dfrac{2}{5}$ bottle remaining

27)
```
   24 men
 + 36 women
 ----------
   60 people in class
```
The men represent $\frac{24}{60}$ or $\frac{2}{5}$ of the students in the class.

29) $\dfrac{80}{160} = \dfrac{1}{2}$ of a dose

30) $\frac{1}{2}$ of 1 teaspoon $= \frac{1}{2}$ teaspoon

Review Set 2 from pages 40–41

1) $8\frac{7}{15}$ **2)** $1\frac{5}{12}$ **3)** $17\frac{7}{24}$ **4)** $1\frac{1}{24}$ **5)** $32\frac{5}{6}$ **6)** $5\frac{7}{12}$ **7)** $1\frac{1}{3}$ **8)** $5\frac{53}{72}$ **9)** 43 **10)** $5\frac{118}{119}$ **11)** $2\frac{8}{15}$ **12)** $\frac{53}{132}$ **13)** $\frac{1}{2}$ **14)** $4\frac{5}{6}$ **15)** $\frac{1}{24}$ **16)** $63\frac{2}{3}$ **17)** $299\frac{4}{5}$ **18)** $\frac{1}{6}$

19) $1\frac{2}{5}$ **20)** $7\frac{1}{16}$ **21)** $7\frac{2}{9}$ **22)** $1\frac{1}{4}$ **23)** $24\frac{6}{11}$ **24)** $\frac{7}{12}$ **25)** $\frac{1}{25}$ **26)** $5\frac{5}{6}$ fluid ounces **27)** $1\frac{1}{8}$ inches **28)** 8 inches **29)** $21\frac{1}{2}$ pints **30)** $13\frac{1}{4}$ pounds

Solutions—Review Set 2

1) $7\frac{4}{5} + \frac{2}{3} = \frac{39}{5} + \frac{2}{3}$

$\frac{39}{5} = \frac{39 \times 3}{5 \times 3} = \frac{117}{15}$

$\frac{2}{3} = \frac{2 \times 5}{3 \times 5} = \frac{10}{15}$

$\frac{117}{15} + \frac{10}{15}$

$\frac{117 + 10}{15} = \frac{127}{15}$

$\frac{127}{15} = 8\frac{7}{15}$

3) $4\frac{2}{3} + 5\frac{1}{24} + 7\frac{1}{2} = \frac{14}{3} + \frac{121}{24} + \frac{15}{2}$

$\frac{14}{3} = \frac{14 \times 8}{3 \times 8} = \frac{112}{24}$

$\frac{15}{2} = \frac{15 \times 12}{2 \times 12} = \frac{180}{24}$

$\frac{112}{24} + \frac{121}{24} + \frac{180}{24} =$

$\frac{112 + 121 + 180}{24} = \frac{413}{24} = 17\frac{5}{24}$

4) $\frac{3}{4} + \frac{1}{8} + \frac{1}{6}$

$\frac{3}{4} = \frac{3 \times 6}{4 \times 6} = \frac{18}{24}$

$\frac{1}{8} = \frac{1 \times 3}{8 \times 3} = \frac{3}{24}$

$\frac{1}{6} = \frac{1 \times 4}{6 \times 4} = \frac{4}{24}$

$\frac{18}{24} + \frac{3}{24} + \frac{4}{24} = \frac{18 + 3 + 4}{24} = \frac{25}{24} = 1\frac{1}{24}$

14) $8\frac{1}{12} - 3\frac{1}{4} = \frac{96}{12} - \frac{13}{4}$

$\frac{13}{4} = \frac{13 \times 3}{4 \times 3} = \frac{39}{12}$

$\frac{96}{12} - \frac{39}{12} = \frac{97 - 39}{12} = \frac{58}{12}$

$\frac{58}{12} = 4\frac{10}{12} = 4\frac{5}{6}$

25) 50 pounds − 48 pounds = 2 pounds lost

$\frac{2}{50} = \frac{1}{25}$ of weight lost

26) $2\frac{1}{2}$ fluid ounces + $3\frac{1}{3}$ fluid ounces =

$2\frac{1}{2} + 3\frac{1}{3} = \frac{5}{2} + \frac{10}{3}$

$\frac{5}{2} = \frac{5 \times 3}{2 \times 3} = \frac{15}{6}$

$\frac{10}{3} = \frac{10 \times 2}{3 \times 2} = \frac{20}{6}$

$\frac{15}{6} + \frac{20}{6} = \frac{15 + 20}{6} = \frac{35}{6}$

$\frac{35}{6} = 5\frac{5}{6}$ fluid ounces

29) 56 pints − $34\frac{1}{2}$ pints $= \frac{56}{1} - \frac{69}{2}$

$\frac{56 \times 2}{1 \times 2} = \frac{112}{2}$

$\frac{112}{2} - \frac{69}{2} = \frac{112 - 69}{2} = \frac{43}{2} = 21\frac{1}{2}$ pints

30) $20\frac{1}{2}$ pounds − $7\frac{1}{4}$ pounds $= \frac{41}{2} - \frac{29}{4}$

$\frac{41 \times 2}{2 \times 2} = \frac{82}{4}$

$\frac{82}{4} - \frac{29}{4} = \frac{82 - 29}{4} = \frac{53}{4} = 13\frac{1}{4}$ pounds

Review Set 3 from pages 45–46

1) $\frac{1}{40}$ **2)** $\frac{36}{125}$ **3)** $\frac{35}{48}$ **4)** $\frac{3}{100}$ **5)** 3 **6)** $1\frac{2}{7}$ **7)** $\frac{4}{5}$ **8)** $6\frac{8}{15}$ **9)** $\frac{1}{2}$ **10)** $23\frac{19}{36}$ **11)** $\frac{3}{32}$ **12)** $254\frac{1}{6}$ **13)** 3 **14)** $1\frac{34}{39}$ **15)** $\frac{3}{14}$ **16)** $\frac{1}{11}$ **17)** $\frac{1}{2}$ **18)** $\frac{1}{30}$ **19)** $3\frac{1}{3}$ **20)** $\frac{3}{20}$ **21)** $\frac{1}{3}$ **22)** $\frac{7}{12}$ **23)** $1\frac{1}{9}$ **24)** 60 calories **25)** 560 seconds **26)** 40 doses **27)** $31\frac{1}{2}$ tablets **28)** 1,275 milliliters **29)** $52\frac{1}{2}$ ounces **30)** 6 full days

Solutions—Review Set 3

3) $\frac{5}{8} \times 1\frac{1}{6} = \frac{5}{8} \times \frac{7}{6} = \frac{35}{48}$

5) $\dfrac{\frac{1}{6}}{\frac{1}{4}} \times \dfrac{\frac{3}{2}}{\frac{2}{3}} = \left(\frac{1}{6} \times \frac{4}{1}\right) \times \left(\frac{3}{1} \times \frac{3}{2}\right) = \frac{\overset{2}{\cancel{4}}}{\underset{3}{\cancel{6}}} \times \frac{9}{2} = \frac{\overset{3}{\cancel{18}}}{\underset{1}{\cancel{6}}} = 3$

16) $\frac{1}{33} \div \frac{1}{3} = \frac{1}{33} \times \frac{3}{1} = \frac{\overset{1}{\cancel{3}}}{\underset{11}{\cancel{33}}} = \frac{1}{11}$

19) $2\frac{1}{2} \div \frac{3}{4} = \frac{5}{2} \div \frac{3}{4} = \frac{5}{\cancel{2}} \times \frac{\overset{2}{\cancel{4}}}{3} = \frac{10}{3} = 3\frac{1}{3}$

27) $3 \times 7 = 21$ doses

$21 \times 1\frac{1}{2} = \frac{21}{1} \times \frac{3}{2} = \frac{63}{2} = 31\frac{1}{2}$ tablets

28) Pitcher is $\frac{1}{3}$ full; $\frac{2}{3}$ was consumed.

$850 \div \frac{2}{3} = \frac{\overset{425}{\cancel{850}}}{1} \times \frac{3}{\underset{1}{\cancel{2}}} = 1,275$ milliliters

30)

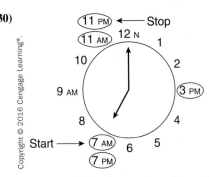

Daily doses would be taken at: 7 AM, 11 AM, 3 PM, 7 PM, and 11 PM for 5 doses/day.

5 doses/day $\times \frac{1}{2}$ fluid ounce/dose $= \frac{5}{2} =$

$2\frac{1}{2}$ fluid ounces/day

16 fluid ounces $\div 2\frac{1}{2}$ fluid ounces/day $= \frac{16}{1} \div \frac{5}{2} =$

$\frac{16}{1} \times \frac{2}{5} = \frac{32}{5} = 6\frac{2}{5}$ days or 6 full days

Review Set 4 from pages 52–53

1) 0.2, two tenths **2)** $\frac{17}{20}$, 0.85 **3)** $1\frac{1}{20}$, one and five hundredths **4)** $\frac{3}{500}$, six thousandths **5)** 10.015, ten and fifteen thousandths **6)** $1\frac{9}{10}$, one and nine tenths **7)** $5\frac{1}{10}$, 5.1 **8)** 0.8, eight tenths **9)** $250\frac{1}{2}$, two hundred fifty and five tenths **10)** 33.03, thirty-three and three hundredths **11)** $\frac{19}{20}$, ninety-five hundredths **12)** 2.75, two and seventy-five hundredths **13)** $7\frac{1}{200}$, 7.005 **14)** 0.084, eighty-four thousandths **15)** $12\frac{1}{8}$, twelve and one hundred twenty-five thousandths **16)** $20\frac{9}{100}$, twenty and nine hundredths **17)** $22\frac{11}{500}$, 22.022 **18)** $\frac{3}{20}$, fifteen hundredths **19)** 1,000.005, one thousand and five thousandths **20)** $4,085\frac{3}{40}$, 4,085.075 **21)** 0.0170 **22)** 0.25 **23)** 0.75 **24)** $\frac{9}{200}$ **25)** 0.12 **26)** 0.063 **27)** False **28)** False **29)** True **30)** 0.8 gram and 1.25 grams

Solutions—Review Set 4

4) $\quad 0.006 = \frac{6}{1,000} = \frac{3}{500}$

8) $\quad \frac{4}{5} = 5\overline{)4.0}^{\,0.8}$

14) $\quad \frac{21}{250} = 250\overline{)21.000}$
$\phantom{14)\quad\frac{21}{250}=250)}\underline{20\,00}$
$\phantom{14)\quad\frac{21}{250}=250)00}1\,000$
$\phantom{14)\quad\frac{21}{250}=250)00}\underline{1\,000}$

15) $\quad 12.125 = 12\frac{125}{1,000} = 12\frac{1}{8}$

18) $\quad 0.15 = \frac{15}{100} = \frac{3}{20}$

30) Safe dosages include amounts greater than or equal to 0.5 gram but less than or equal to 2 grams.
Safe dosages: 0.8 gram and 1.25 grams

Review Set 5 from pages 55–56

1) 22.585 **2)** 44.177 **3)** 12.309 **4)** 11.3 **5)** 175.199 **6)** 25.007 **7)** 0.518 **8)** $9.48 **9)** $18.91 **10)** $22.71 **11)** 6.403 **12)** 0.27 **13)** 4.15 **14)** 1.51 **15)** 10.25 **16)** 2.517 **17)** 374.35 **18)** 604.42 **19)** 27.449 **20)** 23.619 **21)** 0.697 gram **22)** 66.25 milliliters **23)** $2,058.06 **24)** 10.3 grams **25)** 8.1 hours

Solutions—Review Set 5

2)
$$
\begin{array}{r}
7.517 \\
3.200 \\
0.160 \\
+\ 33.300 \\
\hline
44.177
\end{array}
$$

9)
$$
\begin{array}{r}
\overset{8\ 9\ 10}{\$19.0\cancel{0}} \\
-\ 0.09 \\
\hline
\$18.91
\end{array}
$$

25)
$$
\begin{array}{r}
3\text{ h } 20\text{ min} \\
40\text{ min} \\
3\text{ h } 30\text{ min} \\
24\text{ min} \\
+\ 12\text{ min} \\
\hline
6\text{ h } 126\text{ min} = 6\text{ h } + 2\text{ h } 6\text{ min} = 8\text{ h } 6\text{ min } (60\text{ min/h}) \\
= 8\tfrac{6}{60}\text{ h} = 8\tfrac{1}{10}\text{ h} = 8.1\text{ h (hours)}
\end{array}
$$

Review Set 6 from page 60

1) 5.83 **2)** 2.2 **3)** 42.75 **4)** 0.15 **5)** 403.14 **6)** 75,100.75 **7)** 32.86 **8)** 2.78 **9)** 348.58 **10)** 0.02 **11)** 400 **12)** 3.74 **13)** 5 **14)** 2.98 **15)** 4,120 **16)** 5.45 **17)** 272.67 **18)** 1.5 **19)** 50,020 **20)** 300 **21)** 562.50. = 56,250 **22)** 16.0. = 160 **23)** .025. = 0.025 **24)** .032.005 = 0.032005 **25)** .00.125 = 0.00125 **26)** 23.2.5 = 232.5 **27)** 71.7.717 = 71.7717 **28)** 83.1.6 = 831.6 **29)** 0.33. = 33 **30)** 14.106. = 14,106

Solutions—Review Set 6

2) $0.314 \times 7 = 2.198 = 2.20 = 2.2$ **10)** $1.14 \times 0.014 = 0.01596 = 0.02$ **14)** $45.5 \div 15.25 = 2.983 = 2.98$

Practice Problems—Chapter 1 from pages 61–62

1) $\frac{7}{20}$ **2)** 0.375 **3)** LCD = 21 **4)** LCD = 55 **5)** LCD = 18 **6)** LCD = 15 **7)** $3\frac{7}{15}$ **8)** $7\frac{29}{60}$ **9)** $\frac{1}{2}$ **10)** $2\frac{7}{24}$ **11)** $\frac{7}{27}$

12) $10\frac{1}{8}$ **13)** $4\frac{4}{17}$ **14)** $\frac{39}{80}$ **15)** $5\frac{1}{55}$ **16)** $5\frac{5}{18}$ **17)** $2\frac{86}{87}$ **18)** $\frac{3}{20}$ **19)** $\frac{1}{3,125}$ **20)** $\frac{1}{4}$ **21)** $1\frac{5}{7}$ **22)** $16\frac{1}{32}$ **23)** 60.27 **24)** 66.74

25) 42.98 **26)** 4,833.92 **27)** 190.8 **28)** 19.17 **29)** 9.48 **30)** 7.7 **31)** 42.75 **32)** 300 **33)** 12,930.43 **34)** 3,200.63 **35)** 2

36) 150.96 **37)** 9.716. = 9,716 **38)** .50.25 = 0.5025 **39)** 0.25. = 25 **40)** 5.750. = 5,750 **41)** .0.25 = 0.025

42) 11.5.25 = 115.25 **43)** 147 fluid ounces **44)** 138 nurses; 46 maintenance/cleaners; 92 technicians; 92 others **45)** False

46) $1,730.98 **47)** $1.46 **48)** 0.31 gram **49)** 800 milliliters **50)** 2.95 kilograms

Solutions—Practice Problems—Chapter 1

43) $3\frac{1}{2}$ fluid ounces/feeding $\times$ 6 feedings/day =

21 fluid ounces/day, and 21 fluid ounces/day $\times$

7 days/week = 147 fluid ounces in one week

44) $\frac{3}{8} \times \frac{368}{1} = \frac{1,104}{8} = 138$ nurses

$\frac{1}{8} \times \frac{368}{1} = \frac{368}{8} = 46$ maintenance/cleaners

$\frac{1}{4} \times \frac{368}{1} = \frac{368}{4} = 92$ technicians and 92 others

45) $1\frac{2}{32} = 1.0625$; False, it's greater than normal.

46) 40 hours $\times$ $32.66/hour = $1,306.40

6.5 hours overtime $\times$ $65.32 =   + 424.58

(Overtime rate = $32.66 $\times$ 2 = $65.32) $1,730.98

47) A case of 12 boxes with 12 catheters/box =

144 catheters

By case: $975 ÷ 144 = $6.77/catheter

By box: $98.76 ÷ 12 = $8.23/catheter

$8.23

$- 6.77$

$1.46 savings/catheter

48) 0.065 gram/ounce $\times$ 4.75 ounces = 0.31 gram

49) 1,200 milliliters $\times \frac{2}{3} = \frac{\overset{400}{\cancel{1,200}}}{1} \times \frac{2}{\underset{1}{\cancel{3}}} = 800$ milliliters

50)   6.65 kilograms

$- 3.70$ kilograms

2.95 kilograms gained

Review Set 7 from pages 67–68

1) $\frac{1}{50}$ **2)** $\frac{3}{5}$ **3)** $\frac{1}{3}$ **4)** $\frac{4}{7}$ **5)** $\frac{3}{4}$ **6)** 0.5 **7)** 0.15 **8)** 0.14 **9)** 0.07 **10)** 0.24 **11)** 25% **12)** 40% **13)** 12.5% **14)** 70% **15)** 50% **16)** $\frac{9}{20}$ **17)** $\frac{3}{5}$

18) $\frac{1}{200}$ **19)** $\frac{1}{100}$ **20)** $\frac{2}{3}$ **21)** 0.03 **22)** 0.05 **23)** 0.06 **24)** 0.33 **25)** 0.01 **26)** 4:25 **27)** 1:4 **28)** 1:2 **29)** 9:20 **30)** 3:50 **31)** 0.9 **32)** $\frac{1}{5}$

33) 0.25% **34)** 0.5 **35)** $\frac{1}{100}$

Solutions—Review Set 7

1) $3:150 = \frac{3}{150} = \frac{\overset{1}{\cancel{3}}}{\underset{50}{\cancel{150}}} = \frac{1}{50}$

3) $0.05:0.15 = \frac{\overset{1}{\cancel{0.05}}}{\underset{3}{\cancel{0.15}}} = \frac{1}{3}$

7) $\frac{1}{1,000} : \frac{1}{150} = \frac{\frac{1}{1,000}}{\frac{1}{150}} = \frac{1}{1,000} \times \frac{\overset{15}{\cancel{150}}}{1} = \frac{15}{100} = 0.15. = 0.15$

12) $2:5 = \frac{2}{5} = 0.4; 0.4 = 0.40. = 40\%$

13) $0.08:0.64 = \frac{0.08}{0.64} = \frac{1}{8} = 0.125;$

$0.125 = 0.12.5 = 12.5\%$

17) $60\% = \frac{60}{100} = \frac{3}{5}$

18) $0.5\% = \frac{0.5}{100} = 0.5 ÷ 100 = 0.00.5 = 0.005 = \frac{5}{1,000} = \frac{1}{200}$

21) $2.94\% = \frac{2.94}{100} = 2.94 ÷ 100 = 0.02.94 = 0.0294 = 0.03$

30) $6\% = \frac{6}{100} = \frac{3}{50} = 3:50$

31) Convert to decimals and compare:

0.9% = 0.009

0.9   = 0.900 (largest)

1:9   = 0.111

1:90 = 0.011

Review Set 8 from pages 71–72

1) 3 **2)** 3.3 **3)** 1.25 **4)** 5.33 **5)** 0.56 **6)** 1.8 **7)** 0.64 **8)** 12.6 **9)** 40 **10)** 0.48 **11)** 1 **12)** 0.96 **13)** 4.5 **14)** 0.94 **15)** 10 **16)** 0.4 **17)** 1.5

18) 10 **19)** 20 **20)** 1.8

Solutions—Review Set 8

2) $\dfrac{\frac{3}{4}}{\frac{1}{2}} \times 2.2 = X$

$\dfrac{3}{4} \div \dfrac{1}{2} \times \dfrac{2.2}{1} = X$

$\dfrac{3}{\cancel{4}_2} \times \dfrac{\cancel{2}^1}{1} \times \dfrac{2.2}{1} = X$

$\dfrac{6.6}{2} = X$

$X = 3.3$

6) $\dfrac{0.15}{0.1} \times 1.2 = X$

$\dfrac{\cancel{0.15}^3}{\cancel{0.10}_2} \times \dfrac{1.2}{1} = X$

$\dfrac{3}{2} \times \dfrac{1.2}{1} = X$

$\dfrac{3.6}{2} = X$

$X = 1.8$

14) $\dfrac{\cancel{250{,}000}^1}{\cancel{2{,}000{,}000}_8} \times 7.5 = X$

$\dfrac{1}{8} \times \dfrac{7.5}{1} = X$

$\dfrac{7.5}{8} = X$

$X = 0.937$

$X = 0.94$

4) $\dfrac{40\%}{60\%} \times 8 = X$

$\dfrac{\cancel{0.4}^2}{\cancel{0.6}_3} \times 8 = X$

$\dfrac{2}{3} \times \dfrac{8}{1} = X$

$\dfrac{16}{3} = X$

$X = 5.33\overline{3}$

$X = 5.33$

8) $\dfrac{\cancel{1{,}200{,}000}^3}{\cancel{400{,}000}_1} \times 4.2 = X$

$\dfrac{3}{1} \times \dfrac{4.2}{1} = X$

$\dfrac{12.6}{1} = X$

$X = 12.6$

10) $\dfrac{\cancel{30}^3}{\cancel{50}_5} \times 0.8 = X$

$\dfrac{3}{5} \times \dfrac{0.8}{1} = X$

$\dfrac{2.4}{5} = X$

$X = 0.48$

20) $\dfrac{\frac{1}{100}}{\frac{1}{150}} \times 1.2 = X$

$\dfrac{1}{100} \div \dfrac{1}{150} \times \dfrac{1.2}{1} = X$

$\dfrac{1}{\cancel{100}_2} \times \dfrac{\cancel{150}^3}{1} \times \dfrac{1.2}{1} = X$

$\dfrac{1}{2} \times \dfrac{3}{1} \times \dfrac{1.2}{1} = X$

$\dfrac{3.6}{2} = X$

$X = 1.8$

Review Set 9 from pages 75–76

1) 0.25 **2)** 1 **3)** 0.56 **4)** 1,000 **5)** 0.7 **6)** 8 **7)** 21.43 **8)** 500 **9)** 200 **10)** 10.5 **11)** 3 **12)** 0.63 **13)** 10 **14)** 0.67 **15)** 1.25

16) 31.25 **17)** 16.67 **18)** 240 **19)** 0.75 **20)** 2.27 **21)** 1 **22)** 6 **23)** 108 nurses **24)** 72 calories **25)** 81.82 milligrams/hour

Solutions—Review Set 9

4) $\dfrac{0.5}{2} \diagdown \diagup \dfrac{250}{X}$

$0.5X = 500$

$\dfrac{0.5X}{0.5} = \dfrac{500}{0.5}$

$X = 1{,}000$

6) $\dfrac{40}{X} \times 12 = 60$

$\dfrac{40}{X} \times \dfrac{12}{1} = 60$

$\dfrac{480}{X} \diagdown \diagup \dfrac{60}{1}$

$60X = 480$

$\dfrac{60X}{60} = \dfrac{480}{60}$

$X = 8$

9) $\dfrac{15}{500} \times X = 6$

$\dfrac{15X}{500} \diagdown \diagup \dfrac{6}{1}$

$15X = 3{,}000$

$\dfrac{15X}{15} = \dfrac{3{,}000}{15}$

$X = 200$

10) $\dfrac{5}{X} \diagdown \diagup \dfrac{10}{21}$

$10X = 105$

$\dfrac{10X}{10} = \dfrac{105}{10}$

$X = 10.5$

11) $\dfrac{250}{1} \diagdown \diagup \dfrac{750}{X}$

$250X = 750$

$\dfrac{250X}{250} = \dfrac{750}{250}$

$X = 3$

14) $\dfrac{\frac{1}{100}}{1} \diagdown \diagup \dfrac{\frac{1}{150}}{X}$

$\dfrac{1}{100}X = \dfrac{1}{150}$

$\dfrac{\frac{1}{100}X}{\frac{1}{100}} = \dfrac{\frac{1}{150}}{\frac{1}{100}}$

$X = \dfrac{1}{150} \div \dfrac{1}{100}$

$X = \dfrac{1}{\cancel{150}_3} \times \dfrac{\cancel{100}^2}{1}$

$X = \dfrac{2}{3} = 0.666 = 0.67$

22) $\dfrac{25\%}{30\%} = \dfrac{5}{X}$

$\dfrac{0.25}{0.3} \diagdown \diagup \dfrac{5}{X}$

$0.25X = 1.5$

$\dfrac{0.25X}{0.25} = \dfrac{1.5}{0.25}$

$X = 6$

23) $\dfrac{45}{100} \diagdown \diagup \dfrac{X}{240}$

$100X = 10{,}800$

$\dfrac{100X}{100} = \dfrac{10{,}800}{100}$

$X = 108$

Review Set 10 from page 77

1) 1.3 **2)** 4.75 **3)** 56 **4)** 0.43 **5)** 26.67 **6)** 15 **7)** 0.8 **8)** 2.38 **9)** 37.5 **10)** 112.5 **11)** 8 pills **12)** 720 milliliters

13) $3,530.21 **14)** 7.2 ounces **15)** 700 calories

Solutions—Review Set 10

1) $0.25\% = 0.00.25 = 0.0025$; $0.0025 \times 520 = 1.3$

8) $7\% = 0.07. = 0.07$; $0.07 \times 34 = 2.38$

11) $40\% = 0.40. = 0.4$; 0.4×20 pills $= 8$ pills

13) 80% of $\$17,651.07 = 0.8 \times \$17,651.07 = \$14,120.86$

$\$17,651.07$ total bill
$- 14,120.86$ paid by insurance company
$\$3,530.21$ paid by patient

14) $40\% = 0.40. = 0.4$
0.4×18 ounces $= 7.2$ ounces

15) $20\% = 0.20. = 0.2$
$0.2 \times 3,500$ calories $= 700$ calories

Practice Problems—Chapter 2 from pages 78–79

1) 0.4, 40%, $2:5$ **2)** $\frac{1}{20}$, 5%, $1:20$ **3)** 0.17, $\frac{17}{100}$, $17:100$ **4)** 0.25, $\frac{1}{4}$, 25% **5)** 0.06, $\frac{3}{50}$, $3:50$ **6)** 0.17, 17%, $1:6$ **7)** 0.5, $\frac{1}{2}$, $1:2$

8) 0.01, $\frac{1}{100}$, 1% **9)** $\frac{9}{100}$, 9%, $9:100$ **10)** 0.38, 38%, $3:8$ **11)** 0.67, $\frac{2}{3}$, 67% **12)** 0.33, 33%, $1:3$ **13)** $\frac{13}{25}$, 52%, $13:25$

14) 0.45, $\frac{9}{20}$, 45% **15)** 0.86, 86%, $6:7$ **16)** 0.3, $\frac{3}{10}$, 30% **17)** 0.02, 2%, $1:50$ **18)** $\frac{3}{5}$, 60%, $3:5$ **19)** $\frac{1}{25}$, 4%, $1:25$

20) 0.1, $\frac{1}{10}$, $1:10$ **21)** 0.04 **22)** $1:40$ **23)** 7.5% **24)** $\frac{1}{2}$ **25)** $3:4$ **26)** 262.5 **27)** 3.64 **28)** 1.97 **29)** $1:4$ **30)** $1:10$ **31)** 84

32) $90,000$ **33)** 1 **34)** 1.1 **35)** 100 **36)** 39 **37)** 0.75 **38)** 21 **39)** 120 **40)** 90 **41)** 25 grams protein; 6.25 grams fat

42) 231 points **43)** 60 minutes **44)** 50 milliliters **45)** 27 milligrams **46)** 5.4 grams **47)** 283.5 milligrams **48)** 6.5 pounds

49) $\$10.42$ **50)** 6 total doses

Solutions—Practice Problems—Chapter 2

36) $\frac{3}{9} \diagup\!\!\!\!\diagdown \frac{X}{117}$

$9X = 351$

$\frac{9X}{9} = \frac{351}{9}$

$X = 39$

41) $20\% = 0.20. = 0.2$
0.2×125 grams $= 25$ grams (of protein)

$5\% = 0.05. = 0.05$
0.05×125 grams $= 6.25$ grams (of fat)

$\begin{array}{r} 125 \\ \times\ 0.2 \\ \hline 25.0 = 25 \end{array}$

$\begin{array}{r} 125 \\ \times\ 0.05 \\ \hline 6.25 \end{array}$

43) $\frac{90}{27} \diagup\!\!\!\!\diagdown \frac{200}{X}$

$90X = 5,400$

$\frac{90X}{90} = \frac{5,400}{90}$

$X = 60$

45) $45\% = 0.45. = 0.45$
0.45×60 milligrams $= 27$ milligrams

$\begin{array}{r} 60 \\ \times\ 0.45 \\ \hline 300 \\ 240 \\ \hline 27.00 = 27 \end{array}$

46) $\frac{3}{4} = 0.75$

$1\frac{1}{2} = 1.5$

$\frac{2.7}{0.75} \diagup\!\!\!\!\diagdown \frac{X}{1.5}$

$0.75X = 4.05$

$\frac{0.75X}{0.75} = \frac{4.05}{0.75}$

$X = 5.4$

47) $\frac{6.75}{1} \diagup\!\!\!\!\diagdown \frac{X}{42}$

$X = 283.5$

48) $5\% = 0.05. = 0.05$
0.05×130 pounds $= 6.5$ pounds

$\begin{array}{r} 130 \\ \times\ 0.05 \\ \hline 6.50 = 6.5 \end{array}$

49) $17\% = 0.17. = 0.17$; $0.17 \times \$12.56 = \$2.14$

$\begin{array}{r} \$12.56 \\ -\ 2.14 \\ \hline \$10.42 \end{array}$

50) $10\% = 0.10. = 0.1$; $0.1 \times 150 = 15$

$\begin{array}{ll} 150\ \text{milligrams} & \text{first dose} \\ -\ 15\ \text{milligrams} & \\ \hline 135\ \text{milligrams} & \text{second dose} \\ -\ 15\ \text{milligrams} & \\ \hline 120\ \text{milligrams} & \text{third dose} \\ -\ 15\ \text{milligrams} & \\ \hline 105\ \text{milligrams} & \text{fourth dose} \\ -\ 15\ \text{milligrams} & \\ \hline 90\ \text{milligrams} & \text{fifth dose} \\ -\ 15\ \text{milligrams} & \\ \hline 75\ \text{milligrams} & \text{sixth dose} \end{array}$

6 total doses

Section 1—Self-Evaluation from pages 80–82

1) 3.05 **2)** 4,002.5 **3)** 0.63 **4)** 723.27 **5)** LCD = 12 **6)** LCD = 110 **7)** $\frac{11}{12}$ **8)** $\frac{47}{63}$ **9)** 1 **10)** $\frac{1}{2}$ **11)** 45.78 **12)** 0.02 **13)** 59.24 **14)** 0.09 **15)** 12 **16)** $\frac{2}{3}$ **17)** $\frac{1}{10}, \frac{1}{6}, \frac{1}{5}, \frac{1}{3}, \frac{1}{2}$ **18)** $\frac{2}{3}, \frac{3}{4}, \frac{5}{6}, \frac{7}{8}, \frac{9}{10}$ **19)** 0.009, 0.125, 0.1909, 0.25, 0.3 **20)** $\frac{1}{2}$%, 0.9%, 50%, 100%, 500% **21)** 1:3 **22)** 1:600 **23)** 0.01 **24)** 0.9% **25)** $\frac{1}{3}$ **26)** 5:9 **27)** $\frac{1}{20}$ **28)** 1:200 **29)** $\frac{2}{3}$ **30)** 75% **31)** 40% **32)** 0.17 **33)** 1.21 **34)** 1.3 **35)** 2.5 **36)** 100 **37)** 4 **38)** 8.33 **39)** 24 participants **40)** 2 holidays **41)** $2.42 **42)** 12 cans of water **43)** 8 centimeters **44)** 950 milliliters **45)** 23.1 fluid ounces **46)** 17.7 **47)** Milk **48)** 0.049, 0.05, 0.175, 2.25, 2.5, 5, 5.075 **49)** 2.104, 2.06, 2.4 **50)** 0.913

	X
.913	0.913
0.9130	9.130

Solutions—Section 1—Self-Evaluation

16) $\frac{1}{150} \div \frac{1}{100} = \frac{1}{150} \times \frac{100}{1} = \frac{\overset{2}{\cancel{100}}}{\underset{3}{\cancel{150}}} = \frac{2}{3}$

30) $3:4 = \frac{3}{4} = 4\overline{)3.0}^{0.75} = 75\%$

34) $\frac{0.3}{2.6} \diagdown \diagup \frac{0.15}{X}$

$0.3X = 2.6 \times 0.15$

$0.3X = 0.39$

$\frac{0.3X}{0.3} = \frac{0.39}{0.3}$

$X = 1.3$

39) $4\% = 0.\underset{\smile}{04}. = 0.04$

0.04×600 participants = 24 participants

$\begin{array}{r} 600 \\ \times\ 0.04 \\ \hline 24.00 = 24 \end{array}$

Review Set 11 from pages 88–89

1) metric **2)** volume **3)** weight **4)** length **5)** $\frac{1}{1,000}$ or 0.001 **6)** 1,000 **7)** microgram **8)** kilogram **9)** milligram **10)** 1,000 **11)** 1 **12)** 1,000 **13)** 10 **14)** 0.3 g **15)** 1.33 mL **16)** 5 kg **17)** 1.5 mm **18)** 10 mg **19)** microgram **20)** milliliter **21)** milligram **22)** gram **23)** millimeter **24)** kilogram **25)** centimeter

Review Set 12 from page 93

1) 3 quarts **2)** 10 pounds **3)** 10 milliequivalents **4)** $2\frac{1}{2}$ pounds **5)** 10 tablespoons **6)** 75 lb **7)** 30 mEq **8)** 5 T **9)** $1\frac{1}{2}$ t **10)** 14 units **11)** False **12)** False **13)** True **14)** units **15)** 3 **16)** 2 **17)** 1 **18)** 1 **19)** 1 **20)** milliequivalent; mEq

Practice Problems—Chapter 3 from pages 94–96

1) milli **2)** micro **3)** centi **4)** kilo **5)** 1 milligram **6)** 1 kilogram **7)** 1 microgram **8)** 1 centimeter **9)** meter **10)** gram **11)** liter **12)** fluid ounce **13)** ounce **14)** milligram **15)** microgram **16)** pound **17)** milliequivalent **18)** teaspoon **19)** quart **20)** milliliter **21)** pint **22)** tablespoon **23)** millimeter **24)** gram **25)** centimeter **26)** liter **27)** meter **28)** kilogram **29)** pound **30)** 325 mcg **31)** $\frac{1}{2}$ t **32)** 2 t **33)** $\frac{1}{3}$ fl oz **34)** 5,000,000 units **35)** 0.5 L **36)** 0.05 mg **37)** 600 mL **38)** 2.5 cm **39)** 0.08 mL **40)** 5.5 kg **41)** eight and one-quarter fluid ounces **42)** three hundred seventy-five grams **43)** one-half kilogram **44)** two and six-tenths milliliters **45)** twenty milliequivalents **46)** four-tenths liter **47)** three and five-hundredths micrograms **48)** seventeen-hundredths milligram **49)** fourteen and one-half pounds

50) Prevention: This type of error can be prevented by avoiding the use of a decimal point or trailing zero when not necessary. In this instance, the decimal point and zero serve no purpose and can easily be misinterpreted, especially if the decimal point is difficult to see. Question any order that is unclear or unreasonable.

51) Prevention: This type of error can be prevented by asking the prescribing physician for clarification. If you see grains prescribed or if you are unclear as to what the prescriber is ordering, *do not guess—always ask for clarification.* Ideally, grains and other apothecary units will be on the "Do Not Use" list for this health care facility.

Review Set 13 from page 106

1) 0.5 **2)** 15 **3)** 0.008 **4)** 0.01 **5)** 0.06 **6)** 0.3 **7)** 200 **8)** 1,200 **9)** 2.5 **10)** 65 **11)** 5 **12)** 1,500 **13)** 0.1 **14)** 0.25
15) 2,000 **16)** 750 **17)** 5 **18)** 1,000 **19)** 1,000 **20)** 3 **21)** 0.023 **22)** 0.00105 **23)** 0.018 **24)** 400 **25)** 2.625 **26)** 0.5
27) 10,000 **28)** 0.45 **29)** 0.005 **30)** 30,000

Solutions—Review Set 13

2) $\dfrac{1\ g}{1,000\ mg} \diagdown\!\!\diagup \dfrac{0.015\ g}{X\ mg}$

$$X = 1,000 \times 0.015$$
$$X = 15\ mg$$

16) $\dfrac{1\ L}{1,000\ mL} \diagdown\!\!\diagup \dfrac{0.75\ L}{X\ mL}$

$$X = 0.75 \times 1,000$$
$$X = 750\ mL$$

3) $\dfrac{1\ g}{1,000\ mg} \diagdown\!\!\diagup \dfrac{X\ g}{8\ mg}$

$$1,000X = 8$$
$$\dfrac{1,000X}{1,000} = \dfrac{8}{1,000}$$
$$X = 0.008\ g$$

20) $\dfrac{1\ L}{1,000\ mL} \diagdown\!\!\diagup \dfrac{X\ L}{3,000}$

$$1,000X = 3,000$$
$$\dfrac{1,000X}{1,000} = \dfrac{3,000}{1,000}$$
$$X = 3\ L$$

9) $\dfrac{1\ kg}{1,000\ g} \diagdown\!\!\diagup \dfrac{0.0025\ kg}{X\ g}$

$$X = 1,000 \times 0.0025$$
$$X = 2.5\ g$$

23) $\dfrac{1\ mg}{1,000\ mcg} \diagdown\!\!\diagup \dfrac{X\ mg}{18\ mcg}$

$$1,000X = 18$$
$$\dfrac{1,000X}{1,000} = \dfrac{18}{1,000}$$
$$X = 0.018\ mg$$

Review Set 14 from pages 109–111

1) 6; 1 cup = 8 fl oz **2)** 65; 1 t = 5 mL **3)** $\frac{1}{2}$; 1 fl oz = 30 mL **4)** 75; 1 fl oz = 30 mL **5)** $\frac{3}{4}$; 1 qt = 1,000 mL
6) 4; 1 t = 5 mL **7)** 60; 1 T = 15 mL **8)** 19.8; 1 kg = 2.2 lb **9)** 113.64; 1 kg = 2.2 lb **10)** 3; 1 L = 1 qt
11) 121; 1 kg = 2.2 lb **12)** 30; 1 in = 2.5 cm **13)** 2; 1 qt = 1 L **14)** 15; 1 t = 5 mL **15)** 45; 1 kg = 2.2 lb
16) 500; 1 pt = 500 mL **17)** 360; 1 cup = 240 mL **18)** 5; 1 m = 100 cm; 1 in = 2.5 cm; 1 ft = 12 in
19) 12; 1 in = 2.5 cm **20)** 2; 1 fl oz = 30 mL **21)** 80; 1 in = 2.5 cm **22)** 14; 1 in = 2.5 cm **23)** 3; 1 in = 2.5 cm
24) 50; 1 in = 2.5 cm; 1 cm = 10 mm **25)** 88; 1 kg = 2.2 lb **26)** 15.75 or $15\frac{3}{4}$; 1 kg = 2.2 lb **27)** 50; 1 kg = 2.2 lb
28) 7.7; 1 kg = 2.2 lb **29)** 28.64; 1 kg = 2.2 lb **30)** 53.75 **31)** 4; $\frac{1}{2}$ **32)** Yes **33)** 2,430 **34)** 1.25 **35)** 10 **36)** Dissolve
2 teaspoons of Betadine concentrate in 1 pint, or 2 cups, of warm water. **37)** 2 **38)** 3 **39)** 16 **40)** 93.64

Solutions—Review Set 14

4) $\dfrac{1\ fl\ oz}{30\ mL} \diagdown\!\!\diagup \dfrac{2\frac{1}{2}\ fl\ oz}{X\ mL}$

$$X = 30 \times 2.5$$
$$X = 75\ mL$$

6) $\dfrac{1\ t}{5\ mL} \diagdown\!\!\diagup \dfrac{X\ t}{20\ mL}$

$$5X = 20$$
$$\dfrac{5X}{5} = \dfrac{20}{5}$$
$$X = 4\ t$$

11) $\dfrac{1\text{ kg}}{2.2\text{ lb}} \bowtie \dfrac{55\text{ kg}}{X\text{ lb}}$

$X = 2.2 \times 55$

$X = 121\text{ lb}$

15) $\dfrac{1\text{ kg}}{2.2\text{ lb}} \bowtie \dfrac{X\text{ kg}}{99\text{ lb}}$

$2.2X = 99$

$\dfrac{2.2X}{2.2} = \dfrac{99}{2.2}$

$X = 45\text{ kg}$

20) $\dfrac{1\text{ fl oz}}{30\text{ mL}} \bowtie \dfrac{X\text{ fl oz}}{60\text{ mL}}$

$30X = 60$

$\dfrac{30X}{30} = \dfrac{60}{30}$

$X = 2\text{ fl oz}$

24) $\dfrac{1\text{ in}}{2.5\text{ cm}} \bowtie \dfrac{2\text{ in}}{X\text{ cm}}$

$X = 2.5 \times 2$

$X = 5\text{ cm}$

$\dfrac{1\text{ cm}}{10\text{ mm}} \bowtie \dfrac{5\text{ cm}}{X\text{ mm}}$

$X = 50\text{ mm}$

32) $\dfrac{1\text{ kg}}{2.2\text{ lb}} \bowtie \dfrac{108\text{ kg}}{X\text{ lb}}$

$X = 108 \times 2.2$

$X = 237.6\text{ lb}$

$250\text{ lb} - 237.6\text{ lb} = 12.4\text{ lb}$

Yes. He has met weight loss goal of 10 lb.

33) Add up the fluid ounces: 81 fluid ounces

$\dfrac{1\text{ fl oz}}{30\text{ mL}} \bowtie \dfrac{81\text{ fl oz}}{X\text{ mL}}$

$X = 2{,}430\text{ mL}$

34) $\dfrac{1\text{ kg}}{2.2\text{ lb}} \bowtie \dfrac{X\text{ kg}}{55\text{ lb}}$

$2.2X = 55$

$\dfrac{2.2X}{2.2} = \dfrac{55}{2.2}$

$X = 25\text{ kg}$

$\dfrac{0.05\text{ mg}}{1\text{ kg}} \bowtie \dfrac{X\text{ mg}}{25\text{ kg}}$

$X = 0.05 \times 25$

$X = 1.25\text{ mg}$

35) Find the total number of mL per day and the total number of mL per bottle.

mL per day for 4 doses:

$\dfrac{12\text{ mL}}{1\text{ dose}} \bowtie \dfrac{X\text{ mL}}{4\text{ doses}}$

$X = 48\text{ mL}$

mL per bottle:

$\dfrac{1\text{ fl oz}}{30\text{ mL}} \bowtie \dfrac{16\text{ fl oz}}{X\text{ mL}}$

$X = 480\text{ mL (per bottle)}$

How many days will 480 mL (or 16 ounces) last?

$\dfrac{1\text{ day}}{48\text{ mL}} \bowtie \dfrac{X\text{ days}}{480\text{ mL}}$

$48X = 480$

$\dfrac{48X}{48} = \dfrac{480}{48}$

$X = 10\text{ days}$

37) $\dfrac{1\text{ t}}{5\text{ mL}} \bowtie \dfrac{X\text{ t}}{10\text{ mL}}$

$5X = 10$

$\dfrac{5X}{5} = \dfrac{10}{5}$

$X = 2\text{ t}$

38) 1 qt = 32 fl oz (per container)

At 1 feeding every 3 hours, how many feedings does the infant require during 24 hours or per day?

$\dfrac{1\text{ feeding}}{3\text{ hours}} \bowtie \dfrac{X\text{ feedings}}{24\text{ hours}}$

$3X = 24$

$\dfrac{3X}{3} = \dfrac{24}{3}$

$X = 8\text{ feedings}$

How many ounces will the infant consume for 8 feedings or per day?

$\dfrac{1\text{ feeding}}{4\text{ fl oz}} \bowtie \dfrac{8\text{ feedings}}{X\text{ fl oz}}$

$X = 32\text{ fl oz (per day)}$

Each container holds 1 quart or 32 fluid ounces (equivalent: 1 qt = 32 fl oz), so you know she needs 3 containers of formula for 3 days.

Practice Problems—Chapter 4 from pages 113–114

1) 500 **2)** 10 **3)** 0.0075 **4)** 3 **5)** 4,000 **6)** 0.5 **7)** $\frac{1}{2}$ **8)** 0.3 **9)** 70 **10)** 149.6 **11)** 4.46 **12)** 105 **13)** 2.39 **14)** 6.4 **15)** 2

16) 1.63 **17)** 32.05 **18)** 7.99 **19)** 0.008 **20)** 0.45 **21)** 95 **22)** 500 **23)** 600 **24)** 4.05 **25)** 68.18 **26)** $7\frac{1}{2}$ **27)** 10 **28)** 480

29) 2 **30)** 3 **31)** 0.375 **32)** 30 **33)** 1 **34)** 1 **35)** 1 **36)** 1,500 **37)** 45 **38)** $1\frac{1}{2}$ **39)** 4.4 **40)** 0.025 **41)** 4,300 **42)** 0.06

43) 15 **44)** 3 **45)** 250 **46)** 9 **47)** 8 **48)** 840 **49)** 11.55 or $11\frac{1}{2}$

50) Prevention: The nurse didn't use the conversion rules correctly. The nurse divided instead of multiplying. This type of medication error is avoided by double-checking your dosage calculations and asking yourself, "Is this dosage reasonable?" Certainly you know that if there are 1,000 mg in 1 g and you want to give 2 g, then you need *more* than 1,000 milligrams, not less. The correct calculations are:

Convert:

$$\frac{1 \text{ g}}{1,000 \text{ mg}} = \frac{2 \text{ g}}{X \text{ mg}}$$

$$X = 2 \times 1,000$$

$$X = 2,000 \text{ mg}$$

Calculate:

$$\frac{1,000 \text{ mg}}{10 \text{ mL}} = \frac{2,000 \text{ mg}}{X \text{ mL}}$$

$$1,000X = 20,000$$

$$\frac{1,000X}{1,000} = \frac{20,000}{1,000}$$

$$X = 20 \text{ mL}$$

To give 2,000 mg you would need 20 mL of the 1,000 mg per 10 mL supply.

Solutions—Practice Problems—Chapter 4

13) 5 lb 4 oz = 5.25 lb

$$\frac{1 \text{ kg}}{2.2 \text{ lb}} \times \frac{X \text{ kg}}{5.25 \text{ lb}}$$

$$2.2X = 5.25$$

$$\frac{2.2X}{2.2} = \frac{5.25}{2.2}$$

$$X = 2.39 \text{ kg}$$

46) Per bottle:

$$\frac{1 \text{ fl oz}}{30 \text{ mL}} \times \frac{4 \text{ fl oz}}{X \text{ mL}}$$

$$X = 120 \text{ mL}$$

Each dose:

$$\frac{1 \text{ t}}{5 \text{ mL}} \times \frac{2\frac{1}{2} \text{ t}}{X \text{ mL}}$$

$$X = 12.5 \text{ mL}$$

Bottle holds 120 mL; each dose is 12.5 mL.

$$\frac{1 \text{ dose}}{12.5 \text{ mL}} \times \frac{X \text{ doses}}{120 \text{ mL}}$$

$$12.5X = 120$$

$$\frac{12.5X}{12.5} = \frac{120}{12.5}$$

$$X = 9.6 \text{ doses or 9 full doses}$$

47) 1 T per dose = 15 mL per dose

$$\frac{1 \text{ dose}}{15 \text{ mL}} \times \frac{X \text{ doses}}{120 \text{ mL}}$$

$$15X = 120$$

$$\frac{15X}{15} = \frac{120}{15}$$

$$X = 8 \text{ doses}$$

48) 4 + 8 + 6 + 10 = 28 fluid ounces

$$\frac{1 \text{ fl oz}}{30 \text{ mL}} \times \frac{28 \text{ fl oz}}{X \text{ mL}}$$

$$X = 840 \text{ mL}$$

49)

$$\frac{1 \text{ kg}}{1,000 \text{ g}} \times \frac{X \text{ kg}}{5,250 \text{ g}}$$

$$1,000X = 5,250$$

$$\frac{1,000X}{1,000} = \frac{5,250}{1,000}$$

$$X = 5.25 \text{ kg}$$

$$\frac{1 \text{ kg}}{2.2 \text{ lb}} \times \frac{5.25 \text{ kg}}{X \text{ lb}}$$

$$X = 11.55 \text{ or approximately } 11\frac{1}{2} \text{ lb}$$

Review Set 15 from page 118

1) 12:32 AM **2)** 7:30 AM **3)** 4:40 PM **4)** 9:21 PM **5)** 11:59 PM **6)** 12:15 PM **7)** 2:20 AM **8)** 10:10 AM **9)** 1:15 PM **10)** 6:25 PM **11)** 1330 **12)** 0004 **13)** 2145 **14)** 1200 **15)** 2315 **16)** 0345 **17)** 2400 **18)** 1530 **19)** 0620 **20)** 1745 **21)** *zero six twenty-three* **22)** *zero-zero forty-one* **23)** *nineteen zero three* **24)** *twenty-three eleven* **25)** *zero three hundred*

Review Set 16 from pages 120–121

1) 38 **2)** 101.1 **3)** 97.2 **4)** 89.6 **5)** 37 **6)** 37.2 **7)** 39.8 **8)** 104 **9)** 102 **10)** 97.5 **11)** 37.8 **12)** 102.2 **13)** 99.3 **14)** 34.6 **15)** 39.3 **16)** 35.3 **17)** 44.6 **18)** 31.1 **19)** 98.6 **20)** 39.7

Solutions—Review Set 16

1) $°C = \dfrac{°F - 32}{1.8}$

$°C = \dfrac{100.4 - 32}{1.8}$

$°C = \dfrac{68.4}{1.8}$

$°C = 38°$

2) $°F = 1.8°C + 32$

$°F = (1.8 \times 38.4) + 32$

$°F = 69.12 + 32$

$°F = 101.12 = 101.1°$

Practice Problems—Chapter 5 from pages 122–123

1) 2:57 AM **2)** 0310 **3)** 1622 **4)** 8:01 PM **5)** 11:02 AM **6)** 0033 **7)** 0216 **8)** 4:42 PM **9)** 11:56 PM **10)** 0420 **11)** 1931 **12)** 2400 or 0000

13) 0645 **14)** 9:15 AM **15)** 9:07 PM **16)** 6:23 PM **17)** 5:40 AM **18)** 1155 **19)** 2212 **20)** 2106 **21)** 4 h **22)** 7 h **23)** 8 h 30 min **24)** 12 h 15 min

25) 14 h 50 min **26)** 4 h 12 min **27)** 4 h 48 min **28)** 3 h 41 min **29)** 6 h 30 min **30)** 16 h 38 min **31)** False **32)** a. AM; b. PM; c. AM; d. PM

33) 37.6 **34)** 97.7 **35)** 102.6 **36)** 37.9 **37)** 36.7 **38)** 99.3 **39)** 100.8 **40)** 40 **41)** 36.6 **42)** 95.7 **43)** 39.7 **44)** 102.2 **45)** 98.4 **46)** 38.6 **47)** 36.2

48) 37.2, 99 (98.96° rounds to 99.0°F) **49)** True

50) Prevention: Such situations can easily be prevented by accurately applying the complete formula for temperature conversion. Guessing is not acceptable in medical and health care calculations. Temperature conversion charts are readily available in most health care settings, but when they are not, the conversion formulas should be used. It may be wise to try to memorize the common fever temperature conversions between 98.6°F (37°C) and 104°F (40°C).

Solutions—Practice Problems—Chapter 5

24)
$$\begin{array}{r} 2150 \\ -\,0935 \\ \hline 1215 \end{array} = 12\text{ h }15\text{ min}$$

26)   2316 = 11:16 PM, 0328 = 3:28 AM

11:16 PM → 3:16 AM = 4 h

$\dfrac{3\text{:}16 \text{ AM} \to 3\text{:}28 \text{ AM} = 12 \text{ min}}{\text{Total} = 4 \text{ h } 12 \text{ min}}$

28)   4:35 PM → 7:35 PM = 3 h

$\dfrac{7\text{:}35 \text{ PM} \to 8\text{:}16 \text{ PM} = 41 \text{ min}}{\text{Total} = 3 \text{ h } 41 \text{ min}}$

48) $\dfrac{37.6 + 35.5 + 38.1 + 37.6}{4} = \dfrac{148.8}{4} = 37.2°C$ (average)

$°F = (1.8 \times 37.2) + 32 = 98.96 = 99.0 = 99°$

(rounded; zero dropped)

Review Set 17 from pages 133–136

1) 1 mL **2)** Round 1.25 to 1.3 and measure on the mL scale as 1.3 mL **3)** No **4)** 0.5 mL **5)** a) False; b) The size of the drop varies according to the diameter of the tip of the dropper. **6)** No **7)** Measure the oral liquid in a 3 mL syringe, which is not intended for injections. **8)** 5 **9)** Discard the excess prior to injecting the patient. In some cases (such as for controlled substances), the nurse may need a witness to observe the discarding of the excess. **10)** To prevent needlestick injury

11)

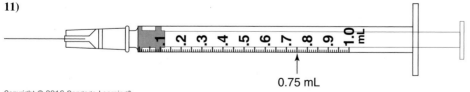

0.75 mL

12)

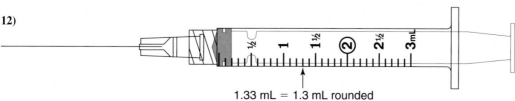

1.33 mL = 1.3 mL rounded

13)

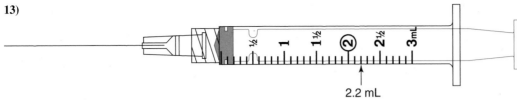

2.2 mL

14)

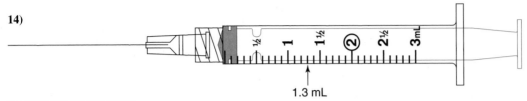

1.3 mL

15)

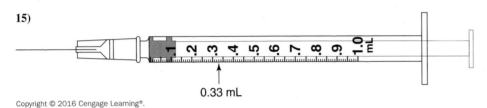

0.33 mL

16)

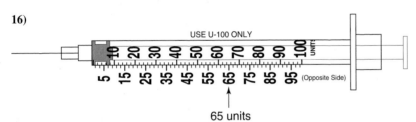

65 units

17)

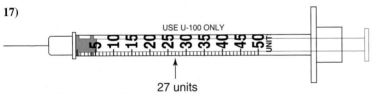

27 units

18)

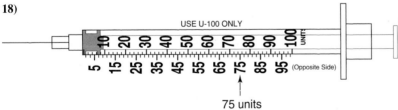

75 units

19)

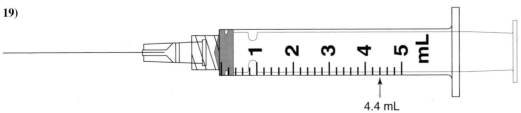

4.4 mL

20)

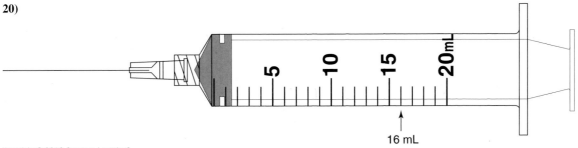

16 mL

21) 0.2 mL **22)** 1 mL **23)** 0.2 mL

Practice Problems—Chapter 6 from pages 138–141

1) 1 **2)** hundredths or 0.01 **3)** No. The tuberculin syringe has a maximum capacity of 1 mL. **4)** Round to 1.3 mL and measure at 1.3 mL. **5)** 30; 1 **6)** 1 mL **7)** 0.75 **8)** False **9)** False **10)** True **11)** to prevent accidental needlesticks during intravenous administration **12)** top ring **13)** 10 **14)** False **15)** 3 mL, 1 mL, and insulin

16)

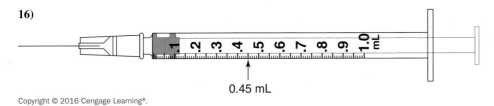

0.45 mL

17)

USE U-100 ONLY

(Opposite Side)

80 units

18)

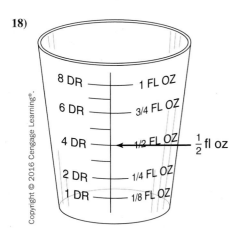

8 DR — 1 FL OZ
6 DR — 3/4 FL OZ
4 DR ◄— 1/2 FL OZ $\frac{1}{2}$ fl oz
2 DR — 1/4 FL OZ
1 DR — 1/8 FL OZ

19)

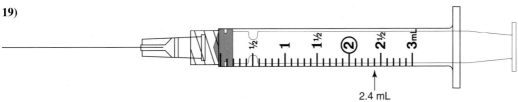

2.4 mL

20)

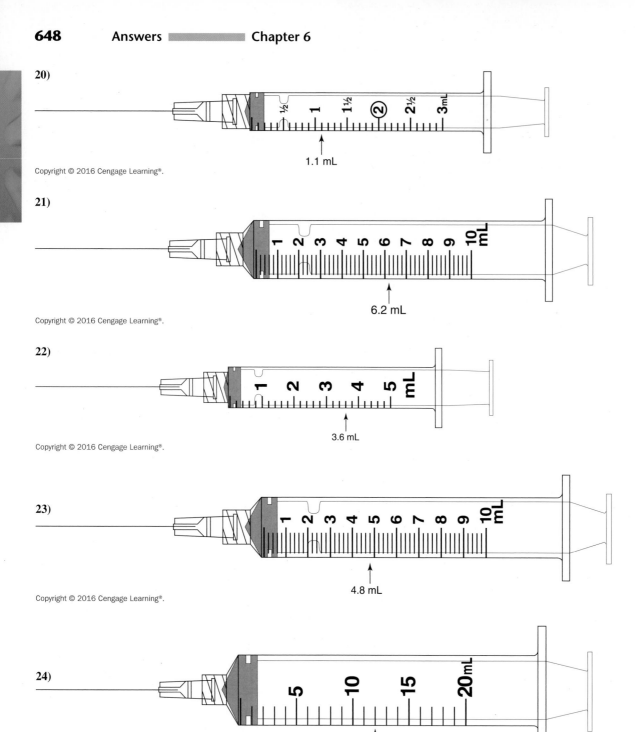

1.1 mL

Copyright © 2016 Cengage Learning®.

21)

6.2 mL

Copyright © 2016 Cengage Learning®.

22)

3.6 mL

Copyright © 2016 Cengage Learning®.

23)

4.8 mL

Copyright © 2016 Cengage Learning®.

24)

12 mL

Copyright © 2016 Cengage Learning®.

25) Prevention: This error could have been avoided by following a simple principle: Don't put oral drugs in syringes intended for injection. Instead, place the medication in an oral syringe to which a needle cannot be attached. In addition, the medication should have been labeled for oral use only. The medication was ordered orally, not by injection. An alert nurse should have noticed the discrepancy. Finally, but just as important, a medication should be administered only by the nurse who prepared it.

26) Prevention: The nurse should ask for assistance to learn how to use unfamiliar equipment. Do not put the patient at risk. The nurse must remove the cap on the oral syringe prior to administering the medication, so that the child cannot choke on the cap.

Review Set 18 from pages 146–147

1) Give 250 milligrams of naproxen orally 2 times a day. **2)** Give 30 units of Humulin N NPH insulin subcutaneously every day 30 minutes before breakfast. **3)** Give 500 milligrams of cefaclor orally immediately, and then give 250 milligrams every 8 hours. **4)** Give 25 micrograms of Synthroid orally once a day. **5)** Give 10 milligrams of Ativan intramuscularly every 4 hours as necessary for agitation. **6)** Give 20 milligrams of furosemide intravenously slowly immediately. **7)** Give 10 milliliters of Mylanta orally after meals and at bedtime. **8)** Instill 2 drops of 1% atropine sulfate ophthalmic in the right eye every 15 minutes for 4 applications. **9)** Give 15 milligrams of morphine sulfate intramuscularly every 3 hours as needed for pain. **10)** Give 0.25 milligram of digoxin orally once a day. **11)** Give 250 milligrams of tetracycline orally 4 times a day. **12)** Give 150 micrograms of nitroglycerin sublingually immediately. **13)** Instill 2 drops of Cortisporin otic suspension in both ears 3 times a day and at bedtime. **14)** The abbreviation t.i.d. means 3 times a day with no specific interval between times. An attempt is made to give the 3 doses during waking hours. The abbreviation q.8h means every 8 hours. These doses would be given around the clock at 8-hour intervals. For example, administration times for t.i.d. might be 0800, 1200, 1700; administration times for q.8h could be 0600, 1400, 2200. **15)** Contact the physician for clarification. **16)** No, q.i.d. orders are given 4 times in 24 hours with no specific interval between times indicated in order, typically during waking hours; whereas q.4h orders are given 6 times in 24 hours at 4-hour intervals. **17)** They are determined by hospital or institutional policy. **18)** patient, drug, dosage, route, frequency, date and time written, signature of physician/prescriber **19)** Parts 1–5: patient's name, drug, dosage, route, frequency **20)** The right patient must receive the right drug in the right amount by the right route at the right time, followed by the right documentation.

Review Set 19 from pages 151–152

1) oral **2)** every other day at 9:00 AM **3)** 7:30 AM, 11:30 AM, 4:30 PM, 10:00 PM **4)** 5 PM **5)** every 6 hours, as needed for severe pain **6)** 09/26/xx at 9:00 AM **7)** sublingual, under the tongue **8)** once a day **9)** 125 **10)** nitroglycerin and ketorolac tromethamine **11)** subcutaneous injection **12)** once **13)** cephalexin **14)** before breakfast (at 7:30 AM) **15)** milliequivalent **16)** cephalexin and K-Dur **17)** Tylenol **18)** twice **19)** 0900 and 2100 **20)** 2400, 0600, 1200, and 1800 **21)** in the "One-Time Medication Dosage" section, lower left corner

Practice Problems—Chapter 7 from pages 153–157

1) twice a day **2)** per rectum **3)** before meals **4)** after **5)** 3 times a day **6)** every 4 hours **7)** when necessary **8)** by mouth, orally **9)** intravenous **10)** 4 times a day **11)** immediately **12)** freely, as desired **13)** after meals **14)** intramuscular **15)** without **16)** noct **17)** gtt **18)** mL **19)** SL **20)** g **21)** q.i.d. **22)** $\bar{c}$ **23)** subcut **24)** t **25)** b.i.d. **26)** q.3h **27)** p.c. **28)** $\bar{a}$ **29)** kg **30)** Give 60 milligrams of Toradol intravenously immediately and every 6 hours when necessary for pain. **31)** Give 300,000 units of procaine penicillin G intravenously 4 times a day. **32)** Give 5 milliliters of Mylanta orally 1 hour before and 1 hour after meals, at bedtime, and every 2 hours as needed at night for gastric upset. **33)** Give 25 milligrams of Librium orally every 6 hours when necessary for agitation. **34)** Give 5,000 units of heparin subcutaneously immediately. **35)** Give 5 milligrams of morphine sulfate intravenously every 4 hours when necessary for moderate to severe pain. **36)** Give 0.25 milligram of digoxin orally every day. **37)** Instill 2 drops of 10% Neo-Synephrine ophthalmic solution in the left eye every 30 minutes for 2 applications. **38)** Give 40 milligrams of Lasix intramuscularly immediately. **39)** Give 4 milligrams of Decadron intravenously twice a day. **40)** 12:00 midnight, 8:00 AM, 4:00 PM **41)** 20 units **42)** subcut: subcutaneous **43)** Give 500 milligrams of Cipro orally every 12 hours. **44)** 8:00 AM, 12:00 noon, 6:00 PM **45)** every 4 hours, as needed for pain **46)** 1 mg **47)** Give 150 milligrams of ranitidine tablets orally twice daily with breakfast and supper. **48)** 1100 **49)** 8

50) Prevention: This error could have been avoided by paying careful attention to the ordered frequency as well as the scheduled times each time a medication was administered.

Review Set 20 from pages 169–172

1) B **2)** D **3)** C **4)** A **5)** E **6)** F **7)** G **8)** 5 mL **9)** oral **10)** A, B, C, D, E, F, G **11)** Filmtab means *film-sealed tablet for extended release of the drug.* **12)** 1 mg/mL **13)** 2 tablets **14)** D **15)** It is a Schedule IV drug. It has limited potential for abuse and is clinically useful. **16)** penicillin G potassium **17)** Pfizerpen **18)** 5,000,000 units per vial; reconstituted to 250,000 units/mL, 500,000 units/mL, or 1,000,000 units/mL **19)** IM or IV **20)** 0049-0520-83 **21)** Pfizer-Roerig **22)** 1 **23)** 1 **24)** 10

Practice Problems—Chapter 8 from pages 174–178

1) 50 mEq per 50 mL (or 1 mEq/mL) **2)** 50 mL **3)** 4,200 mg per 50 mL (or 84 mg/mL) **4)** cefpodoxime proxetil **5)** "Shake bottle to loosen granules. Add approximately half the total amount of distilled water required for constitution (total water = 29 mL). Shake vigorously to wet the granules. Add remaining water and shake vigorously." **6)** Pharmacia **7)** 10 mL **8)** 250 mg per 10 mL (25 mg/mL) **9)** 1 mL **10)** Depo-Provera **11)** medroxyprogesterone acetate **12)** 0009-0626-01 **13)** injection solution **14)** 10 mL **15)** intramuscular **16)** Akrimax Pharmaceuticals, LLC **17)** capsule **18)** 20°–25°C (68°–77°F) **19)** 1 mg per 4 mL (or 0.25 mg/mL) **20)** 1 mg (per 4 mL vial) **21)** I **22)** H **23)** H **24)** H **25)** oral **26)** III **27)** 2% **28)** 2; 20

29) Prevention: This error could have been prevented by carefully comparing the drug label and dosage to the MAR drug and dosage three times while preparing the medication. In this instance, both the incorrect drug and the incorrect dosage strength sent by the pharmacy should have been noted by the nurse. Further, the nurse should have asked for clarification of the order.

30) a) **Prevention:** The nurse should have recognized that the patient was still complaining of signs and symptoms that the medication was ordered to treat. b) If the order was difficult to read, the physician should have been called to clarify the order. Was the dosage of 100 mg a usual dosage for Celexa? The nurse should have consulted a drug guide to ensure that the dosage was appropriate. Also, if the patient wasn't complaining of or diagnosed with depression, the nurse should have questioned why Celexa was ordered.

Review Set 21 from page 197

1) Right patient, right drug, right amount (dosage or dose), right route, right time, right documentation **2)** *NPH insulin 20 units SC daily. NPH insulin 20 units subcut daily* (preferred). The abbreviation SC is included on the ISMP list of error-prone abbreviations and, while not restricted by The Joint Commission, many hospitals have included this on their Do Not Use list. The ISMP recommends "subcut" or "subcutaneously." Know the local policy. **3)** After preparing the drug, just prior to administration **4)** Patient name and date of birth, or patient name and ID number **5)** True **6)** a **7)** Removing medication for more than one patient at a time from the ADC **8)** On the patient identification band and on the medication **9)** Insulin, opiates and narcotics, injectable potassium chloride, and intravenous anticoagulants; high-alert medications **10)** Write the order down on the patient's chart or enter it into the computer record, then read the order back, and finally get confirmation from the prescriber that it is correct. Before administering the medication, verify the safety of the order by consulting a reputable drug reference if you are unfamiliar with the order.

Practice Problems—Chapter 9 from pages 199–200

1) d **2)** False **3)** True **4)** True **5)** True **6)** Patient, drug (or medication), amount (or dosage or dose), route, time, documentation **7)** Prescription, transcription, administration **8)** Upon first contact with the drug, while measuring the dosage, and just prior to administration **9)** 0.75 mg **10)** Write out the order, read it back, and get confirmation from the prescriber. **11)** Any four of these: patient injury; loss of life; increased health care costs; additional technology expenses to prevent error; liability defense; increased length of stay; harm to the nurse involved in regard to his or her personal and professional status, confidence, and practice

12) Prevention: The health care professional originating the order should not have used "q.d." to indicate the frequency of administration. The employee transcribing the order and the nurse signing off on the order both erroneously interpreted the "q.d." notation as "q.i.d." They should have been alert to the risk of errors associated with the use of this notation and should have been especially cautious in transcribing the order correctly.

Section 2—Self-Evaluation from pages 202–207

1) 0.6 g **2)** 4 t **3)** 250,000 units **4)** 0.5 mL **5)** $\frac{1}{2}$ fl oz **6)** four drops **7)** twenty-five hundredths of a milligram

8) one hundred twenty-five micrograms **9)** two tablespoons **10)** twenty-five hundredths of a liter **11)** 0.35; 0.00035

12) 1,200; 1,200,000 **13)** 12; 60 **14)** 150; 0.15 **15)** 3.5 or $3\frac{1}{2}$; 1.59 **16)** 5.62; 2.25 or $2\frac{1}{4}$ **17)** 90; 90,000

18) 11,590; 25.5 or $25\frac{1}{2}$ **19)** 2.5 **20)** 20 **21)** No **22)** 480 **23)** 2335 **24)** 6:44 PM **25)** 0803 **26)** 100.4 **27)** 38.6 **28)** 99

29)

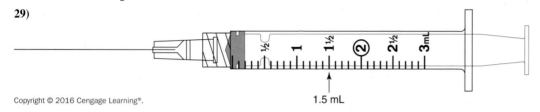

1.5 mL

30)

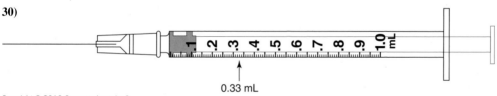

0.33 mL

31)

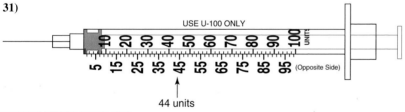

44 units

32)

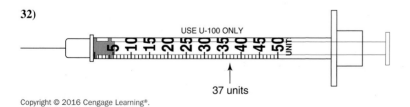

37 units

33)

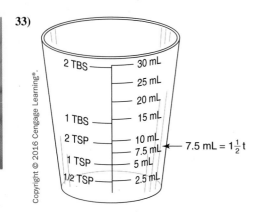

2 TBS — 30 mL
          25 mL
          20 mL
1 TBS — 15 mL
2 TSP — 10 mL
         7.5 mL ← 7.5 mL = $1\frac{1}{2}$ t
1 TSP — 5 mL
1/2 TSP — 2.5 mL

34) nitroglycerin **35)** under the tongue **36)** Give 400 micrograms of nitroglycerin by the sublingual route immediately.

37) 5,000 units per mL **38)** 63323-262-01 **39)** Give 3,750 units of heparin subcutaneously every 8 hours. **40)** neomycin sulfate

41) 125 mg per 5 mL **42)** *heparin 5,000 units subcut daily* **43)** The right patient must receive the right drug, in the right

amount, by the right route, at the right time, with the right documentation. **44)** 250 mcg **45)** c. DOBUTamine – DOPamine

46) 2100 **47)** c. 1.2 mL **48)** acetaminophen (Tylenol); 650 mg; p.o.; q.4h; p.r.n; fever greater than 101°F **49)** b. 0730, 1330,

1830, 2230; e. 7:00 AM, 12:00 PM, 5:00 PM, 10:00 PM

50)

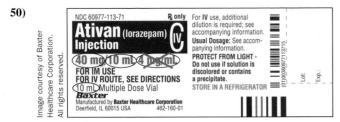

NDC 60977-113-71   ℞ only   For **IV** use, additional
                              dilution is required; see
Ativan (lorazepam)   accompanying information.
Injection   Ⓒⓥ   **Usual Dosage:** See accom-
                              panying information.
40 mg/10 mL (4 mg/mL)   **PROTECT FROM LIGHT -**
FOR IM USE   Do not use if solution is
FOR IV ROUTE, SEE DIRECTIONS discolored or contains
10 mL Multiple Dose Vial   a precipitate.
Baxter   STORE IN A REFRIGERATOR
Manufactured by **Baxter Healthcare Corporation**
Deerfield, IL 60015 USA   462-160-01

Solutions—Section 2—Self-Evaluation

12)
$$\frac{1\,g}{1,000\,mg} \diagdown\!\!\!\diagup \frac{1.2\,g}{X\,mg}$$
$$X = 1,200\ mg$$

$$\frac{1\,mg}{1,000\,mcg} \diagdown\!\!\!\diagup \frac{1,200\,mg}{X\,mcg}$$
$$X = 1,200,000\ mcg$$

15)
$$\frac{16\,oz}{1\,lb} \diagdown\!\!\!\diagup \frac{56\,oz}{X\,lb}$$
$$16X = 56$$
$$\frac{16X}{16} = \frac{56}{16}$$
$$X = 3.5\ lb$$
$$\frac{2.2\,lb}{1\,kg} \diagdown\!\!\!\diagup \frac{3.5\,lb}{X\,kg}$$
$$22X = 3.5$$
$$\frac{2.2X}{2.2} = \frac{3.5}{2.2}$$
$$X = 1.59\ kg$$

20) 2 tabs/dose × 250 mg/tab = 500 mg/dose
500 mg/dose × 4 doses/day = 2,000 mg/day
2,000 mg = 2 g
2 g/day × 10 days = 20 g

21)
$$\frac{16\,oz}{1\,lb} \diagdown\!\!\!\diagup \frac{4\,oz}{X\,lb}$$
$$16X = 4$$
$$\frac{16X}{16} = \frac{4}{16}$$
$$X = 0.25\ lb$$
$$6\ lb\ 4\ oz = 6.25\ lb$$
$$\frac{2.2\,lb}{1\,kg} \diagdown\!\!\!\diagup \frac{6.25\,lb}{X\,kg}$$
$$2.2X = 6.25$$
$$\frac{2.2X}{2.2} = \frac{6.25}{2.2}$$
$$X = 2.84\ kg$$
$$\frac{1,000\,g}{1\,kg} \diagdown\!\!\!\diagup \frac{X\,g}{2.84\,kg}$$
$$X = 2,840\ kg$$

This full-term newborn weighs 2,840 g, which is
more than 2,500 g, the weight considered small for
gestational age.

45) Rationale for correct answer c: The dissimilarities in the LASA drugs are printed in uppercase letters. Rationale for incorrect answers: a) similarities are printed in uppercase letters; b) red type is a recommendation, but all letters are in uppercase; c) underlining is a recommendation, but all letters are in uppercase.

Review Set 22 from pages 228–234

1) 1 **2)** $1\frac{1}{2}$ **3)** $\frac{1}{2}$ **4)** $\frac{1}{2}$ **5)** 3 **6)** 1 **7)** 2 **8)** 2 **9)** I, 2 tablets **10)** H, 2 tablets **11)** G, $1\frac{1}{2}$ tablets **12)** E, 2 tablets **13)** D, 2 tablets **14)** G, 2 tablets **15)** A, 1 capsule **16)** C, 1 tablet

Note: For questions 17 through 30 the *2013 Delmar Nurse's Drug Handbook* was used as reference. Answers may vary slightly if another resource was used.

17) a) Type II diabetes mellitus; b) 0.5 mg, 1 mg, 2 mg tablets; c) 0.5 to 4 mg taken with meals, 16 mg maximum daily dose; d) B and C; e) one 1 mg tablet and one 0.5 mg tablet

18) a) hypertension, edema; b) 12.5 mg capsules, 12.5 mg, 25 mg, 50 mg, 100 mg tablets; c) 12.5 mg to 100 mg per day in one or two daily doses depending on condition; d) A, need to check to see if scored; e) one-half scored tablet

19) a) treat or prevent hypokalemia; b) 8 mEq and 10 mEq extended-release capsules; c) 16 to 24 mEq/day prophylaxis, treatment highly individualized; d) D; e) two 8 mEq capsules

20) a) hypertension; b) 100 mg, 200 mg, 300 mg tablets; c) 100 mg to 400 mg twice a day up to 1,200 to 2,400 mg/day for severe cases; d) F, need to check to see if scored; e) one-half 300 mg scored tablet

21) a) mild to moderate pain, rheumatoid arthritis, and osteoarthritis; b) OTC 100 mg and 200 mg tablets, 200 mg capsules, RX 400 mg, 600 mg, 800 mg tablets; c) 200 mg to 800 mg every 3 to 6 hours depending on condition; d) G; e) two 400 mg tablets

22) a) infections of the skin, urinary tract, and respiratory tract; b) 500 mg capsules, 1 g tablets; c) 1 to 2 g/day in single or 2 divided doses depending on condition; d) E; e) two 500 mg capsules

23) a) moderate to moderately severe pain; b) temporary relief of fever and minor aches and pains; c) 2.5 mg per 325 mg, 2.5 g per 300 mg, 2.5 g per 400 mg, 5 mg per 325 mg, 5 mg per 300 mg, 5 mg per 400 mg, 5 mg per 500 mg, 7.5 mg per 300 mg, 7.5 mg per 325 mg, 7.5 mg per 400 mg, 7.5 mg per 500 mg, 10 mg per 300 mg, 10 mg per 325 mg, 10 mg per 400 mg, 10 mg per 650 mg

24) 1 caplet, capsule, or tablets q.6h as needed for pain; 6 to 12 may be taken per day depending on dosage

25) HYDROcodone—OXYcodone **26)** A **27)** 1200 **28)** 2 **29)** 4,000 mg **30)** No

Solutions—Review Set 22

17) Order: repaglinide 1.5 mg t.i.d. with meals

Convert: order and supply in same unit. No conversion needed.

Think: Look at all the supplied dosages in the drawer. Both 0.5 mg and 1 mg unscored tablets are supplied. Using only 1 mg tablets would require splitting an unscored tablet, which is wrong. Using a combination of dosages will allow administering whole tablets. Use combination of supplied dosages.

Calculate:

1 mg + 0.5 mg = 1.5 mg (verifies estimate)

18) Order: hydrochlorothiazide 12.5 mg p.o. t.i.d.

Supply: 25 mg tablets

Convert: Order and supply in same unit. No conversion needed.

Think: 25 mg scored tablets are supplied; you will need a partial dose of 1 tablet.

Calculate:

$$\frac{25 \text{ mg}}{1 \text{ tablet}} \times \frac{12.5 \text{ mg}}{\text{X tablet(s)}}$$

$$25X = 12.5$$

$$\frac{25X}{25} = \frac{12.5}{25}$$

$$X = \frac{1}{2} \text{ tablet}$$

Discard the leftover $\frac{1}{2}$ tablet in designated container.

19) Order: Klor-Con 16 mEq p.o. daily

Supply: 8 mEq tablets

Convert: Order and supply in same unit, and mEq should not be converted. No conversion needed.

Think: 8 mEq tablets are supplied; you will need more than 1 tablet, or exactly 2 tablets.

Calculate:

$$\frac{8 \text{ mEq}}{1 \text{ tablet}} \times \frac{16 \text{ mEq}}{\text{X tablet(s)}}$$

$$8X = 16$$

$$\frac{8X}{8} = \frac{16}{8}$$

$$X = 2 \text{ tablets}$$

20) Order: Trandate 150 mg p.o. b.i.d.

Supply: 300 mg tablets

Convert: Order and supply in same unit. No conversion needed.

Think: 300 mg scored tablets are supplied; you will need a partial dose of 1 tablet.

Calculate:

$$\frac{300 \text{ mg}}{1 \text{ tablet}} \times \frac{150 \text{ mg}}{\text{X tablet(s)}}$$

$$300X = 150$$

$$\frac{300X}{300} = \frac{150}{300}$$

$$X = \frac{1}{2} \text{ tablet}$$

21) Order: ibuprofen 800 mg p.o. t.i.d.

Supply: 400 mg tablets

Convert: Order and supply in same unit. No conversion needed.

Think: 400 mg tablets are supplied; you will need more than 1 tablet, or exactly 2 tablets.

Calculate:

$$\frac{400 \text{ mg}}{1 \text{ tablet}} \times \frac{800 \text{ mg}}{\text{X tablet(s)}}$$

$$400X = 800$$

$$\frac{400X}{400} = \frac{800}{400}$$

$$X = 2 \text{ tablets}$$

22) Order: cefadroxil monohydrate 1 g p.o. b.i.d.

Supply: 500 mg capsules

Convert: Order expressed in grams and supply is in mg. Conversion needed.

1 g = 1,000 mg (known equivalent)

Think: 500 mg capsules are supplied; you will need more than 1 capsule, or exactly 2 capsules.

Calculate:

$$\frac{500 \text{ mg}}{1 \text{ capsule}} \diagdown \frac{1{,}000 \text{ mg}}{X \text{ capsule(s)}}$$

$$500X = 1{,}000$$

$$\frac{500X}{500} = \frac{1{,}000}{500}$$

$$X = 2 \text{ capsules}$$

30)   Order: oxycodone 5 mg/acetaminophen 325 mg 1 to 2 tablets p.o. q.6h p.r.n., moderate to moderately severe pain

Maximum daily dose of acetaminophen = 4,000 mg

Dose of acetaminophen per tablet = 325 mg

$$\frac{325 \text{ mg}}{1 \text{ tablet}} \diagdown \frac{X \text{ mg}}{2 \text{ tablets}}$$

$$X = 650 \text{ mg (per dose)}$$

$$\frac{650 \text{ mg}}{1 \text{ dose}} \diagdown \frac{X \text{ mg}}{4 \text{ doses}}$$

$$X = 2{,}600 \text{ mg (per day)}$$

2,600 mg per day does not exceed maximum daily dose of 4,000 mg

Review Set 23 from pages 242–250

1) 7.5 **2)** 20 **3)** 2.5 **4)** 1 **5)** 20 **6)** 2 **7)** 7.5 **8)** 3 **9)** 10 **10)** 15 **11)** 7.5 **12)** 5 **13)** 1 **14)** $1\frac{1}{2}$ **15)** 1

Note: For questions 16 through 30 the *2013 Delmar Nurse's Drug Handbook* was used as reference. Answers may vary slightly if another resource was used.

16)   a) broad-spectrum anti-infective, treats variety of infections; b) 250 mg and 500 mg capsules; 125 mg, 187 mg, 250 mg, and 375 mg chewable tablets; 250 mg, 375 mg, and 500 mg extended-release tablets; and 125 mg per 5 mL, 187 mg per 5 mL, 250 mg per 5 mL, and 375 mg per 5 mL strawberry-flavored oral suspension; c) No. Capsules are only in 250 mg and 500 mg doses; d) 250 mg q.8h, may double for severe infections; e) E; f) 4

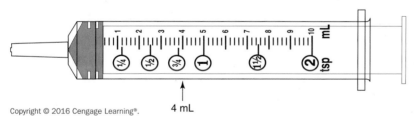

4 mL

17)   a) seizures; b) 250 mg capsules, 250 mg per 5 mL syrup, 100 mg concentrate; c) No; d) 10 to 15 mg/kg/day up to maximum of 60 mg/kg/day; e) B; f) 3

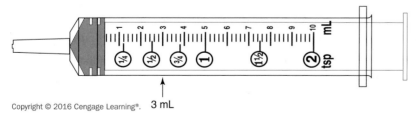

3 mL

18) a) broad-spectrum anti-infective, treats variety of infections; 250 mg and 500 mg capsules; 500 mg and 875 mg tablets; 125 mg, 200 mg, 250 mg, and 400 mg chewable tablets; 775 mg extended-release tablets; 200 mg, 400 mg, and 600 mg tablets for oral suspension; 50 mg/mL, 125 mg per 5 mL, 200 mg per 5 mL, and 250 mg per 5 mL powder for oral suspension; c) Yes; d) 250 mg to 875 mg q.8h to q.12h; e) F; f) 10

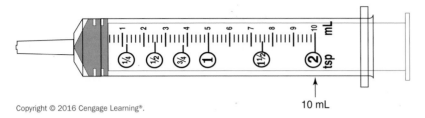

19) a) prevention and treatment of bronchospasm; b) 2 mg and 4 mg tablets, 4 mg and 8 mg extended-release tablets, 2 mg per 5 mL syrup; c) No; d) 2 mg to 4 mg 3 to 4 times a day, maximum 8 mg 4 times a day; e) C; f) 12.5

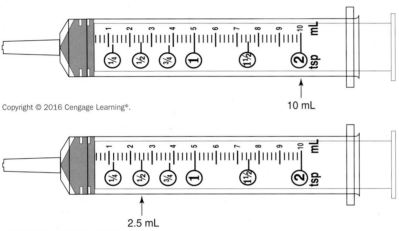

20) a) sedation, anxiety, pruritus; b) 10 mg, 25 mg, and 50 mg tablets, 25 mg, 50 mg, and 100 mg capsules, 10 mg per 5 mL and 25 mg per 5 mL syrup; c) No; d) 50 mg to 100 mg as premedication; e) child; This order for 15 mg is below the recommended adult dosage listed in d. f) D; g) 3

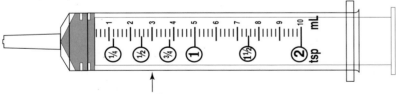

21) a) broad-spectrum anti-infective, treats variety of infections; b) 250 mg and 500 mg capsules; 125 mg, 187 mg, 250 mg, and 375 mg chewable tablets; 250 mg, 375 mg, and 500 mg extended-release tablets; and 125 mg per 5 mL, 187 mg per 5 mL, 250 mg per 5 mL, and 375 mg per 5 mL strawberry-flavored oral suspension; c) No; d) 250 mg q.8h, may double for severe infections; e) child; f) A; g) 4

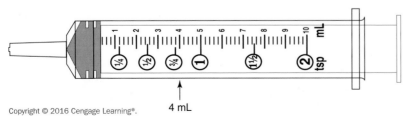

22) a) 10 mL; b) Yes **23)** a) 8 mL; b) Yes **24)** a) 4 mL; b) Yes **25)** a) 7.5 mL; b) No **26)** a) 5 mL; b) Yes

27) a) 10 mL; b) Yes **28)** a) 5 mL; b) Yes **29)** a) 1.5 mL; b) Yes **30)** a) 0.8 mL; b) No

Solutions—Review Set 23

16) Order: cefaclor 300 mg p.o. q.8h

Supply: 375 mg per 5 mL

Convert: Order and supply in same unit. No conversion needed.

Think: Look at all the supplied bottles in refrigerator. There are 2 bottles of cefaclor. The bottle with 375 mg per 5 mL is labeled for Patient #1. 300 mg is a little less than 375 mg, so the amount needed should be a little less than 5 mL.

Calculate:

$$\frac{375 \text{ mg}}{5 \text{ mL}} \times \frac{300 \text{ mg}}{X \text{ mL}}$$

$$375X = 300 \times 5$$

$$375X = 1,500$$

$$\frac{375X}{375} = \frac{1,500}{375}$$

$$X = 4 \text{ mL}$$

17) Order: valproic acid 150 mg p.o. b.i.d.

Supply: 250 mg per 5 mL

Convert: Order and supply in same unit. No conversion needed.

Think: Valproic acid is supplied as 250 mg per 5 mL. 150 mg is a little more than one-half 250 mg, so the amount needed should be a little more than 2.5 mL (a little more than $\frac{1}{2} \times 5$ mL).

$$\frac{250 \text{ mg}}{5 \text{ mL}} \times \frac{150 \text{ mg}}{X \text{ mL}}$$

$$250X = 5 \times 150$$

$$250X = 750$$

$$\frac{250X}{250} = \frac{750}{250}$$

$$X = 3 \text{ mL}$$

18) Order: amoxicillin 500 mg p.o. q.12h

Supply: 250 mg per 5 mL

Convert: Order and supply in same unit. No conversion needed.

Think: Amoxicillin is supplied in 250 mg per 5 mL. 500 mg is twice as much as 250 mg, so the amount needed will be 10 mL (2 × 5 mL).

Calculate:

$$\frac{250 \text{ mg}}{5 \text{ mL}} \times \frac{500 \text{ mg}}{X \text{ mL}}$$

$$250X = 500 \times 5$$

$$250X = 2,500$$

$$\frac{250X}{250} = \frac{2,500}{250}$$

$$X = 10 \text{ mL}$$

19) Order: albuterol sulfate 5 mg p.o. t.i.d.

Supply: 2 mg per 5 mL

Convert: Order and supply in same unit. No conversion needed.

Think: Albuterol is supplied as 2 mg per 5 mL. 5 mg is a little more than twice as large as 2 mg. Will need a little more than 10 mL (a little more than 2 × 5 mL).

Calculate:

$$\frac{2 \text{ mg}}{5 \text{ mL}} \diagdown \frac{5 \text{ mg}}{X \text{ mL}}$$

$$2X = 5 \times 5$$

$$2X = 25$$

$$\frac{2X}{2} = \frac{25}{2}$$

$$X = 12.5 \text{ mL}$$

20) Order: hydroxyzine 15 mg p.o. on call radiology

Supply: 25 mg per 5 mL

Convert: Order and supply in same unit. No conversion needed.

Think: hydroxyzine is supplied in 25 mg per 5 mL. 15 mg is a little more than one-half 25 mg, so the amount needed should be a little more than 2.5 mL (a little more than $\frac{1}{2} \times 5$ mL).

Calculate:

$$\frac{25 \text{ mg}}{5 \text{ mL}} \diagdown \frac{15 \text{ mg}}{X \text{ mL}}$$

$$25X = 15 \times 5$$

$$25X = 75$$

$$\frac{25X}{25} = \frac{75}{25}$$

$$X = 3 \text{ mL}$$

21) Order: cefaclor 100 mg p.o. q.8h

Supply: 125 mg per 5 mL

Convert: Order and supply in same unit. No conversion needed.

Think: Look at all the supplied bottles in refrigerator. There are 2 bottles of cefaclor. The bottle with 125 mg per 5 mL is labeled for Patient #3. 100 mg is a little less than 125 mg, so the amount needed should be a little less than 5 mL.

Calculate:

$$\frac{125 \text{ mg}}{5 \text{ mL}} \diagdown \frac{100 \text{ mg}}{X \text{ mL}}$$

$$125X = 100 \times 5$$

$$125X = 500$$

$$\frac{125X}{125} = \frac{500}{125}$$

$$X = 4 \text{ mL}$$

22) Order: metoclopramide 10 mg p.o. 30 min a.c. and at bedtime

Supply: 5 mg per 5 mL; syringe filled to 10 mL

Convert: Order and supply in same unit. No conversion needed.

Think: 10 mg is twice as large as 5 mg, so the 10 mL amount supplied (2×5 mL) appears to be correct.

Calculate:

$$\frac{5 \text{ mg}}{5 \text{ mL}} \diagdown \frac{10 \text{ mg}}{X \text{ mL}}$$

$$5X = 10 \times 5$$

$$5X = 50$$

$$\frac{5X}{5} = \frac{50}{5}$$

$$X = 10 \text{ mL (verifies pharmacy-supplied dose)}$$

25) Order: furosemide 60 mg p.o. daily

Supply: 40 mg per 5 mL; syringe filled to 8 mL

Convert: Order and supply in same unit. No conversion needed.

Think: 60 mg is $1\frac{1}{2}$ times 40 mg, so the amount needed should be 7.5 mL (1.5 × 5 mL). It appears that the pharmacy supplied too large of a dose.

Calculate:

$$\frac{40 \text{ mg}}{5 \text{ mL}} \diagdown\!\!\!\diagup \frac{60 \text{ mg}}{\text{X mL}}$$

$$40\text{X} = 60 \times 5$$

$$40\text{X} = 300$$

$$\frac{40\text{X}}{40} = \frac{300}{40}$$

$$\text{X} = 7.5 \text{ mL (verifies pharmacy-supplied dose is too large)}$$

Notify pharmacy. Complete medication variance.

28) Order: digoxin 250 mcg p.o. daily

Supply: 0.05 mg per mL; syringe filled to 5 mL

Convert: Order is expressed in mcg, but supply is in mg. Conversion needed. It is best to work without zeros.

1 mg = 1,000 mcg (known equivalent)

$$\frac{1 \text{ mg}}{1,000 \text{ mcg}} \diagdown\!\!\!\diagup \frac{0.05 \text{ mg}}{\text{X mcg}}$$

$$\text{X} = 0.05 \times 1,000$$

$$\text{X} = 50 \text{ mcg}$$

Supply: 50 mcg/mL

Think: 250 mcg is five times 50 mcg, so the amount needed should be 5 mL (5 × 1 mL).

Calculate:

$$\frac{50 \text{ mcg}}{1 \text{ mL}} \diagdown\!\!\!\diagup \frac{250 \text{ mcg}}{\text{X mL}}$$

$$50\text{X} = 250$$

$$\frac{50\text{X}}{50} = \frac{250}{50}$$

$$\text{X} = 5 \text{ mL (verifies pharmacy-supplied dose)}$$

30) Order: acetaminophen 80 mg p.o. q.6h times four doses today

Supply: 100 mg/mL; syringe filled to 1 mL

Convert: Order and supply in same unit. No conversion needed.

Think: 80 mg is a little less than 100 mg, so the amount needed should be a little less than 1 mL. It appears that the pharmacy supplied too large of a dose.

Calculate:

$$\frac{100 \text{ mg}}{1 \text{ mL}} \diagdown\!\!\!\diagup \frac{80 \text{ mg}}{\text{X mL}}$$

$$100\text{X} = 80$$

$$\frac{100\text{X}}{100} = \frac{80}{100}$$

$$\text{X} = 0.8 \text{ mL (verifies pharmacy-supplied dose is too large)}$$

Notify pharmacy. Complete medication variance.

Practice Problems—Chapter 10 from pages 254–264

1) $\frac{1}{2}$ **2)** 2 **3)** $\frac{1}{2}$ **4)** 2.5 **5)** 10 **6)** 2 **7)** 8 **8)** $1\frac{1}{2}$ **9)** 500 mg; 2 **10)** $\frac{1}{2}$ **11)** $1\frac{1}{2}$ **12)** 1 **13)** $1\frac{1}{2}$ **14)** 2 **15)** 2 **16)** 5; $1\frac{1}{2}$ **17)** 7.5

18) 2 **19)** 2 **20)** 1.5 **21)** 0.75; 1 **22)** $\frac{1}{2}$ **23)** 2 **24)** 2 **25)** 2 **26)** 2 **27)** 15 mg and 30 mg; one of each **28)** 2.4 **29)** 2.5

30) 3 **31)** D; 2 tablets **32)** A; 1 capsule **33)** C; 1 tablet **34)** B; 1 capsule **35)** I; 2 tablets **36)** G; 2 tablets **37)** F; 2 tablets

38) H; 1 tablet **39)** M; 2 tablets **40)** L; 2 tablets **41)** E; 30 mL **42)** K; 1 tablet **43)** I; 2 tablets **44)** N; 2 tablets

45) O; 1 tablet **46)** Q; 2 tablets **47)** P; 1 capsule **48)** J; 1 tablet **49)** R; 2 tablets

50) Prevention: This medication error could have been prevented if the nurse had more carefully read the physician's order and the medication label. The doctor's order misled the nurse by noting the volume first and then the drug dosage. If confused by the order, the nurse should have clarified the intent with the physician. By focusing on the volume, the nurse failed to follow the steps in dosage calculation. Had the nurse noted 250 mg as the desired dosage and the supply (or on-hand) dosage as 125 mg per 5 mL, the correct amount to be administered would have been clear. Slow down and take time to compare the order with the labels. Calculate each dose carefully before preparing and administering both solid- and liquid-form medications.

Solutions—Practice Problems—Chapter 10

1)   Order: tolbutamide 250 mg p.o. b.i.d.

Supply: tolbutamide 0.5 g scored tablets

Convert: Order expressed in grams and supply is in mg. Conversion needed. Convert supply to avoid use of decimals.

1 g = 1,000 mg (known equivalent)

$$\frac{1 \text{ g}}{1,000 \text{ mg}} \diagup\!\!\!\!\diagdown \frac{0.5 \text{ g}}{X \text{ mg}}$$

$$X = 0.5 \times 1,000$$

$$X = 500 \text{ mg}$$

Supply: 500 mg scored tablets

Think: 500 mg scored tablets are supplied. You will need less than 1 tablet, or exactly $\frac{1}{2}$ tablet.

Calculate:

$$\frac{500 \text{ mg}}{1 \text{ tablet}} \diagdown\!\!\!\!\diagup \frac{250 \text{ mg}}{X \text{ tablet(s)}}$$

$$500X = 250$$

$$\frac{500X}{500} = \frac{250}{500}$$

$$X = \frac{1}{2} \text{ tablet}$$

Discard the leftover $\frac{1}{2}$ tablet into a designated container.

9)   Order: acetaminophen 1 g p.o. q.6h p.r.n., pain

Supply: 325 mg unscored and 500 mg unscored tablets

Convert: Order expressed in grams and supply is in mg. Conversion needed. Convert supply to avoid use of decimals.

1 g = 1,000 mg (known equivalent)

Think: You must give whole tablets. The equivalent ordered amount of 1,000 mg is a multiple of 500 mg but not of 325 mg. You will need more than one 500 mg tablet, or exactly two tablets.

Calculate:

$$\frac{500 \text{ mg}}{1 \text{ tablet}} \diagdown\!\!\!\!\diagup \frac{1,000 \text{ mg}}{X \text{ tablet(s)}}$$

$$500X = 1,000$$

$$\frac{500X}{500} = \frac{1,000}{500}$$

$$X = 2 \text{ tablets}$$

24)   Order: erythromycin stearate 0.5 g p.o. q.12h

Supply: 250 mg unscored tablets

Convert: Order expressed in grams and supply is in mg. Conversion needed.

1 g = 1,000 mg (known equivalent)

$$\frac{1 \text{ g}}{1,000 \text{ mg}} \diagup\!\!\!\!\diagdown \frac{0.5 \text{ g}}{X \text{ mg}}$$

$$X = 0.5 \times 1,000$$

$$X = 500 \text{ mg}$$

Think: You must give whole tablets. You will need more than 1 tablet, or exactly 2 tablets.

Calculate:

$$\frac{250 \text{ mg}}{1 \text{ tablet}} \diagup\!\!\!\!\diagdown \frac{500 \text{ mg}}{X \text{ tablet(s)}}$$

$$250X = 500$$

$$\frac{250X}{250} = \frac{500}{250}$$

$$X = 2 \text{ tablets}$$

27)   Order: phenobarbital 45 mg p.o. daily

Supply: 15 mg scored, 30 mg scored, 60 mg scored tablets

Convert: No conversion needed.

Think: You will need more than 30 mg but less than 60 mg. Even though tablets are scored, it is best to use whole

tablets whenever possible. Using a combination of 15 mg and 30 mg tablets will give the desired 45 mg dose.

Calculate: 15 mg + 30 mg = 45 mg

Select: One 15 mg tablet and one 30 mg tablet for 45 mg total dosage.

29)   Order: acetaminophen 80 mg p.o. q.4h p.r.n., pain or temperature greater than 102° F

Supply: acetaminophen 160 mg/t

Convert: Equipment chosen is measured in mL and supply volume is in teaspoons. Conversion needed.

1 t = 5 mL (known equivalent)

Supply: 160 mg/5 mL

Think: 80 mg is half of 160 mg. You will need $\frac{1}{2}$ of 5 mL, or exactly 2.5 mL.

Calculate:

$$\frac{160 \text{ mg}}{5 \text{ mL}} \diagup\!\!\!\!\diagdown \frac{80 \text{ mg}}{X \text{ mL}}$$

$$160X = 80 \times 5$$

$$160X = 400$$

$$\frac{160X}{160} = \frac{400}{160}$$

$$X = 2.5 \text{ mL}$$

Review Set 24 from pages 280–289

Note to student: *2013 Delmar Nurse's Drug Handbook* was used as reference. Answers may vary slightly if another
resource was used.

1)   0.75 mL

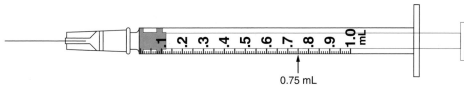

0.75 mL

2)   1 mL

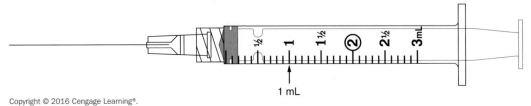

3)   1.7 mL

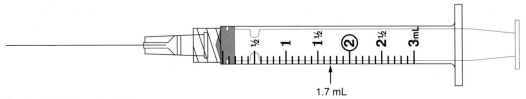

4)   0.63 mL

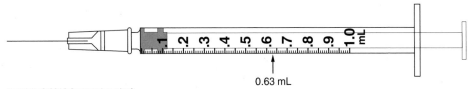

5)   0.2 mL

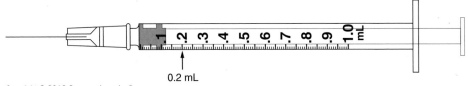

6)   1.7 mL

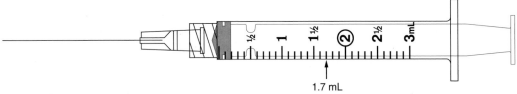

7)   a) treatment of megaloblastic anemias due to folic acid deficiency; b) 5,000 mcg/mL (5 mg/mL); c) deep subcut, IM, IV; d) 250 to 1,000 mcg/day; e) A; f) 0.2 mL;

     g)

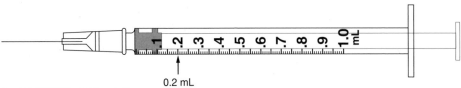

8) a) secondary amenorrhea, abnormal endometrial bleeding, adjunctive treatment for endometrial or renal cancer, contraceptive; b) 104 mg per 0.65 mL, 150 mg/mL, 400 mg/mL; c) subcut, IM; d) 400 mg to 1,000 mg/week, 150 mg q.3 months, 104 mg q.3 months; e) C; f) 2.5 mL;

g)

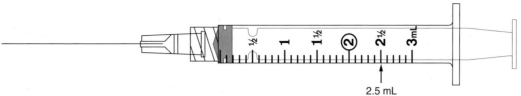

2.5 mL

9) a) nausea and vomiting postoperatively or due to chemotherapy; b) 2 mg/mL, 32 mg per 50 mL (premixed); c) IM, IV; d) 4 mg IV undiluted over 2 to 5 min, 32 mg single dose over 15 min prior to chemotherapy; e) B; f) 1.5 mL;

g)

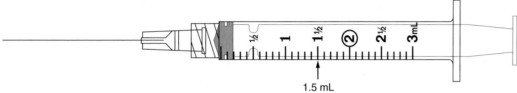

1.5 mL

10) a) serious infections; b) 10 mg/mL, 40 mg/mL; c) IM, IV; d) 1 mg/kg q.8h up to 5 mg/kg/day for life-threatening infection; e) C; f) 1.8 mL;

g)

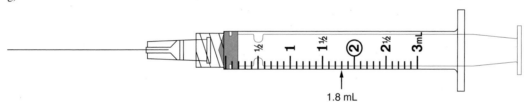

1.8 mL

11) a) serious infections; b) 150 mg/mL; c) IM, IV; d) 600 to 1,200 mg per day in 2 to 4 divided doses; e) A; f) 4 mL;

g)

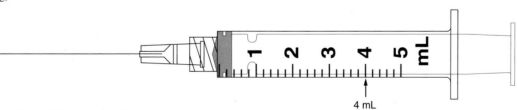

4 mL

12) a) moderate to severe pain; b) 10 mg/mL, 20 mg/mL; c) subcut, IM, IV; d) 10 mg q.3 to 6h single dose not to exceed 20 mg; e) B; f) 0.25 mL;

g)

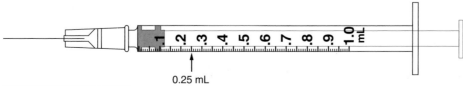

0.25 mL

13) a) prevention and treatment of bronchospasm associated with asthma, bronchitis, and emphysema, preterm labor (investigational); b) 1 mg/mL; c) subcut only; d) 0.25 mg subcut, repeat q.15 to 30 min as needed, do not exceed 0.5 mg in 4 h; e) B; f) 0.25 mL;

g)

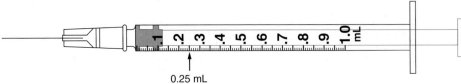

0.25 mL

14) a) treatment of edema associated with CHF, nephrotic syndrome, hepatic disease, and acute pulmonary edema; b) 0.25 mg/mL; c) IM, IV; d) 0.5 mg to 1 mg, may repeat q.3 to 4 h, do not exceed 10 mg/day; e) E; f) 2 mL;

g)

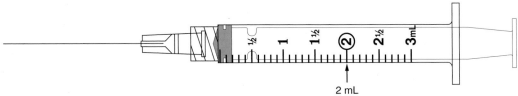

2 mL

15) a) treatment of duodenal and gastric ulcers, hypersecretory conditions, gastroesophageal reflux; b) 1 mg/mL (premixed), 25 mg/mL; c) IM, IV; d) 50 mg q.6 to 8h, dilute 50 mg to a concentration no greater than 2.5 mg/mL; e) D; f) 1.4 mL;

g)

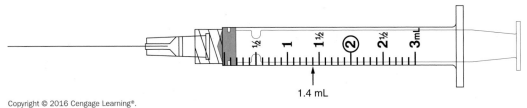

1.4 mL

16) a) treatment of seizures; b) 100 mg/mL; c) IV; d) 10 to 15 mg/kg/day, increase as needed, maximum 60 mg/kg/day; e) A; f) 4.2 mL;

g)

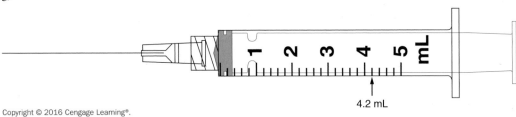

4.2 mL

17) a) oral – hypertension, angina pectoris, and migraine headaches, IV – life-threatening arrhythmias; b) 1 mg/mL; c) IV; d) 1 to 3 mg not to exceed 1 mg per minute; e) F; f) 2 mL;

g)

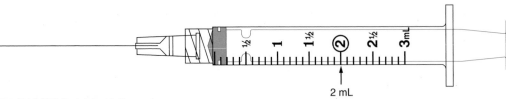

2 mL

18) a) life-threatening ventricular arrhythmias; b) 50 mg/mL, 150 mg per 3 mL, 450 mg per 9 mL, 900 mg per 18 mL;

c) IV; d) initial loading dose 150 mg over 10 minutes then 360 mg over 6 h; e) G; f) 7.2 mL;

g)

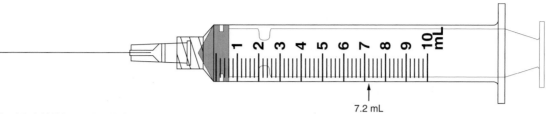

7.2 mL

19) a) short-term prevention and treatment of generalized seizures and status epilepticus; b) 50 mg/mL, 75 mg/mL;

c) IM, IV; d) maintenance 4 to 6 mg/kg/day; e) H; f) 5.6 mL;

g)

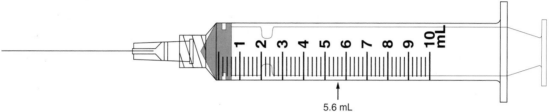

5.6 mL

20) a) hypertension; b) 5 mg/mL; c) IV; d) initially, 20 mg (or 0.25 mg/kg) by slow intravenous injection over a 2-minute period; e) C; f) 3.6 mL;

g)

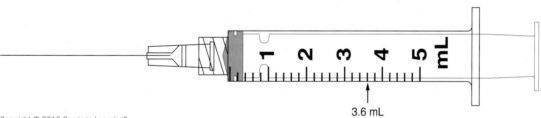

3.6 mL

Solutions Review Set 24

1) Order: Dilaudid 1.5 mg IM q.6h p.r.n., severe pain

Supply: 2 mg/mL

Convert: Order and supply in same unit.

No conversion needed.

Think: 1.5 mg is less than 2 mg but not less than half.

Amount needed will be less than 1 mL but more than half of a mL.

Calculate: $\dfrac{2 \text{ mg}}{1 \text{ mL}} \searrow\nearrow \dfrac{1.5 \text{ mg}}{X \text{ mL}}$

$$2X = 1.5$$

$$\frac{2X}{2} = \frac{1.5}{2}$$

$$X = 0.75 \text{ mL}$$

2) Order: digoxin 0.25 mg IV daily

Supply: 500 mcg/2 mL

Convert: Order expressed in mg, and supply is in mcg. Conversion needed.

Equivalent: 1 mg = 1,000 mcg

$\dfrac{1 \text{ mg}}{1,000 \text{ mcg}} \searrow\nearrow \dfrac{0.25 \text{ mg}}{X \text{ mcg}}$

$$X = 250 \text{ mcg}$$

Order: digoxin 250 mcg

Think: 250 mcg is less than 500 mcg, or exactly half.

Amount needed will be half of 2 mL or 1 mL.

Calculate: $\dfrac{500 \text{ mcg}}{2 \text{ mL}} \diagdown\diagup \dfrac{250 \text{ mcg}}{\text{X mL}}$

$$500\text{X} = 500$$
$$\frac{500\text{X}}{500} = \frac{500}{500}$$
$$\text{X} = 1 \text{ mL}$$

3) Order: ketorolac 25 mg IM q.6h p.r.n., severe pain

Supply: 15 mg/mL

Convert: Order and supply in same unit. No conversion needed.

Think: 25 mg is more than 15 mg, but not twice as much. Amount needed will be more than 1 mL, but less than 2 mL.

Calculate: $\dfrac{15 \text{ mg}}{1 \text{ mL}} \diagdown\diagup \dfrac{25 \text{ mg}}{\text{X mL}}$

$$15\text{X} = 25$$
$$\frac{15\text{X}}{15} = \frac{25}{15}$$
$$\text{X} = 1.66 \text{ mL}$$
$$= 1.7 \text{ mL (verifies estimate)}$$

4) Order: Robinul 125 mcg IM stat

Supply: 0.2 mg/mL

Convert: Order expressed in mcg, and supply is in mg. Conversion needed.

Equivalent: 1 mg = 1,000 mcg

$\dfrac{1 \text{ mg}}{1,000 \text{ mcg}} \diagdown\diagup \dfrac{0.2 \text{ mg}}{\text{X mcg}}$

$$\text{X} = 200 \text{ mcg}$$

Supply: 200 mcg/mL

Think: 125 mcg is less than 200 mcg, but not less than half. Amount needed will be less than 1 mL, but more than half of a mL.

Calculate: $\dfrac{200 \text{ mcg}}{1 \text{ mL}} \diagdown\diagup \dfrac{125 \text{ mcg}}{\text{X mL}}$

$$200\text{X} = 125$$
$$\frac{200\text{X}}{200} = \frac{125}{200}$$
$$\text{X} = 0.625 \text{ mL}$$
$$= 0.63 \text{ mL (verifies estimate)}$$

5) Order: diphenhydramine 10 mg IM q.6h p.r.n., itching

Supply: 50 mg/mL

Convert: Order and supply in same unit. No conversion needed.

Think: 10 mg is quite a bit smaller than 50 mg. Amount needed will be quite a bit less than 1 mL.

Calculate: $\dfrac{50 \text{ mg}}{1 \text{ mL}} \diagdown\diagup \dfrac{10 \text{ mg}}{\text{X mL}}$

$$50\text{X} = 10$$
$$\frac{50\text{X}}{50} = \frac{10}{50}$$
$$\text{X} = 0.2 \text{ mL (verifies estimate)}$$

6) Order: Ativan 3.4 mg IM × 1 dose pre-op

Supply: 2 mg/mL

Convert: Order and supply in same unit. No conversion needed.

Think: 3.4 mg is more than 2 mg, but not twice as much. Amount needed will be more than 1 mL, but less than 2 mL.

Calculate: $\dfrac{2 \text{ mg}}{1 \text{ mL}} \diagdown\diagup \dfrac{3.4 \text{ mg}}{\text{X mL}}$

$$2\text{X} = 3.4$$
$$\frac{2\text{X}}{2} = \frac{3.4}{2}$$
$$\text{X} = 1.7 \text{ mL (verifies estimate)}$$

7) Order: folic acid 1,000 mcg IM daily for 10 days

Supply: 5 mg/mL

Convert: Order expressed in mcg, and supply is in mg. Conversion needed.

Equivalent: 1 mg = 1,000 mcg

$\dfrac{1 \text{ mg}}{1,000 \text{ mcg}} \diagdown\diagup \dfrac{5 \text{ mg}}{\text{X mcg}}$

$$\text{X} = 5,000 \text{ mcg}$$

Supply: 5,000 mcg/mL

Think: 1,000 mcg is quite a bit smaller than 5,000 mg. Amount needed will be quite less than 1 mL.

Calculate: $\dfrac{5,000 \text{ mcg}}{1 \text{ mL}} \diagdown\diagup \dfrac{1,000 \text{ mcg}}{\text{X mL}}$

$$5,000\text{X} = 1,000$$
$$\frac{5,000\text{X}}{5,000} = \frac{1,000}{5,000}$$
$$\text{X} = 0.2 \text{ mL (verifies estimate)}$$

8) Order: medroxyprogesterone acetate 1 g IM stat

Supply: 400 mg/mL

Convert: 1 g = 1,000 mg (known equivalent)

Order: medroxyprogesterone acetate 1,000 mg

Think: 1,000 mg is more than twice as large as 400 mg, but less than 3 times. Amount needed will be more than 2 mL, but less than 3 mL.

Calculate: $\dfrac{400 \text{ mg}}{1 \text{ mL}} \diagdown\diagup \dfrac{1,000 \text{ mg}}{\text{X mL}}$

$$400\text{X} = 1,000$$
$$\frac{400\text{X}}{400} = \frac{1,000}{400}$$
$$\text{X} = 2.5 \text{ mL (verifies estimate)}$$

10) Order: gentamicin 70 mg IV PB q.8h

Supply: 80 mg/2 mL

Convert: Order and supply in same unit. No conversion needed.

Think: 70 mg is slightly less than 80 mg. Amount needed will be slightly less than 2 mL.

Calculate: $\dfrac{80\ mg}{2\ mL} \bowtie \dfrac{70\ mg}{X\ mL}$

$$80X = 140$$
$$\dfrac{80X}{80} = \dfrac{140}{80}$$
$$X = 1.75\ mL$$
$$= 1.8\ mL\ (verifies\ estimate)$$

16) Order: valproate sodium 420 mg IV PB q.12 h

Supply: 500 mg/5 mL

Convert: Order and supply in same unit. No conversion needed.

Think: 420 mg is slightly less than 500 mg. Amount needed will be slightly less than 5 mL.

Calculate: $\dfrac{500\ mg}{5\ mL} \bowtie \dfrac{420\ mg}{X\ mL}$

$$500X = 2,100$$
$$\dfrac{500X}{500} = \dfrac{2,100}{500}$$
$$X = 4.2\ mL$$

20) Order: labetalol 18 mg IV bolus stat

Supply: 5 mg/mL in 20 mL vial

Convert: Order and supply in same unit. No conversion needed.

Think: 18 mg is more than 3 times 5 mg, and closer to but less than 4 times 5 mg. Needed amount will be more than 3 times 1 mL (or more than 3 mL), but less than 4 times 1 mL (or less than 4 mL).

Calculate: $\dfrac{5\ mg}{1\ mL} \bowtie \dfrac{18\ mg}{X\ mL}$

$$5X = 18$$
$$\dfrac{5X}{5} = \dfrac{18}{5}$$
$$X = 3.6\ mL$$

Review Set 25 from pages 318–325

1) A **2)** C **3)** D **4)** B, D **5)** Humulin R, regular, short acting, 100 units/mL, U-100 insulin syringe **6)** Novolin N, NPH, intermediate acting, 100 units/mL, U-100 insulin syringe **7)** NovoLog, aspart, rapid acting, 100 units/mL, U-100 insulin syringe **8)** Humalog, lispro, rapid acting, 100 units/mL, U-100 insulin syringe **9)** Humulin R, regular, short acting, 500 units/mL, 1 mL syringe **10)** Lantus, glargine, long acting, 100 units/mL, U-100 insulin syringe **11)** standard, dual-scale 100 units/mL U-100 insulin syringe; Lo-Dose, 50 units/0.5 mL U-100 insulin syringe; Lo-Dose, 30 units/0.3 mL U-100 insulin syringe **12)** Lo-Dose, 50-unit U-100 insulin syringe **13)** 0.6 **14)** 0.25 **15)** False **16)** 20 **17)** 30,000 **18)** 6,400 **19)** No; order is for 67 units and syringe amount is 68 units **20)** No; order is for Humulin R regular U-100 insulin and drug supplied is Humulin R regular U-500 insulin **21)** Yes **22)** Yes

23)

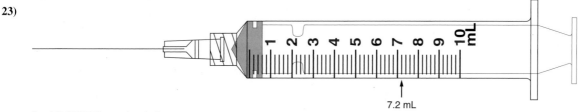

7.2 mL

24)

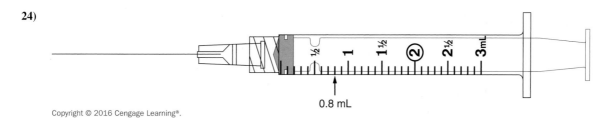

0.8 mL

25)

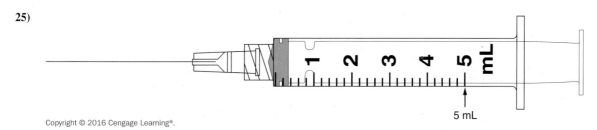

5 mL

26)

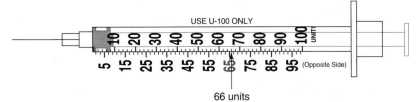

66 units

27)

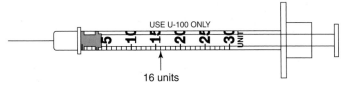

16 units

28)

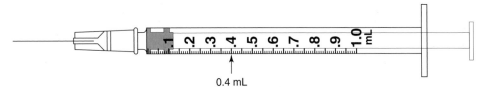

0.4 mL

29)

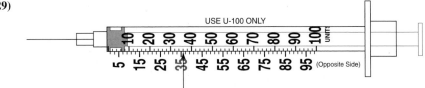

36-unit mark (180 units of U-500 insulin)

30)

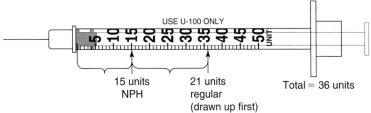

15 units   21 units   Total = 36 units
NPH   regular
             (drawn up first)

31)

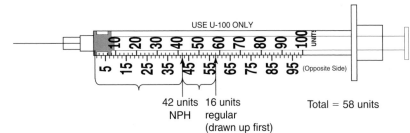

42 units 16 units   Total = 58 units
NPH   regular
          (drawn up first)

32)

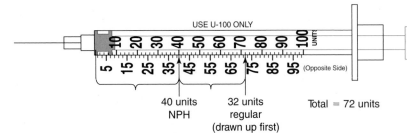

40 units   32 units   Total = 72 units
NPH   regular
                (drawn up first)

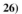

33)

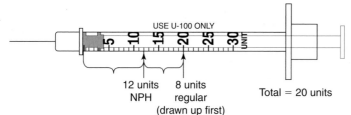

USE U-100 ONLY

12 units NPH   8 units regular (drawn up first)

Total = 20 units

Copyright © 2016 Cengage Learning®.

34) 5

35) 39

36) Before meals (before insulin administration)

37) Blood glucose levels of 160–400 mg/dL

38) Administer 4 units of insulin glulisine (Apidra) U-100 insulin.

39) None; do not administer insulin.

40) Contact the physician immediately for further instructions.

Solutions—Review Set 25

13) Recall that U-100 = 100 units per mL

$$\frac{100 \text{ units}}{1 \text{ mL}} \diagdown\!\!\!\!\diagup \frac{60 \text{ units}}{X \text{ mL}}$$

$$100X = 60$$

$$\frac{100X}{100} = \frac{60}{100}$$

$$X = 0.6 \text{ mL}$$

28) Recall that U-500 = 500 units/mL

$$\frac{500 \text{ units}}{1 \text{ mL}} \diagdown\!\!\!\!\diagup \frac{200 \text{ units}}{X \text{ mL}}$$

$$500X = 200$$

$$\frac{500X}{500} = \frac{200}{500}$$

$$X = 0.4 \text{ mL}$$

Measure 0.4 mL of U-500 insulin in a 1 mL syringe to administer 200 units.

29) U-500 insulin is five times more concentrated than U-100 insulin. To use a U-100 insulin syringe for the more concentrated U-500 insulin, you should divide the units ordered by 5.

$$\frac{180 \text{ units}}{5} = 36\text{-unit mark on U-100 insulin syringe} =$$

180 units of U-500 insulin

You can also use ratio-proportion:

$$\frac{180 \text{ units}}{500 \text{ units}} \diagdown\!\!\!\!\diagup \frac{X \text{ units}}{100 \text{ units}}$$

$$500X = 18,000$$

$$\frac{500X}{500} = \frac{18,000}{500}$$

$$X = 36\text{-unit mark on U-100 insulin syringe} =$$
180 units of U-500 insulin

Teach your patient to draw up U-500 insulin to the 36-unit mark in a U-100 insulin syringe to provide 180 units of U-500 insulin.

Practice Problems—Chapter 11 from pages 328–336

1) 0.4; 1 mL **2)** 1.5; 3 mL **3)** 2.4; 3 mL **4)** 0.6; 1 mL or 3 mL **5)** 2; 3 mL **6)** 10; 10 mL **7)** 0.8; 1 mL or 3 mL

8) 1; 3 mL **9)** 1; 3 mL **10)** 5.6; 10 mL **11)** 1.5; 3 mL **12)** 0.6; 1 mL or 3 mL **13)** 0.6; 1 mL or 3 mL **14)** 1.9; 3 mL

15) 0.6; 1 mL or 3 mL **16)** 0.75; 1 mL **17)** 0.67; 1 mL **18)** 1; 3 mL **19)** 0.3; 1 mL **20)** 1.6; 3 mL **21)** 0.75; 1 mL; The route is IM; the needle may need to be changed to an appropriate gauge and length. **22)** 0.5; 1 mL or 3 mL

23) 0.7; 1 mL or 3 mL **24)** 0.8; 1 mL or 3 mL **25)** 1.3; 3 mL **26)** 1.6; 3 mL **27)** 6; 10 mL **28)** 0.8; 1 mL or 3 mL

29) 1.5; 3 mL **30)** 1.6; 3 mL **31)** 0.7; 1 mL or 3 mL **32)** 0.5; 1 mL or 3 mL **33)** 10; 10 mL **34)** 16; 30-unit Lo-Dose U-100 insulin **35)** 25; 50-unit Lo-Dose U-100 insulin **36)** 5.8; 10 mL

37) 1.5; F

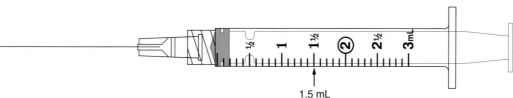

1.5 mL

Copyright © 2016 Cengage Learning®.

38) 1.3; B

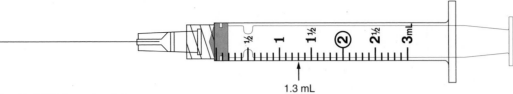

1.3 mL

39) 0.4; H

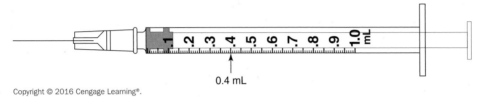

0.4 mL

40) 1.5; A

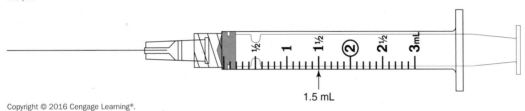

1.5 mL

41) 0.5; J

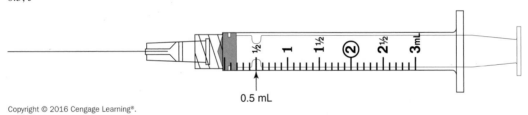

0.5 mL

42) 22; I

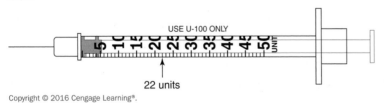

22 units

43) 0.8; C

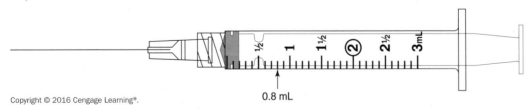

0.8 mL

44) 0.6; G

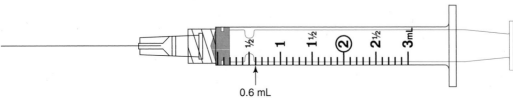

0.6 mL

45)   5; L

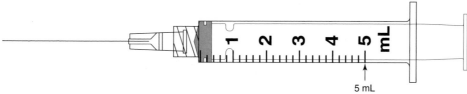

5 mL

46)   0.5; K

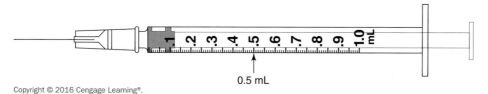

0.5 mL

47)   86; D and M

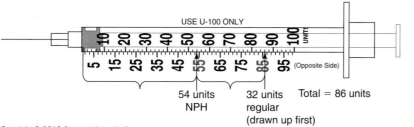

USE U-100 ONLY

(Opposite Side)

54 units NPH   32 units regular (drawn up first)   Total = 86 units

48)   46; E

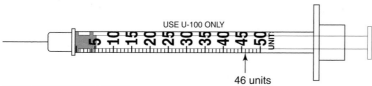

USE U-100 ONLY

46 units

49)   **Prevention:** This error could have been avoided had the nurse been more careful checking the label of the insulin vial and comparing the label to the order. The nurse should have checked the label three times. In addition, the nurse should have asked another nurse to perform an independent verification after each insulin was drawn up, as required. Such hospital policies and procedures are written to protect the patient and the nurse.

50)   **Prevention:** This insulin error should never occur. It is obvious that the nurse did not use Step 2 of the Three-Step Approach. The nurse did not stop to think of the reasonable dosage. If so, the nurse would have realized that the supply dosage of U-100 insulin is 100 units/mL, not 10 units/mL.

  If you are unsure of what you are doing, you need to ask before you act. Insulin should only be given in an insulin syringe. The likelihood of the nurse needing to give insulin in a tuberculin syringe because an insulin syringe is unavailable is almost nonexistent today. The nurse chose the incorrect syringe. Whenever you are in doubt, you should ask for help. Further, if the nurse had asked another nurse to perform an independent verification as required, the error could have been found before the patient received the wrong dosage of insulin. After giving the insulin, it is too late to rectify the error.

Solutions—Practice Problems—Chapter 11

3) Order: digoxin 0.6 mg slow IV push stat

Supply: 500 mcg per 2 mL

Convert: Order expressed in mg, and supply is

in mcg. Conversion needed.

Equivalent: 1 mg = 1,000 mcg

$$\frac{1 \text{ mg}}{1,000 \text{ mcg}} \diagdown \frac{0.6 \text{ mg}}{X \text{ mcg}}$$

$$X = 600 \text{ mcg}$$

Order: digoxin 600 mcg

Calculate: $\frac{500 \text{ mcg}}{2 \text{ mL}} \diagdown \frac{600 \text{ mcg}}{X \text{ mL}}$

$$500X = 1,200$$

$$\frac{500X}{500} = \frac{1,200}{500}$$

$$X = 2.4 \text{ mL}$$

19) Order: hydromorphone 3 mg slow IV push

(over 5–10 min) q.4h p.r.n., severe pain

Supply: 10 mg/mL

Convert: Order and supply in same unit. No conversion

needed.

Calculate: $\frac{10 \text{ mg}}{1 \text{ mL}} \diagdown \frac{3 \text{ mg}}{X \text{ mL}}$

$$10X = 3$$

$$\frac{10X}{10} = \frac{3}{10}$$

$$X = 0.3 \text{ mL}$$

26) Order: digoxin 0.4 mg IV stat

Supply: 500 mcg per 2 mL

Convert: Order expressed in mg, and supply in mcg.

Conversion needed.

Equivalent: 1 mg = 1,000 mcg

$$\frac{1 \text{ mg}}{1,000 \text{ mcg}} \diagdown \frac{0.4 \text{ mg}}{X \text{ mcg}}$$

$$X = 400 \text{ mcg}$$

Order: digoxin 400 mcg

Calculate: $\frac{500 \text{ mcg}}{2 \text{ mL}} \diagdown \frac{400 \text{ mcg}}{X \text{ mL}}$

$$500X = 800$$

$$\frac{500X}{500} = \frac{800}{500}$$

$$X = 1.6 \text{ mL}$$

36) Order: heparin 5,800 units IV bolus ASAP prior to

initiation of continuous heparin infusion

Supply: 1,000 units/mL

Convert: Order and supply in same unit. No conversion

needed.

Calculate: $\frac{1,000 \text{ units}}{1 \text{ mL}} \diagdown \frac{5,800 \text{ units}}{X \text{ mL}}$

$$1,000X = 5,800$$

$$\frac{1,000X}{1,000} = \frac{5,800}{1,000}$$

$$X = 5.8 \text{ mL}$$

45) Order: diltiazem 25 mg slow IV push (over 2 min) stat

Supply: 5 mg/mL

Convert: Order and supply in same unit. No conversion

needed.

Calculate: $\frac{5 \text{ mg}}{1 \text{ mL}} \diagdown \frac{25 \text{ mg}}{X \text{ mL}}$

$$5X = 25$$

$$\frac{5X}{5} = \frac{25}{5}$$

$$X = 5 \text{ mL}$$

46) Order: digoxin 0.125 mg IV daily × 7 days

Supply: 500 mcg/2 mL

Convert: Order expressed in mg, and supply in mcg.

Conversion needed.

Equivalent: 1 mg = 1,000 mcg

$$\frac{1 \text{ mg}}{1,000 \text{ mcg}} \diagdown \frac{0.125 \text{ mg}}{X \text{ mcg}}$$

$$X = 125 \text{ mcg}$$

Order: digoxin 125 mcg

Calculate: $\frac{500 \text{ mcg}}{2 \text{ mL}} \diagdown \frac{125 \text{ mcg}}{X \text{ mL}}$

$$500X = 250$$

$$\frac{500X}{500} = \frac{250}{500}$$

$$X = 0.5 \text{ mL}$$

Review Set 26 from pages 361–375

1)   20; 50; 10; 2

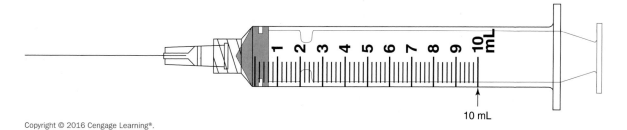

2)   4.8; 100; 5; 1

No reconstitution label is required; all of the medication will be used for 1 dose.

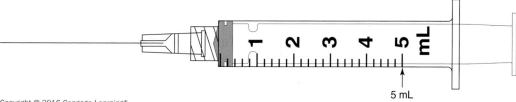

3)   18.2; 250,000; 4

8.2; 500,000; 2

3.2; 1,000,000; 1

Note: 1,000,000; 1. Select this reconstitution concentration because the amount to give is then obvious.

No calculation is necessary.

Five full doses are available in the vial.

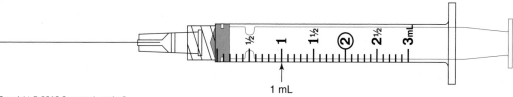

4)   8; 500; 8; 62.5; 2.8; 2

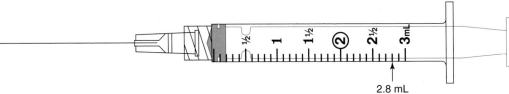

> *2/6/xx, 0800, reconstituted as 62.5 mg/mL. Expires 2/8/xx, 0800. Keep at room temperature and protect from light. G.D.P.*

2.8 mL

5)   20; 50,000; 10

10; 100,000; 5

4; 250,000; 2

1.8; 500,000; 1

Select 500,000 units/mL and give 1 mL. As this is an IV route, the dose would require further dilution before IV administration.

2 doses available

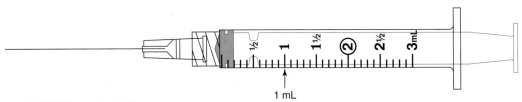

> *2/6/xx, 0800, reconstituted as 500,000 units/mL. Expires 2/13/xx, 0800. Keep refrigerated. G.D.P.*

1 mL

6)   1.2; 40; 0.6; 1

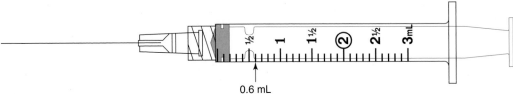

> *2/6/xx, 0800, reconstituted as 40 mg/mL. Expires 2/8/xx, 0800. Store at room temperature. G.D.P.*

0.6 mL

7) 9.6; 1; 10; 100; 7.5; 1; yes; there is a remainder of 2.5 mL available for the next q.12h dose; solution is stable at room temperature for 24 h.

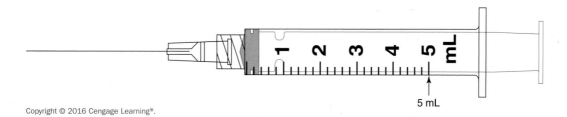

2/6/xx, 0800, reconstituted as IV solution 100 mg/mL. Expires 2/7/xx, 0800. Store at room temperature. Protect from light. G.D.P.

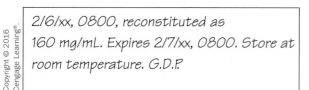

5 mL

2.5 mL

8) 10; 2; 12.5; 160; 9.4; 1

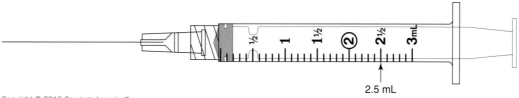

2/6/xx, 0800, reconstituted as 160 mg/mL. Expires 2/7/xx, 0800. Store at room temperature. G.D.P.

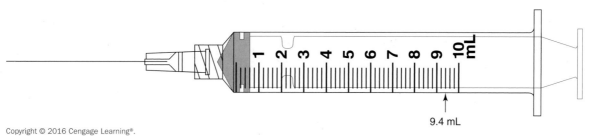

9.4 mL

9) 5; 50; 5; 1

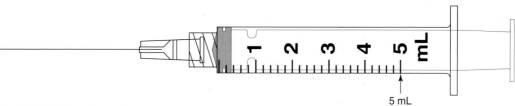

5 mL

10)   2; 225; 1.1; 2

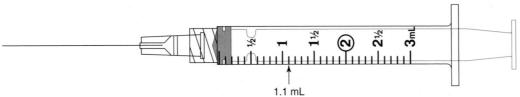

*2/6/xx, 0800, reconstituted as
225 mg/mL. Expires 2/7/xx, 0800, when
kept at room temperature. G.D.P.*

1.1 mL

11)   a. Used mainly for the treatment of leukemias and non-Hodgkin's lymphomas

b. Powder for injection: 100 mg, 500 mg, 1 g, 2 g

c. IV, subcutaneous, or intrathecal

d. Subcut (Adults) Maintenance: 1–1.5 mg/kg q 1–4 wk. (For this patient, 100 kg × 1 mg/kg = 100 mg; 100 kg × 1.5 mg/kg = 150 mg)

e. 10; 50

f. 2

g. The nurse should have a second practitioner independently double-check original order and calculations.

h. Change needles for subcutaneous use.

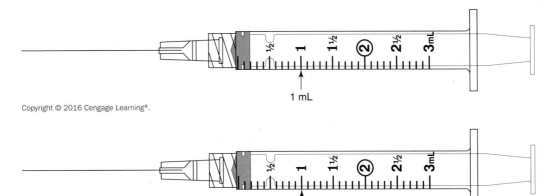

1 mL

1 mL

i. 5

j.

*2/6/xx, 0800, reconstituted as
50 mg/mL. Expires 2/8/xx, 0800. Store at
room temperature. Discard if slight haze
develops. G.D.P.*

12) a. Treatment of various infections caused by unusual organisms

   b. Powder for injection: 100 mg/vial, 200 mg/vial

   c. IV

   d. The usual dosage of intravenous doxycycline is 200 mg on the first day of treatment administered in one or two infusions. Subsequent daily dosage is 100 to 200 mg depending upon the severity of infection, administered in one or two infusions.

   e. 2

   f. 10, 100, 10

   g. 20

   h.

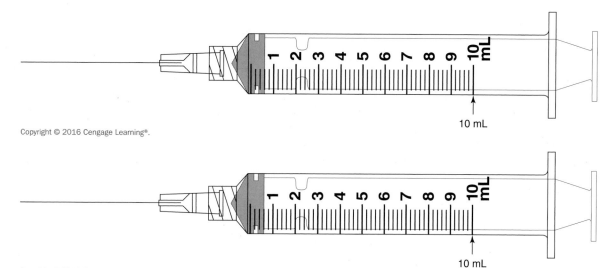

Copyright © 2016 Cengage Learning®.

   i. 5

   j.

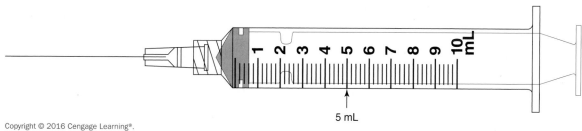

Copyright © 2016 Cengage Learning®.

   k. 2

   l.

2/6/xx, 0800, reconstituted as
10 mg/mL. Expires 2/9/xx, 0800.
Refrigerate and protect from light. G.D.P.

Copyright © 2016 Cengage Learning®.

13) a. Treatment of infections such as skin and skin structure infections, soft-tissue infections, otitis media, sinusitis, respiratory infections, genitourinary infections, meningitis, septicemia. Also endocarditis prophylaxis.

b. 125 mg/vial, 250 mg/vial, 500 mg/vial, 1 g/vial, 2 g/vial, 10 g/vial

c. IM and IV

d. IM, IV: 500 mg to 3 g q.6h (not to exceed 14 g/day)

e. B

f. 3.4, 250

g. 3

h.

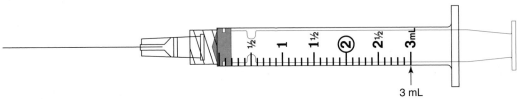

3 mL

i. 1

j. Label specifies that the solution must be used within 1 hour.

14) a. Treatment of a wide variety of infections such as pneumococcal pneumonia, streptococcal pharyngitis, syphilis, gonorrhea strains. Also prevention of rheumatic fever.

b. 5 million units/vial

c. IM, IV

d. IM, IV; most infections: 1–5 million units q.4–6h

e. C

f. 23; 200,000; 7.5

    18; 250,000; 6

    8; 500,000; 3

    3; 1,000,000; 1.5

g. 1,000,000; 1.5. This amount could be easily measured and drawn up in a 3 mL syringe. The 500,000 units per mL reconstitution could also be used, to administer 3 mL with the 3 mL syringe.

h.

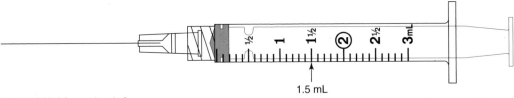

1.5 mL

i. 3 full doses

j.

> 2/6/xx, 0800, reconstituted as
> 1,000,000 units/mL. Expires 2/13/xx,
> 0800. Keep refrigerated. G.D.P.

15) a. Treatment of infections such as skin and skin structure infections, soft-tissue infections, otitis media,

   intra-abdominal infections, sinusitis, respiratory infections, genitourinary infections, meningitis, septicemia.

b. According to the label, each vial contains 1.5 g ampicillin sodium/sulbactam sodium equivalent to 1 g ampicillin

   plus 0.5 g sulbactam.

c. 1.5 g (1 g ampicillin with 500 mg sulbactam), 3 g (2 g ampicillin with 1 g sulbactam), 15 g (10 g ampicillin with

   5 g sulbactam)

d. IM or IV

e. Dosage based on ampicillin component. IM, IV: 1–2 g ampicillin q.6–8h (not to exceed 12 g ampicillin/day).

f. A

g. 2

h. 3.2, 1.5, 4

i. 4, 1.3

j.

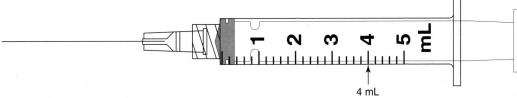

4 mL

Copyright © 2016 Cengage Learning®.

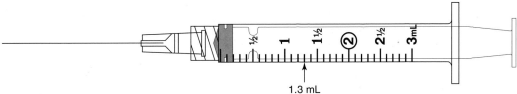

1.3 mL

Copyright © 2016 Cengage Learning®.

k. 3 g (2 g ampicillin with 1 g sulbactam). The nurse should request that the alternate supply dosage be sent up from

   pharmacy for this patient or routinely stocked in the ADC.

l. Label states solution may be stored from 2–8 hours at room temperature and 24–72 hours under refrigeration.

   Remaining solution will be used at next administration in 6 hours. For best results, store in refrigerator and

   discard in 24 hours.

> *2/6/xx, 0800, reconstituted as*
> *1.5 g per 4 mL. Expires 2/7/xx at*
> *0800.*
> *Keep refrigerated. G.D.P.*

Copyright © 2016 Cengage Learning®.

Solutions—Review Set 26

1) Order: 0.5 g

Supply: 50 mg/mL

Convert: 1 g = 1,000 mg (known equivalent)

$$\frac{1 \text{ g}}{1{,}000 \text{ mg}} \diagdown \frac{0.5 \text{ g}}{X \text{ mg}}$$

$$X = 500 \text{ mg}$$

Order: 500 mg

$$\frac{50 \text{ mg}}{1 \text{ mL}} \diagdown \frac{500 \text{ mg}}{X \text{ mL}}$$

$$50X = 500$$

$$\frac{50X}{50} \diagdown \frac{500}{50}$$

$$X = 10 \text{ mL}$$

$$\frac{500 \text{ mg}}{1 \text{ dose}} \diagdown \frac{1{,}000 \text{ mg}}{X \text{ dose(s)}}$$

$$500X = 1{,}000$$

$$\frac{500X}{500} \diagdown \frac{1{,}000}{500}$$

$$X = 2 \text{ doses (per vial)}$$

3) Order: 1,000,000 units

Supply: 250,000 units/mL

$$\frac{250,000 \text{ units}}{1 \text{ mL}} \diagdown \frac{1,000,000 \text{ units}}{X \text{ mL}}$$

$$250,000X = 1,000,000$$

$$\frac{250,000X}{250,000} \diagdown \frac{1,000,000}{250,000}$$

$$X = 4 \text{ mL}$$

Order: 1,000,000 units

Supply: 500,000 units/mL

$$\frac{500,000 \text{ units}}{1 \text{ mL}} \diagdown \frac{1,000,000 \text{ units}}{X \text{ mL}}$$

$$500,000X = 1,000,000$$

$$\frac{500,000X}{500,000} = \frac{1,000,000}{500,000}$$

$$X = 2 \text{ mL}$$

Order: 1,000,000 units

Supply: 1,000,000 units/mL

It is obvious that the dose is 1 mL.

$$\frac{1,000,000 \text{ units}}{1 \text{ dose}} \diagdown \frac{5,000,000 \text{ units}}{X \text{ doses}}$$

$$1,000,000X = 5,000,000$$

$$\frac{1,000,000X}{1,000,000} \diagdown \frac{5,000,000}{1,000,000}$$

$$X = 5 \text{ doses (per vial)}$$

4) Order: 175 mg

Supply: 500 mg per 8 mL

$$\frac{500 \text{ mg}}{8 \text{ mL}} \diagdown \frac{X \text{ mg}}{1 \text{ mL}}$$

$$8X = 500$$

$$\frac{8X}{8} = \frac{500}{8}$$

$$X = 62.5 \text{ mg}$$

$$\frac{62.5 \text{ mg}}{1 \text{ mL}} \diagdown \frac{175 \text{ mg}}{X \text{ mL}}$$

$$62.5X = 175$$

$$\frac{62.5X}{62.5} = \frac{175}{62.5}$$

$$X = 2.8 \text{ mL}$$

$$\frac{175 \text{ mg}}{1 \text{ dose}} = \frac{500 \text{ mg}}{X \text{ doses}}$$

$$175X = 500$$

$$\frac{175X}{175} = \frac{500}{175}$$

$$X = 2.85 \text{ or 2 full doses (per vial)}$$

7) Order: 750 mg

Supply: 100 mg/mL

$$\frac{100 \text{ mg}}{1 \text{ mL}} \diagdown \frac{750 \text{ mg}}{X \text{ mL}}$$

$$100X = 750$$

$$\frac{100X}{100} = \frac{750}{100}$$

$$X = 7.5 \text{ mL}$$

$$\frac{750 \text{ mg}}{1 \text{ dose}} \diagdown \frac{1,000 \text{ mg}}{X \text{ doses}}$$

$$750X = 1,000$$

$$\frac{750X}{750} = \frac{1,000}{750}$$

$$X = 1.33 \text{ doses (per vial or 1 full dose)}$$

9) Order: 250 mg

Supply: 250 mg per 5 mL

$$\frac{250 \text{ mg}}{5 \text{ mL}} \diagdown \frac{X \text{ mg}}{1 \text{ mL}}$$

$$5X = 250$$

$$\frac{5X}{5} = \frac{250}{5}$$

$$X = 50 \text{ mg (50 mg/mL)}$$

You will give all of the 250 mg reconstituted with 5 mL diluent; give 5 mL. One full dose is available.

Review Set 27 from pages 380–381

1) 160 mL hydrogen peroxide (solute) + 320 mL saline (solvent) = 480 mL $\frac{1}{3}$ strength solution

2) 1 fl oz hydrogen peroxide + 3 fl oz saline = 4 fl oz $\frac{1}{4}$ strength solution

3) 180 mL hydrogen peroxide + 60 mL saline = 240 mL $\frac{3}{4}$ strength solution

4) 8 fl oz hydrogen peroxide + 8 fl oz saline = 16 fl oz $\frac{1}{2}$ strength solution

5) 300 mL Ensure + 600 mL water = 900 mL $\frac{1}{3}$ strength Ensure; one 12 fl oz can. Discard 2 fl oz (60 mL).

6) 6 fl oz (180 mL) Isomil + 18 fl oz (540 mL) water = 24 fl oz (720 mL) $\frac{1}{4}$ strength Isomil; one 6 fl oz can. None discarded.

7) 1,200 mL needed for daily supply. 800 mL Sustacal + 400 mL water = 1,200 mL $\frac{2}{3}$ strength Sustacal; three 10 fl oz cans. Discard 100 mL.

8) 13 fl oz Ensure + 13 fl oz water = 26 fl oz $\frac{1}{2}$ strength Ensure; one 12 fl oz can + one 4 fl oz can. Discard 3 fl oz (90 mL).

9)   1,000 mL needed for daily supply. 500 mL Sustacal + 500 mL water = 1,000 mL $\frac{1}{2}$ strength Sustacal; two 10 fl oz cans. Discard 100 mL.

10)   36 fl oz Isomil + 12 fl oz water = 48 fl oz $\frac{3}{4}$ strength Isomil; use three 12 fl oz cans. None discarded.

11)   4 fl oz Ensure + 2 fl oz water = 6 fl oz $\frac{2}{3}$ strength Ensure; use one 4 fl oz can. None discarded.

12)   4 fl oz Ensure + 12 fl oz water = 16 fl oz (1 pt) $\frac{1}{4}$ strength Ensure; use one 4 fl oz can. None discarded.

Solutions—Review Set 27

1) $\frac{1}{3}$ ⤬ $\frac{\text{X mL}}{480 \text{ mL}}$

$3X = 480$

$\frac{3X}{3} = \frac{480}{3}$

$X = 160$ mL (solute)

480 mL (total solution) − 160 mL (solute)

$= 320$ mL (solvent)

5) $\frac{1}{3}$ ⤬ $\frac{\text{X mL}}{900 \text{ mL}}$

$3X = 900$

$\frac{3X}{3} = \frac{900}{3}$

$X = 300$ mL (Ensure)

900 mL (total solution) − 300 mL (Ensure)

$= 600$ mL (water)

$\frac{1 \text{ fl oz}}{30 \text{ mL}}$ ⤬ $\frac{12 \text{ fl oz}}{\text{X mL}}$

$X = 360$ mL (per can)

360 mL (full can) − 300 mL (Ensure needed)

$= 60$ mL (discarded)

6)   4 fl oz q.4h = 4 × 6 = 24 fl oz per 24 h

$\frac{1}{4}$ ⤬ $\frac{\text{X fl oz}}{24 \text{ fl oz}}$

$4X = 24$

$\frac{4X}{4} = \frac{24}{4}$

$X = 6$ fl oz (Isomil)

24 fl oz (total solution) − 6 fl oz (Isomil) = 18 fl oz (water); use one 6 fl oz can.

12) $\frac{1}{4}$ ⤬ $\frac{\text{X fl oz}}{16 \text{ fl oz}}$

$4X = 16$

$\frac{4X}{4} = \frac{16}{4}$

$X = 4$ fl oz (Ensure)

16 fl oz (total solution) − 4 fl oz (Ensure) = 12 fl oz (water); use one 4 fl oz can Ensure. None discarded.

Practice Problems—Chapter 12 from pages 383–390

1)   3.375; 5; 3.7; 5 mL **2)** 2; 3 mL **3)** 1.5; 3 mL **4)** 9; 1; 10 mL **5)** 1.8; 3 mL; 2 (Dilute further for IV administration.)

> *2/6/xx, 0800, reconstituted as 280 mg/mL.*
>
> *Expires 2/13/xx, 0800. Keep refrigerated. G.D.P.*

6) 3.8; 5 mL; 1 **7)** 2; 225; 1.3; 3 mL; 1; Yes **8)** 8; 500; 8; 62.5; 3.2; 5; 2; Yes **9)** 19.2; 100; 12.5; 20 mL; 1; Yes **10)** 3; 1,000,000; 0.5; 3 mL; 10; Yes **11)** 0.9; 250; 0.8; 3; 1; No, it would be too difficult to withdraw the small remainder for the next dose. **12)** 29; 20; 10; 5; Yes **13)** 2; 225; 1.8; 3 mL; 1; Yes **14)** 3.2; 1,000,000; 2; 3 mL; 2; Yes **15)** 1.8; 500,000; 2; 3 mL; 1; No

16)   2 fl oz hydrogen peroxide + 14 fl oz normal saline = 16 fl oz of the $\frac{1}{8}$ strength solution

17)   120 mL hydrogen peroxide + 200 mL normal saline = 320 mL of the $\frac{3}{8}$ strength solution

18)   50 mL hydrogen peroxide + 30 mL normal saline = 80 mL of the $\frac{5}{8}$ strength solution

19)   12 fl oz hydrogen peroxide + 6 fl oz normal saline = 18 fl oz of the $\frac{2}{3}$ strength solution

20)   14 fl oz hydrogen peroxide + 2 fl oz normal saline = 16 fl oz (1 pt) of the $\frac{7}{8}$ strength solution

21)   250 mL hydrogen peroxide + 750 mL normal saline = 1,000 mL (1 L) of the $\frac{1}{4}$ strength solution

22)   30 mL Enfamil + 90 mL water = 120 mL of the $\frac{1}{4}$ strength Enfamil; one 3 fl oz bottle. Discard 2 fl oz (60 mL).

23)   270 mL Sustacal + 90 mL water = 360 mL of the $\frac{3}{4}$ strength Sustacal; one 10 fl oz can. Discard 1 fl oz (30 mL).

24)   300 mL Ensure + 150 mL water = 450 mL of the $\frac{2}{3}$ strength Ensure; two 8 fl oz cans. Discard 6 fl oz (180 mL).

25) 36 fl oz Enfamil + 60 fl oz water = 96 fl oz of the $\frac{3}{8}$ strength Enfamil; six 6 fl oz bottles. None discarded.

26) 20 mL Ensure + 140 mL water = 160 mL of the $\frac{1}{8}$ strength Ensure; one 4 fl oz can. Discard 100 mL.

27) 275 mL Ensure + 275 mL water = 550 mL of the $\frac{1}{2}$ strength Ensure; one 12 fl oz can. Discard 85 mL.

28) 2 cans are needed; $1\frac{1}{2}$ cans are used (12 fl oz Enfamil)

29) 36

30) **Prevention:** This type of error could have been prevented had the nurse read the label carefully for the correct amount of diluent for the dosage of medication to be prepared. Had the nurse read the label carefully before the medication was prepared, medication charges, valuable time, and health care resources would have been saved. Additionally, if the nurse had used Step 2 (Think) of the Three-Step Approach, the nurse would have realized earlier (before preparing it) that 4 mL would be an unreasonable volume for an IM injection.

Solutions—Practice Problems—Chapter 12

1) Concentration is 3.375 g per 5 mL

Order: 2.5 g

Supply: 3.375 g per 5 mL

$$\frac{3.375 \text{ mg}}{5 \text{ mL}} \diagdown \frac{2.5 \text{ g}}{X \text{ mL}}$$

$$3.375X = 12.5$$

$$\frac{3.375X}{3.375} = \frac{12.5}{3.375}$$

$$X = 3.70 \text{ mL} = 3.7 \text{ mL}$$

4) Order: 900 mg

Supply: 100 mg/mL

$$\frac{100 \text{ mg}}{1 \text{ mL}} \diagdown \frac{900 \text{ mg}}{X \text{ mL}}$$

$$100X = 900$$

$$\frac{100X}{100} = \frac{900}{100}$$

$$X = 9 \text{ mL}$$

Vial has 1 g Rocephin. Order is for 900 mg/dose.

$$\frac{900 \text{ mg}}{1 \text{ dose}} \diagdown \frac{1{,}000 \text{ mg}}{X \text{ doses}}$$

$$900X = 1{,}000$$

$$\frac{900X}{900} = \frac{1{,}000}{900}$$

$$X = 1.1 \text{ doses (per vial or 1 full dose per vial)}$$

6) Order: 375 mg

Supply: 100 mg/mL

$$\frac{100 \text{ mg}}{1 \text{ mL}} \diagdown \frac{375 \text{ mg}}{X \text{ mL}}$$

$$100X = 375$$

$$\frac{100X}{100} = \frac{375}{100}$$

$$X = 3.75 \text{ mL} = 3.8 \text{ mL}$$

$$\frac{375 \text{ mg}}{1 \text{ dose}} \diagdown \frac{500 \text{ mg}}{X \text{ doses}}$$

$$375X = 500$$

$$\frac{375X}{375} = \frac{500}{375}$$

$$X = 1.3 \text{ doses (per vial or 1 full dose per vial)}$$

8) Order: 200 mg

Supply: 500 mg per 8 mL

$$\frac{500 \text{ mg}}{8 \text{ mL}} \diagdown \frac{X \text{ mg}}{1 \text{ mL}}$$

$$8X = 500$$

$$\frac{8X}{8} = \frac{500}{8}$$

$$X = 62.5 \text{ mg}$$

Supply: 62.5 mg/mL

$$\frac{62.5 \text{ mg}}{1 \text{ mL}} \diagdown \frac{200 \text{ mg}}{X \text{ mL}}$$

$$62.5X = 200$$

$$\frac{62.5X}{62.5} = \frac{200}{62.5}$$

$$X = 3.2 \text{ mL}$$

$$\frac{200 \text{ mg}}{1 \text{ dose}} \diagdown \frac{500 \text{ mg}}{X \text{ doses}}$$

$$200X = 500$$

$$\frac{200X}{200} = \frac{500}{200}$$

$$X = 2.5 \text{ doses (per vial or 2 full doses per vial)}$$

9) Order: 1.25 g

Supply: 100 mg/mL

$$\frac{1{,}000 \text{ mg}}{1 \text{ g}} \diagdown \frac{X \text{ mg}}{1.25 \text{ g}}$$

$$X = 1{,}250 \text{ mg}$$

$$\frac{100 \text{ mg}}{1 \text{ mL}} \diagdown \frac{1{,}250 \text{ mg}}{X \text{ mL}}$$

$$100X = 1{,}250$$

$$\frac{100X}{100} = \frac{1{,}250}{100}$$

$$X = 12.5 \text{ mL}$$

$$\frac{1{,}250 \text{ mg}}{1 \text{ dose}} \diagdown \frac{2{,}000 \text{ mg}}{X \text{ doses}}$$

$$1{,}250X = 2{,}000$$

$$\frac{1{,}250X}{1{,}250} = \frac{2{,}000}{1{,}250}$$

$$X = 1.6 \text{ doses (per vial or 1 full dose per vial)}$$

11)   Order: 200 mg

Supply: 250 mg/mL

$$\frac{250 \text{ mg}}{1 \text{ mL}} \diagdown\diagup \frac{200 \text{ mg}}{\text{X mL}}$$

$$250\text{X} = 200$$

$$\frac{250\text{X}}{250} = \frac{200}{250}$$

$$\text{X} = 0.8 \text{ mL}$$

$$\frac{200 \text{ mg}}{1 \text{ dose}} \diagdown\diagup \frac{250 \text{ mg}}{\text{X doses}}$$

$$200\text{X} = 250$$

$$\frac{200\text{X}}{200} = \frac{250}{200}$$

$$\text{X} = 1.25 \text{ doses (per vial or 1 full dose per vial)}$$

15)   Order: 1,000,000 units

Supply: 50,000 units/mL

$$\frac{50,000 \text{ units}}{1 \text{ mL}} \diagdown\diagup \frac{1,000,000 \text{ units}}{\text{X mL}}$$

$$50,000\text{X} = 1,000,000$$

$$\frac{50,000\text{X}}{50,000} = \frac{1,000,000}{50,000}$$

$$\text{X} = 20 \text{ mL (too much for an IM dose)}$$

Order: 1,000,000 units

Supply: 100,000 units/mL

$$\frac{100,000 \text{ units}}{1 \text{ mL}} \diagdown\diagup \frac{1,000,000 \text{ units}}{\text{X mL}}$$

$$100,000\text{X} = 1,000,000$$

$$\frac{100,000\text{X}}{100,000} = \frac{1,000,000}{100,000}$$

$$\text{X} = 10 \text{ mL (too much for an IM dose)}$$

Order: 1,000,000 units

Supply: 250,000 units/mL

$$\frac{250,000 \text{ units}}{1 \text{ mL}} \diagdown\diagup \frac{1,000,000 \text{ units}}{\text{X mL}}$$

$$250,000\text{X} = 1,000,000$$

$$\frac{250,000\text{X}}{250,000} = \frac{1,000,000}{250,000}$$

X = 4 mL (too much for an IM dose; 3 mL or less

is preferred)

Order: 1,000,000 units

Supply: 500,000 units/mL

$$\frac{500,000 \text{ units}}{1 \text{ mL}} \diagdown\diagup \frac{1,000,000 \text{ units}}{\text{X mL}}$$

$$500,000\text{X} = 1,000,000$$

$$\frac{500,000\text{X}}{500,000} = \frac{1,000,000}{500,000}$$

$$\text{X} = 2 \text{ mL (acceptable IM dose)}$$

22)   12 mL every hour for 10 hours = 12 × 10 = 120 mL

total:

$$\frac{1}{4} \diagdown\diagup \frac{\text{X mL}}{120 \text{ mL}}$$

$$4\text{X} = 120$$

$$\frac{4\text{X}}{4} = \frac{120}{4}$$

$$\text{X} = 30 \text{ mL (Enfamil)}$$

120 mL (solution) − 30 mL (Enfamil) = 90 mL

(water); one 3 fl oz bottle = 90 mL

90 mL (full bottle) − 30 mL (Enfamil needed) =

60 mL (1 fl oz = 30 mL; 2 fl oz = 60 mL; therefore,

2 fl oz discarded)

28) $$\frac{1}{4} \diagdown\diagup \frac{\text{X fl oz}}{48 \text{ fl oz}}$$

$$4\text{X} = 48$$

$$\frac{4\text{X}}{4} = \frac{48}{4}$$

$$\text{X} = 12 \text{ fl oz (Enfamil)}$$

$$\frac{1 \text{ can}}{8 \text{ fl oz}} \diagdown\diagup \frac{\text{X cans}}{12 \text{ fl oz}}$$

$$8\text{X} = 12$$

$$\frac{8\text{X}}{8} = \frac{12}{8}$$

$$\text{X} = 1\tfrac{1}{2} \text{ cans}$$

Need $1\tfrac{1}{2}$ cans (8 fl oz/can) of Enfamil for each infant.

29)   48 fl oz (solution) − 12 fl oz (Enfamil)

= 36 fl oz (water)

Review Set 28 from pages 412–420

1) 25; 312.5; 78.1; 625; 156.3; Yes **2)** 10 **3)** 2.2; 110; 55; Yes **4)** 0.55 **5)** 15; 120; Yes **6)** 6; 8 **7)** 320; 480; Yes **8)** 15

9) 20; 500; 125; 1,000; 250; Yes **10)** 5 **11)** 3.4; 51; 17; No

12)   The dosage of kanamycin sulfate 34 mg IV q.8h is higher than the recommended dosage. Therefore, the ordered

dosage is not safe. The prescribing practitioner should be called and the order questioned.

13)   120; 60; 7.5; Yes

14) 7.5; $1\frac{1}{2}$

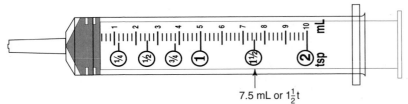

7.5 mL or $1\frac{1}{2}$ t

15) 32.7; 818; 205; 1,635; 409; Yes

16) 1.6

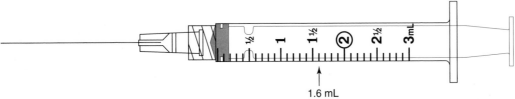

1.6 mL

17) 17.7; 354; 118; 708; 236; No

18) The dosage ordered of 100 mg q.8h does not fall within the recommended dosage range of 118 to 236 mg/dose. It is an underdosage and would not produce a therapeutic effect. The physician should be called for clarification.

19) 25; 375; 125; 625; 208.3; No

20) The ordered dosage of 100 mg q.8h does not fall within the recommended dosage range of 125 to 208.3 mg q.8h. It is an underdosage, and the physician should be called for clarification.

21) 13.6; Yes

22) 1.4

23) 272; 136; 544; 272; Yes

24) 1.7

25) Treatment of serious infections and less serious infections when penicillins or other less toxic drugs are contraindicated; 10 mg/mL, 40 mg/mL; IM or IV; 1 to 2 mg/kg q.8h or 4 to 6.6 mg/kg q.24h; 364; 600; Yes

26) D; 9.4

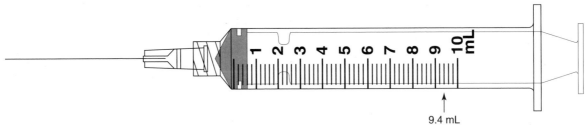

9.4 mL

27) Treatment of serious infections and less serious infections when penicillins or other less toxic drugs are contraindicated; 10 mg/mL, 40 mg/mL; IM or IV; 2.5 mg/kg/dose q.8h or 5 to 7.5 mg/kg/dose q.24h; 12; Yes

28) A; 1.2

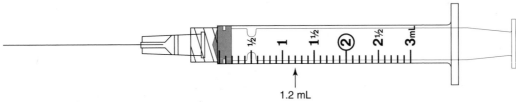

1.2 mL

29) Treatment of potentially life-threatening infections when less toxic anti-infectives are contraindicated; 500 mg, 750 mg, 1 g vial, 5 g vial, 10 g vial; IV; 40 mg/kg/day divided q.6–8h; 656; 164; 219; No

30) The dosage ordered is too high; therefore, neither of the supply dosages is appropriate. It is imperative to consult with the physician before proceeding. To administer the order would deliver 1,980 mg/day or approximately 2 g/day, which is the recommended adult dosage. The 3-year-old child for whom this medication is ordered should have a maximum dosage of 656 mg/day. Perhaps the physician ordered an adult dosage by mistake. Perhaps the physician intended to divide the dosage and administer it q.6h, which would deliver 165 mg per dose. Perhaps this is simply a calculation or prescription error. Regardless, catching this error would avoid the potential of serious harm to this child. Let this be you!

Solutions—Review Set 28

1) $\dfrac{1 \text{ kg}}{2.2 \text{ lb}} \times \dfrac{X \text{ kg}}{55 \text{ lb}}$

$2.2X = 55$

$\dfrac{2.2X}{2.2} = \dfrac{55}{2.2}$

$X = 25 \text{ kg}$

Minimum daily dosage:

$12.5 \text{ mg/kg/day} \times 25 \text{ kg} = 312.5 \text{ mg/day, or:}$

$\dfrac{12.5 \text{ mg}}{1 \text{ kg}} \times \dfrac{X \text{ mg}}{25 \text{ kg}}$

$X = 312.5 \text{ mg/day}$

$312.5 \text{ mg} \div 4 \text{ doses} = 78.12 \text{ mg/dose} = 78.1 \text{ mg/dose}$

Maximum daily dosage:

$25 \text{ mg/kg/day} \times 25 \text{ kg} = 625 \text{ mg/day or}$

$\dfrac{25 \text{ mg}}{1 \text{ kg}} \times \dfrac{X \text{ mg}}{25 \text{ kg}}$

$X = 625 \text{ mg/day}$

$625 \text{ mg} \div 4 \text{ doses} = 156.25 \text{ mg/dose} = 156.3 \text{ mg/dose}$

Yes, dosage is safe.

2) $\dfrac{62.5 \text{ mg}}{5 \text{ mL}} \times \dfrac{125 \text{ mg}}{X \text{ mL}}$

$62.5X = 625$

$\dfrac{62.5X}{62.5} = \dfrac{625}{62.5}$

$X = 10 \text{ mL}$

3) $\dfrac{1 \text{ kg}}{1,000 \text{ g}} \times \dfrac{X \text{ kg}}{2,200 \text{ g}}$

$1,000X = 2,200$

$\dfrac{1,000X}{1,000} = \dfrac{2,200}{1,000}$

$X = 2.2 \text{ kg}$

Dose: $50 \text{ mg/kg/day} \times 2.2 \text{ kg} = 110 \text{ mg/day, or:}$

$\dfrac{1 \text{ kg}}{50 \text{ mg}} \times \dfrac{2.2 \text{ kg}}{X \text{ mg}}$

$X = 110 \text{ mg (per day)}$

$110 \text{ mg} \div 2 \text{ doses} = 55 \text{ mg/dose}$

Yes, dosage is safe.

4) $1 \text{ g} = 1,000 \text{ mg}$

$\dfrac{1,000 \text{ mg}}{10 \text{ mL}} \times \dfrac{55 \text{ mg}}{X \text{ mL}}$

$1,000X = 550$

$\dfrac{1,000X}{1,000} = \dfrac{550}{1,000}$

$X = 0.55 \text{ mL}$

6) $\dfrac{100 \text{ mg}}{5 \text{ mL}} \times \dfrac{120 \text{ mg}}{X \text{ mL}}$

$100X = 600$

$\dfrac{100X}{100} = \dfrac{600}{100}$

$X = 6 \text{ mL}$

$\dfrac{6 \text{ mL}}{1 \text{ dose}} \times \dfrac{50 \text{ mL}}{X \text{ doses}}$

$6X = 50$

$\dfrac{6X}{6} = \dfrac{50}{6}$

$X = 8.3 \text{ doses} = 8 \text{ full doses}$

7) Minimum dosage: $10 \text{ mg/kg/dose} \times 32 \text{ kg} = 320 \text{ mg/dose, or:}$

$\dfrac{10 \text{ mg}}{1 \text{ kg}} \times \dfrac{X \text{ mg}}{32 \text{ kg}}$

$X = 320 \text{ mg (per dose)}$

Maximum dosage:

$15 \text{ mg/kg/dose} \times 32 \text{ kg} = 480 \text{ mg/dose, or:}$

$\dfrac{15 \text{ mg}}{1 \text{ kg}} \times \dfrac{X \text{ mg}}{32 \text{ kg}}$

$X = 480 \text{ mg (per dose)}$

Dosage is the *maximum* dosage (480 mg) and is safe.

8) $\dfrac{160 \text{ mg}}{5 \text{ mL}} \times \dfrac{480 \text{ mg}}{X \text{ mL}}$

$160X = 2,400$

$\dfrac{160X}{160} = \dfrac{2,400}{160}$

$X = 15 \text{ mL}$

11)

$$\frac{1 \text{ lb}}{16 \text{ oz}} \times \frac{X \text{ lb}}{8 \text{ oz}}$$

$$16X = 8$$

$$\frac{16X}{16} = \frac{8}{16}$$

$$X = \frac{1}{2} \text{ lb}$$

$$7 \text{ lb } 8 \text{ oz} = 7\frac{1}{2} \text{ lb}$$

$$\frac{1 \text{ kg}}{2.2 \text{ lb}} \times \frac{X \text{ kg}}{7.5 \text{ lb}}$$

$$2.2X = 7.5$$

$$\frac{2.2X}{2.2} = \frac{7.5}{2.2}$$

$$X = 3.40 \text{ kg} = 3.4 \text{ kg}$$

15 mg/kg/day × 3.4 kg = 51 mg/day, or:

$$\frac{15 \text{ mg}}{1 \text{ kg}} \times \frac{X \text{ mg}}{3.4 \text{ kg}}$$

$$X = 51 \text{ mg (per day)}$$

51 mg ÷ 3 doses = 17 mg/dose, if administered q.8h

Ordered dosage of 34 mg q.8h exceeds recommended dosage and is not safe.

15)

$$\frac{1 \text{ kg}}{2.2 \text{ lb}} \times \frac{X \text{ kg}}{72 \text{ lb}}$$

$$2.2X = 72$$

$$\frac{2.2X}{2.2} = \frac{72}{2.2}$$

$$X = 32.72 \text{ kg} = 32.7 \text{ kg}$$

Minimum daily dosage:

25 mg/kg/day × 32.7 kg = 817.5 mg/day = 818 mg/day; or

$$\frac{25 \text{ mg}}{1 \text{ kg}} \times \frac{X \text{ mg}}{32.7 \text{ kg}}$$

$$X = 817.65 \text{ mg} = 818 \text{ mg (per day)}$$

Minimum single dosage:

818 mg ÷ 4 doses = 204.5 mg/dose = 205 mg/dose

Maximum daily dosage:

50 mg/kg/day × 32.7 kg = 1,635 mg/day; or

$$\frac{50 \text{ mg}}{1 \text{ kg}} \times \frac{X \text{ mg}}{32.7 \text{ kg}}$$

$$X = 1,635 \text{ mg (per day)}$$

Maximum single dosage:

1,635 mg ÷ 4 doses = 408.7 mg/dose = 409 mg/dose

Yes, dosage is safe.

16) Order: 400 mg

Supply: 250 mg/mL

$$\frac{250 \text{ mg}}{1 \text{ mL}} \times \frac{400 \text{ mg}}{X \text{ mL}}$$

$$250X = 400$$

$$\frac{250X}{250} = \frac{400}{250}$$

$$X = 1.6 \text{ mL}$$

17)

$$\frac{1 \text{ kg}}{2.2 \text{ lb}} \times \frac{X \text{ mg}}{39 \text{ lb}}$$

$$2.2X = 39$$

$$\frac{2.2X}{2.2} = \frac{39}{2.2}$$

$$X = 17.72 \text{ kg} = 17.7 \text{ kg}$$

Minimum daily dosage:

20 mg/kg/day × 17.7 kg = 354 mg/day, or:

$$\frac{20 \text{ mg}}{1 \text{ kg}} \times \frac{X \text{ mg}}{17.7 \text{ kg}}$$

$$X = 354 \text{ mg (per day)}$$

Minimum single dosage:

354 mg ÷ 3 doses = 118 mg/dose

Maximum daily dosage:

40 mg/kg/day × 17.7 kg = 708 mg/day, or:

$$\frac{40 \text{ mg}}{1 \text{ kg}} \times \frac{X \text{ mg}}{17.7 \text{ kg}}$$

$$X = 708 \text{ mg (per day)}$$

Maximum single dosage:

708 mg ÷ 3 doses = 236 mg/dose

The dosage of 100 mg q.8h is not safe. It is an underdosage, and would not produce a therapeutic effect, because the recommended dosage range is 118–236 mg/dose.

21)

$$\frac{1 \text{ kg}}{2.2 \text{ lb}} \times \frac{X \text{ kg}}{30 \text{ lb}}$$

$$2.2X = 30$$

$$\frac{2.2X}{2.2} = \frac{30}{2.2}$$

$$X = 13.63 \text{ kg} = 13.6 \text{ kg}$$

13.6 kg × 10 mcg/kg = 136 mcg or,

$$\frac{10 \text{ mcg}}{1 \text{ kg}} \times \frac{X \text{ mcg}}{13.6 \text{ kg}}$$

$$X = 136 \text{ mcg}$$

22) Order: 136 mcg

Supply: 0.1 mg/mL

$$\frac{1 \text{ mg}}{1,000 \text{ mcg}} \times \frac{0.1 \text{ mg}}{X \text{ mcg}}$$

$$X = 100 \text{ mcg}$$

$$\frac{100 \text{ mcg}}{1 \text{ mL}} \times \frac{136 \text{ mcg}}{X \text{ mL}}$$

$$100X = 136$$

$$\frac{100X}{100} = \frac{136}{100}$$

$$X = 1.36 = 1.4 \text{ mL}$$

23) Minimum daily dosage:

13.6 kg × 20 mcg/kg/day = 272 mcg/day or,

$$\frac{20 \text{ mcg}}{1 \text{ kg}} \diagdown\diagup \frac{X \text{ mcg}}{13.6 \text{ kg}}$$

X = 272 mcg/day

272 mcg/day ÷ 2 doses/day = 136 mcg/dose

Maximum daily dosage:

13.6 kg × 40 mcg/kg/day = 544 mcg/day or,

$$\frac{40 \text{ mcg}}{1 \text{ kg}} \diagdown\diagup \frac{X \text{ mcg}}{13.6 \text{ kg}}$$

X = 544 mcg/day

544 mcg/day ÷ 2 doses/day = 272 mcg/dose

24) Order: 170 mcg

Supply: 0.1 mg/mL

$$\frac{1 \text{ mg}}{1,000 \text{ mcg}} \diagdown\diagup \frac{0.1 \text{ mg}}{X \text{ mcg}}$$

X = 100 mcg

$$\frac{100 \text{ mcg}}{1 \text{ mL}} \diagdown\diagup \frac{170 \text{ mcg}}{X \text{ mL}}$$

100X = 170

$$\frac{100X}{100} = \frac{170}{100}$$

X = 1.7 mL

25) $$\frac{1 \text{ kg}}{2.2 \text{ lb}} \diagdown\diagup \frac{X \text{ kg}}{200 \text{ lb}}$$

2.2X = 200

$$\frac{2.2X}{2.2} = \frac{200}{2.2}$$

X = 90.9 kg

Minimum single dosage:

90.9 kg × 4 mg/kg = 363.6 mg = 364 mg or,

$$\frac{4 \text{ mg}}{1 \text{ kg}} \diagdown\diagup \frac{X \text{ mg}}{90.9 \text{ kg}}$$

X = 363.6 = 364 mg

Maximum single dosage:

90.9 kg × 6.6 mg/kg = 599.94 mg = 600 mg or,

$$\frac{6.6 \text{ mg}}{1 \text{ kg}} \diagdown\diagup \frac{X \text{ mg}}{90.9 \text{ kg}}$$

X = 599.94 = 600 mg

26) $$\frac{40 \text{ mg}}{1 \text{ mL}} \diagdown\diagup \frac{375 \text{ mg}}{X \text{ mL}}$$

40X = 375

$$\frac{40X}{40} = \frac{375}{40}$$

X = 9.375 = 9.4 mL

Practice Problems—Chapter 13 from pages 422–434

1) 5.5 **2)** 3.8 **3)** 1.6 **4)** 2.3 **5)** 15.5 **6)** 3 **7)** 23.6 **8)** 0.9 **9)** 240 **10)** 80 **11)** 19.5; 39; 48.8; Yes

12) 1

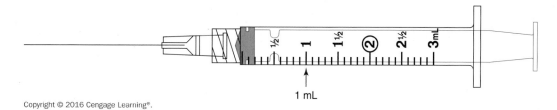

13) 7.3; 3.7; 14.6; Yes

14) 1

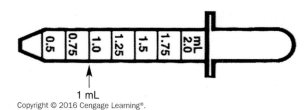

15) 18.2; 182; 91; 364; 182; Yes

16) 7.5

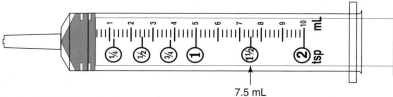

17) 29.1; 291; 145.5; 1,746; 873; Yes

18) 3

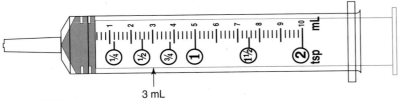

3 mL

19) 2.5; 125,000; 125,000; Yes

20) 18; 20; 250,000; 0.5

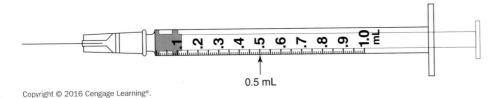

0.5 mL

21) 18.6; 372; 124; 744; 248; Yes

22) 6

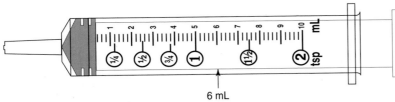

6 mL

23) 13.9; 556; 185.3; Yes, the ordered dosage is reasonably safe.

24) 5

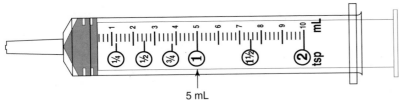

5 mL

25) 10; 0.1; Yes

26) 0.25

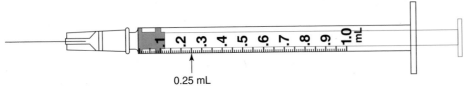

0.25 mL

27) 28; 35; Yes

28) 3.5

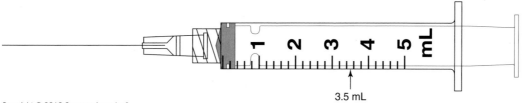

3.5 mL

29) 9.1; 455; 227.5; 682.5; 341.3; No

30) The ordered dosage of 1 g is not safe. The recommended q.12h dosage range for a child of this weight is 227.5 to
     341.3 mg/dose. The physician should be called for clarification.

31) 25.1; 0.05; Yes

32) 0.25

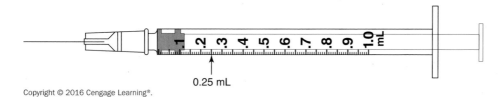

0.25 mL

     Route is IM; may need to change needle to appropriate gauge and length.

33) 8.2; 1,200; 1.2; 410; 615; Yes

34) 9.6; 10; 100; 6

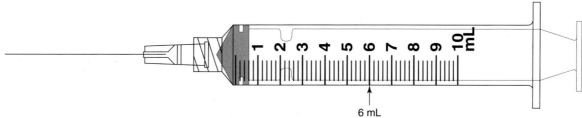

6 mL

35) 20.5; 512.5; 256.3; No

36) The dosage ordered is not safe. It is too low compared to the recommended dosage. Call the prescriber and clarify
     the order.

37) 8.2; 164; 54.7; No

38) Dosage ordered is not safe. Call the prescriber for clarification, because the ordered dosage is higher than the recom-
     mended dosage.

39) 20.5; 200; 400; No

40) The dosage ordered is not safe based on the recommended maximum daily dosage and on the frequency of the order.
     Call the prescriber for clarification.

41) 23.2; 348; 174; Yes, dosage is reasonably safe.

42) 3.5

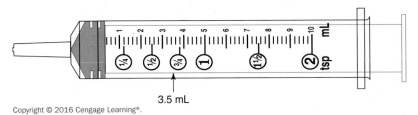

3.5 mL

43) 0.25

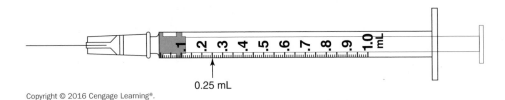

0.25 mL

44) 3.5

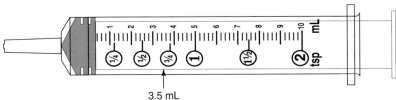

3.5 mL

45) 500,000; 0.9

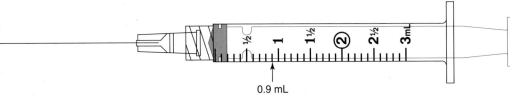

0.9 mL

46) Dosage is not safe; this child is ordered a total of 2 mg/day, which is too high. The prescriber should be called to clarify.

47) The ordered dosage of 1 mg IM stat is too high when compared to the recommended dosage range for a child of this weight. The order should be clarified with the prescriber.

48) 0.76; Route is IM. The needle may need to be changed to appropriate gauge and length.

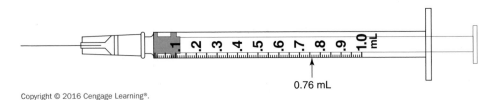

0.76 mL

49) #45 (penicillin G potassium) and #48 (cefazolin). (Note: #43 methylprednisolone is a single-dose vial. Check package insert to determine if storage after mixing is safe.)

50) **Prevention:** The child should have received 75 mg a day and no more than 25 mg per dose. The child received more than four times the safe dosage of tobramycin. Had the nurse calculated the safe dosage, the error would have been caught sooner, the resident would have been consulted, and the dosage could have been adjusted before the child ever received the first dose. The pharmacist also should have caught the error but did not. In this scenario, the resident, pharmacist, and nurse all committed medication errors. If the resident had not noticed the error, one can only wonder how many doses the child would have received. The nurse is the last safety net for the patient when it comes to a dosage error, because the nurse administers the drug.

In addition, the nurse has to reconcile the fact that she actually gave the overdose. The nurse is responsible for whatever dosage is administered and must verify the safety of the order and the patient's Six Rights. We are all accountable for our actions. Taking shortcuts in administering medications to children can be disastrous. The time the nurse saved by not calculating the safe dosage was more than lost in the extra monitoring, not to mention the cost of follow-up to the medication error and, *most importantly,* the risk to the child.

Solutions—Practice Problems—Chapter 13

1) $\dfrac{1 \text{ kg}}{2.2 \text{ lb}} \times \dfrac{X \text{ kg}}{12 \text{ lb}}$

    $2.2X = 12$

    $\dfrac{2.2X}{2.2} = \dfrac{12}{2.2}$

    $X = 5.45 \text{ kg} = 5.5 \text{ kg}$

2) $8 \text{ lb } 4 \text{ oz} = 8\frac{4}{16} \text{ lb} = 8\frac{1}{4} \text{ lb} = 8.25 \text{ lb}$

    $\dfrac{1 \text{ kg}}{2.2 \text{ lb}} \times \dfrac{X \text{ kg}}{8.25 \text{ lb}}$

    $2.2X = 8.25$

    $\dfrac{2.2X}{2.2} = \dfrac{8.25}{2.2}$

    $X = 3.75 \text{ kg} = 3.8 \text{ kg}$

3) $\dfrac{1 \text{ kg}}{1{,}000 \text{ g}} \times \dfrac{X \text{ kg}}{1{,}570 \text{ g}}$

    $1{,}000X = 1{,}570$

    $\dfrac{1{,}000 X}{1{,}000} = \dfrac{1{,}570}{1{,}000}$

    $X = 1.57 \text{ kg} = 1.6 \text{ kg}$

6) $1 \text{ lb} = 16 \text{ oz}$

    $\dfrac{1 \text{ lb}}{16 \text{ oz}} \times \dfrac{X \text{ lb}}{10 \text{ oz}}$

    $16X = 10$

    $\dfrac{16X}{16} = \dfrac{10}{16}$

    $X = 0.625 \text{ lb}$

    $6 \text{ lb } 10 \text{ oz} = 6.625 \text{ lb}$

    $\dfrac{1 \text{ kg}}{2.2 \text{ lb}} \times \dfrac{X \text{ kg}}{6.625 \text{ lb}}$

    $2.2X = 6.625$

    $\dfrac{2.2 X}{2.2} = \dfrac{6.625}{2.2}$

    $X = 3.01 \text{ kg} = 3 \text{ kg}$

17) $\dfrac{1 \text{ kg}}{2.2 \text{ lb}} \times \dfrac{X \text{ kg}}{64 \text{ lb}}$

    $2.2X = 64$

    $\dfrac{2.2X}{2.2} = \dfrac{64}{2.2}$

    $X = 29.09 \text{ kg} = 29.1 \text{ kg}$

Minimum daily dosage:

$10 \text{ mg/kg/day} \times 29.1 \text{ kg} = 291 \text{ mg/day}$, or:

$\dfrac{10 \text{ mg}}{1 \text{ kg}} \times \dfrac{X \text{ mg}}{29.1 \text{ kg}}$

    $X = 291 \text{ mg (per day)}$

Minimum single dose (based on b.i.d.):

$291 \text{ mg per 2 doses} = 145.5 \text{ mg/dose}$

Maximum daily dosage:

$60 \text{ mg/kg/day} \times 29.1 \text{ kg} = 1{,}746 \text{ mg/day}$

Maximum single dosage (based on 60 mg/kg/day):

$1{,}746 \text{ mg} \div 2 \text{ doses} = 873 \text{ mg/dose}$

Dosage ordered is safe. Child will receive 300 mg in a 24-hour period in divided doses of 150 mg b.i.d. This falls within the allowable dosage range of 145.5 mg/dose to 873 mg/dose. Because the daily dosage exceeds 250 mg, the order is appropriately divided.

18) $\dfrac{250 \text{ mg}}{5 \text{ mL}} \times \dfrac{150 \text{ mg}}{X \text{ mL}}$

    $250X = 750$

    $\dfrac{250X}{250} = \dfrac{750}{250}$

    $X = 3 \text{ mL}$

19) $\dfrac{1 \text{ kg}}{1{,}000 \text{ g}} \times \dfrac{X \text{ kg}}{2{,}500 \text{ g}}$

    $1{,}000X = 2{,}500$

    $\dfrac{1{,}000X}{1{,}000} = \dfrac{2{,}500}{1{,}000}$

    $X = 2.5 \text{ kg}$

Recommended daily dosage:

$50{,}000 \text{ units/kg/day} \times 2.5 \text{ kg} = 125{,}000 \text{ units/day}$, or:

$\dfrac{50{,}000 \text{ units}}{1 \text{ kg}} \times \dfrac{X \text{ units}}{2.5 \text{ kg}}$

    $X = 125{,}000 \text{ units (per day)}$

Recommended daily and single dosage:

125,000 units/dose

Ordered dosage is safe.

20) Select 250,000 units/mL concentration because the amount to give will be an exact measurement in the 1 mL syringe; this will require you to add 18 mL of diluent.

Total solution volume after reconstitution:

$$\frac{250,000\ units}{1\ mL} \diagup\diagdown \frac{5,000,000\ units}{X\ mL}$$

$$250,000X = 5,000,000$$

$$\frac{250,000X}{250,000} = \frac{5,000,000}{250,000}$$

$$X = 20\ mL$$

$$\frac{250,000\ units}{1\ mL} \diagup\diagdown \frac{125,000\ units}{X\ mL}$$

$$250,000X = 125,000$$

$$\frac{250,000X}{250,000} = \frac{125,000}{250,000}$$

$$X = 0.5\ mL$$

23)
$$\frac{1\ kg}{2.2\ lb} \diagup\diagdown \frac{X\ kg}{30.5\ lb}$$

$$2.2X = 30.5$$

$$\frac{2.2X}{2.2} = \frac{30.5}{2.2}$$

$$X = 13.86\ kg = 13.9\ kg$$

Recommended daily dosage (for otitis media):

40 mg/kg/day × 13.9 kg = 556 mg/day, or:

$$\frac{40\ mg}{1\ kg} \diagup\diagdown \frac{X\ mg}{13.9\ kg}$$

$$X = 556\ mg\ (per\ day)$$

Recommended single dosage: 556 mg ÷ 3 doses = 185.33 mg = 185.3 mg

The ordered dosage of 187 mg p.o. is reasonably safe for this child.

24) Order: 187 mg

Supply: 187 mg per 5 mL

Think: It is obvious that you want to give 5 mL.

$$\frac{187\ mg}{5\ mL} \diagup\diagdown \frac{187\ mg}{X\ mL}$$

$$187X = 935$$

$$\frac{187X}{187} = \frac{935}{187}$$

$$X = 5\ mL$$

If we use the exact recommended single dosage of 185.3 mg/dose, the calculation would be:

$$\frac{187\ mg}{5\ mL} \diagup\diagdown \frac{185.3\ mg}{X\ mL}$$

$$187X = 926.5$$

$$\frac{187X}{187} = \frac{926.5}{187}$$

X = 4.95 mL; which we would round up to 5 mL to measure in the pediatric oral syringe; therefore, as stated above, the ordered dosage is reasonably safe.

25)
$$\frac{1\ kg}{2.2\ lb} \diagup\diagdown \frac{X\ kg}{22\ lb}$$

$$2.2X = 22$$

$$\frac{2.2X}{2.2} = \frac{22}{2.2}$$

$$X = 10\ kg$$

0.01 mg/kg/dose × 10 kg = 0.1 mg/dose, or:

$$\frac{1\ kg}{10\ mg} \diagup\diagdown \frac{0.01\ kg}{X\ mg}$$

$$X = 0.1\ mg\ (per\ dose)$$

$$\frac{1\ mg}{1,000\ mcg} \diagup\diagdown \frac{0.1\ mg}{X\ mcg}$$

$$X = 100\ mcg\ (per\ dose)$$

Ordered dosage is safe.

29)
$$\frac{1\ kg}{2.2\ lb} \diagup\diagdown \frac{X\ kg}{20\ lb}$$

$$2.2X = 20$$

$$\frac{2.2X}{2.2} = \frac{20}{2.2}$$

$$X = 9.09\ kg = 9.1\ kg$$

Recommended minimum daily dosage:

50 mg/kg/day × 9.1 kg = 455 mg/day, or:

$$\frac{50\ mg}{1\ kg} \diagup\diagdown \frac{X\ mg}{9.1\ kg}$$

$$X = 455\ mg\ (per\ day)$$

Recommended minimum single dosage:

455 mg ÷ 2 doses = 227.5 mg/dose

Recommended maximum daily dosage:

75 mg/kg/day × 9.1 kg = 682.5 mg/day, or:

$$\frac{75\ mg}{1\ kg} \diagup\diagdown \frac{X\ mg}{9.1\ kg}$$

$$X = 682.5\ mg/day$$

Maximum single dosage:

682.5 mg ÷ 2 doses = 341.25 mg = 341.3 mg/dose

The dosage ordered (1 g q.12 h) is not safe. The recommended range for a child of this weight is 227.5−341.3 mg/dose. The physician should be called for clarification.

41)
$$\frac{1\ kg}{2.2\ lb} \diagup\diagdown \frac{X\ kg}{51\ lb}$$

$$2.2X = 51$$

$$\frac{2.2X}{2.2} = \frac{51}{2.2}$$

$$X = 23.18\ kg = 23.2\ kg$$

Recommended daily dosage:

15 mg/kg/day × 23.2 kg = 348 mg/day, or:

$$\frac{15\ mg}{1\ kg} \diagup\diagdown \frac{X\ mg}{23.2\ kg}$$

$$X = 348\ mg\ (per\ day)$$

Recommended single dosage:

348 mg ÷ 2 doses = 174 mg/dose

Ordered dosage of 175 mg is reasonably safe as an oral medication and should be given.

43) $\dfrac{1 \text{ kg}}{2.2 \text{ lb}} \bowtie \dfrac{X \text{ kg}}{95 \text{ lb}}$

$2.2X = 95$

$\dfrac{2.2X}{2.2} = \dfrac{95}{2.2}$

$X = 43.18 \text{ kg} = 43.2 \text{ kg}$

$0.5 \text{ mg/kg/day} \times 43.2 \text{ kg} = 21.6 \text{ mg/day}$, or:

$\dfrac{0.5 \text{ mg}}{1 \text{ kg}} \bowtie \dfrac{X \text{ mg}}{43.2 \text{ kg}}$

$X = 21.6 \text{ mg}$ (per day, minimum)

Because the recommended dosage is not less than 21.6 mg/day and the order is for 10 mg q.6h for a total of 40 mg/day, the order is safe.

$\dfrac{40 \text{ mg}}{1 \text{ mL}} \bowtie \dfrac{10 \text{ mg}}{X \text{ mL}}$

$40X = 10$

$\dfrac{40X}{40} = \dfrac{10}{40}$

$X = 0.25 \text{ mL}$

Review Set 29 from page 437

1) 0.05; 1 L = 1,000 mL 2) 0.3; 1 kg = 1,000 g 3) 38.2; 1 kg = 2.2 lb 4) $2\frac{1}{2}$; 1 fl oz = 30 mL 5) 0.75; 1 L = 1,000 mL
6) 45; 1 fl oz = 30 mL 7) 0.625; 1 mg = 1,000 mcg 8) $\frac{1}{2}$; 1 t = 5 mL 9) 600; 1 kg = 1,000 g 10) 3; 1 in = 2.5 cm
11) 16,000; 1 g = 1,000 mg 12) $\frac{1}{2}$; 1 fl oz = 30 mL 13) 0.2; 1 lb = 16 oz 14) 2; 1 qt = 1 L 15) 33; 1 kg = 2.2 lb
16) 5; 1 fl oz = 30 mL 17) 1; 1 t = 5 mL 18) 8; 1 L = 1,000 mL; 1 qt = 1 L; 1 qt = 32 fl oz 19) 3; 1 t = 5 mL
20) 0.25; 1 mg = 1,000 mcg

Solutions—Review Set 29

3) lb → kg; Smaller ↑ Larger → (÷)

84 lb ÷ 2.2 lb/kg = 84 lb $\times \dfrac{1 \text{ kg}}{2.2 \text{ lb}}$ = 38.18 kg = 38.2 kg

5) mL → L; Smaller ↑ Larger → (÷)

750 mL ÷ 1,000 mL/L = 750 mL $\times \dfrac{1 \text{ L}}{1,000 \text{ mL}}$ = 0.75 L

or, .750. mL = 0.750 L = 0.75 L

9) kg → g; Larger ↓ Smaller (×)

0.6 kg × 1,000 g/kg = 600 g

or, 0.600. kg = 600 g

18) mL → L; Smaller ↑ Larger (÷)

2,000 mL ÷ 1,000 mL/L = 2,000 mL $\times \dfrac{1 \text{ L}}{1,000 \text{ mL}}$ = 2 L

or, 2.000. mL = 2.0 L = 2 L

L → fl oz; Larger ↓ Smaller (×)

2 L × 32 fl oz/L = 64 fl oz

1 cup = 8 fl oz

fl oz → cups; Smaller ↑ Larger (÷)

64 fl oz ÷ 8 fl oz/cup = $\dfrac{64}{8}$ = 8 cups, or eight 8 fl oz glasses

Review Set 30 from pages 440–441

1) 2 2) 2.5 3) 0.8 4) 1.3 5) 7.5 6) 0.6 7) $1\frac{1}{2}$ 8) 3 9) 30 10) 1.6 11) 3 12) 0.5 13) $2\frac{1}{2}$ 14) 250 mg; $\frac{1}{2}$ of 250 mg tab
15) 2.4 16) 2 17) 18 18) 1.3 19) 16 20) 7

Solutions—Review Set 30

2) Order: 150 mg

Supply: 300 mg per 5 mL

$\dfrac{D}{H} \times Q = \dfrac{\overset{1}{\cancel{150}} \text{ mg}}{\underset{2}{\cancel{300}} \text{ mg}} \times 5 \text{ mL} = \dfrac{5}{2} \text{ mL} = 2.5 \text{ mL}$

5) Order: 450 mg

Supply: 300 mg per 5 mL

$\dfrac{D}{H} \times Q = \dfrac{\overset{3}{\cancel{450}} \text{ mg}}{\underset{2}{\cancel{300}} \text{ mg}} \times 5 \text{ mL} = \dfrac{15}{2} \text{ mL} = 7.5 \text{ mL}$

6) Order: 2.4 mg

Supply: 4 mg per 1 mL

$\dfrac{D}{H} \times Q = \dfrac{2.4 \text{ mg}}{4 \text{ mg}} \times 1 \text{ mL} = 0.6 \text{ mL}$

9) Order: 160 mg

Supply: 80 mg per 15 mL

$\dfrac{D}{H} \times Q = \dfrac{\overset{2}{\cancel{160}} \text{ mg}}{\underset{1}{\cancel{80}} \text{ mg}} \times 15 \text{ mL} = \dfrac{30}{1} \text{ mL} = 30 \text{ mL}$

16) Order: 0.15 mg

Supply: 75 mcg/tab

mg → mcg; Larger ↓ Smaller → (×); or move 3 decimal places to the right.

Conversion factor: 1,000 mcg/mg

0.15 mg × 1,000 mcg/mg = 150 mg,

or 0.150. mg = 150 mcg

$\dfrac{D}{H} \times Q = \dfrac{\overset{2}{\cancel{150}} \text{ mcg}}{\underset{1}{\cancel{75}} \text{ mcg}} \times 1 \text{ tab} = 2 \text{ tab}$

18)   Order: 100 mg

       Supply: 80 mg per 1 mL

$$\frac{D}{H} \times Q = \frac{100 \text{ mg}}{80 \text{ mg}} \times 1 \text{ mL} = 1.25 \text{ mL} = 1.3 \text{ mL}$$

19)   Order: 8 mg

       Supply: 2.5 mg per 5 mL

$$\frac{D}{H} \times Q = \frac{8 \text{ mg}}{2.5 \text{ mg}} \times 5 \text{ mL} = \frac{40}{2.5} \text{ mL} = 16 \text{ mL}$$

Review Set 31 from pages 451–452

1) 0.5   **2)** 3   **3)** 34   **4)** 12   **5)** 10   **6)** 13   **7)** $1\frac{1}{2}$ **8)** 2   **9)** 2   **10)** 3   **11)** 1.7   **12)** 0.91   **13)** 0.31   **14)** 7.5   **15)** 0.75   **16)** 6   **17)** 3.2   **18)** 1.2   **19)** 4.4   **20)** 6.2

Solutions—Review Set 31

1) $X \text{ mL} = \frac{1 \text{ mL}}{10,000 \text{ units}} \times 5,000 \text{ units} = 0.5 \text{ mL}$

3) $X \text{ mL} = \frac{5 \text{ mL}}{250 \text{ mg}} \times \frac{15 \text{ mg}}{1 \text{ kg}} \times \frac{1 \text{ kg}}{2.2 \text{ lb}} \times 250 \text{ lb} = 34 \text{ mL}$

6) $X \text{ mL} = \frac{5 \text{ mL}}{250 \text{ mg}} \times \frac{1,000 \text{ mg}}{1 \text{ g}} \times \frac{0.01 \text{ g}}{1 \text{ kg}} \times \frac{1 \text{ kg}}{2.2 \text{ lb}} \times 143 \text{ lb} = 13 \text{ mL}$

11) $X \text{ mL} = \frac{1 \text{ mL}}{0.2 \text{ mg}} \times \frac{1 \text{ mg}}{1,000 \text{ mcg}} \times \frac{4 \text{ mcg}}{1 \text{ kg}} \times \frac{1 \text{ kg}}{2.2 \text{ lb}} \times 185 \text{ lb} = 1.68 \text{ mL} = 1.7 \text{ mL}$

12) $X \text{ mL} = \frac{1 \text{ mL}}{10,000 \text{ units}} \times \frac{150 \text{ units}}{1 \text{ kg}} \times \frac{1 \text{ kg}}{2.2 \text{ lb}} \times 133 \text{ lb} = 0.906 \text{ mL} = 0.91 \text{ mL}$

13) $X \text{ mL} = \frac{1 \text{ mL}}{2 \text{ mg}} \times \frac{1 \text{ mg}}{1,000 \text{ mcg}} \times \frac{50 \text{ mcg}}{1 \text{ kg}} \times \frac{1 \text{ kg}}{2.2 \text{ lb}} \times 27 \text{ lb} = 0.306 \text{ mL} = 0.31 \text{ mL}$

15) $X \text{ mL} = \frac{1 \text{ mL}}{0.2 \text{ mg}} \times \frac{1 \text{ mg}}{1,000 \text{ mcg}} \times 150 \text{ mcg} = 0.75 \text{ mL}$

17) $X \text{ mL} = \frac{1 \text{ mL}}{2 \text{ mg}} \times \frac{1 \text{ mg}}{1,000 \text{ mcg}} \times \frac{80 \text{ mcg}}{1 \text{ kg}} \times 80 \text{ kg} = 3.2 \text{ mL}$

19) $X \text{ mL} = \frac{5 \text{ mL}}{375 \text{ mg}} \times \frac{990 \text{ mg}}{1 \text{ day}} \times \frac{1 \text{ day}}{24 \text{ h}} \times 8 \text{ h} = 4.4 \text{ mL (per dose)}$

Practice Problems—Chapter 14 from pages 454–456

1) 45   **2)** 2   **3)** 2   **4)** $\frac{1}{2}$ **5)** 2.5   **6)** 16   **7)** 1.4   **8)** 0.7   **9)** 2.3   **10)** 0.13 (measured in a 1 mL syringe)   **11)** 1.6   **12)** 1.5   **13)** 1.3   **14)** 2.5   **15)** 1.6   **16)** 7.5   **17)** 1.6   **18)** 2   **19)** 8   **20)** 4.5   **21)** 30   **22)** 1.4   **23)** 0.4   **24)** 20   **25)** 12

26) Prevention: This type of calculation error occurred because the nurse set up the formula incorrectly. In this instance, the nurse placed the *have-on-hand dosage* (H) in the numerator and the *desired dosage* (D) in the denominator. The *desired dosage* should be in the numerator and the *dosage you have on hand* should be placed in the denominator.

$$\frac{D \text{ (desired)}}{H \text{ (have)}} \times Q \text{ (quantity)} = X \text{ (amount)}$$

$$\frac{D}{H} \times Q = \frac{50 \text{ mg}}{125 \text{ mg}} \times 5 \text{ mL} = \frac{\overset{2}{250}}{\underset{1}{125}} \text{ mL} = \frac{2}{1} \text{ mL} = 2 \text{ mL}$$

In addition, **think first.** Then use the $\frac{D}{H} \times Q$ formula to calculate the dosage.

Solutions—Practice Problems—Chapter 14

1)   Formula Method

       Order: 30 g

       Supply: 3.33 g per 5 mL

$$\frac{D}{H} \times Q = \frac{30 \text{ g}}{3.33 \text{ g}} \times 5 \text{ mL} = 45 \text{ mL}$$

Dimensional Analysis

$$X \text{ mL} = \frac{5 \text{ mL}}{3.33 \text{ g}} \times 30 \text{ g} = 45 \text{ mL}$$

2) Formula Method

Order: 500,000 units

Supply: 5,000,000 units per 20 mL

$$\frac{D}{H} \times Q = \frac{\overset{1}{\cancel{500,000 \text{ units}}}}{\underset{10}{\cancel{5,000,000 \text{ units}}}} \times 20 \text{ mL} = \frac{20}{10} \text{ mL} = 2 \text{ mL}$$

Dimensional Analysis

$$X \text{ mL} = \frac{20 \text{ mL}}{5,000,000 \text{ units}} \times 500,000 \text{ units} = 2 \text{ mL}$$

6) Formula Method

Order: 40 mg

Supply: 12.5 mg per 5 mL

$$\frac{D}{H} \times Q = \frac{40 \text{ mg}}{12.5 \text{ mg}} \times 5 \text{ mL} = \frac{200}{12.5} \text{ mL} = 16 \text{ mL}$$

Dimensional Analysis

$$X \text{ mL} = \frac{5 \text{ mL}}{12.5 \text{ mg}} \times 40 \text{ mg} = 16 \text{ mL}$$

7) Formula Method

Order: 350,000 units

Supply: 500,000 units per 2 mL

$$\frac{D}{H} \times Q = \frac{\overset{7}{\cancel{350,000 \text{ units}}}}{\underset{10}{\cancel{500,000 \text{ units}}}} \times 2 \text{ mL} = \frac{14}{10} \text{ mL} = 1.4 \text{ mL}$$

Dimensional Analysis

$$X \text{ mL} = \frac{2 \text{ mL}}{500,000 \text{ units}} \times 350,000 \text{ units} = 1.4 \text{ mL}$$

8) Formula Method

Order: 3.5 mg

Supply: 10 mg per 2 mL

$$\frac{D}{H} \times Q = \frac{3.5 \text{ mg}}{10 \text{ mg}} \times 2 \text{ mL} = \frac{7}{10} \text{ mL} = 0.7 \text{ mL}$$

Dimensional Analysis

$$X \text{ mL} = \frac{2 \text{ mL}}{10 \text{ mg}} \times 3.5 \text{ mg} = 0.7 \text{ mL}$$

9) Formula Method

Order: 90 mg

Supply: 80 mg per 2 mL

$$\frac{D}{H} \times Q = \frac{90 \text{ mg}}{80 \text{ mg}} \times 2 \text{ mL} = \frac{180}{80} \text{ mL} =$$

2.25 mL = 2.3 mL (measured in a 3 mL syringe)

Dimensional Analysis

$$X \text{ mL} = \frac{2 \text{ mL}}{80 \text{ mg}} \times 90 \text{ mg} = 2.25 \text{ mL} = 2.3 \text{ mL}$$

13) Formula Method

Order: 500 mg

Supply: 1 g per 2.5 mL = 1,000 mg per 2.5 mL

$$\frac{D}{H} \times Q = \frac{\overset{1}{\cancel{550 \text{ mg}}}}{\underset{2}{\cancel{1,000 \text{ mg}}}} \times 2.5 \text{ mL} = \frac{2.5}{2} \text{ mL} =$$

1.25 mL = 1.3 mL (measured in a 3 mL syringe)

Dimensional Analysis

$$X \text{ mL} = \frac{2.5 \text{ mL}}{1 \text{ g}} \times \frac{1 \text{ g}}{1,000 \text{ mg}} \times 500 \text{ mg} =$$

1.25 mL = 1.3 mL

16) Formula Method

Order: 10 mEq

Supply: 20 mEq per 15 mL

$$\frac{D}{H} \times Q = \frac{\overset{1}{\cancel{10 \text{ mEq}}}}{\underset{2}{\cancel{20 \text{ mEq}}}} \times 15 \text{ mL} = \frac{15}{2} \text{ mL} = 7.5 \text{ mL}$$

Dimensional Analysis

$$X \text{ mL} = \frac{15 \text{ mL}}{20 \text{ mEq}} \times 10 \text{ mEq} = 7.5 \text{ mL}$$

18) Formula Method

Order: 150 mcg

Supply: 0.075 mg/tab

mg → mcg; Larger ↓ Smaller → (×)

Conversion factor: 1,000 mcg/mg

0.075 mg × 1,000 mcg/mg = 75 mg, or 0.075 mg = 75 mcg

$$\frac{D}{H} \times Q = \frac{\overset{2}{\cancel{150 \text{ mcg}}}}{\underset{1}{\cancel{75 \text{ mcg}}}} \times 1 \text{ tab} = 2 \text{ tab}$$

Dimensional Analysis

$$X \text{ tab} = \frac{1 \text{ tab}}{0.075 \text{ mg}} \times \frac{1 \text{ mg}}{1,000 \text{ mcg}} \times 150 \text{ mcg} =$$

$$\frac{150}{75} = 2 \text{ tab}$$

Section 3—Self-Evaluation from pages 457–470

1) C; 2 **2)** F; 1 **3)** G; 2 **4)** B; 2 **5)** H; 12 **6)** I; 2 **7)** E; 2 **8)** K; $1\frac{1}{2}$ **9)** M; 1.25 **10)** L; 7.5 **11)** E; 4 **12)** C; 3.5 **13)** G; 0.2
14) A; 2 **15)** D; 1.5 **16)** F; 0.75 **17)** B; 0.75 **18)** H; 0.75
19)

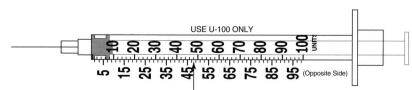

48 units

20)

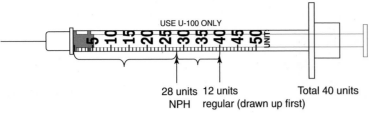

USE U-100 ONLY

28 units NPH   12 units regular (drawn up first)   Total 40 units

21)   4.8; 5; 100; 5

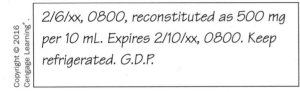

5 mL

22)   10; 10; 500; 10; 8; 1

2/6/xx, 0800, reconstituted as 500 mg per 10 mL. Expires 2/10/xx, 0800. Keep refrigerated. G.D.P.

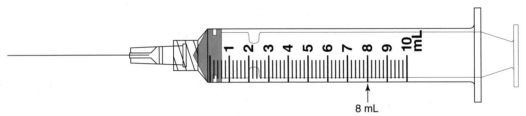

8 mL

23)   2.4; 2.5; 100; 1.5

2/6/xx, 0800, reconstituted as 100 mg/mL. Expires 2/9/xx, 0800. Keep refrigerated. G.D.P.

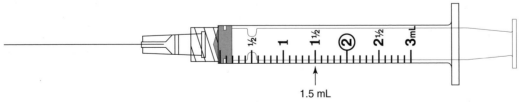

1.5 mL

24) 2.5; 3; 330; 2.3

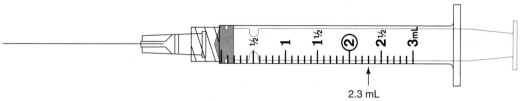

2/6/xx, 0800, reconstituted as
330 mg/mL. Expires 2/7/xx, 0800.
Store at room temperature. G.D.P.

2.3 mL

25) 8; 8; 62.5; 4; 2

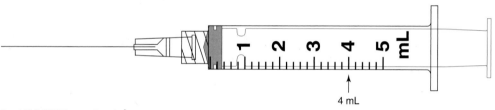

2/6/xx, 0800, reconstituted as
62.5 mg/mL. Expires 2/8/xx, 0800. Keep
at controlled room temperature 20–25°C
(66-77°F). G.D.P.

4 mL

26) 29; 50; 100; 5; 20; 5

2/6/xx, 0800, reconstituted as
100 mg per 5 mL. Expires 2/20/xx, 0800.
Keep refrigerated. G.D.P.

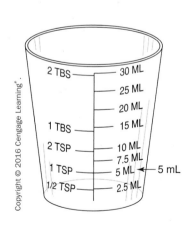

5 mL

27) 10

28) No; the medication supplied will be used up before it expires. It is good for 14 days under refrigeration. The medication is to be given every 12 hours; therefore, 10 doses will be administered in 5 days.

29) 120; 240 **30)** 180; 60 **31)** 120 **32)** 1 **33)** 3 **34)** 540

35) 0.75

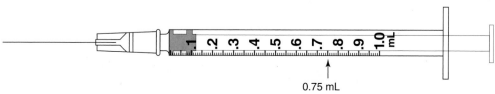

0.75 mL

36)   113; 150; 25; 3

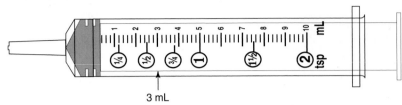

3 mL

37)   Order of 100 mg t.i.d. is too high. The maximum recommended dosage is 100 mg/day for this child. The order is not safe. The physician should be called for clarification.

38)   Order is too high, and the maximum recommended dosage for this child is 292 mg/day. This order would deliver 748 mg/day. Recommended dosage is also 3 times daily, and this order is for 4 times/daily. This order is not safe. The physician should be called for clarification.

39)   a) Order is too high and is not safe. Recommended dosage is 109.5 mg/day or 36.5 mg/dose. The physician should be called for clarification.

      b) 500

40)   **Prevention:** This type of calculation error occurred because the nurse set up the ratio and proportion incorrectly. In this instance the nurse mixed up the values for desired dosage and the dosage on hand.

$$\frac{125 \text{ mg}}{5 \text{ mL}} \times \frac{50 \text{ mg}}{X \text{ mL}}$$

$$125X = 250$$

$$\frac{125X}{125} = \frac{250}{125}$$

$$X = 2 \text{ mL}$$

In addition, **think first.** Then use ratio-proportion to calculate the dosage.

41)   0.015; 1 g = 1,000 mg **42)** 52.3; 1 kg = 2.2 lb **43)** 0.625; 1 mg = 1,000 mcg **44)** 300; 1 g = 1,000 mg **45)** 7

46)   1.5 **47)** 10 **48)** 2 **49)** 3 **50)** 3.8 **51)** 1 mL **52)** a, b, c, d **53)** c

54)   Gather information about the drug.

      Inject 2 mL air into the vial of sterile water.

      Withdraw 2 mL sterile water.

      Add 2 mL sterile water to the antibiotic powder.

      Mix the powder and sterile water.

      Withdraw 1 mL antibiotic solution.

55)   B

Solutions—Section 3—Self-Evaluation

5) $$\frac{20 \text{ mEq}}{15 \text{ mL}} \times \frac{16 \text{ mEq}}{X \text{ mL}}$$

$$20X = 240$$

$$\frac{20X}{20} = \frac{240}{20}$$

$$X = 12 \text{ mL}$$

7) $$\frac{1 \text{ mg}}{1,000 \text{ mcg}} \times \frac{0.05 \text{ mg}}{X \text{ mcg}}$$

$$X = 50 \text{ mcg}$$

$$\frac{25 \text{ mcg}}{1 \text{ tab}} \times \frac{50 \text{ mcg}}{X \text{ tab}}$$

$$25X = 50$$

$$\frac{25X}{25} = \frac{50}{25}$$

$$X = 2 \text{ tab}$$

Label N (Synthroid 100 mcg/tab) is not selected because it is best to give whole tablets when possible rather than splitting a tablet in half.

8) Order: 45 mg

Supply: 30 mg/tab

$$\frac{30\ mg}{1\ tab} \diagdown\!\!\!\!\!\diagup \frac{45\ mg}{X\ tab}$$

$$30X = 45$$

$$\frac{30X}{30} = \frac{45}{30}$$

$$X = 1.5\ tab = 1\tfrac{1}{2}\ tab$$

9) Order: 12.5 mg

Supply: 10 mg/mL

$$\frac{10\ mg}{1\ mL} \diagdown\!\!\!\!\!\diagup \frac{12.5\ mg}{X\ mL}$$

$$10X = 12.5$$

$$\frac{10X}{10} = \frac{12.5}{10}$$

$$X = 1.25\ mL$$

Answer should be left as 1.25 mL and not rounded because the dropper supplied with the medication will measure 1.25 mL. Notice the picture of the dropper on the label.

13) Order: 200 mcg

Supply: 1 mg/mL = 1,000 mcg/mL

$$\frac{1,000\ mcg}{1\ mL} \diagdown\!\!\!\!\!\diagup \frac{200\ mcg}{X\ mL}$$

$$1,000X = 200$$

$$\frac{1,000X}{1,000} = \frac{200}{1,000}$$

$$X = 0.2\ mL$$

17) Order: 7.5 mg

Supply: 10 mg/mL

$$\frac{10\ mg}{1\ mL} \diagdown\!\!\!\!\!\diagup \frac{7.5\ mg}{X\ mL}$$

$$10X = 7.5$$

$$\frac{10X}{10} = \frac{7.5}{10}$$

$$X = 0.75\ mL$$

22) Order: 400 mg

Supply: 500 mg per 10 mL

$$\frac{500\ mg}{10\ mL} \diagdown\!\!\!\!\!\diagup \frac{400\ mg}{X\ mL}$$

$$500X = 4,000$$

$$\frac{500X}{500} = \frac{4,000}{500}$$

$$X = 8\ mL$$

$$\frac{400\ mg}{1\ dose} \diagdown\!\!\!\!\!\diagup \frac{500\ mg}{X\ dose}$$

$$400X = 500$$

$$\frac{400X}{400} = \frac{500}{400}$$

$$X = 1.25\ doses\ (1\ full\ available)$$

25) Order: 250 mg

Supply: 500 mg/8 mL = 62.5 mg/mL

$$\frac{62.5\ mg}{1\ mL} \diagdown\!\!\!\!\!\diagup \frac{250\ mg}{X\ mL}$$

$$62.5X = 250$$

$$\frac{62.5X}{62.5} = \frac{250}{62.5}$$

$$X = 4\ mL$$

500 mg vial:

$$\frac{250\ mg}{1\ dose} \diagdown\!\!\!\!\!\diagup \frac{500\ mg}{X\ dose}$$

$$250X = 500$$

$$\frac{250X}{250} = \frac{500}{250}$$

$$X = 2\ doses\ (available)$$

29) $$\frac{1}{3} \diagdown\!\!\!\!\!\diagup \frac{X\ mL}{360\ mL}$$

$$3X = 360$$

$$\frac{3X}{3} = \frac{360}{3}$$

$$X = 120\ mL\ (hydrogen\ peroxide)$$

360 mL (total) − 120 mL (solute) = 240 mL (solvent)

31) $$\frac{1\ fl\ oz}{30\ mL} \diagdown\!\!\!\!\!\diagup \frac{8\ fl\ oz}{X\ mL}$$

$$X = 240\ mL$$

$$\frac{2}{3} \diagdown\!\!\!\!\!\diagup \frac{240\ mL}{X\ mL}$$

$$2X = 720$$

$$\frac{2X}{2} = \frac{720}{2}$$

$$X = 360\ mL\ (total\ quantity)$$

360 mL (total) − 240 mL (Ensure) = 120 mL (water)

33) 9 infants require 4 fl oz each; 4 fl oz × 9 = 36 fl oz total

$$\frac{1}{2} \diagdown\!\!\!\!\!\diagup \frac{X\ fl\ oz}{36\ fl\ oz}$$

$$2X = 36$$

$$\frac{2X}{2} = \frac{36}{2}$$

$$X = 18\ fl\ oz\ (Isomil)$$

$$\frac{8\ fl\ oz}{1\ can} \diagdown\!\!\!\!\!\diagup \frac{18\ fl\ oz}{X\ can}$$

$$8X = 18$$

$$\frac{8X}{8} = \frac{18}{8}$$

$$X = 2\tfrac{1}{4}\ cans\ (you\ would\ need\ to\ open\ 3\ cans)$$

34) 36 fl oz total solution − 18 fl oz solute (Isomil) =

18 fl oz solvent (water)

$$\frac{30\ mL}{1\ fl\ oz} \diagdown\!\!\!\!\!\diagup \frac{X\ mL}{18\ fl\ oz}$$

$$X = 540\ mL\ (water)$$

36) $$\frac{1\ kg}{2.2\ lb} \diagdown\!\!\!\!\!\diagup \frac{X\ kg}{15}$$

$$2.2X = 15$$

$$\frac{2.2X}{2.2} = \frac{15}{2.2}$$

$$X = 6.81\ kg = 6.8\ kg$$

Minimum daily dosage:

20 mg/kg/day × 6.8 kg = 136 mg/day

Minimum single dosage:

136 mg ÷ 3 doses = 45.3 mg/dose

Maximum daily dosage:

40 mg/kg/day × 6.8 kg = 272 mg/day

Maximum single dosage:

272 mg ÷ 3 doses = 90.7 mg/dose

Dosage ordered is safe.

$$\frac{125 \text{ mg}}{5 \text{ mL}} \diagdown\!\!\!\diagup \frac{75 \text{ mg}}{\text{X mL}}$$

$$125X = 375$$

$$\frac{125X}{125} = \frac{375}{125}$$

$$X = 3 \text{ mL}$$

37) Recommended dosage:

5 mg/kg/day × 20 kg = 100 mg/day, or:

$$\frac{5 \text{ mg}}{1 \text{ kg}} \diagdown\!\!\!\diagup \frac{\text{X mg}}{20 \text{ kg}}$$

$$X = 100 \text{ mg (per day)}$$

100 mg ÷ 3 doses = 33.33 mg/dose = 33.3 mg/dose

Order of 100 mg t.i.d. is not safe. It is higher than the recommended dosage of 33.3 mg/dose.

38)
$$\frac{1 \text{ kg}}{2.2 \text{ lb}} \diagdown\!\!\!\diagup \frac{\text{X kg}}{16 \text{ lb}}$$

$$2.2X = 16$$

$$\frac{2.2X}{2.2} = \frac{16}{2.2}$$

$$X = 7.27 \text{ kg} = 7.3 \text{ kg}$$

Recommended dosage:

40 mg/kg/day × 7.3 kg = 292 mg/day, or:

$$\frac{40 \text{ mg}}{1 \text{ kg}} \diagdown\!\!\!\diagup \frac{\text{X mg}}{7.3 \text{ kg}}$$

$$X = 292 \text{ mg/day}$$

Ordered dosage is not safe. The child would receive 187 mg/dose × 4 doses/day or a total of 748 mg per day, which is over the recommended dosage of 292 mg/day.

39a)
$$\frac{1 \text{ kg}}{2.2 \text{ lb}} \diagdown\!\!\!\diagup \frac{\text{X kg}}{16 \text{ lb}}$$

$$2.2X = 16$$

$$\frac{2.2X}{2.2} = \frac{16}{2.2}$$

$$X = 7.27 \text{ kg} = 7.3 \text{ kg}$$

Recommended dosage:

15 mg/kg/day × 7.3 kg = 109.5 mg/day, or:

$$\frac{15 \text{ mg}}{1 \text{ kg}} \diagdown\!\!\!\diagup \frac{\text{X mg}}{7.3 \text{ kg}}$$

$$X = 109.5 \text{ mg/day}$$

109.5 mg ÷ 3 doses = 36.5 mg/dose

Dosage ordered is 60 mg q.8h, which is over the recommended dosage of 36.5 mg/dose. Although the total daily dosage is within limits, the q.8h dosage is too high and is not safe.

39b)
$$\frac{1 \text{ kg}}{2.2 \text{ lb}} \diagdown\!\!\!\diagup \frac{\text{X kg}}{275 \text{ lb}}$$

$$2.2X = 275$$

$$\frac{2.2X}{2.2} = \frac{275}{2.2}$$

$$X = 125 \text{ kg}$$

15 mg/kg/day × 125 kg = 1,875 mg/day, or:

$$\frac{15 \text{ mg}}{1 \text{ kg}} \diagdown\!\!\!\diagup \frac{\text{X mg}}{125 \text{ kg}}$$

$$X = 1,875 \text{ mg (per day)}$$

Because 1,875 mg/day or 1.9 g/day exceeds the recommended maximum dosage of 1.5 g/day, you would expect the order for this adult to be the maximum recommended dosage of 1.5 g/day or 1,500 mg/day. This could be divided into 3 doses of 0.5 mg q.8h or 500 mg q.8h.

41) Equivalent: 1 g = 1,000 mg; Conversion factor:

1,000 mg/g

15 mg ÷ 1,000 mg/g = 15 m̶g̶ × $\frac{1 \text{ g}}{1,000 \text{ m̶g̶}}$ = 0.015 g

or, .015. mg = 0.015 g

45) Order: 175 mg

Supply: 25 mg/mL

Formula Method

$$\frac{\overset{7}{\cancel{175 \text{ m̶g̶}}}}{\underset{1}{\cancel{25 \text{ m̶g̶}}}} \times 1 \text{ mL} = 7 \text{ mL}$$

Dimensional Analysis

$$X \text{ mL} = \frac{1 \text{ mL}}{25 \text{ m̶g̶}} \times 175 \text{ m̶g̶} = 7 \text{ mL}$$

48) Order: 600 mcg

Supply: 0.3 mg/tab

Formula Method

Equivalent: 1 mg = 1,000 mcg; Conversion factor:

1,000 mcg/mg

0.3 m̶g̶ × 1,000 mcg/m̶g̶ = 300 mcg

$$\frac{600 \text{ m̶c̶g̶}}{300 \text{ m̶c̶g̶}} \times 1 \text{ tab} = X \text{ tab}$$

$$X = 2 \text{ tabs}$$

Dimensional Analysis

$$X \text{ tab} = \frac{1 \text{ tab}}{0.3 \text{ m̶g̶}} \times \frac{1 \text{ m̶g̶}}{1,000 \text{ m̶c̶g̶}} \times 600 \text{ m̶c̶g̶} =$$

$$\frac{600}{300} \text{ tab} = 2 \text{ tab}$$

Review Set 32 from pages 477–479

1) C; sodium chloride 0.9%, 0.9 g per 100 mL; 308 mOsm/L; isotonic

2) E; dextrose 5%, 5 g per 100 mL; 252 mOsm/L; isotonic

3) G; dextrose 5%, 5 g per 100 mL; sodium chloride 0.9%, 0.9 g per 100 mL; 560 mOsm/L; hypertonic

4) D; dextrose 5%, 5 g per 100 mL, sodium chloride 0.45%, 0.45 g per 100 mL; 406 mOsm/L; hypertonic

5) A; dextrose 5%, 5 g per 100 mL, sodium chloride 0.225%, 0.225 g per 100 mL; 329 mOsm/L; isotonic

6) H; dextrose 5%, 5 g per 100 mL; sodium lactate 0.31 g per 100 mL, NaCl 0.6 g per 100 mL; KCl 0.03 g per 100 mL; CaCl 0.02 g per 100 mL; 525 mOsm/L; hypertonic

7) B; dextrose 5%, 5 g per 100 mL; sodium chloride 0.45%; 0.45 g per 100 mL; potassium chloride 20 mEq per liter (0.149 g per 100 mL); 447 mOsm/L; hypertonic

8) F; sodium chloride 0.45%, 0.45 g per 100 mL; 154 mOsm/L; hypotonic

Review Set 33 from page 481

1) 50; 9 **2)** 25; 2.25 **3)** 25 **4)** 6.75 **5)** 25; 1.125 **6)** 150; 27 **7)** 50; 1.125 **8)** 36; 2.7 **9)** 100; 4.5 **10)** 3.375

Solutions—Review Set 33

1) D_5NS = 5 g dextrose per 100 mL

   and 0.9 g NaCl per 100 mL

   Dextrose:

   $$\frac{5\text{ g}}{100\text{ mL}} \diagtimes \frac{X\text{ g}}{1{,}000\text{ mL}}$$

   $$100X = 5{,}000$$

   $$\frac{100X}{100} = \frac{5{,}000}{100}$$

   $$X = 50\text{ g (dextrose)}$$

   NaCl:

   $$\frac{0.9\text{ g}}{100\text{ mL}} \diagtimes \frac{X\text{ g}}{1{,}000\text{ mL}}$$

   $$100X = 900$$

   $$\frac{100X}{100} = \frac{900}{100}$$

   $$X = 9\text{ g (NaCl)}$$

7) $D_{10}\frac{1}{4}NS$ = 10 g dextrose per 100 mL

   and 0.225 g NaCl per 100 mL

   $0.5\text{ L} = 0.5\text{ L} \times 1{,}000\text{ mL/L} = 500\text{ mL}$

   Dextrose:

   $$\frac{10\text{ g}}{100\text{ mL}} \diagtimes \frac{X\text{ g}}{500\text{ mL}}$$

   $$100X = 5{,}000$$

   $$\frac{100X}{100} = \frac{5{,}000}{100}$$

   $$X = 50\text{ g (dextrose)}$$

   NaCl:

   $$\frac{0.225\text{ g}}{100\text{ mL}} \diagtimes \frac{X\text{ g}}{500\text{ mL}}$$

   $$100X = 112.5$$

   $$\frac{100X}{100} = \frac{112.5}{100}$$

   $$X = 1.125\text{ g (NaCl)}$$

Review Set 34 from page 492

1) 100 **2)** 120 **3)** 83 **4)** 200 **5)** 120 **6)** 125 **7)** 125 **8)** 200 **9)** 75 **10)** 125 **11)** 63 **12)** 24 **13)** 150 **14)** 125 **15)** 42

Solutions—Review Set 34

1) $1\text{ L} = 1{,}000\text{ mL}$

   $$\frac{\text{Total mL}}{\text{Total h}} = \frac{1{,}000\text{ mL}}{10\text{ h}} = 100\text{ mL/h}$$

3) $$\frac{\text{Total mL}}{\text{Total h}} = \frac{2{,}000\text{ mL}}{24\text{ h}} = 83.3\text{ mL/h} = 83\text{ mL/h}$$

4) $$\frac{100\text{ mL}}{30\text{ min}} \diagtimes \frac{X\text{ mL/h}}{60\text{ min/h}}$$

   $$30X = 6{,}000$$

   $$\frac{30X}{30} = \frac{6{,}000}{30}$$

   $$X = 200\text{ mL/h}$$

5)
$$\frac{30 \text{ mL}}{15 \text{ min}} \diagdown \frac{X \text{ mL/h}}{60 \text{ min/h}}$$

$$15X = 1,800$$

$$\frac{15X}{15} = \frac{1,800}{15}$$

$$X = 120 \text{ mL/h}$$

6)
$$\frac{1 \text{ L}}{1,000 \text{ mL}} \diagdown \frac{2.5 \text{ L}}{X \text{ mL}}$$

$$X = 2,500 \text{ mL}$$

$$\frac{\text{Total mL}}{\text{Total h}} = \frac{2,500 \text{ mL}}{20 \text{ h}} = 125 \text{ mL/h}$$

Review Set 35 from pages 494–495

1) 15 **2)** 10 **3)** 60 **4)** 60 **5)** 10

Review Set 36 from pages 497–498

1) $\frac{V}{T} \times C = R$ **2)** 21 **3)** 50 **4)** 33 **5)** 25 **6)** 83 **7)** 42 **8)** 50 **9)** 50 **10)** 80 **11)** 20 **12)** 30 **13)** 17 **14)** 55 **15)** 40

Solutions—Review Set 36

1) $\frac{V}{T} \times C = R$ or $\frac{\text{Volume}}{\text{Time in min}} \times \text{Drop factor} = \text{Rate}$

Volume in mL divided by *time* in minutes, multiplied by the *drop factor calibration* in drops per milliliter, equals the flow *rate* in drops per minute.

2) $\frac{V}{T} \times C = \frac{125 \text{ mL}}{\underset{6}{60} \text{ min}} \times \overset{1}{10} \text{ gtt/mL} = \frac{125 \text{ gtt}}{6 \text{ min}} = 20.8 \text{ gtt/min}$
$= 21 \text{ gtt/min}$

3) $\frac{V}{T} \times C = \frac{50 \text{ mL}}{\underset{1}{60} \text{ min}} \times \overset{1}{60} \text{ gtt/mL} = 50 \text{ gtt/min}$

Recall that when drop factor is 60 mL/h, then number of mL/h = number of gtt/min.

4) $\frac{V}{T} \times C = \frac{100 \text{ mL}}{\underset{3}{60} \text{ min}} \times \overset{1}{20} \text{ gtt/mL} = \frac{100 \text{ gtt}}{3 \text{ min}} = 33.3 \text{ gtt/min}$
$= 33 \text{ gtt/min}$

6) Two 500 mL units of blood = 1,000 mL total volume

$\text{mL/h} = \frac{1,000 \text{ mL}}{4 \text{ h}} = 250 \text{ mL/h}$

$\frac{V}{T} \times C = \frac{250 \text{ mL}}{\underset{3}{60} \text{ min}} \times \overset{1}{20} \text{ gtt/mL}$

$= \frac{250 \text{ gtt}}{3 \text{ min}} = 83.3 \text{ gtt/min} = 83 \text{ gtt/min}$

7) $\frac{\text{Total mL}}{\text{Total h}} = \frac{1,000 \text{ mL}}{6 \text{ h}} = 166.6 \text{ mL/h} = 167 \text{ mL/h}$

$\frac{V}{T} \times C = \frac{167 \text{ mL}}{\underset{4}{60} \text{ min}} \times \overset{1}{15} \text{ gtt/mL} = \frac{167 \text{ gtt}}{4 \text{ min}}$

$= 41.7 \text{ gtt/min} = 42 \text{ gtt/min}$

9) $\frac{V}{T} \times C = \frac{150 \text{ mL}}{\underset{3}{45} \text{ min}} \times \overset{1}{15} \text{ gtt/mL} = \frac{\overset{50}{150} \text{ gtt}}{\underset{1}{3} \text{ min}} = 50 \text{ gtt/min}$

Review Set 37 from pages 500–501

1) 60 **2)** 1 **3)** 3 **4)** 4 **5)** 6 **6)** $\frac{\text{mL/h}}{\text{Drop factor constant}} = \text{gtt/min}$ **7)** 50 **8)** 42 **9)** 28 **10)** 60 **11)** 8 **12)** 31 **13)** 28 **14)** 25 **15)** 11

Solutions—Review Set 37

4) $\frac{60}{15} = 4$

7) $\frac{\text{mL/h}}{\text{Drop factor constant}} = \text{gtt/min}; \frac{200 \text{ mL/h}}{4} = 50 \text{ gtt/min}$

8) $\frac{\text{mL/h}}{\text{Drop factor constant}} = \text{gtt/min}; \frac{125 \text{ mL/h}}{3} = 41.6 \text{ gtt/min}$
$= 42 \text{ gtt/min}$

9) $\frac{\text{mL/h}}{\text{Drop factor constant}} = \text{gtt/min}; \frac{165 \text{ mL/h}}{6} = 27.5 \text{ gtt/min}$
$= 28 \text{ gtt/min}$

10) $\frac{\text{mL/h}}{\text{Drop factor constant}} = \text{gtt/min}; \frac{60 \text{ mL/h}}{1} = 60 \text{ gtt/min}$

(Set the flow rate at the same number of gtt/min as the number of mL/h when the drop factor is 60 gtt/mL, because the drop factor constant is 1.)

14) 0.5 L = 500 mL; $\frac{500 \text{ mL}}{20 \text{ h}} = 25 \text{ mL/h}$; When the drop factor is 60 gtt/mL, number of mL/h = number of gtt/min, so the rate is 25 gtt/min

15) $\frac{650 \text{ mL}}{10 \text{ h}} = 65 \text{ mL/h}$

$\frac{\text{mL/h}}{\text{Drop factor constant}} = \text{gtt/min}; \frac{65 \text{ mL/h}}{6} = 10.8 \text{ gtt/min}$
$= 11 \text{ gtt/min}$

Review Set 38 from pages 504–506

1) 125; 31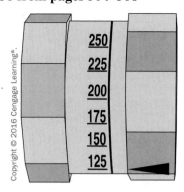

2) 100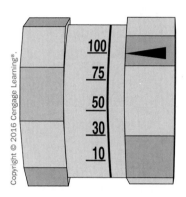

3) 100; 33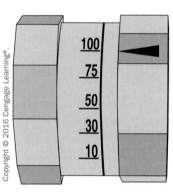

4) 50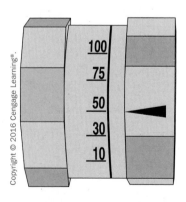

5) 125; 31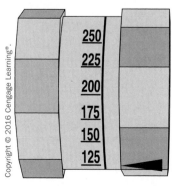

6) 125; 125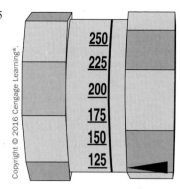

7) 35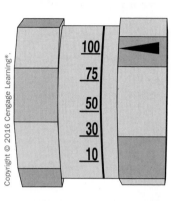

8) 17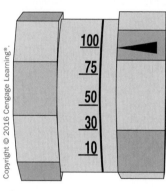

9) 25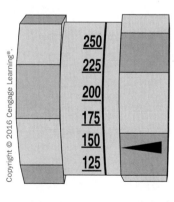

10) 125; 42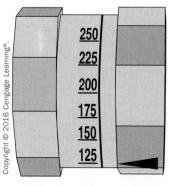

Solutions—Review Set 38

1) $\dfrac{\text{Total mL}}{\text{Total h}} = \dfrac{3{,}000 \text{ mL}}{24 \text{ h}} = 125 \text{ mL/h}$

$\dfrac{V}{T} \times C = \dfrac{125 \text{ mL}}{\underset{4}{60} \text{ min}} \times \overset{1}{15} \text{ gtt/mL} = \dfrac{125 \text{ gtt}}{4 \text{ min}} = 31.2 \text{ gtt/min} = 31 \text{ gtt/min}$

7) $\dfrac{\text{mL/h}}{\text{Drop factor constant}} = \text{gtt/min}; \dfrac{105 \text{ mL/h}}{3} = 35 \text{ gtt/min}$

8) $\dfrac{\text{mL/h}}{\text{Drop factor constant}} = \text{gtt/min}; \dfrac{100 \text{ mL/h}}{6} = 16.6 \text{ gtt/min} = 17 \text{ gtt/min}$

Review Set 39 from pages 509–512

1) 42; 6; 142; 47; 12%; reset to 47 gtt/min (12% increase is acceptable)

2) 42; 2; 180; 45; 7%; reset to 45 gtt/min (7% increase is acceptable)

3) 42; 4; 200; 67; 60%; recalculated rate is 67 gtt/min; 60% increase is unacceptable—consult physician

4) 28; 4; 188; 31; 11%; reset to 31 gtt/min (11% increase is acceptable)

5) 21; 4; 188; 31; 48%; 48% increase is unacceptable—consult physician

6) 31; 1,350; 10; 135; 34; 10%; reset to 34 gtt/min (10% increase is acceptable)

7) 50; 3; 233; 78; 56%; 56% increase is unacceptable—consult physician

8) 33; 3; 83; 28; −15%; −15% slower is acceptable, IV is ahead of schedule, slow rate to 28 gtt/min and observe patient's condition

9) 13; 10; 60; 15; 15%; reset to 15 gtt/min (15% increase is acceptable)

10) 100; 5; 100; 100; 0%; IV is on time, so no adjustment is needed

Solutions—Review Set 39

1) $\dfrac{V}{T} \times C = \dfrac{125 \text{ mL}}{\underset{3}{60} \text{ min}} \times \overset{1}{20} \text{ gtt/mL} = \dfrac{125 \text{ gtt}}{3 \text{ min}} = 41.6 \text{ gtt/min} = 42 \text{ gtt/min (ordered rate)}$

$12 \text{ h} - 6 \text{ h} = 6 \text{ h}$

$\dfrac{\text{Remaining volume}}{\text{Remaining hours}} = \text{Recalculated mL/h}; \dfrac{850 \text{ mL}}{6 \text{ h}} = 141.6 \text{ mL/h} = 142 \text{ mL/h}$

$\dfrac{V}{T} \times C = \dfrac{142 \text{ mL}}{\underset{3}{60} \text{ min}} \times \overset{1}{20} \text{ gtt/mL} = \dfrac{142 \text{ gtt}}{3 \text{ min}} = 47.3 \text{ gtt/min} = 47 \text{ gtt/min (adjusted rate)}$

$\dfrac{\text{Adjusted gtt/min} - \text{Ordered gtt/min}}{\text{Ordered gtt/min}} = \% \text{ of variation}; \dfrac{47 - 42}{42} = \dfrac{5}{42} = 0.119 = 0.12 = 12\% \text{ (within the acceptable \% of variation)};$

reset rate to 47 gtt/min

3) $\dfrac{V}{T} \times C = \dfrac{125 \text{ mL}}{\underset{3}{60} \text{ min}} \times \overset{1}{20} \text{ gtt/mL} = \dfrac{125 \text{ gtt}}{3 \text{ min}} = 41.6 \text{ gtt/min} = 42 \text{ gtt/min (ordered rate)}$

$8 \text{ h} - 4 \text{ h} = 4 \text{ h}$

$\dfrac{800 \text{ mL}}{4 \text{ h}} = 200 \text{ mL/h}; \dfrac{V}{T} \times C = \dfrac{200 \text{ mL}}{\underset{3}{60} \text{ min}} \times \overset{1}{20} \text{ gtt/mL} = \dfrac{200 \text{ gtt}}{3 \text{ min}} = 66.6 \text{ gtt/min} = 67 \text{ gtt/min (adjusted rate)}$

$\dfrac{\text{Adjusted gtt/min} - \text{Ordered gtt/min}}{\text{Ordered gtt/min}} = \% \text{ of variation}; \dfrac{67 - 42}{42} = \dfrac{25}{42} = 0.595 = 0.6 = 60\% \text{ faster};$

unacceptable % of variation—call physician for a revised order

6) $\dfrac{V}{T} \times C = \dfrac{125 \text{ mL}}{\underset{4}{60} \text{ min}} \times \overset{1}{15} \text{ gtt/mL} = \dfrac{125 \text{ gtt}}{4 \text{ min}} = 31.2 \text{ gtt/min} = 31 \text{ gtt/min (ordered rate)}$

$2{,}000 \text{ mL} - 650 \text{ mL} = 1{,}350 \text{ mL remaining}; 16 \text{ h} - 6 \text{ h} = 10 \text{ h}$

$\dfrac{1{,}350 \text{ mL}}{10 \text{ h}} = 135 \text{ mL/h}; \dfrac{V}{T} \times C = \dfrac{135 \text{ mL}}{\underset{4}{60} \text{ min}} \times \overset{1}{15} \text{ gtt/mL} = \dfrac{135 \text{ gtt}}{4 \text{ min}} = 33.7 \text{ gtt/min} = 34 \text{ gtt/min}$

$\dfrac{\text{Adjusted gtt/min} - \text{Ordered gtt/min}}{\text{Ordered gtt/min}} = \% \text{ of variation}; \dfrac{34 - 31}{31} = \dfrac{3}{31} = 0.096 = 0.10 = 10\% \text{ (within acceptable \% of variation)};$

reset rate to 34 gtt/min

8) $\dfrac{V}{T} \times C = \dfrac{100 \text{ mL}}{\underset{3}{60} \text{ min}} \times \overset{1}{20} \text{ gtt/mL} = \dfrac{100 \text{ gtt}}{3 \text{ min}} = 33.3 \text{ gtt/min} = 33 \text{ gtt/min (ordered rate)}$

$5 \text{ h} - 2 \text{ h} = 3 \text{ h}$

$$\frac{250 \text{ mL}}{3 \text{ h}} = 83.3 \text{ mL/h} = 83 \text{ mL/h};$$

$$\frac{V}{T} \times C = \frac{83 \text{ mL}}{\underset{3}{60 \text{ min}}} \times \overset{1}{20} \text{ gtt/mL} = \frac{83 \text{ gtt}}{3 \text{ min}} = 27.6 \text{ gtt/min} = 28 \text{ gtt/min (adjusted rate)}$$

$$\frac{\text{Adjusted gtt/min} - \text{Ordered gtt/min}}{\text{Ordered gtt/min}} = \% \text{ of variation}; \frac{28 - 33}{33} = \frac{-5}{33} = -0.151 = -0.15 = -15\%$$

(Remember that the minus sign indicates the IV is ahead of schedule and rate must be decreased.) Within the acceptable % of variation.

Slow IV to 28 gtt/min and closely monitor patient.

Review Set 40 from pages 517–518

1) 133 **2)** 133 **3)** 50 **4)** 200 **5)** 100 **6)** 25 **7)** 50 **8)** 200 **9)** 150 **10)** 167 **11)** 133 **12)** 25 **13)** 120 **14)** 56 **15)** 200 **16)** 12; 3; 1 **17)** 3; 3; 0.25 **18)** 0.6; 2.4; 0.06 **19)** 2; 18; 10; 2.5 **20)** 1.5; 0.75; 0.19

Solutions—Review Set 40

1) $\frac{V}{T} \times C = \frac{100 \text{ mL}}{\underset{3}{45 \text{ min}}} \times \overset{4}{60} \text{ gtt/mL} = \frac{400 \text{ gtt}}{3 \text{ min}} = 133.3 \text{ gtt/min}$

$= 133 \text{ gtt/min}$

2) $\frac{100 \text{ mL}}{45 \text{ min}} \times \frac{X \text{ mL/h}}{60 \text{ min/h}}$

$45X = 6,000$

$\frac{45X}{45} = \frac{6,000}{45}$

$X = 133.3 \text{ mL/h} = 133 \text{ mL/h}$

3) $\frac{V}{T} \times C = \frac{50 \text{ mL}}{\underset{1}{15 \text{ min}}} \times \overset{1}{15} \text{ gtt/mL} = 50 \text{ gtt/min}$

4) $\frac{50 \text{ mL}}{15 \text{ min}} \times \frac{X \text{ mL/h}}{60 \text{ min/h}}$

$15X = 3,000$

$\frac{15X}{15} = \frac{3,000}{15}$

$X = 200 \text{ mL/h}$

11) $\frac{V}{T} \times C = \frac{100 \text{ mL}}{\underset{3}{15 \text{ min}}} \times \overset{4}{20} \text{ gtt/mL} = \frac{400 \text{ gtt}}{3 \text{ min}} = 133.3 \text{ gtt/min}$

$= 133 \text{ gtt/min}$

16) $\frac{10 \text{ mg}}{1 \text{ mL}} \times \frac{120 \text{ mg}}{X \text{ mL}}$

$10X = 120$

$\frac{10X}{10} = \frac{120}{10}$

$X = 12 \text{ mL}$

$\frac{40 \text{ mg}}{1 \text{ min}} \times \frac{120 \text{ mg}}{X \text{ min}}$

$40X = 120$

$\frac{40X}{40} = \frac{120}{40}$

$X = 3 \text{ min}$

Administer 12 mL over at least 3 min.

1 min = 60 sec

3 min × 60 sec/min = 180 sec

$\frac{12 \text{ mL}}{180 \text{ sec}} \times \frac{X \text{ mL}}{15 \text{ sec}}$

$180X = 180$

$\frac{180X}{180} = \frac{180}{180}$

$X = 1 \text{ mL (per 15 sec)}$

17) $\frac{250 \text{ mg}}{5 \text{ mL}} \times \frac{150 \text{ mg}}{X \text{ mL}}$

$250X = 750$

$\frac{250X}{250} = \frac{750}{250}$

$X = 3 \text{ mL}$

$\frac{50 \text{ mg}}{1 \text{ min}} \times \frac{150 \text{ mg}}{X \text{ min}}$

$50X = 150$

$\frac{50X}{50} = \frac{150}{50}$

$X = 3 \text{ min}$

Administer 3 mL over 3 min.

1 min = 60 sec

3 min × 60 sec/min = 180 sec

$\frac{3 \text{ mL}}{180 \text{ sec}} \times \frac{X \text{ mL}}{15 \text{ sec}}$

$180X = 45$

$\frac{180X}{180} = \frac{45}{180}$

$X = 0.25 \text{ mL (per 15 sec)}$

18) $\frac{10 \text{ mg}}{1 \text{ mL}} \times \frac{6 \text{ mg}}{X \text{ mL}}$

$10X = 6$

$\frac{10X}{10} = \frac{6}{10}$

$X = 0.6 \text{ mL}$

$\frac{2.5 \text{ mg}}{1 \text{ min}} \times \frac{6 \text{ mg}}{X \text{ min}}$

$2.5X = 6$

$\frac{2.5X}{2.5} = \frac{6}{2.5}$

$X = 2.4 \text{ min}$

1 min = 60 sec

2.4 min × 60 sec/min = 144 sec

$\frac{0.6 \text{ mL}}{144 \text{ sec}} \times \frac{X \text{ mL}}{15 \text{ sec}}$

$144X = 9$

$\frac{144X}{144} = \frac{9}{144}$

$X = 0.062 \text{ mL} = 0.06 \text{ mL (per 15 sec)}$

Review Set 41 from pages 520–521

1) 5 h and 33 min **2)** 10 h **3)** 6 h and 24 min **4)** 12; 0400 the next morning **5)** 16; 0730 the next morning **6)** 3,000 **7)** 260 **8)** 300 **9)** 600
10) 360; 2400 (midnight)

Solutions—Review Set 41

1)

$$\frac{\text{Total volume}}{\text{mL/h}} = \text{Total h}$$

$$\frac{500 \text{ mL}}{90 \text{ mL/h}} = 5.55 \text{ h}$$

$$0.55 \text{ h} \times 60 \text{ min/h} = 33 \text{ min}$$

$$5.55 \text{ h} = 5 \text{ h and } 33 \text{ min}$$

2)

$$\frac{\text{Total volume}}{\text{mL/h}} = \text{Total h}$$

$$\frac{\overset{10}{1,000} \text{ mL}}{\underset{1}{100} \text{ mL/h}} = 10 \text{ h}$$

4)

$$\frac{\text{Total volume}}{\text{mL/h}} = \text{Total h}$$

$$\frac{1,200 \text{ mL}}{100 \text{ mL/h}} = 12 \text{ h}$$

$$2400 \text{ h} - 1600 \text{ h} = 8 \text{ h (until midnight)}$$

$$12 \text{ h} - 8 \text{ h} = 4 \text{ h (into next day)}$$

Completion time = 0400 (the next morning)

Hint: Go back to Chapter 5, Figure 5-1, and look at the 24-hour clock.

5)

$$\frac{\text{Total volume}}{\text{mL/h}} = \text{Total h}$$

$$\frac{\overset{16}{2,000} \text{ mL}}{\underset{1}{125} \text{ mL/h}} = 16 \text{ h}$$

$$2400 \text{ h} = 23 \text{ h and } 60 \text{ min}$$

$$23 \text{ h } 60 \text{ min} - 15 \text{ h } 30 \text{ min} = 8 \text{ h } 30 \text{ min (until midnight)}$$

$$16 \text{ h} = 15 \text{ h and } 60 \text{ min}$$

$$15 \text{ h } 60 \text{ min} - 8 \text{ h } 30 \text{ min} = 7 \text{ h } 30 \text{ min (into the next day)}$$

Completion time = 0730 (the next morning)

6) Total hours × mL/h = Total mL

$$24 \text{ h} \times 125 \text{ mL/h} = 3,000 \text{ mL}$$

7) Total hours × mL/h = Total mL

$$4 \text{ h} \times 65 \text{ mL/h} = 260 \text{ mL}$$

Practice Problems—Chapter 15 from pages 523–528

1) 17 **2)** 42 **3)** 42 **4)** 8 **5)** 125 **6)** Assess your patient and the pump. If the pump is programmed at 125 mL/h and is plugged in, discontinue the IV pump and confer with your supervisor to implement your backup plan. **7)** 31 **8)** 42 **9)** Assess patient. If stable, recalculate and reset to 50 gtt/min; observe patient closely. **10)** 3,000 **11)** Abbott Laboratories **12)** 15 gtt/mL **13)** 4

14) $\text{mL/h} = \frac{500 \text{ mL}}{4 \text{ h}} = 125 \text{ mL/h}$

$$\frac{\text{mL/h}}{\text{Drop factor constant}} = \text{gtt/min}; \frac{125 \text{ mL/h}}{4} = 31.2 \text{ gtt/min} = 31 \text{ gtt/min}$$

15) $\frac{V}{T} \times C = \frac{125 \text{ mL}}{\underset{4}{60} \text{ min}} \times \overset{1}{15} \text{ gtt/mL} = \frac{125 \text{ gtt}}{4 \text{ min}} = 31.2 \text{ gtt/min} = 31 \text{ gtt/min}$

16) 1930 (or 7:30 PM) **17)** 250 **18)** Recalculate 210 mL to infuse over remaining 2 hours. Reset IV to 26 gtt/min and observe patient closely. **19)** 125 **20)** 100 **21)** Dextrose 2.5% (2.5 g per 100 mL) and NaCl 0.45% (0.45 g per 100 mL) **22)** 25; 4.5 **23)** 5; 2; 0.4; 0.2 **24)** 3.5; 7; 2; 0.5 **25)** 6; 3; 0.5; 0.25 **26)** 10; 5; 0.5; 0.13 **27)** 225; 38 **28)** 75; 75 **29)** 125; 42 **30)** 100; 25 **31)** 150; 50 **32)** 14 **33)** 21 **34)** 28 **35)** 83 **36)** 17 **37)** 25 **38)** 33 **39)** 100 **40)** 33 **41)** 50 **42)** 67 **43)** 200 **44)** 8 **45)** 11 **46)** 15 **47)** 45 **48)** 62.5 mL. The IV will finish in less than 30 minutes. IV will run out. Advise relief nurse to monitor IV, discontinue bag when complete, and plan to flush and cap the saline lock. **49)** 1250 (or 12:50 PM)

50) Prevention: This error could have been prevented had the nurse carefully inspected the IV tubing package to determine the drop factor and stopped to think about why so much IV fluid would be administered in just 8 hours. Every IV tubing set has the drop factor printed on the package, so it is not necessary to memorize or guess the drop factor. The IV calculation should have looked like this:

$$\frac{V}{T} \times C = \frac{125 \text{ mL}}{\underset{3}{60} \text{ min}} \times \overset{1}{20} \text{ gtt/mL} = \frac{125 \text{ gtt}}{3 \text{ min}} = 41.6 \text{ gtt/min} = 42 \text{ gtt/min}$$

With the infusion set of 20 gtt/mL, a flow rate of 42 gtt/min would infuse 125 mL/h. At the 125 gtt/min rate the nurse calculated, the patient received three times the IV fluid ordered hourly. Thus, the patient actually received 375 mL/h of IV fluids.

Solutions—Practice Problems—Chapter 15

1) 100 mL/h = 100 mL per 60 min

$$\frac{V}{T} \times C = \frac{100 \text{ mL}}{\underset{6}{60} \text{ min}} \times \overset{1}{10} \text{ gtt/mL} = \frac{100 \text{ gtt}}{6 \text{ min}} = 16.6 \text{ gtt/min}$$

$$= 17 \text{ gtt/min}$$

2) $\dfrac{\text{Total mL}}{\text{Total h}} = \dfrac{1,000 \text{ mL}}{24 \text{ h}} = 41.6 \text{ mL/h} = 42 \text{ mL/h}$

drop factor is 60 gtt/mL; 42 mL/h = 42 gtt/min

5) 1800 − 1000 = 800, or 8 h

$$\frac{\text{Total mL}}{\text{Total h}} = \frac{1,000 \text{ mL}}{8 \text{ h}} = 125 \text{ mL/h}$$

6) After 1 h, there should be 875 mL remaining (1,000 mL − 125 mL = 875 mL). Patient received 200 mL in one hour, a rate of 200 mL/h; a rate of 60% more than ordered. The IV is running too fast and is ahead of schedule. Assess your patient and the pump. Confirm that the IV pump is correctly programmed for 125 mL/h, and check to be sure that it is plugged in. If so, consider that it may need recalibration or that it has a mechanical or electrical failure. Discontinue the IV pump and confer with your supervisor to implement your backup plan: replace the IV pump with another one or with a straight gravity-flow IV system until another IV pump can be located.

7) 1,000 mL + 2,000 mL = 3,000 mL;

$$\frac{\text{Total mL}}{\text{Total h}} = \frac{3,000 \text{ mL}}{24 \text{ h}} = 125 \text{ mL/h}$$

$$\frac{V}{T} \times C = \frac{125 \text{ mL}}{\underset{4}{60} \text{ min}} \times \overset{1}{15} \text{ gtt/mL} = \frac{125 \text{ gtt}}{4 \text{ min}} = 31.2 \text{ gtt/min}$$

$$= 31 \text{ gtt/min}$$

8) $\dfrac{V}{T} \times C = \dfrac{125 \text{ mL}}{\underset{3}{60} \text{ min}} \times \overset{1}{20} \text{ gtt/mL} = \dfrac{125 \text{ gtt}}{3 \text{ min}} = 41.6 \text{ gtt/min}$

$$= 42 \text{ gtt/min}$$

9) $\dfrac{\text{Total mL}}{\text{Total h}} = \dfrac{1,000 \text{ mL}}{6 \text{ h}} = 166.6 \text{ mL/h} = 167 \text{ mL/h}$

$$\frac{V}{T} \times C = \frac{167 \text{ mL}}{\underset{4}{60} \text{ min}} \times \overset{1}{15} \text{ gtt/mL} = \frac{167 \text{ gtt}}{4 \text{ min}} = 41.7 \text{ gtt/min}$$

$$= 42 \text{ gtt/min}$$

6 h − 2 h = 4 h remaining; $\dfrac{\text{Total mL}}{\text{Total h}} = \dfrac{\overset{200}{800} \text{ mL}}{\underset{1}{4} \text{ h}} = 200 \text{ mL/h}$

$$\frac{V}{T} \times C = \frac{200 \text{ mL}}{\underset{4}{60} \text{ min}} \times \overset{1}{15} \text{ gtt/mL} = \frac{\overset{50}{200} \text{ gtt}}{\underset{1}{4} \text{ min}} = 50 \text{ gtt/min}$$

$$\frac{\text{Adjusted gtt/min } - \text{ Ordered gtt/min}}{\text{Ordered gtt/min}} = \% \text{ variation;}$$

$$\frac{50 - 42}{42} = \frac{8}{42} = 0.19 = 19\% \text{ increase;}$$

within safe limits of 25% variance

Reset infusion rate to 50 gtt/min.

10) q.4h = 6 times per 24 h; 6 × 500 mL = 3,000 mL

13) $\dfrac{60}{15} = 4$

16) 1530 + 4 h = 1530 + 0400 = 1930; 1930 − 1200 = 7:30 PM

17) $\dfrac{\text{Total mL}}{\text{Total h}} = \dfrac{500 \text{ mL}}{4 \text{ h}} = 125 \text{ mL/h}$

1730 − 1530 = 200, or 2 h

125 mL/h × 2 h = 250 mL

18) $\dfrac{\text{Total mL}}{\text{Total h}} = \dfrac{210 \text{ mL}}{2 \text{ h}} = 105 \text{ mL/h}$

$$\frac{V}{T} \times C = \frac{105 \text{ mL}}{\underset{4}{60} \text{ min}} \times \overset{1}{15} \text{ gtt/mL} = \frac{105 \text{ gtt}}{4 \text{ min}} = 26.2 \text{ gtt/min}$$

$$= 26 \text{ gtt/min}$$

$$\frac{\text{Adjusted gtt/min } - \text{ Ordered gtt/min}}{\text{Ordered gtt/min}} = \% \text{ of variation:}$$

$$\frac{26 - 31}{31} = \frac{-5}{31} = -0.161 = -0.16 = -16\% \text{ decrease;}$$

within safe limits

Reset infusion rate to 26 gtt/min.

19) $\dfrac{\text{Total mL}}{\text{Total h}} = \dfrac{500 \text{ mL}}{4 \text{ h}} = 125 \text{ mL/h}$

20) $\dfrac{50 \text{ mL}}{30 \text{ min}} \diagdown\diagup \dfrac{X \text{ mL/h}}{60 \text{ min/h}}$

$$30X = 3,000$$

$$\frac{30X}{30} = \frac{3,000}{30}$$

$$X = 100 \text{ mL/h}$$

22) Dextrose 5% = 5 g per 100 mL; NaCl 0.9% = 0.9 g per 100 mL

Dextrose: NaCl:

$$\frac{5 \text{ g}}{100 \text{ mL}} \diagdown\diagup \frac{X \text{ g}}{500 \text{ mL}} \qquad \frac{0.9 \text{ g}}{100 \text{ mL}} \diagdown\diagup \frac{X \text{ g}}{500 \text{ mL}}$$

$$100X = 2,500 \qquad\qquad 100X = 450$$

$$\frac{100X}{100} = \frac{2,500}{100} \qquad\quad \frac{100X}{100} = \frac{450}{100}$$

$$X = 25 \text{ g (dextrose)} \qquad X = 4.5 \text{ g (NaCl)}$$

23) $\dfrac{2 \text{ mg}}{1 \text{ min}} = \dfrac{10 \text{ mg}}{X \text{ min}}$

$$2X = 10$$

$$\frac{2X}{2} = \frac{10}{2}$$

$$X = 5 \text{ min}$$

$$\frac{\text{Dosage on hand}}{\text{Amount on hand}} = \frac{\text{Dosage desired}}{X \text{ Amount desired}}$$

$$\frac{5 \text{ mg}}{1 \text{ mL}} = \frac{10 \text{ mg}}{X \text{ mL}}$$

$$5X = 10$$

$$\frac{5X}{5} = \frac{10}{5}$$

$$X = 2 \text{ mL}$$

Administer 2 mL over 5 min, or

$$\frac{2 \text{ mL}}{5 \text{ min}} = \frac{X \text{ mL}}{1 \text{ min}}$$

$$5X = 2$$

$$\frac{5X}{5} = \frac{2}{5}$$

$$X = 0.4 \text{ mL (per min)}$$

1 min = 60 sec

$$\frac{0.4 \text{ mL}}{60 \text{ sec}} = \frac{X \text{ mL}}{30 \text{ sec}}$$

$$60X = 12$$

$$\frac{60X}{60} = \frac{12}{60}$$

$$X = 0.2 \text{ mL (per 30 sec)}$$

24) $\dfrac{10 \text{ mg}}{1 \text{ min}} = \dfrac{35 \text{ mg}}{X \text{ min}}$

$10X = 35$

$\dfrac{10X}{10} = \dfrac{35}{10}$

$X = 3.5 \text{ min}$

$\dfrac{\text{Dosage on hand}}{\text{Amount on hand}} = \dfrac{\text{Dosage desired}}{X \text{ Amount desired}}$

$\dfrac{5 \text{ mg}}{1 \text{ mL}} = \dfrac{35 \text{ mg}}{X \text{ mL}}$

$5X = 35$

$\dfrac{5X}{5} = \dfrac{35}{5}$

$X = 7 \text{ mL}$

Administer 7 mL over 3.5 min, or

$\dfrac{7 \text{ mL}}{3.5 \text{ min}} = \dfrac{X \text{ mL}}{1 \text{ min}}$

$3.5X = 7$

$\dfrac{3.5X}{3.5} = \dfrac{7}{3.5}$

$X = 2 \text{ mL (per min)}$

$1 \text{ min} = 60 \text{ sec}$

$\dfrac{2 \text{ mL}}{60 \text{ sec}} = \dfrac{X \text{ mL}}{15 \text{ sec}}$

$60X = 30$

$\dfrac{60X}{60} = \dfrac{30}{60}$

$X = 0.5 \text{ mL (per 15 sec)}$

32) $\dfrac{\text{Total mL}}{\text{Total h}} = \dfrac{1{,}000 \text{ mL}}{12 \text{ h}} = 83.3 \text{ mL/h} = 83 \text{ mL/h};$

$\dfrac{V}{T} \times C = \dfrac{83 \text{ mL}}{\underset{6}{60} \text{ min}} \times \overset{1}{10} \text{ gtt/mL} = \dfrac{83 \text{ gtt}}{6 \text{ min}}$

$= 13.8 \text{ gtt/min} = 14 \text{ gtt/min}$

33) $\dfrac{V}{T} \times C = \dfrac{83 \text{ mL}}{\underset{4}{60} \text{ min}} \times \overset{1}{15} \text{ gtt/mL} = \dfrac{83 \text{ gtt}}{4 \text{ min}}$

$= 20.7 \text{ gtt/min} = 21 \text{ gtt/min}$

34) $\dfrac{V}{T} \times C = \dfrac{83 \text{ mL}}{\underset{3}{60} \text{ min}} \times \overset{1}{20} \text{ gtt/mL} = \dfrac{83 \text{ gtt}}{3 \text{ min}}$

$= 27.6 \text{ gtt/min} = 28 \text{ gtt/min}$

35) $\dfrac{V}{T} \times C = \dfrac{83 \text{ mL}}{\underset{1}{60} \text{ min}} \times \overset{1}{60} \text{ gtt/mL} = 83 \text{ gtt/min}$

Remember: If the drop factor is 60 gtt/mL, then number
of mL/h = number of gtt/min, so 83 mL/h = 83 gtt/min.

48) Think: Flow rate is 125 mL/h. You will be gone 30 min, or $\frac{1}{2}$ hour.

$125 \text{ mL/h} \times 0.5 \text{ h} = 62.5 \text{ mL}$

Alert your relief nurse that the IV will likely run out before
you return and to prepare to discontinue the bag and flush and
cap the saline lock.

49) $\dfrac{400 \text{ mL}}{75 \text{ mL/h}} = 5\frac{1}{3} \text{ h or 5 h and 20 min}$

$0730 + 0520 = 1250 \text{ (or 12:50 PM)}$

Review Set 42 from page 533

1) 0.68 **2)** 2.35 **3)** 0.69 **4)** 1.4 **5)** 2.03 **6)** 1 **7)** 1.67 **8)** 0.4 **9)** 1.69 **10)** 0.52 **11)** 1.11 **12)** 0.78 **13)** 0.15 **14)** 0.78 **15)** 0.39 **16)** 0.64
17) 0.25 **18)** 1.08 **19)** 0.5 **20)** 0.88

Solutions—Review Set 42

1) Household: BSA (m²) $= \sqrt{\dfrac{\text{ht (in)} \times \text{wt (lb)}}{3{,}131}} = \sqrt{\dfrac{36 \times 40}{3{,}131}} = \sqrt{\dfrac{1{,}440}{3{,}131}} = \sqrt{0.459916} = 0.678 \text{ m}^2 = 0.68 \text{ m}^2$

2) Metric: BSA (m²) $= \sqrt{\dfrac{\text{ht (cm)} \times \text{wt (kg)}}{3{,}600}} = \sqrt{\dfrac{190 \times 105}{3{,}600}} = \sqrt{\dfrac{19{,}950}{3{,}600}} = \sqrt{5.541666} = 2.354 \text{ m}^2 = 2.35 \text{ m}^2$

Review Set 43 from pages 535–537

1) 1,640,000 **2)** 5.9; 11.8 **3)** 735 **4)** 15.84; 63.36 **5)** 250 **6)** 0.49; 122.5; Yes; 2.5 **7)** 0.89; 2.9; Yes; 1.2 **8)** 66; 22; Yes
9) 198; Yes; 990 **10)** 612; 612; 1,224; 2,448 **11)** 8.1; 24.7 **12)** 67–167.5; 33.5–83.8; Yes **13)** 8–14.4; Yes **14)** 0.82; 2,050; Yes; 2.7;
102.7; 51 **15)** 1.62; 4,050; Yes; 5.4; 105.4; 53

Solutions—Review Set 43

1) $2{,}000{,}000 \text{ units/m}^2 \times 0.82 \text{ m}^2 = 1{,}640{,}000 \text{ units}$

2) $10 \text{ mg/m}^2/\text{day} \times 0.59 \text{ m}^2 = 5.9 \text{ mg/day}$
(minimum safe dosage)
$20 \text{ mg/m}^2/\text{day} \times 0.59 \text{ m}^2 = 11.8 \text{ mg/day}$
(maximum safe dosage)

3) $500 \text{ mg/m}^2 \times 1.47 \text{ m}^2 = 735 \text{ mg}$

4) $6 \text{ mg/m}^2/\text{day} \times 2.64 \text{ m}^2 = 15.84 \text{ mg/day}$
$15.84 \text{ mg/day} \times 4 \text{ days} = 63.36 \text{ mg}$

6) Household: BSA (m²) = $\sqrt{\dfrac{\text{ht (in)} \times \text{wt (lb)}}{3{,}131}} = \sqrt{\dfrac{30 \times 25}{3{,}131}}$

$= \sqrt{\dfrac{750}{3{,}131}} = \sqrt{0.23954} = 0.489 \text{ m}^2 = 0.49 \text{ m}^2$

250 mg/m² × 0.49 m² = 122.5 mg; dosage is safe

$\dfrac{50 \text{ mg}}{1 \text{ mL}} \Large\times \normalsize \dfrac{122.5 \text{ mg}}{\text{X mL}}$

50X = 122.5

$\dfrac{50\text{X}}{50} = \dfrac{122.5}{50}$

X = 2.45 mL = 2.5 mL

8) 150 mg/m²/day × 0.44 m² = 66 mg/day

$\dfrac{66 \text{ mg}}{3 \text{ doses}}$ = 22 mg/dose; dosage is safe

9) 900 mg/m²/day × 0.22 m² = 198 mg/day; dosage is safe

198 mg/day × 5 days = 990 mg

10) 600 mg/m² × 1.02 m² = 612 mg, initially

300 mg/m² × 1.02 m² = 306 mg (per q.4h dose)

306 mg × 2 doses = 612 mg (for 2 q.4h doses)

q.12h is 2 doses/day and

2 doses/day × 2 days = 4 doses

306 mg × 4 doses = 1,224 mg (for 4 q.12h doses)

612 mg + 612 mg + 1,224 mg = 2,448 mg (total)

11) 10 mg/m² × 0.81 m² = 8.1 mg (bolus)

30.5 mg/m²/day × 0.81 m² = 24.7 mg/day

14) Metric: BSA (m²) = $\sqrt{\dfrac{\text{ht (cm)} \times \text{wt (kg)}}{3{,}600}} = \sqrt{\dfrac{100 \times 24}{3{,}600}}$

$= \sqrt{\dfrac{2{,}400}{3{,}600}} = \sqrt{0.666666} = 0.816 \text{ m}^2 = 0.82 \text{ m}^2$

2,500 units/m² × 0.82 m² = 2,050 units; dosage is safe

$\dfrac{750 \text{ units}}{1 \text{ mL}} \Large\times \normalsize \dfrac{2{,}050 \text{ units}}{\text{X mL}}$

750X = 2,050

$\dfrac{750\text{X}}{750} = \dfrac{2{,}050}{750}$

X = 2.73 = 2.7 mL

2.7 mL (Oncaspar) + 100 mL (D₅W) = 102.7 mL (total volume)

$\dfrac{102.7 \text{ mL}}{2 \text{ h}}$ = 51.3 mL/h = 51 mL/h

15) Metric: BSA (m²) = $\sqrt{\dfrac{\text{ht (cm)} \times \text{wt (kg)}}{3{,}600}} = \sqrt{\dfrac{162 \times 58.2}{3{,}600}}$

$= \sqrt{\dfrac{9{,}428.4}{3{,}600}} = \sqrt{2.619} = 1.618 \text{ m}^2 = 1.62 \text{ m}^2$

2,500 units/m² × 1.62 m² = 4,050 units; dosage is safe

$\dfrac{750 \text{ units}}{1 \text{ mL}} \Large\times \normalsize \dfrac{4{,}050 \text{ units}}{\text{X mL}}$

750X = 4,050

$\dfrac{750\text{X}}{750} = \dfrac{4{,}050}{750}$

X = 5.4 mL

5.4 mL (Oncaspar) + 100 mL (D₅W) = 105.4 mL (total volume)

$\dfrac{105.4 \text{ mL}}{2 \text{ h}}$ = 52.7 mL/h = 53 mL/h

Review Set 44 from pages 540–541

1) 87; 2; 48 **2)** 75; 3; 57 **3)** 120; 3; 22 **4)** 80; 6; 44 **5)** 60; 1; 31; 180 **6)** 2; 23 **7)** 2; 8 **8)** 12; 45 **9)** 7.2; 36.8 **10)** 7.5; 88.5

Solutions—Review Set 44

1) Total volume: 50 mL + 15 mL = 65 mL

$\dfrac{\text{V}}{\text{T}} \times \text{C} = \dfrac{65 \text{ mL}}{45 \text{ min}} \times 60 \text{ gtt/mL} = \dfrac{260 \text{ gtt}}{3 \text{ min}}$

= 86.6 gtt/min = 87 gtt/min

$\dfrac{60 \text{ mg}}{2 \text{ mL}} \Large\times \normalsize \dfrac{60 \text{ mg}}{\text{X mL}}$

60X = 120

$\dfrac{60\text{X}}{60} = \dfrac{120}{60}$

X = 2 mL (medication)

Volume IV fluid to add to chamber:

50 mL − 2 mL = 48 mL

4) Total volume: 50 mL + 30 mL = 80 mL

80 mL per 60 min = 80 mL/h

$\dfrac{1 \text{ g}}{10 \text{ mL}} \Large\times \normalsize \dfrac{0.6 \text{ g}}{\text{X mL}}$

X = 6 mL (medication)

Volume IV fluid to add to chamber:

50 mL − 6 mL = 44 mL

6) $\dfrac{50 \text{ mL}}{60 \text{ min}} \Large\times \normalsize \dfrac{\text{X mL}}{30 \text{ min}}$

60X = 1,500

$\dfrac{60\text{X}}{60} = \dfrac{1{,}500}{60}$

X = 25 mL (total volume)

$\dfrac{125 \text{ mg}}{1 \text{ mL}} \Large\times \normalsize \dfrac{250 \text{ mg}}{\text{X mL}}$

125X = 250

$\dfrac{125\text{X}}{125} = \dfrac{250}{125}$

X = 2 mL (medication)

Volume IV fluid to add to chamber:

25 mL − 2 mL = 23 mL.

8) $\dfrac{85 \text{ mL}}{60 \text{ min}} \diagup\!\!\!\!\diagdown \dfrac{X \text{ mL}}{40 \text{ min}}$

$\qquad 60X = 3{,}400$

$\qquad \dfrac{60X}{60} = \dfrac{3{,}400}{60}$

$\qquad\qquad X = 56.6 \text{ mL} = 57 \text{ mL (total volume)}$

$\dfrac{50 \text{ mg}}{1 \text{ mL}} \diagup\!\!\!\!\diagdown \dfrac{600 \text{ mg}}{X \text{ mL}}$

$\qquad 50X = 600$

$\qquad \dfrac{50X}{50} = \dfrac{600}{50}$

$\qquad\qquad X = 12 \text{ mL (medication)}$

Volume IV fluid to add to chamber:

57 mL − 12 mL = 45 mL

9) $\dfrac{66 \text{ mL}}{60 \text{ min}} \diagup\!\!\!\!\diagdown \dfrac{X \text{ mL}}{40 \text{ min}}$

$\qquad 60X = 2{,}640$

$\qquad \dfrac{60X}{60} = \dfrac{2{,}640}{60}$

$\qquad\qquad X = 44 \text{ mL (total volume)}$

$\dfrac{1{,}000 \text{ mg}}{10 \text{ mL}} \diagup\!\!\!\!\diagdown \dfrac{720 \text{ mg}}{X \text{ mL}}$

$\qquad 1{,}000X = 7{,}200$

$\qquad \dfrac{1{,}000X}{1{,}000} = \dfrac{7{,}200}{1{,}000}$

$\qquad\qquad X = 7.2 \text{ mL (medication)}$

Volume IV fluid to add to chamber:

44 mL − 7.2 mL = 36.8 mL

Hint: Add the medication to the volume-control chamber, and fill with IV fluid to the 44 mL mark. The chamber measures whole (not fractional) mL.

10) $48 \text{ mL/}\cancel{h} \times 2 \,\cancel{h} = 96 \text{ mL (total volume)}$

$\dfrac{100 \text{ mg}}{10 \text{ mL}} \diagup\!\!\!\!\diagdown \dfrac{75 \text{ mg}}{X \text{ mL}}$

$\qquad 100X = 750$

$\qquad \dfrac{100X}{100} = \dfrac{750}{100}$

$\qquad\qquad X = 7.5 \text{ mL}$

Volume IV fluid to add to chamber:

96 mL − 7.5 mL = 88.5 mL

Review Set 45 from page 545

1) 4 **2)** 25 **3)** 1,600; 67 **4)** 1,150; 48 **5)** 1,800; 75 **6)** 350; 15 **7)** 3.5 or 4; 11.6 or 12 **8)** 2.6 or 3; 65 **9)** 2.3 or 2; 35 **10)** This order should be questioned, because normal saline is an isotonic solution and appears to be a continuous infusion for this child. This solution does not contribute enough electrolytes for the child, and water intoxication may result.

Solutions—Review Set 45

1) $\dfrac{100 \text{ mg}}{1 \text{ mL}} \diagup\!\!\!\!\diagdown \dfrac{400 \text{ mg}}{X \text{ mL}}$

$\qquad 100X = 400$

$\qquad \dfrac{100X}{100} = \dfrac{400}{100}$

$\qquad\qquad X = 4 \text{ mL}$

3) $100 \text{ mL/kg/day} \times 10 \text{ kg} = 1{,}000 \text{ mL/day for first 10 kg}$

$ 50 \text{ mL/kg/day} \times 10 \text{ kg} = 500 \text{ mL/day for next 10 kg}$

$ \underline{20 \text{ mL/kg/day} \times 5 \text{ kg} = 100 \text{ mL/day for remaining 5 kg}}$

$\qquad\qquad\qquad \text{Total} = 1{,}600 \text{ mL/day or per 24 h}$

$\qquad\qquad\qquad\qquad \dfrac{1{,}600 \text{ mL}}{24 \text{ h}} = 66.6 \text{ mL/h} = 67 \text{ mL/h}$

4) $100 \text{ mL/kg/day} \times 10 \text{ kg} = 1{,}000 \text{ mL/day for first 10 kg}$

$ \underline{50 \text{ mL/kg/day} \times 3 \text{ kg} = 150 \text{ mL/day for next 3 kg}}$

$\qquad\qquad\qquad \text{Total} = 1{,}150 \text{ mL/day or per 24 h}$

$\qquad\qquad\qquad\qquad \dfrac{1{,}150 \text{ mL}}{24 \text{ h}} = 47.9 \text{ mL/h} = 48 \text{ mL/h}$

5) $\dfrac{1 \text{ kg}}{2.2 \text{ lb}} \diagup\!\!\!\!\diagdown \dfrac{X \text{ kg}}{77 \text{ lb}}$

$\qquad 2.2X = 77$

$\qquad \dfrac{2.2X}{2.2} = \dfrac{77}{2.2}$

$\qquad\qquad X = 35 \text{ kg}$

$100 \text{ mL/kg/day} \times 10 \text{ kg} = 1{,}000 \text{ mL/day for first 10 kg}$

$50 \text{ mL/kg/day} \times 10 \text{ kg} = 500 \text{ mL/day for next 10 kg}$

$\underline{20 \text{ mL/kg/day} \times 15 \text{ kg} = 300 \text{ mL/day for remaining 15 kg}}$

$\qquad\qquad \text{Total} = 1{,}800 \text{ mL/day or per 24 h}$

$\qquad\qquad\qquad \dfrac{1{,}800 \text{ mL}}{24 \text{ h}} = 75 \text{ mL/h}$

7) $\dfrac{100 \text{ mg}}{1 \text{ mL}} \diagup\!\!\!\!\diagdown \dfrac{350 \text{ mg}}{X \text{ mL}}$

$\qquad 100X = 350$

$\qquad \dfrac{100X}{100} = \dfrac{350}{100}$

$\qquad\qquad X = 3.5 \text{ or } 4 \text{ mL}$

$\qquad\qquad \text{(min. dilution volume)}$

$\dfrac{30 \text{ mg}}{1 \text{ mL}} \diagup\!\!\!\!\diagdown \dfrac{350 \text{ mg}}{X \text{ mL}}$

$\qquad 30X = 350$

$\qquad \dfrac{30X}{30} = \dfrac{350}{30}$

$\qquad\qquad X = 11.6 \text{ or } 12 \text{ mL}$

$\qquad\qquad \text{(max. dilution volume)}$

Practice Problems—Chapter 16 from pages 547–552

1) 1.17; 1.8–2.3; Yes; 2; 0.5 **2)** 0.51; 41; 0.82 **3)** 0.43; 108 **4)** 2.2 **5)** 0.7 **6)** 350 **7)** one of each (one 100 mg capsule and one 250 mg capsule)
8) 0.8; 2,000 **9)** 2.7 **10)** No **11)** 1.3; 26 **12)** 13 **13)** 1.69 **14)** 1.11 **15)** 0.32 **16)** 1.92 **17)** 1.63 **18)** 0.69 **19)** 1.67 **20)** 0.52 **21)** 560,000 **22)** 1,085;
1.09 **23)** 1.9–3.8 **24)** 8 **25)** 40 **26)** 45; 90; 4.2; 25.8 **27)** 58.8 **28)** 60; 60; 1.9; 43.1 **29)** 22.8 **30)** 10; 33 **31)** 200 **32)** 6.2; 37.8 **33)** 130.2
34) 1,000; 42 **35)** 1,520; 63 **36)** 1,810; 75 **37)** 1,250; 52 **38)** 240; 10 **39)** 1,500–1,875; 250–312.5; Yes; 2.8 **40)** 35; 2.8; 32.2 **41)** 12.3; 1,230; 308;
Yes; 6.2 **42)** 23; 6.2; 16.8 **43)** 330–495; 110–165; Yes; 3.3 **44)** 25; 3.3; 21.7 **45)** 1,800–2,700; 300–450; No; exceeds maximum dose; do not give
dosage ordered. **46)** Consult physician before further action. **47)** 25; 2,500,000–6,250,000; 416,667–1,041,667 **48)** Yes; 2.6 **49)** 20; 2.6; 17.4
50) Prevention: The nurse made several assumptions in trying to calculate and prepare this chemotherapy quickly. The recording of the
weights as 20/.45 was confusing. The nurse interpreted the 20/.45 notation to indicate the patient's weight in pounds or kilograms, as was done
in the adult unit. Notice the period before the 45, which later the physician stated was the calculated BSA, 0.45 m². Because no unit of measure
was identified, it was unclear what those numbers really meant. Never assume; always ask for clarification when notation is unclear. Additionally, the actual volume drawn up was probably small in comparison to most adult dose volumes that this nurse prepares. The amount of 1.6 mL
likely seemed reasonable to the nurse. Finally, this is an instance in which the person giving the medication, the physician, prevented a medication error by stopping and thinking what was a reasonable amount for this child and questioning the actual calculation of the dose. Remember:
The person who administers the medication is the last point at which a potential error can be avoided.

Solutions—Practice Problems—Chapter 16

1) Household: $BSA\ (m^2) = \sqrt{\dfrac{ht\ (in) \times wt\ (lb)}{3,131}} = \sqrt{\dfrac{50 \times 85}{3,131}}$

$= \sqrt{\dfrac{4,250}{3,131}} = \sqrt{1.357393} = 1.165\ m^2 = 1.17\ m^2$

Recommended dosage range:

$1.5\ mg/m^2 \times 1.17\ m^2 = 1.8\ mg$

$2\ mg/m^2 \times 1.17\ m^2 = 2.3\ mg$

Ordered dosage is safe.

$\dfrac{1\ mg}{1\ mL} \diagdown \dfrac{2\ mg}{X\ mL}$

$X = 2\ mL$

Give 2 mL/min.

$\dfrac{2\ mL}{60\ sec} \diagdown \dfrac{X\ mL}{15\ sec}$

$60X = 30$

$\dfrac{60X}{60} = \dfrac{30}{60}$

$X = 0.5\ mL\ (per\ 15\ sec)$

2) $BSA = 0.51\ m^2$

$80\ mg/m^2/day \times 0.51\ m^2 = 40.8\ mg/day$
$= 41\ mg/day$

$\dfrac{50\ mg}{1\ mL} \diagdown \dfrac{41\ mg}{X\ mL}$

$50X = 41$

$\dfrac{50X}{50} = \dfrac{41}{50}$

$X = 0.82\ mL$

3) $BSA = 0.43\ m^2$

$250\ mcg/m^2/day \times 0.43\ m^2 = 107.5\ mcg/day$
$= 108\ mcg/day$

4) $\dfrac{50\ mcg}{1\ mL} \diagdown \dfrac{108\ mcg}{X\ mL}$

$50X = 108$

$\dfrac{50X}{50} = \dfrac{108}{50}$

$X = 2.16\ mL = 2.2\ mL$

6) $0.5\ g/m^2 \times 0.7\ m^2 = 0.35\ g$

$0.35\ g = 0.350. = 350\ mg$

8) $BSA = 0.8\ m^2$

$2,500\ units/m^2 \times 0.8\ m^2 = 2,000\ units$

9) $\dfrac{750\ units}{1\ mL} \diagdown \dfrac{2,000\ units}{X\ mL}$

$750X = 2,000$

$\dfrac{750X}{750} = \dfrac{2,000}{750}$

$X = 2.66\ mL = 2.7\ mL$

10) Dose amount exceeds child maximum IM volume per injection site; give in 2 injections.

11) Metric: $BSA\ (m^2) = \sqrt{\dfrac{ht\ (cm) \times wt\ (kg)}{3,600}}$

$= \sqrt{\dfrac{140 \times 43.5}{3,600}} = \sqrt{\dfrac{6.090}{3,600}}$

$= \sqrt{1.691666} = 1.30\ m^2 = 1.3\ m^2$

$20\ mg/m^2 \times 1.3\ m^2 = 26\ mg$

12)

$$\frac{2 \text{ mg}}{1 \text{ mL}} \times \frac{26 \text{ mg}}{X \text{ mL}}$$

$$2X = 26$$

$$\frac{2X}{2} = \frac{26}{2}$$

$$X = 13 \text{ mL}$$

13) 1 ft = 12 in

$$\frac{1 \text{ ft}}{12 \text{ in}} \times \frac{5 \text{ ft}}{X \text{ in}}$$

$$X = 60 \text{ in}$$

Convert 5 ft 6 in to total in: 60 in + 6 in = 66 in

Household: BSA (m^2) = $\sqrt{\dfrac{\text{ht (in)} \times \text{wt (lb)}}{3,131}} = \sqrt{\dfrac{66 \times 136}{3,131}}$

$$= \sqrt{\frac{8,976}{3,131}} = \sqrt{2.866815} = 1.693 \text{ m}^2 = 1.69 \text{ m}^2$$

15) Metric: BSA (m^2) = $\sqrt{\dfrac{\text{ht (cm)} \times \text{wt (kg)}}{3,600}} = \sqrt{\dfrac{60 \times 6}{3,600}}$

$$= \sqrt{\frac{360}{3,600}} = \sqrt{0.1} = 0.316 \text{ m}^2 = 0.32 \text{ m}^2$$

19) 1 in = 2.5 cm

$$\frac{1 \text{ in}}{2.5 \text{ cm}} \times \frac{64 \text{ in}}{X \text{ cm}}$$

$$X = 160 \text{ cm}$$

Metric: BSA (m^2) = $\sqrt{\dfrac{\text{ht (cm)} \times \text{wt (kg)}}{3,600}} = \sqrt{\dfrac{160 \times 63}{3,600}}$

$$= \sqrt{\frac{10,080}{3,600}} = \sqrt{2.8} = 1.673 \text{ m}^2 = 1.67 \text{ m}^2$$

22) 500 mg/m^2 × 2.17 m^2 = 1,085 mg

1,085 mg = 1.085. = 1.085 g = 1.09 g

24) 6 mg/m^2 × 1.34 m^2 = 8.04 mg = 8 mg

25) 8 mg/day × 5 days = 40 mg

26) Total volume = 30 mL + 15 mL = 45 mL

IV pump flow rate if time is less than 1 h:

$$\frac{45 \text{ mL}}{30 \text{ min}} \times \frac{X \text{ mL/h}}{60 \text{ min/h}}$$

$$30X = 2,700$$

$$\frac{30X}{30} = \frac{2,700}{30}$$

$$X = 90 \text{ mL}$$

$$\frac{500 \text{ mg}}{5 \text{ mL}} \times \frac{420 \text{ mg}}{X \text{ mL}}$$

$$500X = 2,100$$

$$\frac{500X}{500} = \frac{2,100}{500}$$

$$X = 4.2 \text{ mL (medication)}$$

30 mL (total solution) − 4.2 mL (med) = 25.8 mL (D$_5$NS)

Note: Add 4.2 mL med to chamber and fill with D$_5$NS to 30 mL.

27) 4.2 mL/dose × 2 doses/day = 8.4 mL/day

8.4 mL/day × 7 days = 58.8 mL (total)

28) Total volume: 45 mL + 15 mL = 60 mL

Flow rate: $\dfrac{60 \text{ mL}}{60 \text{ min}}$ = 60 mL/h

$$\frac{75 \text{ mg}}{0.5 \text{ mL}} \times \frac{285 \text{ mg}}{X \text{ mL}}$$

$$75X = 142.5$$

$$\frac{75X}{75} = \frac{142.5}{75}$$

$$X = 1.9 \text{ mL (medication)}$$

Volume of IV fluid: 45 mL − 1.9 mL = 43.1 mL

29) 1.9 mL/dose × 3 doses/day = 5.7 mL/day

5.7 mL/day × 4 days = 22.8 mL (total)

30)

$$\frac{50 \text{ mg}}{1 \text{ mL}} \times \frac{500 \text{ mg}}{X \text{ mL}}$$

$$50X = 500$$

$$\frac{50X}{50} = \frac{500}{50}$$

$$X = 10 \text{ mL (medication)}$$

$$\frac{65 \text{ mL}}{60 \text{ min}} \times \frac{X \text{ mL}}{40 \text{ min}}$$

$$60X = 2,600$$

$$\frac{60X}{60} = \frac{2,600}{60}$$

$$X = 43.3 \text{ mL} = 43 \text{ mL}$$

43 mL (total solution) − 10 mL (med) =

33 mL (D$_5$ 0.33% NaCl)

31) 10 mL/dose × 4 doses/day = 40 mL/day

40 mL/day × 5 days = 200 mL

35) 100 mL/kg/day × 10 kg = 1,000 mL/day for first 10 kg

50 mL/kg/day × 10 kg = 500 mL/day for next 10 kg

20 mL/kg/day × 1 kg = 20 mL/day for remaining 1 kg

Total = 1,520 mL/day or per 24 h

$$\frac{1,520 \text{ mL}}{24 \text{ h}} = 63.3 \text{ mL/h} = 63 \text{ mL/h}$$

36)

$$\frac{1 \text{ kg}}{2.2 \text{ lb}} \times \frac{X \text{ kg}}{78 \text{ lb}}$$

$$2.2X = 78$$

$$\frac{2.2X}{2.2} = \frac{78}{2.2}$$

$$X = 35.45 \text{ kg} = 35.5 \text{ kg}$$

100 mL/kg/day × 10 kg = 1,000 mL/day for first 10 kg

50 mL/kg/day × 10 kg = 500 mL/day for next 10 kg

20 mL/kg/day × 15.5 kg = 310 mL/day for remaining 15.5 kg

Total = 1,810 mL/day or per 24 h

$$\frac{1,810 \text{ mL}}{24 \text{ h}} = 75.4 \text{ mL/h} = 75 \text{ mL/h}$$

38) $2,400 \text{ g} = 2.400. = 2.4 \text{ kg}$

$100 \text{ mL/kg/day} \times 2.4 \text{ kg} = 240 \text{ mL/day or } 240 \text{ mL/24 h}$

$\dfrac{240 \text{ mL}}{24 \text{ h}} = 10 \text{ mL/h}$

39)   Safe daily dosage range:

$100 \text{ mg/kg} \times 15 \text{ kg} = 1,500 \text{ mg}$

$125 \text{ mg/kg} \times 15 \text{ kg} = 1,875 \text{ mg}$

Safe single dosage range:

$\dfrac{1,500 \text{ mg}}{6 \text{ doses}} = 250 \text{ mg/dose}$

$\dfrac{1,875 \text{ mg}}{6 \text{ doses}} = 312.5 \text{ mg/dose}$

Yes, the dosage is safe.

$1 \text{ g} = 1,000 \text{ mg}$

$\dfrac{1,000 \text{ mg}}{10 \text{ mL}} \bowtie \dfrac{275 \text{ mg}}{X \text{ mL}}$

$1,000X = 2,750$

$\dfrac{1,000X}{1,000} = \dfrac{2,750}{1,000}$

$X = 2.75 \text{ mL} = 2.8 \text{ mL (med)}$

40)   IV fluid volume:

$\dfrac{53 \text{ mL}}{60 \text{ min}} \bowtie \dfrac{X \text{ mL}}{40 \text{ min}}$

$60X = 2,120$

$\dfrac{60X}{60} = \dfrac{2,120}{60}$

$X = 35.3 \text{ mL} = 35 \text{ mL}$

$35 \text{ mL (total)} - 2.8 \text{ mL (med)} = 32.2 \text{ mL (D}_5 \text{ 0.45\% NaCl)}$

45)   Safe daily dosage range:

$200 \text{ mg/kg} \times 9 \text{ kg} = 1,800 \text{ mg}$

$300 \text{ mg/kg} \times 9 \text{ kg} = 2,700 \text{ mg}$

Safe single dosage range:

$\dfrac{1,800 \text{ mg}}{6 \text{ doses}} = 300 \text{ mg/dose}$

$\dfrac{2,700 \text{ mg}}{6 \text{ doses}} = 450 \text{ mg/dose}$

Dosage is *not* safe; exceeds maximum safe dosage.

Do not give dosage ordered; consult with physician.

47) $\dfrac{1 \text{ kg}}{2.2 \text{ lb}} \bowtie \dfrac{X \text{ kg}}{55 \text{ lb}}$

$2.2X = 55$

$\dfrac{2.2X}{2.2} = \dfrac{55}{2.2}$

$X = 25 \text{ kg}$

Safe daily dosage:

$100,000 \text{ units/kg} \times 25 \text{ kg} = 2,500,000 \text{ units}$

$250,000 \text{ units/kg} \times 25 \text{ kg} = 6,250,000 \text{ units}$

Safe single dosage:

$\dfrac{2,500,000 \text{ units}}{6 \text{ doses}} = 416,666.6 \text{ units/dose}$

$= 416,667 \text{ units/dose}$

$\dfrac{6,250,000 \text{ units}}{6 \text{ doses}} = 1,041,666.6 \text{ units/dose}$

$= 1,041,667 \text{ units/dose}$

48)   Yes, dosage is safe.

$\dfrac{200,000 \text{ units}}{1 \text{ mL}} \bowtie \dfrac{525,000 \text{ units}}{X \text{ mL}}$

$200,000X = 525,000$

$\dfrac{200,000X}{200,000} = \dfrac{525,000}{200,000}$

$X = 2.62 \text{ mL} = 2.6 \text{ mL}$

49) $\dfrac{60 \text{ mL}}{60 \text{ min}} \bowtie \dfrac{X \text{ mL}}{20 \text{ min}}$

$60X = 1,200$

$\dfrac{60X}{60} = \dfrac{1,200}{60}$

$X = 20 \text{ mL}$

$20 \text{ mL (total)} - 2.6 \text{ mL (med)} = 17.4 \text{ mL (D}_5\text{NS)}$

Review Set 46 from pages 569–571

1) 40 **2)** 14 **3)** 10 **4)** 19 **5)** 48; Consult physician; per policy, you may be directed to stop this infusion if physician does not respond immediately. **6)** 16 **7)** 75; 6,000; 6; 1,350; 14 **8)** 6,000; 6; 300; 3; 17 **9)** 3,000; 3; 150; 1.5; 19 **10)** Continue the rate at 19 mL/h. **11)** Yes; 10 **12)** 25 **13)** no bolus required **14)** 8 **15)** Hold insulin infusion × 60 min and check blood glucose every 15 min until greater than or equal to 80 mg/dL.

Solutions—Review Set 46

1)
$$\frac{25,000 \text{ units}}{1,000 \text{ mL}} \times \frac{1,000 \text{ units/h}}{\text{X mL/h}}$$

$$25,000\text{X} = 1,000,000$$

$$\frac{25,000\text{X}}{25,000} = \frac{1,000,000}{25,000}$$

$$\text{X} = 40 \text{ mL/h}$$

4)
$$\frac{40,000 \text{ units}}{500 \text{ mL}} \times \frac{1,500 \text{ units/h}}{\text{X mL/h}}$$

$$40,000\text{X} = 750,000$$

$$\frac{40,000\text{X}}{40,000} = \frac{750,000}{40,000}$$

$$\text{X} = 18.7 \text{ mL/h} = 19 \text{ mL/h}$$

5)
$$\frac{25,000 \text{ units}}{1,000 \text{ mL}} \times \frac{1,200 \text{ units/h}}{\text{X mL/h}}$$

$$25,000\text{X} = 1,200,000$$

$$\frac{25,000\text{X}}{25,000} = \frac{1,200,000}{25,000}$$

$$\text{X} = 48 \text{ mL/h}$$

The IV is infusing too rapidly. The physician should be called immediately for further action.

6)
$$\frac{25,000 \text{ units}}{500 \text{ mL}} \times \frac{800 \text{ units/h}}{\text{X mL/h}}$$

$$25,000\text{X} = 400,000$$

$$\frac{25,000\text{X}}{25,000} = \frac{400,000}{25,000}$$

$$\text{X} = 16 \text{ mL/h}$$

7)
$$\frac{1 \text{ kg}}{2.2 \text{ lb}} \times \frac{\text{X kg}}{165 \text{ lb}}$$

$$2.2\text{X} = 165$$

$$\frac{2.2\text{X}}{2.2} = \frac{165}{2.2}$$

$$\text{X} = 75 \text{ kg}$$

Initial heparin bolus:
80 units/kg × 75 kg = 6,000 units

$$\frac{1,000 \text{ units}}{1 \text{ mL}} \times \frac{6,000 \text{ units}}{\text{X mL}}$$

$$1,000\text{X} = 6,000$$

$$\frac{1,000\text{X}}{1,000} = \frac{6,000}{1,000}$$

$$\text{X} = 6 \text{ mL}$$

Initial heparin infusion rate:
18 units/kg/h × 75 kg = 1,350 units/h

$$\frac{25,000 \text{ units}}{250 \text{ mL}} \times \frac{1,350 \text{ units/h}}{\text{X mL/h}}$$

$$25,000\text{X} = 337,500$$

$$\frac{25,000\text{X}}{25,000} = \frac{337,500}{25,000}$$

$$\text{X} = 13.5 \text{ mL/h}$$

$$= 14 \text{ mL/h (on infusion pump)}$$

8) Rebolus: 80 units/kg × 75 kg = 6,000 units

$$\frac{1,000 \text{ units}}{1 \text{ mL}} \times \frac{6,000 \text{ units}}{\text{X mL}}$$

$$1,000\text{X} = 6,000$$

$$\frac{1,000\text{X}}{1,000} = \frac{6,000}{1,000}$$

$$\text{X} = 6 \text{ mL}$$

Reset infusion rate:

4 units/kg/h × 75 kg = 300 units/h (increase)

$$\frac{25,000 \text{ units}}{250 \text{ mL}} \times \frac{300 \text{ units/h}}{\text{X mL/h}}$$

$$25,000\text{X} = 75,000$$

$$\frac{25,000\text{X}}{25,000} = \frac{75,000}{25,000}$$

$$\text{X} = 3 \text{ mL/h (increase)}$$

14 mL/h + 3 mL/h = 17 mL/h

Reset infusion rate to 17 mL/h.

9) Rebolus: 40 units/kg × 75 kg = 3,000 units

$$\frac{1,000 \text{ units}}{1 \text{ mL}} \times \frac{3,000 \text{ units}}{\text{X mL}}$$

$$1,000\text{X} = 3,000$$

$$\frac{1,000\text{X}}{1,000} = \frac{3,000}{1,000}$$

$$\text{X} = 3 \text{ mL}$$

Reset infusion rate:

2 units/kg/h × 75 kg = 150 units/h (increase)

$$\frac{25,000 \text{ units}}{250 \text{ mL}} \times \frac{150 \text{ units/h}}{\text{X mL/h}}$$

$$25,000\text{X} = 37,500$$

$$\frac{25,000\text{X}}{25,000} = \frac{37,500}{25,000}$$

$$\text{X} = 1.5 \text{ mL/h (increase)}$$

17 mL/h + 1.5 mL/h = 18.5 mL/h = 19 mL/h

(on infusion pump)

Reset infusion rate to 19 mL/h.

12)
$$\frac{100 \text{ units}}{100 \text{ mL}} \times \frac{25 \text{ units/h}}{\text{X mL/h}}$$

$$100\text{X} = 2,500$$

$$\frac{100\text{X}}{100} = \frac{2,500}{100}$$

$$\text{X} = 25 \text{ mL/h}$$

14)
$$\frac{100 \text{ units}}{100 \text{ mL}} \times \frac{8 \text{ units/h}}{\text{X mL/h}}$$

$$100\text{X} = 800$$

$$\frac{100\text{X}}{100} = \frac{800}{100}$$

$$\text{X} = 8 \text{ mL/h}$$

Review Set 47 from pages 581–582

1) 2; 120 **2)** 1; 60 **3)** 1.5; 90 **4)** 90; 360; 0.4; 24 **5)** 1,050; 0.66; 39.6 **6)** 142–568 **7)** 0.14–0.57 **8)** Yes **9)** 4 **10)** Yes **11)** 100; 25 **12)** 1 **13)** 0.025 **14)** 25 **15)** Yes

Solutions—Review Set 47

1)
$$\frac{2{,}000 \text{ mg}}{1{,}000 \text{ mL}} \times \frac{4 \text{ mg/min}}{X \text{ mL/min}}$$

$$2{,}000X = 4{,}000$$

$$\frac{2{,}000X}{2{,}000} = \frac{4{,}000}{2{,}000}$$

$$X = 2 \text{ mL/min}$$

$$\frac{2 \text{ mL}}{1 \text{ min}} \times \frac{X \text{ mL/h}}{60 \text{ min/h}}$$

$$X = 120 \text{ mL/h}$$

2)
$$\frac{500 \text{ mg}}{250 \text{ mL}} \times \frac{2 \text{ mg/min}}{X \text{ mL/min}}$$

$$500X = 500$$

$$\frac{500X}{500} = \frac{500}{500}$$

$$X = 1 \text{ mL/min}$$

$$\frac{1 \text{ mL}}{1 \text{ min}} \times \frac{X \text{ mL/h}}{60 \text{ min/h}}$$

$$X = 60 \text{ mL/h}$$

3)
$$\frac{2{,}000 \text{ mcg}}{500 \text{ mL}} \times \frac{6 \text{ mcg/min}}{X \text{ mL/min}}$$

$$2{,}000X = 3{,}000$$

$$\frac{2{,}000X}{2{,}000} = \frac{3{,}000}{2{,}000}$$

$$X = 1.5 \text{ mL/min}$$

$$\frac{1.5 \text{ mL}}{1 \text{ min}} \times \frac{X \text{ mL/h}}{60 \text{ min/h}}$$

$$X = 90 \text{ mL/h}$$

4)
$$\frac{1 \text{ kg}}{2.2 \text{ lb}} \times \frac{X \text{ kg}}{198 \text{ lb}}$$

$$2.2X = 198$$

$$\frac{2.2X}{2.2} = \frac{198}{2.2}$$

$$X = 90 \text{ kg}$$

$$4 \text{ mcg/kg/min} \times 90 \text{ kg} = 360 \text{ mcg/min}$$

$$\frac{1{,}000 \text{ mcg}}{1 \text{ mg}} \times \frac{360 \text{ mcg/min}}{X \text{ mg/min}}$$

$$1{,}000X = 360$$

$$\frac{1{,}000X}{1{,}000} = \frac{360}{1{,}000}$$

$$X = 0.36 \text{ mg/min}$$

$$\frac{450 \text{ mg}}{500 \text{ mL}} \times \frac{0.36 \text{ mg/min}}{X \text{ mL/min}}$$

$$450X = 180$$

$$\frac{450X}{450} = \frac{180}{450}$$

$$X = 0.4 \text{ mL/min}$$

$$\frac{0.4 \text{ mL}}{1 \text{ min}} \times \frac{X \text{ mL/h}}{60 \text{ min/h}}$$

$$X = 24 \text{ mL/h}$$

5)
$$15 \text{ mcg/kg/min} \times 70 \text{ kg} = 1{,}050 \text{ mcg/min}$$

$$\frac{1 \text{ mg}}{1{,}000 \text{ mcg}} \times \frac{X \text{ mg/min}}{1{,}050 \text{ mcg/min}}$$

$$1{,}000X = 1{,}050$$

$$\frac{1{,}000X}{1{,}000} = \frac{1{,}050}{1{,}000}$$

$$X = 1.05 \text{ mg/min}$$

$$\frac{800 \text{ mg}}{500 \text{ mL}} \times \frac{1.05 \text{ mg/min}}{X \text{ mL/min}}$$

$$800X = 525$$

$$\frac{800X}{800} = \frac{525}{800}$$

$$X = 0.656 \text{ mL/min} = 0.66 \text{ mL/min}$$

$$\frac{0.66 \text{ mL}}{1 \text{ min}} \times \frac{X \text{ mL/h}}{60 \text{ min/h}}$$

$$X = 39.6 \text{ mL/h} = 40 \text{ mL/h}$$

6)
$$\frac{1 \text{ kg}}{2.2 \text{ lb}} \times \frac{X \text{ kg}}{125 \text{ lb}}$$

$$2.2X = 125$$

$$\frac{2.2X}{2.2} = \frac{125}{2.2}$$

$$X = 56.8 \text{ kg}$$

Minimum: $2.5 \text{ mcg/kg/min} \times 56.8 \text{ kg} = 142 \text{ mcg/min}$

Maximum: $10 \text{ mcg/kg/min} \times 56.8 \text{ kg} = 568 \text{ mcg/min}$

7) Minimum:
$$\frac{1 \text{ mg}}{1{,}000 \text{ mcg}} \times \frac{X \text{ mg/min}}{142 \text{ mcg/min}}$$

$$1{,}000X = 142$$

$$\frac{1{,}000X}{1{,}000} = \frac{142}{1{,}000}$$

$$X = 0.142 \text{ mg/min} = 0.14 \text{ mg/min}$$

Maximum:
$$\frac{1 \text{ mg}}{1{,}000 \text{ mcg}} \times \frac{X \text{ mg/min}}{568 \text{ mcg/min}}$$

$$1{,}000X = 568$$

$$\frac{1{,}000X}{1{,}000} = \frac{568}{1{,}000}$$

$$X = 0.568 \text{ mg/min} = 0.57 \text{ mg/min}$$

8)
$$\frac{500 \text{ mg}}{500 \text{ mL}} \times \frac{X \text{ mg/h}}{15 \text{ mL/h}}$$

$$500X = 7{,}500$$

$$\frac{500X}{500} = \frac{7{,}500}{500}$$

$$X = 15 \text{ mg/h}$$

$$\frac{15 \text{ mg}}{60 \text{ min}} \times \frac{X \text{ mg}}{1 \text{ min}}$$

$$60X = 15$$

$$\frac{60X}{60} = \frac{15}{60}$$

$$X = 0.25 \text{ mg (per min) or } 0.25 \text{ mg/min}$$

Yes, the order is within the safe range of 0.14–0.57 mg/min.

9)

$$\frac{2,000 \text{ mg}}{500 \text{ mL}} \bowtie \frac{X \text{ mg/h}}{60 \text{ mL/h}}$$

$$500X = 120,000$$

$$\frac{500X}{500} = \frac{120,000}{500}$$

$$X = 240 \text{ mg/h}$$

$$\frac{240 \text{ mg}}{60 \text{ min}} \bowtie \frac{X \text{ mg}}{1 \text{ min}}$$

$$60X = 240$$

$$\frac{60X}{60} = \frac{240}{60}$$

$$X = 4 \text{ mg (per min) or 4 mg/min}$$

10) Yes, 4 mg/min is within the normal range of 2–6 mg/min.

11) Bolus:

$$\frac{2 \text{ g}}{30 \text{ min}} \bowtie \frac{X \text{ g}}{60 \text{ min}}$$

$$30X = 120$$

$$X = 4 \text{ g (per 60 min) or 4 g/h}$$

$$\frac{20 \text{ g}}{500 \text{ mL}} \bowtie \frac{4 \text{ g/h}}{X \text{ mL/h}}$$

$$20X = 2,000$$

$$\frac{20X}{20} = \frac{2,000}{20}$$

$$X = 100 \text{ mL/h}$$

Continuous:

$$\frac{20 \text{ g}}{500 \text{ mL}} \bowtie \frac{1 \text{ g/h}}{X \text{ mL/h}}$$

$$20X = 500$$

$$\frac{20X}{20} = \frac{500}{20}$$

$$X = 25 \text{ mL/h}$$

12)

$$\frac{1 \text{ unit}}{1,000 \text{ milliunits}} \bowtie \frac{X \text{ units}}{1 \text{ milliunit}}$$

$$1,000X = 1$$

$$\frac{1,000X}{1,000} = \frac{1}{1,000}$$

$$X = 0.001 \text{ units}$$

$$\frac{15 \text{ units}}{250 \text{ mL}} \bowtie \frac{0.001 \text{ units/min}}{X \text{ mL/min}}$$

$$15X = 0.25$$

$$\frac{15X}{15} = \frac{0.25}{15}$$

$$X = 0.0166 \text{ mL/min} = 0.017 \text{ mL/min}$$

$$\frac{0.017 \text{ mL}}{1 \text{ min}} \bowtie \frac{X \text{ mL/h}}{60 \text{ min/h}}$$

$$X = 1.02 \text{ mL/h} = 1 \text{ mL/h}$$

13)

$$\frac{10 \text{ mg}}{1,000 \text{ mL}} \bowtie \frac{X \text{ mg/h}}{150 \text{ mL/h}}$$

$$1,000X = 1,500$$

$$\frac{1,000X}{1,000} = \frac{1,500}{1,000}$$

$$X = 1.5 \text{ mg/h}$$

$$\frac{1.5 \text{ mg}}{60 \text{ min}} \bowtie \frac{X \text{ mg}}{1 \text{ min}}$$

$$60X = 1.5$$

$$\frac{60X}{60} = \frac{1.5}{60}$$

$$X = 0.025 \text{ mg (per min) or 0.025 mg/min}$$

14)

$$\frac{1 \text{ mg}}{1,000 \text{ mcg}} \bowtie \frac{0.025 \text{ mg/min}}{X \text{ mcg/min}}$$

$$X = 25 \text{ mcg/min}$$

Review Set 48 from pages 584–586

1) 33; 19 **2)** 40; 42 **3)** 25; 32 **4)** 50; 90 **5)** 50; 40 **6)** 100; 100 **7)** 200; 76 **8)** 200; 122 **9)** 17; 21 **10)** 120; 112

Solutions—Review Set 48

1) **Step 1**   IV PB rate: $\frac{V}{T} \times C = \frac{100 \text{ mL}}{\overset{30 \text{ min}}{3}} \times \overset{1}{10} \text{ gtt/mL} =$

$\frac{100}{3}$ gtt/min = 33.3 gtt/min = 33 gtt/min

Step 2   Total IV PB time: q.4h = 6 times per 24 h; 6 × 30 min = 180 min;
180 min ÷ 60 min/h = 180 min × 1 h/60 min = 3 h

Step 3   Total IV PB volume: 6 × 100 mL = 600 mL

Step 4   Total regular IV volume: 3,000 mL − 600 mL = 2,400 mL

Step 5   Total regular IV time: 24 h − 3 h = 21 h

Step 6   Regular IV rate:

$\frac{2,400 \text{ mL}}{21 \text{ h}}$ = 114.2 mL/h = 114 mL/h

$\frac{\text{mL/h}}{\text{Drop factor constant}}$ = gtt/min; $\frac{114 \text{ mL/h}}{6}$ = 19 gtt/min

2) **Step 1**   IV PB rate: When drop factor is 60 gtt/mL, then mL/h = gtt/min. Rate is 40 gtt/min.

Step 2   Total IV PB time: q.i.d. = 4 times per 24 h; 4 × 1 h = 4 h

Step 3   Total IV PB volume: 4 × 40 mL = 160 mL

Step 4   Total regular IV volume: 1,000 mL − 160 mL = 840 mL

Step 5   Total regular IV time: 24 h − 4 h = 20 h

Step 6   Total regular IV rate: mL/h = $\frac{840 \text{ mL}}{20 \text{ h}}$ = 42 mL/h. When drop factor is 60 gtt/mL, then

mL/h = gtt/min. Rate is 42 gtt/min.

3)   **Step 1**   IV PB rate: $\frac{V}{T} \times C = \frac{50 \text{ mL}}{\overset{}{\underset{2}{30 \text{ min}}}} \times \overset{1}{15} \text{ gtt/mL} = \frac{\overset{25}{50}}{\underset{1}{2}} \text{ gtt/min} = 25 \text{ gtt/min}$

Step 2   Total IV PB time: q.6h = 4 times per 24 h; 4 × 30 min = 120 min;

120 min ÷ 60 min/h = 120 min × 1 h/60 min = 2 h

Step 3   Total IV PB volume: 4 × 50 mL = 200 mL

Step 4   Total regular IV volume: 3,000 mL − 200 mL = 2,800 mL

Step 5   Total regular IV time: 24 h − 2 h = 22 h

Step 6   Total regular IV rate:

$\frac{2,800 \text{ mL}}{22 \text{ h}}$ = 127.2 mL/h = 127 mL/h

$\frac{\text{mL/h}}{\text{Drop factor constant}}$ = gtt/min; $\frac{127 \text{ mL/h}}{4}$ = 31.7 gtt/min = 32 gtt/min

4)   **Step 1**   IV PB rate: 50 mL/h or 50 gtt/min (because drop factor is 60 gtt/mL)

Step 2   Total IV PB time: q.6h = 4 times per 24 h; 4 × 1 h = 4 h

Step 3   Total IV PB volume: 4 × 50 mL = 200 mL

Step 4   Total regular IV volume: 2,000 mL − 200 mL = 1,800 mL

Step 5   Total regular IV time: 24 h − 4 h = 20 h

Step 6   Regular IV rate: $\frac{1,800 \text{ mL}}{20 \text{ h}}$ = 90 mL/h or 90 gtt/min (because drop factor is 60 gtt/mL)

5)   **Step 1**   IV PB rate: 50 mL/h or 50 gtt/min (because drop factor is 60 gtt/mL)

Step 2   IV PB time: q.8h = 3 times per 24 h; 3 × 1 h = 3 h

Step 3   IV PB volume: 3 × 50 mL = 150 mL

Step 4   Total regular IV volume: 1,000 mL − 150 mL = 850 mL

Step 5   Total regular IV time: 24 h − 3 h = 21 h

Step 6   Regular IV rate: $\frac{850 \text{ mL}}{21 \text{ h}}$ = 40.4 mL/h = 40 mL/h or 40 gtt/min (because drop factor is 60 gtt/mL)

6)   **Step 1**   IV PB rate

$\frac{50 \text{ mL}}{30 \text{ min}} \times \frac{X \text{ mL}}{60 \text{ min}}$

30X = 3,000

$\frac{30X}{30} = \frac{3,000}{30}$

X = 100 mL (per 60 min) or 100 mL/h

Step 2   IV PB time: q.6h = 4 times per 24 h; 4 × 30 min = 120 min;

120 min ÷ 60 min/h = 120 min × 1 h/60 min = 2 h

Step 3   IV PB volume: 4 × 50 mL = 200 mL

Step 4   Total regular IV volume: 2,400 mL − 200 mL = 2,200 mL

Step 5   Total regular IV time: 24 h − 2 h = 22 h

Step 6   Regular IV rate: $\frac{2,200 \text{ mL}}{22 \text{ h}}$ = 100 mL/h

7)   **Step 1**   IV PB rate:

$\frac{100 \text{ mL}}{30 \text{ min}} \times \frac{X \text{ mL}}{60 \text{ min}}$

30X = 6,000

$\frac{30X}{30} = \frac{6,000}{30}$

X = 200 mL (per 60 min) or 200 mL/h

Step 2   IV PB time: q.8h = 3 times per 24 h; 3 × 30 min = 90 min;

90 min ÷ 60 min/h = 90 min × 1 h/60 min = $1\frac{1}{2}$ h

Step 3   IV PB volume: 3×100 mL $= 300$ mL

Step 4   Total regular IV volume: $2,000$ mL $- 300$ mL $= 1,700$ mL

Step 5   Total regular IV time: 24 h $- 1\frac{1}{2}$ h $= 22\frac{1}{2}$ h

Step 6   Regular IV rate: $\frac{1,700 \text{ mL}}{22.5 \text{ h}} = 75.5$ mL/h $= 76$ mL/h

8)   **Step 1**   IV PB rate

$$\frac{50 \text{ mL}}{15 \text{ min}} \diagdown\!\!\!\diagup \frac{X \text{ mL}}{60 \text{ min}}$$

$$15X = 3,000$$

$$\frac{15X}{15} = \frac{3,000}{15}$$

$$X = 200 \text{ mL (per 60 min) or 100 mL/h}$$

Step 2   IV PB time: q.6h $= 4$ times per 24 h; 4×15 min $= 60$ min $= 1$ h

Step 3   IV PB volume: 4×50 mL $= 200$ mL

Step 4   Total regular IV volume: $3,000$ mL $- 200$ mL $= 2,800$ mL

Step 5   Total regular IV time: 24 h $- 1$ h $= 23$ h

Step 6   Regular IV rate: $\frac{2,800 \text{ mL}}{23 \text{ h}} = 121.7$ mL/h $= 122$ mL/h

Practice Problems—Chapter 17 from pages 587–593

1) 12 **2)** 50 **3)** 63 **4)** 35 **5)** 6; 15 **6)** 60 **7)** 45 **8)** 60 **9)** 24 **10)** Yes **11)** 17; 22 **12)** 100; 127 **13)** 102 **14)** 8 mEq **15)** 2 **16)** 15 **17)** 50 **18)** 25 **19)** 7.4 **20)** 12; 18 **21)** 150; 50 **22)** 2 **23)** 35 **24)** 8 **25)** 63 **26)** 80 **27)** 0.4 **28)** 4 **29)** 4 **30)** 100 **31)** 0.2; 200 **32)** 30 **33)** 200; 50 **34)** 5 **35)** 550 **36)** 2,450 **37)** 19 **38)** 129 **39)** 13; 39 **40)** Yes; 10 **41)** 12 **42)** No **43)** 4 **44)** Give $\frac{1}{2}$ amp of 50 mL of 50% dextrose, hold insulin for 60 minutes, and check blood glucose every 15 minutes until equal to or greater than 80. **45)** 100; 80 **46)** 8,000; 1,000; 8 **47)** 18; 1,800; 100; 18 **48)** 6; 40; 4,000; 4; increase; 2; 200; 2; 20 **49)** Decrease rate by 2 units/kg/h; 18

STANDARD WEIGHT-BASED HEPARIN PROTOCOL WORKSHEET

Round patient's total body weight to nearest 10 kg: __100__ kg.
DO NOT change the weight based on daily measurements.

FOUND ON THE ORDER FORM
Initial Bolus (80 units/kg): __8,000__ units __8__ mL
Initial Infusion Rate (18 units/kg/h): __1,800__ units/h __18__ mL/h

Make adjustments to the heparin drip rate as directed by the order form.
ALL DOSES ARE ROUNDED TO THE NEAREST 100 UNITS.

Date	Time	aPTT	Bolus	Rate Change Units/h	mL/h	New Rate	RN 1	RN 2
5/10/xx	1730	37 sec	4,000 units (4 mL)	+200 units/h	+2 mL/h	20 mL/h	G.P.	M.S.
5/10/xx	2330	77 sec		−200 units/h	−2 mL/h	18 mL/h	G.P.	M.S.

Signatures   Initials

G.Pickar, R.N.   G.P.

M.Smith, R.N.   M.S.

50) **Prevention:** The nurse who prepares any IV solution with an additive should *carefully* compare the order and medication three times: before beginning to prepare the dose, after the dosage is prepared, and just before it is administered to the patient. Further, the nurse should verify the safety of the dosage using the Three-Step Approach (convert, think, and calculate). It was clear that the nurse realized the error when a colleague questioned what was being prepared and the nurse verified the actual order. Also, taking the time to do the calculation on paper helps the nurse to "see" the answer and avoid a potentially life-threatening error. The prescriber should also write out units and milliunits (U and mU are not permitted abbreviations). The nurse should contact the prescriber to clarify an order when unacceptable notation is used.

Solutions—Practice Problems—Chapter 17

1)
$$\frac{25,000 \text{ units}}{250 \text{ mL}} \diagdown \frac{1,200 \text{ units/h}}{X \text{ mL/h}}$$

$$25,000X = 300,000$$

$$\frac{25,000X}{25,000} = \frac{300,000}{25,000}$$

$$X = 12 \text{ mL/h}$$

2)
$$\frac{100 \text{ mg}}{1,000 \text{ mL}} \diagdown \frac{5 \text{ mg/h}}{X \text{ mL/h}}$$

$$100X = 5,000$$

$$\frac{100X}{100} = \frac{5,000}{100}$$

$$X = 50 \text{ mL/h}$$

3)
$$\frac{4,000 \text{ mg}}{500 \text{ mL}} \diagdown \frac{500 \text{ mg/h}}{X \text{ mL/h}}$$

$$4,000X = 250,000$$

$$\frac{4,000X}{4,000} = \frac{250,000}{4,000}$$

$$X = 62.5 \text{ mL/h} = 63 \text{ mL/h}$$

4)
$$\frac{20,000 \text{ units}}{500 \text{ mL}} \diagdown \frac{1,400 \text{ units/h}}{X \text{ mL/h}}$$

$$20,000X = 700,000$$

$$\frac{20,000X}{20,000} = \frac{700,000}{20,000}$$

$$X = 35 \text{ mL/h}$$

5)
$$\frac{1 \text{ L}}{1,000 \text{ mL}} \diagdown \frac{1.5 \text{ L}}{X \text{ mL}}$$

$$X = 1,500 \text{ mL}$$

$$\frac{4 \text{ mL}}{1 \text{ min}} \diagdown \frac{1,500 \text{ mL}}{X \text{ min}}$$

$$4X = 1,500$$

$$\frac{4X}{4} = \frac{1,500}{4}$$

$$X = 375 \text{ min}$$

$$\frac{60 \text{ min}}{1 \text{ h}} \diagdown \frac{375 \text{ min}}{X \text{ h}}$$

$$60X = 375$$

$$\frac{60X}{60} = \frac{375}{60}$$

$$X = 6.25 \text{ h} = 6\frac{1}{4} \text{ h} = 6 \text{ h } 15 \text{ min}$$

6)
$$\frac{2,000 \text{ mg}}{500 \text{ mL}} \diagdown \frac{4 \text{ mg/min}}{X \text{ mL/min}}$$

$$2,000X = 2,000$$

$$\frac{2,000X}{2,000} = \frac{2,000}{2,000}$$

$$X = 1 \text{ mL/min}$$

which is the same as 60 mL per 60 min or 60 mL/h

7)
$$\frac{1,000 \text{ mg}}{250 \text{ mL}} \diagdown \frac{3 \text{ mg/min}}{X \text{ mL/min}}$$

$$1,000X = 750$$

$$\frac{1,000X}{1,000} = \frac{750}{1,000}$$

$$X = 0.75 \text{ mL/min}$$

$$\frac{0.75 \text{ mL}}{1 \text{ min}} \diagdown \frac{X \text{ mL/h}}{60 \text{ min/h}}$$

$$X = 45 \text{ mL/h}$$

8)
$$\frac{1,000 \text{ mg}}{500 \text{ mL}} \diagdown \frac{2 \text{ mg/min}}{X \text{ mL/min}}$$

$$1,000X = 1,000$$

$$\frac{1,000X}{1,000} = \frac{1,000}{1,000}$$

$$X = 1 \text{ mL/min}$$

which is the same as 60 mL per 60 min or 60 mL/h

9) 5 mcg/kg/min × 80 kg = 400 mcg/min

$$\frac{1 \text{ mg}}{1,000 \text{ mcg}} \diagdown \frac{X \text{ mg/min}}{400 \text{ mcg/min}}$$

$$1,000X = 400$$

$$\frac{1,000X}{1,000} = \frac{400}{1,000}$$

$$X = 0.4 \text{ mg/min}$$

$$\frac{250 \text{ mg}}{250 \text{ mL}} \diagdown \frac{0.4 \text{ mg/min}}{X \text{ mL/min}}$$

$$250X = 100$$

$$\frac{250X}{250} = \frac{100}{250}$$

$$X = 0.4 \text{ mL/min}$$

$$\frac{0.4 \text{ mL}}{1 \text{ min}} \diagdown \frac{X \text{ mL/h}}{60 \text{ min/h}}$$

$$X = 24 \text{ mL/h}$$

10)
$$\frac{2,000 \text{ mg}}{1,000 \text{ mL}} \diagdown \frac{X \text{ mg/h}}{75 \text{ mL/h}}$$

$$1,000X = 150,000$$

$$\frac{1,000X}{1,000} = \frac{150,000}{1,000}$$

$$X = 150 \text{ mg/h}$$

$$\frac{150 \text{ mg}}{60 \text{ min}} \diagdown \frac{X \text{ mg}}{1 \text{ min}}$$

$$60X = 150$$

$$\frac{60X}{60} = \frac{150}{60}$$

$$X = 2.5 \text{ mg (per min)} = 2.5 \text{ mg/min}$$

within normal range of 1 to 4 mg/min

11) IV PB flow rate: $\dfrac{mL/h}{drop\ factor\ constant} = \dfrac{100\ mL/h}{6} =$

16.6 gtt/min = 17 gtt/min

Total IV PB time: q.6h × 1 h = 4 × 1 h = 4 h

Total IV PB volume: 4 × 100 mL = 400 mL

Total regular IV volume: 3,000 mL − 400 mL = 2,600 mL

Total regular IV time: 24 h − 4 h = 20 h

Regular IV rate: mL/h = $\dfrac{2,600\ mL}{20\ h}$ = 130 mL/h;

$\dfrac{mL/h}{drop\ factor\ constant} = \dfrac{130\ mL/h}{6}$ = 21.6 gtt/min = 22 gtt/min

12) IV PB rate:

$\dfrac{50\ mL}{30\ min} \diagup\!\!\!\!\diagdown \dfrac{X\ mL}{60\ min}$

30X = 3,000

$\dfrac{30X}{30} = \dfrac{3,000}{30}$

X = 100 mL; 100 mL per 60 min = 100 mL/h

Total IV PB time: q.i.d. × 30 min = 4 × 30 min =

120 min;

$\dfrac{60\ min}{1\ h} \diagup\!\!\!\!\diagdown \dfrac{120\ min}{X\ h}$

60X = 120

$\dfrac{60X}{60} = \dfrac{120}{60}$

X = 2 h

Total IV PB volume: 4 × 50 mL = 200 mL

Total regular IV volume: 3,000 mL − 200 mL = 2,800 mL

Total regular IV time: 24 h − 2 h = 22 h

Regular IV rate: $\dfrac{2,800\ mL}{22\ h}$ = 127.2 mL/h = 127 mL/h

13) $\dfrac{1\ kg}{2.2\ lb} \diagup\!\!\!\!\diagdown \dfrac{X\ kg}{125\ lb}$

2.2X = 125

$\dfrac{2.2X}{2.2} = \dfrac{125}{2.2}$

X = 56.8 kg

3 mcg/kg/min × 56.8 kg = 170.4 mcg/min

$\dfrac{1\ mg}{1,000\ mcg} \diagup\!\!\!\!\diagdown \dfrac{X\ mg/min}{170.4\ mcg/min}$

1,000X = 170.4

$\dfrac{1,000X}{1,000} = \dfrac{170.4}{1,000}$

X = 0.17 mg/min

$\dfrac{50\ mg}{500\ mL} \diagup\!\!\!\!\diagdown \dfrac{0.17\ mg/min}{X\ mL/min}$

50X = 85

$\dfrac{50X}{50} = \dfrac{85}{50}$

X = 1.7 mL/min

$\dfrac{1.7\ mL}{1\ min} \diagup\!\!\!\!\diagdown \dfrac{X\ mL/h}{60\ min/h}$

X = 102 mL/h

14) 1,000 mL − 800 mL = 200 mL infused

$\dfrac{40\ mEq}{1,000\ mL} \diagup\!\!\!\!\diagdown \dfrac{X\ mEq}{200\ mL}$

1,000X = 8,000

$\dfrac{1,000X}{1,000} = \dfrac{8,000}{1,000}$

X = 8 mEq

15) $\dfrac{125\ mL}{60\ min}$ = 2 mL/min

16) $\dfrac{100\ mL}{1\ h} \diagup\!\!\!\!\diagdown \dfrac{1,500\ mL}{X\ h}$

100X = 1,500

$\dfrac{100X}{100} = \dfrac{1,500}{100}$

X = 15 h

17) $\dfrac{40\ mEq}{1,000\ mL} \diagup\!\!\!\!\diagdown \dfrac{2\ mEq/h}{X\ mL/h}$

40X = 2,000

$\dfrac{40X}{40} = \dfrac{2,000}{40}$

X = 50 mL/h

18) $\dfrac{50,000\ units}{1,000\ mL} \diagup\!\!\!\!\diagdown \dfrac{1,250\ units/h}{X\ mL/h}$

50,000X = 1,250,000

$\dfrac{50,000X}{50,000} = \dfrac{1,250,000}{50,000}$

X = 25 mL/h

19) $\dfrac{5\ mg}{1\ mL} \diagup\!\!\!\!\diagdown \dfrac{37\ mg}{X\ mL}$

5X = 37

$\dfrac{5X}{5} = \dfrac{37}{5}$

X = 7.4 mL

20) $\dfrac{1\ unit}{1,000\ milliunits} \diagup\!\!\!\!\diagdown \dfrac{10\ units}{X\ milliunits}$

X = 10,000 milliunits

$\dfrac{10,000\ milliunits}{500\ mL} \diagup\!\!\!\!\diagdown \dfrac{4\ milliunits/min}{X\ mL/min}$

10,000X = 2,000

$\dfrac{10,000X}{10,000} = \dfrac{2,000}{10,000}$

X = 0.2 mL/min (for first 20 minutes)

$\dfrac{0.2\ mL}{1\ min} \diagup\!\!\!\!\diagdown \dfrac{X\ mL/h}{60\ min/h}$

X = 12 mL/h

$\dfrac{10,000\ milliunits}{500\ mL} \diagup\!\!\!\!\diagdown \dfrac{6\ milliunits/min}{X\ mL/min}$

10,000X = 3,000

$\dfrac{10,000X}{10,000} = \dfrac{3,000}{10,000}$

X = 0.3 mL/min (for next 20 minutes)

$\dfrac{0.3\ mL}{1\ min} \diagup\!\!\!\!\diagdown \dfrac{X\ mL/h}{60\ min/h}$

X = 18 mL/h

21) Bolus:

$$\frac{3 \text{ g}}{30 \text{ min}} \diagdown\diagup \frac{X \text{ g/h}}{60 \text{ min/h}}$$

$$\frac{30X}{30} = \frac{180}{30}$$

$$X = 6 \text{ g/h}$$

$$\frac{20 \text{ g}}{500 \text{ mL}} \diagdown\diagup \frac{6 \text{ g/h}}{X \text{ mL/h}}$$

$$20X = 3,000$$

$$\frac{20X}{20} = \frac{3,000}{20}$$

$$X = 150 \text{ mL/h}$$

Continuous infusion:

$$\frac{20 \text{ g}}{500 \text{ mL}} \diagdown\diagup \frac{2 \text{ g/h}}{X \text{ mL/h}}$$

$$20X = 1,000$$

$$\frac{20X}{20} = \frac{1,000}{20}$$

$$X = 50 \text{ mL/h}$$

24) $\dfrac{\overset{8}{4,000} \text{ mg}}{\underset{1}{500} \text{ mL}} = 8 \text{ mg/mL}$

25) $\dfrac{4,000 \text{ mg}}{500 \text{ mL}} \diagdown\diagup \dfrac{500 \text{ mg/h}}{X \text{ mL/h}}$

$$4,000X = 250,000$$

$$\frac{4,000X}{4,000} = \frac{250,000}{4,000}$$

$$X = 62.5 \text{ mL/h} = 63 \text{ mL/h}$$

26) $\dfrac{1 \text{ unit}}{1,000 \text{ milliunits}} \diagdown\diagup \dfrac{80 \text{ units}}{X \text{ milliunits}}$

$$X = 80,000 \text{ milliunits}$$

$$\frac{80,000 \text{ milliunits}}{1,000 \text{ mL}} \diagdown\diagup \frac{X \text{ milliunits}}{1 \text{ mL}}$$

$$1,000X = 80,000$$

$$\frac{1,000X}{1,000} = \frac{80,000}{1,000}$$

$$X = 80 \text{ milliunits (per mL) or 80 milliunits/mL}$$

28) $\dfrac{1 \text{ mg}}{1,000 \text{ mcg}} \diagdown\diagup \dfrac{4 \text{ mg}}{X \text{ mcg}}$

$$X = 4,000 \text{ mcg}$$

$$\frac{4,000 \text{ mcg}}{1,000 \text{ mL}} \diagdown\diagup \frac{X \text{ mcg}}{1 \text{ mL}}$$

$$1,000X = 4,000$$

$$\frac{1,000X}{1,000} = \frac{4,000}{1,000}$$

$$X = 4 \text{ mcg (per mL) or 4 mcg/mL}$$

31) $\dfrac{20 \text{ mg}}{100 \text{ mL}} \diagdown\diagup \dfrac{X \text{ mg}}{1 \text{ mL}}$

$$100X = 20$$

$$\frac{100X}{100} = \frac{20}{100}$$

$$X = 0.2 \text{ mg (per mL) or 0.2 mg/mL}$$

$$\frac{1 \text{ mg}}{1,000 \text{ mcg}} \diagdown\diagup \frac{0.2 \text{ mg/mL}}{X \text{ mcg/mL}}$$

$$X = 200 \text{ mcg (per mL) or 200 mcg/mL}$$

32) $1 \text{ mcg/kg/min} \times 100 \text{ kg} = 100 \text{ mcg/min}$

$$\frac{20,000 \text{ mcg}}{100 \text{ mL}} \diagdown\diagup \frac{100 \text{ mcg/min}}{X \text{ mL/min}}$$

$$20,000X = 10,000$$

$$\frac{20,000X}{20,000} = \frac{10,000}{20,000}$$

$$X = 0.5 \text{ mL/min}$$

$$\frac{0.5 \text{ mL}}{1 \text{ min}} \diagdown\diagup \frac{X \text{ mL/h}}{60 \text{ min/h}}$$

$$X = 30 \text{ mL/h}$$

33) IV PB rates:

$$\frac{100 \text{ mL}}{30 \text{ min}} \diagdown\diagup \frac{X \text{ mL}}{60 \text{ min}}$$

$$30X = 6,000$$

$$\frac{30X}{30} = \frac{6,000}{30}$$

$$X = 200 \text{ mL (per 60 min)}$$

$200 \text{ mL per 60 min} = 200 \text{ mL/h (ampicillin)}$

gentamicin: 50 mL/h

34) ampicillin: q.6h $\times$ 30 min = 4 $\times$ 30 min = 120 min;

$$\frac{60 \text{ min}}{1 \text{ h}} \diagdown\diagup \frac{120 \text{ min}}{X \text{ h}}$$

$$60X = 120$$

$$\frac{60X}{60} = \frac{120}{60}$$

$$X = 2 \text{ h}$$

gentamicin: q.8h $\times$ 1 h = 3 $\times$ 1 h = 3 h

Total IV PB time: 2 h + 3 h = 5 h

35) ampicillin: 4 d̶o̶s̶e̶s̶ $\times$ 100 mL/d̶o̶s̶e̶ = 400 mL

gentamicin: 3 d̶o̶s̶e̶s̶ $\times$ 50 mL/d̶o̶s̶e̶ = 150 mL

Total IV PB volume: 400 mL + 150 mL = 550 mL

36) 3,000 mL − 550 mL = 2,450 mL

37) 24 h − 5 h = 19 h

38) $\dfrac{2,450 \text{ mL}}{19 \text{ h}} = 128.9 \text{ mL/h} = 129 \text{ mL/h}$

39) $\dfrac{1 \text{ kg}}{2.2 \text{ lb}} \diagdown\diagup \dfrac{X \text{ kg}}{190 \text{ lb}}$

$$2.2X = 190$$

$$\frac{2.2X}{2.2} = \frac{190}{2.2}$$

$$X = 86.36 \text{ kg} = 86.4 \text{ kg}$$

$4 \text{ mcg/kg/min} \times 86.4 \text{ kg} = 345.6 \text{ mcg/min}$

$$\frac{345.6 \text{ mcg}}{1 \text{ min}} \diagdown\diagup \frac{X \text{ mcg/h}}{60 \text{ min/h}}$$

$$X = 20,736 \text{ mcg/h}$$

$$\frac{1 \text{ mg}}{1,000 \text{ mcg}} \diagdown\diagup \frac{X \text{ mg}}{20,736 \text{ mcg}}$$

$$1,000X = 20,736$$

$$\frac{1,000X}{1,000} = \frac{20,736}{1,000}$$

$$X = 20.7 \text{ mg/h} = 21 \text{ mg/h}$$

$$\frac{800 \text{ mg}}{500 \text{ mL}} \diagtimes \frac{21 \text{ mg/h}}{X \text{ mL/h}}$$

$$800X = 10,500$$

$$\frac{800X}{800} = \frac{10,500}{800}$$

$$X = 13.1 \text{ mL/h} = 13 \text{ mL/h (initial rate)}$$

$$12 \text{ mcg/kg/min} \times 86.4 \text{ kg} = 1,036.8 \text{ mcg/min}$$

$$\frac{1,036.8 \text{ mcg}}{1 \text{ min}} \diagtimes \frac{X \text{ mcg/h}}{60 \text{ min/h}}$$

$$X = 62,208 \text{ mcg/h}$$

$$\frac{1 \text{ mg}}{1,000 \text{ mcg}} \diagtimes \frac{X \text{ mg}}{62,208 \text{ mcg}}$$

$$1,000X = 62,208$$

$$\frac{1,000X}{1,000} = \frac{62,208}{1,000}$$

$$X = 62 \text{ mg/h}$$

$$\frac{800 \text{ mg}}{500 \text{ mL}} \diagtimes \frac{62 \text{ mg/h}}{X \text{ mL/h}}$$

$$800X = 31,000$$

$$\frac{800X}{800} = \frac{31,000}{800}$$

$$X = 38.7 \text{ mL/h} = 39 \text{ mL/h (after titration)}$$

41) $\dfrac{\text{Dosage on hand}}{\text{Amount on hand}} = \dfrac{\text{Dosage desired/h}}{X \text{ Amount desired/h}}$

$$\frac{100 \text{ units}}{100 \text{ mL}} \diagtimes \frac{12 \text{ units/h}}{X \text{ mL/h}}$$

$$100X = 1,200$$

$$\frac{100}{100} = \frac{1,200}{100}$$

$$X = 12 \text{ mL/h}$$

43) $\dfrac{\text{Dosage on hand}}{\text{Amount on hand}} = \dfrac{\text{Dosage desired/h}}{X \text{ Amount desired/h}}$

$$\frac{100 \text{ units}}{100 \text{ mL}} \diagtimes \frac{4 \text{ units/h}}{X \text{ mL/h}}$$

$$100X = 400$$

$$\frac{100}{100} = \frac{400}{100}$$

$$X = 4 \text{ mL/h}$$

45) $\dfrac{1 \text{ kg}}{2.2 \text{ lb}} \diagtimes \dfrac{X \text{ kg}}{225 \text{ lb}}$

$$2.2X = 225$$

$$\frac{2.2X}{2.2} = \frac{225}{2.2}$$

$$X = 102.27 \text{ kg} = 100 \text{ kg (rounded to nearest 10 kg)}$$

80 units/kg bolus dosage

46) 80 units/kg $\times$ 100 kg = 8,000 units

1,000 units/mL

$$\frac{1,000 \text{ units}}{1 \text{ mL}} \diagtimes \frac{8,000 \text{ units}}{X \text{ mL}}$$

$$1,000X = 8,000$$

$$\frac{1,000X}{1,000} = \frac{8,000}{1,000}$$

$$X = 8 \text{ mL}$$

47) 18 units/kg/h $\times$ 100 kg = 1,800 units/h

$$\frac{25,000 \text{ units}}{250 \text{ mL}} \diagtimes \frac{X \text{ units}}{1 \text{ mL}}$$

$$250X = 25,000$$

$$\frac{250X}{250} = \frac{25,000}{250}$$

$$X = 100 \text{ units (per mL)}$$

$$\frac{100 \text{ units}}{1 \text{ mL}} \diagtimes \frac{1,800 \text{ units/h}}{X \text{ mL/h}}$$

$$100X = 1,800$$

$$\frac{100X}{100} = \frac{1,800}{100}$$

$$X = 18 \text{ mL/h}$$

48) q.6h

40 units/kg $\times$ 100 kg = 4,000 units

$$\frac{1,000 \text{ units}}{1 \text{ mL}} \diagtimes \frac{4,000 \text{ units}}{X \text{ mL}}$$

$$1,000X = 4,000$$

$$\frac{1,000X}{1,000} = \frac{4,000}{1,000}$$

$$X = 4 \text{ mL}$$

Increase rate: 2 units/kg/h $\times$ 100 kg = 200 units/h

Increase rate:

$$\frac{100 \text{ units}}{1 \text{ mL}} \diagtimes \frac{200 \text{ units/h}}{X \text{ mL/h}}$$

$$100X = 200$$

$$\frac{100X}{100} = \frac{200}{100}$$

$$X = 2 \text{ mL/h (increase)}$$

18 mL/h + 2 mL/h = 20 mL/h (new infusion rate)

49) Decrease rate by 2 units/kg/h

2 units/kg/h $\times$ 100 kg = 200 units/h (decrease)

$$\frac{100 \text{ units}}{1 \text{ mL}} \diagtimes \frac{200 \text{ units/h}}{X \text{ mL/h}}$$

$$100X = 200$$

$$\frac{100X}{100} = \frac{200}{100}$$

$$X = 2 \text{ mL/h (decrease)}$$

20 mL/h − 2 mL/h = 18 mL/h (new infusion rate)

Section 4—Self-Evaluation from pages 594–600

1) 0.9% NaCl **2)** 0.9 g NaCl per 100 mL **3)** 0.45 g NaCl per 100 mL **4)** 50 **5)** 4.5 **6)** 2.25 **7)** 75 **8)** 6.75 **9)** mL/h

10) 83 mL/h

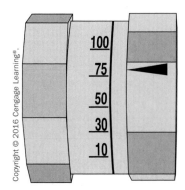

11) 21 **12)** 4 **13)** Approximately 2000 hours; approximately 8:00 PM **14)** Give a total of 3,000 mL IV solution per day, to include normal saline (0.9% NaCl) with 20 milliequivalents of potassium chloride added per liter (1,000 mL) *and* an IV piggyback solution of 250 mg cefazolin added to 100 mL of normal saline (0.9% NaCl) over 30 min administered every 8 hours. To administer the order each day, give 900 mL NS with KCl over $7\frac{1}{2}$ hours × 3 administrations and 100 mL NS with cafazolin over $\frac{1}{2}$ hour × 3 administrations **15)** 120 **16)** 200 **17)** Reset rate to 118 gtt/min, if policy and patient's condition permit. **18)** 1,410 **19)** 59 **20)** 120 **21)** 5 **22)** 0.48 **23)** 1.3 **24)** 1.04 **25)** 0.5 **26)** 18.5–37.5 **27)** Yes **28)** 18.5 **29)** 37 mL **30)** 120 **31)** 18.5 **32)** 0.8 **33)** 1.6 **34)** Yes **35)** 1.6 **36)** 18; 2 **37)** 7.5 **38)** 43 **39)** 200 **40)** 43 **41)** 200 **42)** 50 **43)** 12 **44)** 15 **45)** 0.13 **46)** 8 **47)** 80 **48)** 20.5 **49)** 61.4 **50)** 37.5 **51)** protamine sulfate **52)** a, c, and d **53)** b

54)   1—Record weight in kilograms.

2—Check aPTT test results.

3—Administer bolus, if required.

4—Start continuous infusion, if required.

5—Check aPTT test results.

6—Administer rebolus, if required.

7—Adjust infusion rate, if required.

55)   D:50,000 units per 5 mL (10,000 units/mL) is the best and only reasonable choice.

Solutions—Section 4—Self-Evaluation

4) D_5 0.45% NaCl = 5% dextrose = 5 g dextrose per 100 mL

$$\frac{5 \text{ g}}{100 \text{ mL}} \diagup\!\!\!\diagdown \frac{X \text{ g}}{1,000 \text{ mL}}$$

$$100X = 5,000$$

$$\frac{100X}{100} = \frac{5,000}{100}$$

$$X = 50 \text{ g}$$

5) D_5 0.45% NaCl = 0.45% NaCl = 0.45 g NaCl per 100 mL

$$\frac{0.45 \text{ g}}{100 \text{ mL}} \diagup\!\!\!\diagdown \frac{X \text{ g}}{1,000 \text{ mL}}$$

$$100X = 450$$

$$\frac{100X}{100} = \frac{450}{100}$$

$$X = 4.5 \text{ g}$$

10) $\frac{2,000 \text{ mL}}{24 \text{ h}} = 83.3$ mL/h = 83 mL/h

11)   83 mL/h = 83 mL/60 min

$$\frac{V}{T} \times C = \frac{83 \text{ mL}}{\overset{4}{\cancel{60} \text{ min}}} \times \overset{1}{\cancel{15}} \text{ gtt/mL} = \frac{83}{4} =$$

20.75 gtt/min = 21 gtt/min

13)   1 L = 1,000 mL

$$\frac{V}{T} \times C = R: \frac{1,000 \text{ mL}}{T} \times 15 \text{ gtt/mL} = 21 \text{ gtt/min}$$

$$\frac{1,000}{T} \times 15 = 21$$

$$\frac{15,000}{T} \diagup\!\!\!\diagdown \frac{21}{1}$$

$$21T = 15,000$$

$$\frac{21T}{21} = \frac{15,000}{21}$$

$$T = 714.2 \text{ min} = 714 \text{ min}$$

$$\frac{60 \text{ min}}{1 \text{ h}} \diagdown \frac{714 \text{ min}}{X \text{ h}}$$

$$60X = 714$$

$$\frac{60X}{60} = \frac{714}{60}$$

$$X = 11.9 \text{ h} = 12 \text{ h}$$

0800 hours
+ 1200 hours

2000 hours (24-hour clock) = 8 PM (traditional time)

Because of rounding the IV will run out 6 min sooner than exactly 12 h later. Also, more simply, if 2,000 mL is ordered to be infused in 24 h, then 1,000 mL should be infused in 12 h. 12 hours after 0800 or 8 AM is 2000 or 8 PM.

15) On fluid restriction of 3,000 mL/day

IV PB total volume: 100 mL × 3 = 300 mL

IV PB total time: 30 min × 3 = 90 min = $1\frac{1}{2}$ h

Regular IV total volume: 3,000 mL − 300 mL = 2,700 mL

Regular IV total time: 24 h − $1\frac{1}{2}$ h = $22\frac{1}{2}$ h (22.5 h)

$$\frac{2,700 \text{ mL}}{22.5 \text{ h}} = 120 \text{ mL/h}$$

16) $$\frac{100 \text{ mL}}{30 \text{ min}} \diagdown \frac{X \text{ mL/h}}{60 \text{ min/h}}$$

$$30X = 6,000$$

$$\frac{30X}{30} = \frac{6,000}{30}$$

$$X = 200 \text{ mL/h}$$

17) 1,200 mL ÷ 100 mL/h = 1,200 mL × 1 h/100 mL = 12 h

2200 hours (current time)
− 1530 hours (start time)

0630 = 6 h 30 min (elapsed time)

6 h 30 min = $6\frac{1}{2}$ h = 6.5 h;

6.5 h × 100 mL/h = 650 mL (expected to be infused)

1,200 mL − 650 mL = 550 mL (should be remaining)

After $6\frac{1}{2}$ h, 650 mL should have been infused, with 550 mL remaining. IV is behind schedule.

$$\frac{\text{Remaining volume}}{\text{Remaining time}} = \frac{650 \text{ mL}}{5.5 \text{ h}} = 118 \text{ mL/h (adjusted rate)}$$

$$\frac{\text{Adjusted gtt/min} - \text{Ordered gtt/min}}{\text{Ordered gtt/min}} = \% \text{ of variation;}$$

$$\frac{118 - 100}{100} = \frac{18}{100} = 0.18 = 18\% \text{ (variance is safe)}$$

If policy and patient's condition permit, reset rate to 118 mL/h.

18) $$\frac{1 \text{ kg}}{2.2 \text{ lb}} \diagdown \frac{X \text{ kg}}{40 \text{ lb}}$$

$$2.2X = 40$$

$$\frac{2.2X}{2.2} = \frac{40}{2.2}$$

$$X = 18.18 \text{ kg} = 18.2 \text{ kg}$$

First 10 kg: 100 mL/kg/day × 10 kg =   1,000 mL/day

Remaining 8.2 kg: 50 mL/kg/day × 8.2 kg =   410 mL/day

1,410 mL/day

19) $$\frac{1,410 \text{ mL}}{24 \text{ h}} = 58.7 \text{ mL/h} = 59 \text{ mL/h}$$

20) 1,185 g = 1.185. = 1.185 kg = 1.2 kg

First 10 kg: 100 mL/kg/day × 1.2 kg = 120 mL/day

21) $$\frac{120 \text{ mL}}{24 \text{ h}} = 5 \text{ mL/h}$$

22) Household:

$$\text{BSA (m}^2) = \sqrt{\frac{\text{ht (in)} \times \text{wt (lb)}}{3,131}} = \sqrt{\frac{30 \times 24}{3,131}} = \sqrt{\frac{720}{3,131}}$$

$$= \sqrt{0.229958} = 0.479 \text{ m}^2 = 0.48 \text{ m}^2$$

23) Metric:

$$\text{BSA (m}^2) = \sqrt{\frac{\text{ht (cm)} \times \text{wt (kg)}}{3,600}} = \sqrt{\frac{155 \times 39}{3,600}}$$

$$= \sqrt{\frac{6,045}{3,600}} = \sqrt{1.679166} = 1.295 \text{ m}^2 = 1.3 \text{ m}^2$$

26) Minimum safe dosage: 37 mg/m² × 0.5 m² = 18.5 mg

Maximum safe dosage: 75 mg/m² × 0.5 m² = 37.5 mg

28) $$\frac{1 \text{ mg}}{1 \text{ mL}} \diagdown \frac{18.5 \text{ mg}}{X \text{ mL}}$$

$$X = 18.5 \text{ mL}$$

29) $$\frac{1 \text{ mg}}{2 \text{ mL}} \diagdown \frac{18.5 \text{ mg}}{X \text{ mL}}$$

$$X = 37 \text{ mL}$$

30) $$\frac{18.5 \text{ mg}}{37 \text{ mL}} \diagdown \frac{1 \text{ mg/min}}{X \text{ mL/min}}$$

$$18.5X = 37$$

$$\frac{18.5X}{18.5} = \frac{37}{18.5}$$

$$X = 2 \text{ mL/min}$$

$$\frac{2 \text{ mL}}{1 \text{ min}} \diagdown \frac{X \text{ mL/h}}{60 \text{ min/h}}$$

$$X = 120 \text{ mL/h}$$

31) Think: At 1 mg/min, 18.5 mg will infuse in 18.5 min.

$$\frac{1 \text{ mg}}{1 \text{ min}} \diagdown \frac{18.5 \text{ mg}}{X \text{ min}}$$

$$X = 18.5 \text{ min}$$

33) 2 mg/m² × 0.8 m² = 1.6 mg

36) $$\frac{125 \text{ mg}}{1 \text{ mL}} \diagdown \frac{250 \text{ mg}}{X \text{ mL}}$$

$$125X = 250$$

$$\frac{125X}{125} = \frac{250}{125}$$

$$X = 2 \text{ mL (Ancef)}$$

$$\frac{40 \text{ mL}}{60 \text{ min}} \diagdown \frac{X \text{ mL}}{30 \text{ min}}$$

$$60X = 1,200$$

$$\frac{60X}{60} = \frac{1,200}{60}$$

$$X = 20 \text{ mL}$$

20 mL (total IV solution) − 2 mL (Ancef) = 18 mL (NS)

37) $\dfrac{100 \text{ mg}}{1 \text{ mL}} \diagup\!\!\!\!\!\diagdown \dfrac{750 \text{ mg}}{X \text{ mL}}$

$100X = 750$

$\dfrac{100X}{100} = \dfrac{750}{100}$

$X = 7.5 \text{ mL}$

7.5 mL IV solution to be used with the 750 mg of Timentin for minimal dilution.

38) Total IV PB volume: $100 \text{ mL} \times 6 = 600 \text{ mL}$

Regular IV volume: $1,500 \text{ mL} - 600 \text{ mL} = 900 \text{ mL}$

Total IV PB time of q.4h $\times$ 30 min: $6 \times 30 \text{ min} = 180 \text{ min}$;

$\dfrac{60 \text{ min}}{1 \text{ h}} \diagup\!\!\!\!\!\diagdown \dfrac{180 \text{ min}}{X \text{ h}}$

$60X = 180$

$\dfrac{60X}{60} = \dfrac{180}{60}$

$X = 3 \text{ h}$

Total regular IV time: $24 \text{ h} - 3 \text{ h} = 21 \text{ h}$

Regular IV rate: $\text{mL/h} = \dfrac{900 \text{ mL}}{21 \text{ h}} = 42.8 \text{ mL/h} = 43 \text{ mL/h}$

or 43 gtt/min (because drop factor is 60 gtt/mL)

39) $\dfrac{100 \text{ mL}}{30 \text{ min}} \diagup\!\!\!\!\!\diagdown \dfrac{X \text{ mL}}{60 \text{ min}}$

$30X = 6,000$

$\dfrac{30X}{30} = \dfrac{6,000}{30}$

$X = 200 \text{ mL/h}$ or 200 gtt/min (because drop factor is 60 gtt/mL)

40) See #38, Regular IV rate calculated at 43 mL/h.

41) See #39, IV PB rate calculated at 200 mL/h.

42) $\dfrac{40 \text{ mEq}}{1,000 \text{ mL}} \diagup\!\!\!\!\!\diagdown \dfrac{2 \text{ mEq/h}}{X \text{ mL/h}}$

$40X = 2,000$

$\dfrac{40X}{40} = \dfrac{2,000}{40}$

$X = 50 \text{ mL/h}$

43) $1 \text{ L} = 1,000 \text{ mL}$

$1 \text{ mg} = 1,000 \text{ mcg}$

$\dfrac{1 \text{ mg}}{1,000 \text{ mcg}} \diagup\!\!\!\!\!\diagdown \dfrac{25 \text{ mg}}{X \text{ mcg}}$

$X = 25,000 \text{ mcg}$

25 mg per L = 25,000 mcg per 1,000 mL

$\dfrac{25,000 \text{ mcg}}{1,000 \text{ mL}} \diagup\!\!\!\!\!\diagdown \dfrac{X \text{ mcg}}{1 \text{ mL}}$

$10,000X = 25,000$

$\dfrac{1,000X}{1,000} = \dfrac{25,000}{1,000}$

$X = 25 \text{ mcg/mL}$

$\dfrac{25 \text{ mcg}}{1 \text{ mL}} \diagup\!\!\!\!\!\diagdown \dfrac{5 \text{ mcg/min}}{X \text{ mL/min}}$

$25X = 5$

44) $1 \text{ L} = 1,000 \text{ mL}$

$1 \text{ unit} = 1,000 \text{ milliunits}$

$\dfrac{1 \text{ unit}}{1,000 \text{ milliunits}} \diagup\!\!\!\!\!\diagdown \dfrac{15 \text{ units}}{X \text{ milliunits}}$

$X = 15,000 \text{ milliunits}$

$\dfrac{15,000 \text{ milliunits}}{1,000 \text{ mL}} \diagup\!\!\!\!\!\diagdown \dfrac{X \text{ milliunits}}{1 \text{ mL}}$

$1,000X = 15,000$

$\dfrac{1,000X}{1,000} = \dfrac{15,000}{1,000}$

$X = 15 \text{ milliunits/mL}$

45) $\dfrac{15 \text{ milliunits}}{1 \text{ mL}} \diagup\!\!\!\!\!\diagdown \dfrac{2 \text{ milliunits/min}}{X \text{ mL/min}}$

$15X = 2$

$\dfrac{15X}{15} = \dfrac{2}{15}$

$X = 0.13 \text{ mL/min}$

46) $\dfrac{0.13 \text{ mL}}{1 \text{ min}} \diagup\!\!\!\!\!\diagdown \dfrac{X \text{ mL/h}}{60 \text{ min/h}}$

$X = 7.8 \text{ mL/h} = 8 \text{ mL/h}$

47) $\dfrac{15 \text{ milliunits}}{1 \text{ mL}} \diagup\!\!\!\!\!\diagdown \dfrac{20 \text{ milliunits/min}}{X \text{ mL/min}}$

$15X = 20$

$\dfrac{15X}{15} = \dfrac{20}{15}$

$X = 1.33 \text{ mL/min}$

$\dfrac{1.33 \text{ mL}}{1 \text{ min}} \diagup\!\!\!\!\!\diagdown \dfrac{X \text{ mL/h}}{60 \text{ min/h}}$

$X = 79.8 \text{ mL/h} = 80 \text{ mL/h}$

48) $\dfrac{1 \text{ kg}}{2.2 \text{ lb}} \diagup\!\!\!\!\!\diagdown \dfrac{X \text{ kg}}{150 \text{ lb}}$

$2.2X = 150$

$\dfrac{2.2X}{2.2} = \dfrac{150}{2.2}$

$X = 68.18 \text{ kg} = 68.2 \text{ kg}$

4 mcg/kg/min $\times$ 68.2 kg = 272.8 mcg/min = 273 mcg/min

$\dfrac{273 \text{ mcg}}{1 \text{ min}} \diagup\!\!\!\!\!\diagdown \dfrac{X \text{ mcg/h}}{60 \text{ min/h}}$

$X = 16,380 \text{ mcg/h}$

$\dfrac{1 \text{ L}}{1,000 \text{ mL}} \diagup\!\!\!\!\!\diagdown \dfrac{0.5 \text{ L}}{X \text{ mL}}$

$X = 500 \text{ mL}$

$\dfrac{400 \text{ mg}}{500 \text{ mL}} \diagup\!\!\!\!\!\diagdown \dfrac{X \text{ mg}}{1 \text{ mL}}$

$500X = 400$

$\dfrac{500X}{500} = \dfrac{400}{500}$

$X = 0.8 \text{ mg (per mL)}$

$$\frac{1 \text{ mg}}{1,000 \text{ mcg}} \diagdown\!\!\!\!\diagup \frac{0.8 \text{ mg}}{X \text{ mcg}}$$

$$X = 800 \text{ mcg (per mL)}$$

$$\frac{800 \text{ mcg}}{1 \text{ mL}} \diagdown\!\!\!\!\diagup \frac{16,380 \text{ mcg/h}}{X \text{ mL/h}}$$

$$800X = 16,380$$

$$\frac{800X}{800} = \frac{16,380}{800}$$

$$X = 20.47 \text{ mL/h} = 20.5 \text{ mL/h}$$

49) $12 \text{ mcg/kg/min} \times 68.2 \text{ kg} = 818.4 \text{ mcg/min} =$

818 mcg/min

$$\frac{818 \text{ mcg}}{1 \text{ min}} \diagdown\!\!\!\!\diagup \frac{X \text{ mcg/h}}{60 \text{ min/h}}$$

$$X = 49,080 \text{ mcg/h}$$

$$\frac{800 \text{ mcg}}{1 \text{ mL}} \diagdown\!\!\!\!\diagup \frac{49,080 \text{ mcg/h}}{X \text{ mL/h}}$$

$$800X = 49,080$$

$$\frac{800X}{800} = \frac{49,080}{800}$$

$$X = 61.35 \text{ mL/h} = 61.4 \text{ mL/h}$$

50) $\dfrac{10,000 \text{ units}}{500 \text{ mL}} \diagdown\!\!\!\!\diagup \dfrac{750 \text{ units/h}}{X \text{ mL/h}}$

$$10,000X = 375,000$$

$$\frac{10,000X}{10,000} = \frac{375,000}{10,000}$$

$$X = 37.5 \text{ mL/h}$$

Comprehensive Skills Evaluation from pages 609–625

1) 80   **2)** 0500; 09/04/xx   **3)** 1,920   **4)** 1.6; 38.4   **5)** a) immediately b) one time only

6)   a) 1; 4; 5; 1; 0.25

     b) Fill syringe with 1 mL of digoxin and 4 mL of normal saline.

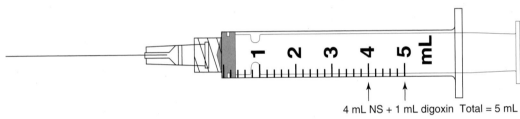

4 mL NS + 1 mL digoxin   Total = 5 mL

7)   e

8)   a) 2; 2; 0.5

     b)

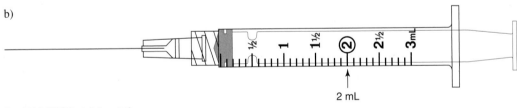

2 mL

9) $\frac{1}{2}$ **10)** 1   **11)** 2   **12)** a) 2 b) 4 hours later, if she complains again of a headache   **13)** digoxin for injection and tablets, furosemide for injection, nitroglycerin, and potassium chloride in 5% dextrose and 0.45% sodium chloride IV solution   **14)** 80

15)   a) 5

     b)

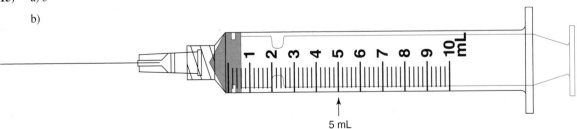

5 mL

16) 30

17) a) Yes; dosage ordered is at the maximum of the recommended range of 250 mcg/min to 500 mcg/min for

   Mrs. Smith, who weighs 110 lb, or 50 kg.

   b) 5

   c)

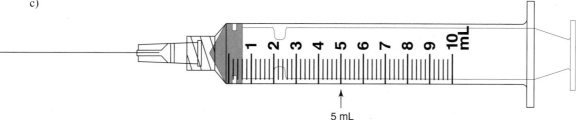

5 mL

18) 18.6 **19)** 30,000; 30 **20)** 60 **21)** a) Yes, the recommended dosage for this child is 225 mg/day in 3 divided doses, or 75 mg/dose. This is the same as the order. b) 2; 23; 40 **22)** Yes, safe dosage for this child is 300 mg/dose, which is the same as the order. **23)** a) 6 b) 44 c) 1,200 **24)** a) 1,700 b) 70.8 c) No. The ordered rate of 50 mL per hour is less than the recommended hourly maintenance IV rate. **25)** 3.2

26)

2/6/xx, 0800, reconstituted as 1.5 g
in 4 mL. Expires 2/7/xx, 0800, keep
refrigerated. G.D.P.

27) 1.3

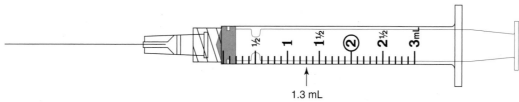

1.3 mL

28) 103

29) a) 2

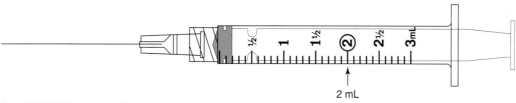

2 mL

   b) 60

30) a) 56.8 b) 4,544 c) 4.5 d) 1,022; 10.2 **31)** a) Decrease rate by 2 units/kg/h. b) 114; 1.1 c) 9.1

32) 8; 0.08; Insulin should be administered with an insulin syringe. This question and answer are provided to evaluate your understanding of the insulin syringe and insulin concentration. 8 units of U-100 insulin equals a volume of 0.08 mL.

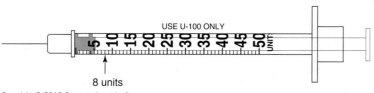

8 units

33)   a) 60

      b)

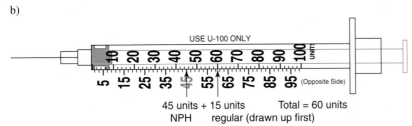

45 units + 15 units   Total = 60 units
NPH   regular (drawn up first)

34) 20   **35)** 720; 960   **36)** 730; 30   **37)** 1.43   **38)** a) 14.3–28.6 b) Yes; the dosage ordered is within the allowable range.

39) a) 0.5 b) 56; 5.6; 1.4   **40)** 50; 4.5   **41)** 6; 44   **42)** Yes; the recommended amount of IV fluid to safely dilute this med is 15–60 mL. The order calls for 50 mL total, or 44 mL of IV fluid.   **43)** a) 1,600,000 b) Yes, the minimum daily dosage is 1,500,000 units/day, and the maximum is 2,500,000 units/day. The ordered dosage falls within this range. c) 1.8; 500,000 d) 0.8 e) Contact the prescriber when an order is not within the recommended range (this order did fall within the safe range).

>
> 1/14/xx; 0800, reconstituted as
> 500,000 units/mL. Expires 1/21/xx; 0800.
> Keep refrigerated. G.D.P.

44) 101   **45)** 2145   **46)** 0.5; 0.13   **47)** 15   **48)** 230

49) Prevention: The frequency of this order is missing and the route is unclear. If the student actually gave this medication in the eye, it would cause a severe reaction. The medication particles could scratch the eye or cause a worse reaction, such as blindness.

     To prevent this from occurring, the student nurse should always ensure that each medication order is complete. Every order should include the name of the drug, the dose, the route, and the time (with the patient, prescriber, and licensure identified). When any of these are missing, the order should be clarified. Further, the "O.D." abbreviation is obsolete and discouraged by The Joint Commission. The student nurse should also look up medications and know the safe use for each medication ordered. Had this student looked up digoxin in a drug guide, the student would have discovered that the medication is never given in the eye.

50) Prevention: The student nurse took the correct action with this order. The nurses who had given the medication previously should have looked up the medication if they were unfamiliar with it, to safely identify whether it was ordered with an appropriate route, correct dosage, and correct frequency. There was also an error made by the pharmacist who supplied the medication to the nursing unit. It is extremely important to be familiar with the medications being given. If there's a question or any doubt, the medication should be looked up in a drug guide and/or the prescriber should be questioned. Also, close reading of the label and matching it to the order is extremely important. Remember the Six Rights of medication administration. Ideally, packaging by the pharmacy using "Tall Man" lettering would further enhance patient safety and alert the nurse to select the correct drug.

Solutions—Comprehensive Skills Evaluation

1)   80 mL/h = 80 gtt/min (because drop factor is 60 gtt/mL)

2) $\dfrac{1,000 \text{ mL}}{80 \text{ mL/h}} = 12.5 \text{ h} = 12 \text{ h } 30 \text{ min}$

     1630 hours + 12 h 30 min later = 0500 hours the next day (09/04/xx)

3)   80 mL/h × 24 h = 1,920 mL

4) $\dfrac{20 \text{ mEq}}{1,000 \text{ mL}} \diagdown\!\!\!\!\diagup \dfrac{X \text{ mEq/h}}{80 \text{ mL/h}}$

     1,000X = 1,600

     $\dfrac{1,000X}{1,000} = \dfrac{1,600}{1,000}$

     X = 1.6 mEq/h

     1.6 mEq/h × 24 h = 38.4 mEq (per day)

6) 0.25 mg is ordered and the supply dosage is

0.25 mg/mL. It is obvious that the nurse should give

1 mL. 1 mL added to 4 mL NS = 5 mL total solution.

$$\frac{\overset{1}{\cancel{5}} \text{ mL}}{\underset{1}{\cancel{5}} \text{ min}} = 1 \text{ mL/min}$$

$$\frac{1 \text{ mL}}{60 \text{ sec}} \diagdown \frac{X \text{ mL}}{15 \text{ sec}}$$

$$60X = 15$$

$$\frac{60X}{60} = \frac{15}{60}$$

$$X = 0.25 \text{ mL (per 15 sec)}$$

7) The total amount of fluid is too small for an IV PB.

8) $$\frac{10 \text{ mg}}{1 \text{ mL}} \diagdown \frac{20 \text{ mg}}{X \text{ mL}}$$

$$10X = 20$$

$$\frac{10X}{10} = \frac{20}{10}$$

$$X = 2 \text{ mL}$$

$$\frac{40 \text{ mg}}{2 \text{ min}} \diagdown \frac{20 \text{ mg}}{X \text{ min}}$$

$$40X = 40$$

$$\frac{40X}{40} = \frac{40}{40}$$

$$X = 1 \text{ min} \quad \text{Give 2 mL over 1 min}$$

$$\frac{2 \text{ mL}}{60 \text{ sec}} \diagdown \frac{X \text{ mL}}{15 \text{ sec}}$$

$$60X = 30$$

$$\frac{60X}{60} = \frac{30}{60}$$

$$X = 0.5 \text{ mL} \quad \text{Give 0.5 mL over 15 sec}$$

9) 1 mg = 1,000 mcg (known equivalent)

$$\frac{1 \text{ mg}}{1,000 \text{ mcg}} \diagdown \frac{0.125 \text{ mg}}{X \text{ mcg}}$$

$$X = 125 \text{ mcg}$$

$$\frac{250 \text{ mcg}}{1 \text{ tab}} \diagdown \frac{125 \text{ mcg}}{X \text{ tab}}$$

$$250X = 125$$

$$\frac{250X}{250} \diagdown \frac{125}{250}$$

$$X = 0.5 \text{ tablet} = \tfrac{1}{2} \text{ tablet}$$

0.125 mg ordered daily means you will need to give

$\tfrac{1}{2}$ tablet per 24 h.

10) $$\frac{20 \text{ mg}}{1 \text{ tab}} \diagdown \frac{20 \text{ mg}}{X \text{ tab}}$$

$$20X = 20$$

$$\frac{20X}{20} = \frac{20}{20}$$

$$X = 1 \text{ tablet}$$

11) $$\frac{6.5 \text{ mg}}{1 \text{ cap}} \diagdown \frac{13 \text{ mg}}{X \text{ cap}}$$

$$6.5X = 13$$

$$\frac{6.5X}{6.5} = \frac{13}{6.5}$$

$$X = 2 \text{ capsules}$$

12) 1 g = 1,000 mg

$$\frac{500 \text{ mg}}{1 \text{ tab}} \diagdown \frac{1,000 \text{ mg}}{X \text{ tab}}$$

$$500X = 1,000$$

$$\frac{500X}{500} = \frac{1,000}{500}$$

$$X = 2 \text{ tablets}$$

14) Order is for 80 mL/h—this is the setting for the

insulin pump.

15) $$\frac{10 \text{ mg}}{1 \text{ mL}} \diagdown \frac{50 \text{ mg}}{X \text{ mL}}$$

$$10X = 50$$

$$\frac{10X}{10} = \frac{50}{10}$$

$$X = 5 \text{ mL}$$

16) 2 g = 2,000 mg

$$\frac{2,000 \text{ mg}}{500 \text{ mL}} \diagdown \frac{2 \text{ mg/min}}{X \text{ mL/min}}$$

$$2,000X = 1,000$$

$$\frac{2,000X}{2,000} = \frac{1,000}{2,000}$$

$$X = 0.5 \text{ mL/min}$$

$$\frac{0.5 \text{ mL}}{1 \text{ min}} \diagdown \frac{X \text{ mL/h}}{60 \text{ min/h}}$$

$$X = 30 \text{ mL/h}$$

17) $$\frac{1 \text{ kg}}{2.2 \text{ lb}} \diagdown \frac{X \text{ kg}}{110 \text{ lb}}$$

$$2.2X = 110$$

$$\frac{2.2X}{2.2} = \frac{110}{2.2}$$

$$X = 50 \text{ kg}$$

Minimum: 5 mcg/kg/min $\times$ 50 kg = 250 mcg/min

Maximum: 10 mcg/kg/min $\times$ 50 kg = 500 mcg/min

Ordered dosage is safe.

$$\frac{80 \text{ mg}}{1 \text{ mL}} \diagdown \frac{400 \text{ mg}}{X \text{ mL}}$$

$$80X = 400$$

$$\frac{80X}{80} = \frac{400}{80}$$

$$X = 5 \text{ mL}$$

18) $$\frac{1 \text{ mg}}{1,000 \text{ mcg}} \diagdown \frac{X \text{ mg/min}}{500 \text{ mcg/min}}$$

$$1,000X = 500$$

$$\frac{1,000X}{1,000} = \frac{500}{1,000}$$

$$X = 0.5 \text{ mg/min}$$

$$\frac{400 \text{ mg}}{250 \text{ mL}} \diagdown \frac{0.5 \text{ mg/min}}{X \text{ mL/min}}$$

$$400X = 125$$

$$\frac{400X}{400} = \frac{125}{400}$$

$$X = 0.312 \text{ mL/min} = 0.31 \text{ mL/min}$$

$$\frac{0.31 \text{ mL}}{1 \text{ min}} \diagdown \frac{X \text{ mL/h}}{60 \text{ min/h}}$$

$$X = 18.6 \text{ mL/h (program in tenths of mL)}$$

19)

$$\frac{500 \text{ mcg}}{1 \text{ min}} \diagdown\!\!\!\!\diagup \frac{X \text{ mcg/h}}{60 \text{ min/h}}$$

$$X = 30{,}000 \text{ mcg/h}$$

$$\frac{1 \text{ mg}}{1{,}000 \text{ mcg}} \diagdown\!\!\!\!\diagup \frac{X \text{ mg/h}}{30{,}000 \text{ mcg/h}}$$

$$1{,}000X = 30{,}000$$

$$\frac{1{,}000X}{1{,}000} = \frac{30{,}000}{1{,}000}$$

$$X = 30 \text{ mg/h}$$

20)

$$\frac{2{,}000 \text{ mg}}{500 \text{ mL}} \diagdown\!\!\!\!\diagup \frac{4 \text{ mg/min}}{X \text{ mL/min}}$$

$$2{,}000X = 2{,}000$$

$$\frac{2{,}000X}{2{,}000} = \frac{2{,}000}{2{,}000}$$

$$X = 1 \text{ mL/min}$$

$$\frac{1 \text{ mL}}{1 \text{ min}} \diagdown\!\!\!\!\diagup \frac{X \text{ mL/h}}{60 \text{ min/h}}$$

$$X = 60 \text{ mL/h}$$

21)

$$\frac{1 \text{ kg}}{2.2 \text{ lb}} \diagdown\!\!\!\!\diagup \frac{X \text{ kg}}{33 \text{ lb}}$$

$$2.2X = 33$$

$$\frac{2.2X}{2.2} = \frac{33}{2.2}$$

$$X = 15 \text{ kg}$$

$$15 \text{ mg/kg/day} \times 15 \text{ kg} = 225 \text{ mg/day}$$

Maximum:

$$\frac{225 \text{ mg}}{3 \text{ doses}} \diagdown\!\!\!\!\diagup \frac{X \text{ mg}}{1 \text{ dose}}$$

$$3X = 225$$

$$\frac{3X}{3} = \frac{225}{3}$$

$$X = 75 \text{ mg (per dose)}$$

The order is safe. It is obvious you want to give 2 mL.

25 mL (total IV solution) − 2 mL (Kantrex) = 23 mL

($D_5 \frac{1}{2}$ NS)

25 mL (total solution) + 15 mL (flush) = 40 mL

(total in 1 h)

40 mL over 1 h is 40 mL/h.

22)

$$\frac{2.2 \text{ lb}}{1 \text{ kg}} \diagdown\!\!\!\!\diagup \frac{66 \text{ lb}}{X \text{ kg}}$$

$$2.2X = 66$$

$$\frac{2.2X}{2.2} = \frac{66}{2.2}$$

$$X = 30 \text{ kg}$$

$$40 \text{ mg/kg/day} \times 30 \text{ kg} = 1{,}200 \text{ mg/day}$$

$$\frac{1{,}200 \text{ mg}}{4 \text{ doses}} \diagdown\!\!\!\!\diagup \frac{X \text{ mg}}{1 \text{ dose}}$$

$$4X = 1{,}200$$

$$\frac{4X}{4} = \frac{1{,}200}{4}$$

$$X = 300 \text{ mg/dose}$$

23)

$$\frac{500 \text{ mg}}{10 \text{ mL}} \diagdown\!\!\!\!\diagup \frac{300 \text{ mg}}{X \text{ mL}}$$

$$500X = 3{,}000$$

$$\frac{500X}{500} = \frac{3{,}000}{500}$$

$$X = 6 \text{ mL}$$

50 mL (total IV volume) − 6 mL (vancomycin) =

44 mL ($D_5 \frac{1}{2}$ NS); 50 mL/h̶ × 24 h̶ = 1,200 mL

24) Child weighs 30 kg.

100 mL/k̶g̶/day × 10 k̶g̶ = 1,000 mL/day

(for first 10 kg)

50 mL/k̶g̶/day × 10 k̶g̶ = 500 mL/day

(for next 10 kg)

20 mL/k̶g̶/day × 10 k̶g̶ = 200 mL/day

(for remaining 10 kg)

Total: 1,000 mL/day + 500 mL/day + 200 mL/day

= 1,700 mL/day or per 24 h

1,700 mL ÷ 24 h = 70.83 mL/h = 70.8 mL/h

The ordered rate is less than the recommended daily rate of maintenance fluids. The nurse should consider possible clinical reasons for the difference and consult the physician as needed for clarification.

25) The vial size is 1.5 g. Choose the diluent that corresponds to the vial chosen. Adding 3.2 mL will yield a total of 4.0 mL containing 1.5 g.

27)

$$\frac{1 \text{ g}}{1{,}000 \text{ mg}} \diagdown\!\!\!\!\diagup \frac{1.5 \text{ g}}{X \text{ mg}}$$

$$X = 1{,}500 \text{ mg}$$

$$\frac{1{,}500 \text{ mg}}{4 \text{ mL}} \diagdown\!\!\!\!\diagup \frac{500 \text{ mg}}{X \text{ mL}}$$

$$1{,}500X = 2{,}000$$

$$\frac{1{,}500X}{1{,}500} = \frac{2{,}000}{1{,}500}$$

$$X = 1.33 \text{ mL} = 1.3 \text{ mL}$$

28) 50 mL (total IV PB) + 1.3 mL (med) = 51.3 mL

(total to infuse in 30 min)

$$\frac{51.3 \text{ mL}}{30 \text{ min}} \diagdown\!\!\!\!\diagup \frac{X \text{ mL/h}}{60 \text{ min/h}}$$

$$30X = 3{,}078$$

$$\frac{30X}{30} \diagdown\!\!\!\!\diagup \frac{3{,}078}{30}$$

$$X = 102.6 \text{ mL/h} = 103 \text{ mL/h}$$

29)

$$\frac{5{,}000 \text{ units}}{1 \text{ mL}} \diagdown\!\!\!\!\diagup \frac{10{,}000 \text{ units}}{X \text{ mL}}$$

$$5{,}000X = 10{,}000$$

$$\frac{5{,}000X}{5{,}000} = \frac{10{,}000}{5{,}000}$$

$$X = 2 \text{ mL}$$

$$\frac{10{,}000 \text{ units}}{500 \text{ mL}} \diagdown\!\!\!\!\diagup \frac{1{,}200 \text{ units/h}}{X \text{ mL/h}}$$

$$10{,}000X = 600{,}000$$

$$\frac{10{,}000X}{10{,}000} = \frac{600{,}000}{10{,}000}$$

$$X = 60 \text{ mL/h}$$

30)

$$\frac{1 \text{ kg}}{2.2 \text{ lb}} \diagdown\!\!\!\!\diagup \frac{X \text{ kg}}{125 \text{ lb}}$$

$$2.2X = 125$$

$$\frac{2.2X}{2.2} = \frac{125}{2.2}$$

$$X = 56.81 \text{ kg} = 56.8 \text{ kg}$$

80 units/kg × 56.8 kg = 4,544 units

$$\frac{1{,}000 \text{ units}}{1 \text{ mL}} \diagdown\!\!\!\!\diagup \frac{4{,}544 \text{ units}}{X \text{ mL}}$$

$$1{,}000X = 4{,}544$$

$$\frac{1{,}000X}{1{,}000} = \frac{4{,}544}{1{,}000}$$

$$X = 4.544 \text{ mL} = 4.5 \text{ mL}$$

18 units/kg/h × 56.8 kg = 1,022.4 units/h
= 1,022 units/h

$$\frac{25{,}000 \text{ units}}{250 \text{ mL}} \diagdown\!\!\!\!\diagup \frac{1{,}022 \text{ units/h}}{X \text{ mL/h}}$$

$$25{,}000X = 255{,}500$$

$$\frac{25{,}000X}{25{,}000} = \frac{255{,}500}{25{,}000}$$

$$X = 10.22 \text{ mL/h} = 10.2 \text{ mL/h}$$

31) Decrease rate by 2 units/kg/h.

2 units/kg/h × 56.8 kg = 113.6 units/h =
114 units/h (decrease)

$$\frac{25{,}000 \text{ units}}{250 \text{ mL}} \diagdown\!\!\!\!\diagup \frac{114 \text{ units/h}}{X \text{ mL/h}}$$

$$25{,}000X = 28{,}500$$

$$\frac{25{,}000X}{25{,}000} = \frac{28{,}500}{25{,}000}$$

$$X = 1.14 \text{ mL/h} = 1.1 \text{ mL/h}$$

1,022 units/h − 114 units/h = 908 units/h

$$\frac{25{,}000 \text{ units}}{250 \text{ mL}} \diagdown\!\!\!\!\diagup \frac{908 \text{ units/h}}{X \text{ mL/h}}$$

$$25{,}000X = 227{,}000$$

$$\frac{25{,}000X}{25{,}000} = \frac{227{,}000}{25{,}000}$$

$$X = 9.08 \text{ mL/h} = 9.1 \text{ mL/h}$$
$$\text{or } 10.2 \text{ mL/h} = 1.1 \text{ mL/h} = 9.1 \text{ mL/h}$$

32)

$$\frac{100 \text{ units}}{1 \text{ mL}} \diagdown\!\!\!\!\diagup \frac{8 \text{ units}}{X \text{ mL}}$$

$$100X = 8$$

$$\frac{100X}{100} = \frac{8}{100}$$

$$X = 0.08 \text{ mL}$$

Insulin should be administered with an insulin syringe. This question and solution are provided to evaluate your understanding of the insulin syringe and insulin concentration. 8 units of U-100 insulin equals a dose volume of 0.08 mL.

33) 15 units + 45 units = 60 units

34) U-100 insulin: 100 units/mL

$$\frac{100 \text{ units}}{1 \text{ mL}} \diagdown\!\!\!\!\diagup \frac{300 \text{ units}}{X \text{ mL}}$$

$$100X = 300$$

$$\frac{100X}{100} = \frac{300}{100}$$

$$X = 3 \text{ mL}$$

Total IV volume: 150 mL (NS) + 3 mL (insulin) =
153 mL

$$\frac{300 \text{ units}}{153 \text{ mL}} \diagdown\!\!\!\!\diagup \frac{X \text{ units/h}}{10 \text{ mL/h}}$$

$$153X = 3{,}000$$

$$\frac{153X}{153} = \frac{3{,}000}{153}$$

$$X = 19.6 \text{ units/h} = 20 \text{ units/h}$$

35)

$$\frac{1 \text{ fl oz}}{30 \text{ mL}} \diagdown\!\!\!\!\diagup \frac{8 \text{ fl oz}}{X \text{ mL}}$$

$$X = 240 \text{ mL}$$

$$\frac{1}{4} \diagdown\!\!\!\!\diagup \frac{240}{X \text{ mL}}$$

$$X = 960 \text{ mL (total volume of reconstituted}$$
$$\tfrac{1}{4} \text{ strength Isomil)}$$

960 mL (total solution) − 240 mL (solute or Isomil) =
720 mL (solvent or water)

36)

$$\frac{1 \text{ kg}}{2.2 \text{ lb}} \diagdown\!\!\!\!\diagup \frac{X \text{ kg}}{16 \text{ lb}}$$

$$2.2X = 16$$

$$\frac{2.2X}{2.2} = \frac{16}{2.2}$$

$$X = 7.27 \text{ kg} = 7.3 \text{ kg}$$

730 mL ÷ 24 h = 30.4 mL/h = 30 mL/h

37)

$$\frac{1 \text{ ft}}{12 \text{ in}} \diagdown\!\!\!\!\diagup \frac{5 \text{ ft}}{X \text{ in}}$$

$$X = 60 \text{ in}$$

60 in + 2 in = 62 in

Household:
$$\text{BSA (m}^2) = \sqrt{\frac{\text{ht (in)} \times \text{wt (lb)}}{3{,}131}} = \sqrt{\frac{62 \times 103}{3{,}131}} =$$
$$\sqrt{\frac{6{,}386}{3{,}131}} = \sqrt{2.039603} = 1.428 \text{ m}^2 = 1.43 \text{ m}^2$$

38) 10 mg/m² × 1.43 m² = 14.3 mg
20 mg/m² × 1.43 m² = 28.6 mg

Yes, the order is safe.

39) Concentration: 40 mg per 80 mL

$$\frac{40 \text{ mg}}{80 \text{ mL}} \diagdown\!\!\!\!\diagup \frac{X \text{ mg}}{1 \text{ mL}}$$

$$80X = 40$$

$$\frac{80X}{80} = \frac{40}{80}$$

$$X = 0.5 \text{ mg (per mL) or } 0.5 \text{ mg/mL}$$

$$\frac{0.5 \text{ mg}}{1 \text{ mL}} \diagdown\!\!\!\!\diagup \frac{28 \text{ mg}}{X \text{ mL}}$$

$$0.5X = 28$$

$$\frac{0.5X}{0.5} = \frac{28}{0.5}$$

$$X = 56 \text{ mL}$$

$$\frac{56 \text{ mL}}{10 \text{ min}} \diagdown\diagup \frac{X \text{ mL}}{1 \text{ min}}$$

$$10X = 56$$

$$\frac{10X}{10} = \frac{56}{10}$$

$$X = 5.6 \text{ mL (per min) or } 5.6 \text{ mL/min}$$

or 5.6 mL per 60 sec

$$\frac{5.6 \text{ mL}}{60 \text{ sec}} \diagdown\diagup \frac{X \text{ mL}}{15 \text{ sec}}$$

$$60X = 84$$

$$\frac{60X}{60} = \frac{84}{60}$$

$$X = 1.4 \text{ mL (per 15 sec)}$$

40)   Dextrose: NaCl:

$$\frac{5 \text{ g}}{100 \text{ mL}} \diagdown\diagup \frac{X \text{ g}}{1,000 \text{ mL}} \qquad \frac{0.45 \text{ g}}{100 \text{ mL}} \diagdown\diagup \frac{X \text{ g}}{1,000 \text{ mL}}$$

$$100X = 5,000 \qquad\qquad 100X = 450$$

$$\frac{100X}{100} = \frac{5,000}{100} \qquad\qquad \frac{100X}{100} = \frac{450}{100}$$

$$X = 50 \text{ g} \qquad\qquad\qquad X = 4.5 \text{ g}$$

41) $$\frac{100 \text{ mg}}{1 \text{ mL}} \diagdown\diagup \frac{600 \text{ mg}}{X \text{ mL}}$$

$$100X = 600$$

$$\frac{100X}{100} = \frac{600}{100}$$

$$X = 6 \text{ mL}$$

50 mL (total fluid) − 6 mL (med) = 44 mL (IV fluid). Note: Add the med to the chamber and then add IV fluid up to the 50 mL mark.

42)   Maximal dilution:

$$\frac{10 \text{ mg}}{1 \text{ mL}} \diagdown\diagup \frac{600 \text{ mg}}{X \text{ mL}}$$

$$10X = 600$$

$$\frac{10X}{10} = \frac{600}{10}$$

$$X = 60 \text{ mL (per 600 mg)}$$

Minimal dilution:

$$\frac{40 \text{ mg}}{1 \text{ mL}} \diagdown\diagup \frac{600 \text{ mg}}{X \text{ mL}}$$

$$40X = 600$$

$$\frac{40X}{40} = \frac{600}{40}$$

$$X = 15 \text{ mL (per 600 mg)}$$

43)   400,000 units/dose × 4 doses/day = 1,600,000 units/day

Minimum: 150,000 units/kg/day × 10 kg = 1,500,000 units/day

Maximum: 250,000 units/kg/day × 10 kg = 2,500,000 units/day

Reconstitute with 1.8 mL for a concentration of 500,000 units/mL. This concentration is selected because it will be further diluted.

$$\frac{500,000 \text{ units}}{1 \text{ mL}} \diagdown\diagup \frac{400,000 \text{ units}}{X \text{ mL}}$$

$$500,000X = 400,000$$

$$\frac{500,000X}{500,000} = \frac{400,000}{500,000}$$

$$X = 0.8 \text{ mL (penicillin)}$$

44)   100 mL (NS) + 0.8 mL (penicillin) = 100.8 or 101 mL to be infused in 60 min or 1 h. Set IV pump at 101 mL/h.

45) $$\frac{125 \text{ mL}}{1 \text{ h}} \diagdown\diagup \frac{1,000 \text{ mL}}{X \text{ h}}$$

$$125X = 1,000$$

$$\frac{125X}{125} = \frac{1,000}{125}$$

$$X = 8 \text{ h}$$

The primary IV will infuse for 8 hours. The IV PB will infuse for 30 minutes. Therefore, the primary IV will be interrupted by the IV PB and then will resume. The IV will be completely infused in 8 hours and 30 min.

1:15 PM + 8 h 30 min = 1315 + 0830 = 2145

46) $$\frac{25 \text{ mg}}{1 \text{ mL}} \diagdown\diagup \frac{12.5 \text{ mg}}{X \text{ mL}}$$

$$25X = 12.5$$

$$\frac{25X}{25} = \frac{12.5}{25}$$

$$X = 0.5 \text{ mL}$$

Think: Although the recommendation is "not to exceed 25 mg/min," which is 1 mL of the dosage you have on hand, you don't have to give it that rapidly. The order requires 12.5 mg or half the maximum allowable amount to give in 1 min. Use the dose amount (0.5 mL) and administer that over 1 min (60 sec).

Give 0.5 mL/min or

$$\frac{0.5 \text{ mL}}{60 \text{ sec}} \diagdown\diagup \frac{X \text{ mL}}{15 \text{ sec}}$$

$$60X = 7.5$$

$$\frac{60X}{60} = \frac{7.5}{60}$$

$$X = 0.125 \text{ mL} = 0.13 \text{ mL (per 15 sec)}$$

47) $$\frac{100 \text{ mg}}{1 \text{ mL}} \diagdown\diagup \frac{1,500 \text{ mg}}{X \text{ mL}}$$

$$100X = 1,500$$

$$\frac{100X}{100} = \frac{1,500}{100}$$

$$X = 15 \text{ mL}$$

48)   100 mL (IV PB) 1 15 mL (med) 5 115 mL (total to infuse in 30 min)

$$\frac{115 \text{ mL}}{30 \text{ min}} \diagdown\diagup \frac{X \text{ mL/h}}{60 \text{ min/h}}$$

$$30X = 6,900$$

$$\frac{30X}{30} = \frac{6,900}{30}$$

$$X = 230 \text{ mL/h}$$

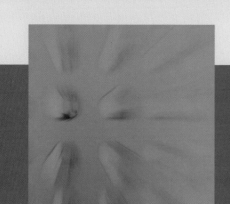

Appendix A: Study Guide

CHAPTER 3—SYSTEMS OF MEASUREMENT

Base Units in the Metric System

Weight: gram (g)
Volume: liter (L)
Length: meter (m)

Metric Prefixes

micro-   one millionth *or* 0.000001 *or* $\frac{1}{1,000,000}$ of the base unit

milli-   one thousandth *or* 0.001 *or* $\frac{1}{1,000}$ of the base unit

centi-   one hundredth *or* 0.01 *or* $\frac{1}{100}$ of the base unit

deci-   one tenth *or* 0.1 *or* $\frac{1}{10}$ of the base unit

kilo-   one thousand *or* 1,000 times the base unit

SI Metric System

	Unit	Abbreviation	Equivalent
Weight	**gram** (base unit)	g	**1 g** = 1,000 mg = 1,000,000 mcg
	milligram	mg	0.001 g = **1 mg** = 1,000 mcg
	microgram	mcg	0.000001 g = 0.001 mg = **1 mcg**
	kilogram	kg	**1 kg** = 1,000 g
Volume	**liter** (base unit)	L	**1 L** = 1,000 mL
	deciliter	dL	0.1 L = **1 dL**
	milliliter	mL	0.001 L = **1 mL**
Length	**meter** (base unit)	m	**1 m** = 100 cm = 1,000 mm
	centimeter	cm	0.01 m = **1 cm** = 10 mm
	millimeter	mm	0.001 m = 0.1 cm = **1 mm**

Frequently Used Household Units

Abbreviation	Unit
gtt	drop
t	teaspoon
T	tablespoon
fl oz	fluid ounce
cup	cup
pt	pint
qt	quart
oz	ounce (weight)
lb	pound
in	inch

CHAPTER 4—CONVERSIONS

Approximate Equivalents: Metric and Household

1 t = 5 mL

$1 \text{ T} = 3 \text{ t} = 15 \text{ mL} = \frac{1}{2} \text{ fl oz}$

1 fl oz = 30 mL = 6 t

1 L = 1 qt = 32 fl oz = 2 pt = 4 cups

1 pt = 16 fl oz = 2 cups

1 cup = 8 fl oz = 240 mL

1 kg = 2.2 lb

1 in = 2.5 cm

Converting Using the Ratio-Proportion Method

In a proportion, the ratio for a known equivalent equals the ratio for an unknown equivalent. To use the ratio-proportion method to convert from one unit to another:

1. Recall the equivalents.

2. Set up a proportion of two equivalent ratios.

3. Cross-multiply to solve for the unknown quantity, X.

EXAMPLE ■

Convert 0.3 g to mg.

Equivalent: 1 g = 1,000 mg

$$\frac{1 \text{ g}}{1,000 \text{ mg}} \diagdown \frac{0.3 \text{ g}}{X \text{ mg}}$$

$$X = 1,000 \times 0.3$$

$$X = 300 \text{ mg}$$

$$0.3 \text{ g} = 300 \text{ mg}$$

CHAPTER 5—CONVERSIONS FOR TIME AND TEMPERATURE

Converting Between Traditional and International Time

- International time is designated by 0001 through 1259 for 12:01 AM through 12:59 PM and 1300 through 2400 for 1:00 PM through 12:00 midnight.

- Between the hours of 1:00 PM (1300) and 12:00 AM (2400), **add 1200** to traditional time to find the equivalent international time; **subtract 1200** from international time to convert to equivalent traditional time.

Comparison of Traditional and International Time

AM	Int'l. Time	PM	Int'l. Time
12:00 midnight	2400	12:00 noon	1200
1:00	0100	1:00	1300
2:00	0200	2:00	1400
3:00	0300	3:00	1500
4:00	0400	4:00	1600
5:00	0500	5:00	1700
6:00	0600	6:00	1800
7:00	0700	7:00	1900
8:00	0800	8:00	2000
9:00	0900	9:00	2100
10:00	1000	10:00	2200
11:00	1100	11:00	2300

Converting Between Celsius and Fahrenheit Temperature Scales

$$°C = \frac{°F - 32}{1.8}$$

$$°F = 1.8°C + 32$$

CHAPTER 7—INTERPRETING DRUG ORDERS

Seven Parts of a Drug Order

1. Name of **patient**

2. Name of **drug**

3. **Dosage** of drug

4. **Route** by which the drug is to be administered

5. **Frequency, time, and special instructions** related to administration of drug

6. **Date and time** the order was written

7. **Signature and licensure** of the person writing the order

Medical Abbreviations

Abbreviation	Interpretation
Route:	
IM	intramuscular
IV	intravenous
IV PB	intravenous piggyback
subcut	subcutaneous
SL	sublingual, under the tongue
ID	intradermal
GT	gastrostomy tube
NG	nasogastric tube
NJ	nasojejunal tube
p.o.	by mouth, orally
p.r.	per rectum, rectally
Frequency:	
a.c.	before meals
p.c.	after meals
ad. lib.	as desired, freely
p.r.n.	when necessary
stat	immediately
b.i.d.	twice a day
t.i.d.	3 times a day
q.i.d.	4 times a day
min	minute
h	hour
q.h	every hour
q.2h	every 2 hours
q.4h	every 4 hours
q.6h	every 6 hours
q.8h	every 8 hours
q.12h	every 12 hours
General:	
$\bar{a}$	before
$\bar{p}$	after
$\bar{c}$	with
$\bar{s}$	without
q	every
qs	quantity sufficient
aq	water
NPO	nothing by mouth
gtt	drop
tab	tablet
cap	capsule
et	and
noct	night

CHAPTER 9—PREVENTING MEDICATION ERRORS

"Do Not Use" List of Medical Abbreviations

Do Not Use	Safe to Use
U, u	units
IU	international units
Q.D., QD, q.d., qd	daily
Q.O.D., QOD, q.o.d., qod	every other day
Trailing zero (X.0 mg)	no trailing zero (X mg)
Lack of leading zero (.X mg)	add 0 before decimal point for amounts less than 1 (0.X mg)
MS	morphine sulfate or magnesium sulfate
MSO_4 and $MgSO_4$	morphine sulfate or magnesium sulfate

Six Rights of Safe and Accurate Medication Administration

The *right patient* must receive the *right drug* in the *right amount* by the *right route* at the *right time* followed by the *right documentation.*

CHAPTERS 10 & 11—ORAL AND PARENTERAL DOSAGE OF DRUGS

Three-Step Approach to Dosage Calculations

Step 1: **Convert**—Ensure that all measurements are in the same system of measurement.
Step 2: **Think**—Estimate what is a *reasonable amount* of the drug to administer.
Step 3: **Calculate**—Use the ratio-proportion method to calculate the amount to give.

Dosage Calculations: Ratio-Proportion Method

$$\frac{\text{Dosage on hand}}{\text{Amount on hand}} = \frac{\text{Dosage desired}}{\text{X Amount desired}}$$

CHAPTER 12—RECONSTITUTION OF SOLUTIONS

Important Definitions

- **Reconstitution:** the process of mixing and diluting solutions
- **Solute:** a substance to be dissolved or diluted
- **Solvent:** a substance (liquid) that dissolves another substance to prepare a solution; diluent
- **Solution:** the resulting mixture of a solute plus a solvent

Fractions That Express the Strength of a Solution

- The numerator of the fraction expresses the number of parts of the solute.
- The denominator of the fraction is the total number of parts of the solution.
- The difference between the denominator (total solution) and the numerator (parts of the solute) is the number of parts of the solvent.

Formulas for Preparing Solutions

1. **Ratio for desired solution strength** $= \dfrac{\text{X Amount of solute}}{\text{Quantity of desired solution}}$

2. Quantity of desired solution $-$ Amount of solute $=$ Amount of solvent

CHAPTER 13—PEDIATRIC AND ADULT DOSAGES BASED ON BODY WEIGHT

Body Weight Method for Calculating Safe Dosages

1. Convert the patient's weight from pounds to kilograms (rounded to nearest tenths): 1 kg = 2.2 lb

2. Calculate the safe dosage in mg/kg for a patient of this weight:
    Multiply mg/kg by patient's weight in kg: **mg/kg × kg = X mg**

3. Compare the ordered dosage to the recommended dosage, and decide if dosage is safe.

4. If safe, calculate the amount to give and administer the dose; if the dosage seems unsafe, consult with the prescribing practitioner before administering the drug.

Note: The dosage per kg may be **mg/kg, mcg/kg, g/kg, mEq/kg, units/kg, milliunits/kg.**

CHAPTER 14—ALTERNATIVE DOSAGE CALCULATION METHODS: FORMULA AND DIMENSIONAL ANALYSIS

Conversion-Factor Method

To convert from a larger to a smaller unit, multiply by the conversion factor:

Larger ↓ Smaller → Multiply (×)   2 m̶g̶ × 1,000 mcg/m̶g̶ = 2.000. = 2,000 mcg

To convert from a smaller to a larger unit, divide by the conversion factor:

Smaller ↑ Larger → Divide (÷)   450 g ÷ 1,000 g/kg = 450 g̶ × 1 kg/1,000 g̶ = .450. = 0.45 kg

Dosage Calculations: Formula Method

$\dfrac{\text{D}}{\text{H}} \times \text{Q} = \text{X}$ $\dfrac{\text{D (desired)}}{\text{H (have)}} \times \text{Q (quantity)} = \text{X (amount)}$

Dosage Calculations: Dimensional Analysis Method

Amount-to-give ratio = Supply-dosage ratio × Conversion-factor ratio × Ordered-dosage ratio

1. Write the unknown X and the unit of measure for *amount-to-give ratio* on the left side of the equation, followed by equal sign (=).

2. Units in the numerator on the left side of the equal sign are the same units that are placed in the numerator of the first ratio on the right side of the equation.

3. When multiplying, if the units in a numerator and the units in a denominator are the same, they cancel each other out.

4. Set up the rest of the ratios so that the units cancel out, leaving only the *amount-to-give* unit.

CHAPTER 15—INTRAVENOUS SOLUTIONS, EQUIPMENT, AND CALCULATIONS

Common IV Component Abbreviations

D = Dextrose
W = Water
S = Saline
NaCl = Sodium Chloride
NS = Normal Saline (0.9% NaCl)
RL = Ringer's Lactate
LR = Lactated Ringer's

Solution strength expressed as a percent (%) indicates the number of g per 100 mL:

$$\frac{\text{\# of g solute}}{\text{100 mL solution}}$$

Osmolarity of Solutions

Hypotonic: less than 250 mOsm/L
Isotonic: 250–375 mOsm/L
Hypertonic: greater than 375 mOsm/L

IV Rate by Electronic Infusion Pump (mL/h)

$$\frac{\text{Total mL ordered}}{\text{Total h ordered}} = \text{mL/h (rounded to a whole number or tenths, depending on equipment)}$$

If infusion time is less than 1 hour, then $\frac{\text{Total mL ordered}}{\text{Total min ordered}} = \frac{\text{X mL/h}}{\text{60 min/h}}$

Flow Rate for Manually-Regulated IV (gtt/min)

Drop factor = gtt/mL
Macrodrop factors: 10, 15, or 20 gtt/mL
Microdrop factor: 60 gtt/mL

Calculating IV Flow Rate for Manually-Regulated IV in gtt/min: Formula Method

$$\frac{\text{V}}{\text{T}} \times \text{C} = \text{R} \qquad \frac{\text{Volume (mL)}}{\text{Time (min)}} \times \text{Calibration or drop factor (gtt/mL)} = \text{Rate (gtt/min)}$$

Shortcut Method to Calculate IV Flow Rate in gtt/min

To use shortcut method, remember drop factor constants: 10 gtt/mL = $\frac{60}{10}$ = **6**

15 gtt/mL = $\frac{60}{15}$ = **4**

20 gtt/mL = $\frac{60}{20}$ = **3**

60 gtt/mL = $\frac{60}{60}$ = **1**

$$\frac{\text{mL/h}}{\text{Drop factor constant}} = \textbf{gtt/min}$$ *(Do not use shortcut method if time is less than 1 hour, unless the rate is first converted to mL/h.)*

Adjusting IV Flow Rates (as allowed by agency policy)

Step 1: $\dfrac{\text{Remaining volume}}{\text{Remaining hours}} = \text{Recalculated mL/h}$

Step 2: $\dfrac{V}{T} \times C = R \text{ (gtt/min)}$

Step 3: $\dfrac{\text{Adjusted rate } - \text{ Ordered rate}}{\text{Ordered rate}} = \% \text{ Variation (maximum 25\% variation)}$

Calculating IV Infusion Time

$\dfrac{\text{Total mL}}{\text{mL/h}} = \text{Total hours}$

Calculating IV Infusion Volume

$\text{Total hours} \times \text{mL/h} = \text{Total mL}$

CHAPTER 16—BODY SURFACE AREA AND ADVANCED PEDIATRIC CALCULATIONS

Calculating Body Surface Area (BSA): Formula Method

*Using **metric** measurement of height and weight:* $\text{BSA (m}^2) = \sqrt{\dfrac{\text{ht (cm)} \times \text{wt (kg)}}{3{,}600}}$

*Using **household** measurement of height and weight:* $\text{BSA (m}^2) = \sqrt{\dfrac{\text{ht (in)} \times \text{wt (lb)}}{3{,}131}}$

Dosage Calculations Using BSA

1. Determine BSA in m^2.
2. Calculate safe dosage based on BSA: $\text{mg/m}^2 \times m^2 = X \text{ mg}$.
3. Compare the ordered dosage to the recommended dosage, and decide if dosage is safe.
4. If the dosage is safe, calculate the amount to give and administer dose. If dosage seems unsafe, consult with the ordering practitioner before administering the drug.

Note: The dosage per m^2 may be mg/m^2, mcg/m^2, g/m^2, mEq/m^2, units/m^2, milliunits/m^2.

Calculation of Daily Volume for Pediatric Maintenance Fluids

- 100 mL/kg/day for first 10 kg of body weight
- 50 mL/kg/day for next 10 kg of body weight
- 20 mL/kg/day for each kg above 20 kg of body weight

CHAPTER 17—ADVANCED ADULT INTRAVENOUS CALCULATIONS

Actions for the Administration of Critical Intravenous Medications (e.g., Heparin and Insulin)

Action 1: Calculate bolus.
Action 2: Calculate initial continuous infusion flow rate.
Action 3: Calculate rebolus and/or adjust continuous infusion flow rate.

Action 1: Calculation of the Heparin Bolus

1. Calculate the dosage (units) of the heparin bolus based on patient's weight (kg):

   units/kg × kg = units

2. Calculate the volume (mL) of the bolus to prepare using ratio-proportion:

   $$\frac{\textbf{Dosage on hand}}{\textbf{Amount on hand}} = \frac{\textbf{Dosage desired}}{\textbf{X Amount desired}}$$

Action 2: Calculation of Initial Continuous Flow Rate of the IV Heparin Solution (mL/h)

1. Calculate the dosage (units/h) of the initial continuous infusion based on patient's weight (kg):

   units/kg/h × kg = units/h

2. Calculate the continuous infusion rate (mL/h) using ratio-proportion:

   $$\frac{\textbf{Dosage on hand}}{\textbf{Amount on hand}} = \frac{\textbf{Dosage desired/h}}{\textbf{X Amount desired/h}}$$

Action 3: Calculation of the Heparin Rebolus and Adjustment of Continuous Infusion Rate

1. Calculate the dose (units) of the heparin bolus based on aPTT results and patient's weight (kg):

   units/kg × kg = units

2. Calculate the volume (mL) of the bolus to prepare using ratio-proportion:

   $$\frac{\textbf{Dosage on hand}}{\textbf{Amount on hand}} = \frac{\textbf{Dosage desired}}{\textbf{X Amount desired}}$$

3. Calculate the dosage (units/h) of the continuous infusion adjustment based on aPTT results and patient's weight (kg): **units/kg/h × kg = units/h**

4. Calculate the adjustment to the hourly infusion rate (mL/h) using ratio-proportion:

   $$\frac{\textbf{Dosage on hand}}{\textbf{Amount on hand}} = \frac{\textbf{Dosage desired/h}}{\textbf{X Amount desired/h}}$$

5. Calculate the new hourly infusion rate (mL/h):

   Current rate (mL/h) ± adjustment (mL/h) = new rate (mL/h)

Calculation of the Insulin Bolus and Continuous Flow Rate

The insulin bolus is based on blood glucose level.

$$\frac{\text{Dosage on hand}}{\text{Amount on hand}} = \frac{\text{Dosage desired/h}}{\text{X Amount desired/h}}$$

Note: This rule applies to other drugs ordered in **units/h, milliunits/h, mg/h, mcg/h, g/h,** or **mEq/h.**

Calculation of the Flow Rate for IV Medications Ordered in mg/min

Step 1:   Calculate the dosage in mL/min: $\dfrac{\text{Dosage on hand}}{\text{Amount of solution on hand}} = \dfrac{\text{Dosage desired/min}}{\text{X Amount desired/min}}$

Step 2:   Calculate the flow rate in mL/h of the volume to administer per minute:

$$\frac{\text{Volume on hand}}{\text{Min to be infused}} = \frac{\text{X volume to be infused/h}}{\text{60 min/h}}$$

Or, **mL/min × 60 min/h = mL/h**

Calculation of the Flow Rate for IV Medications Ordered in mg/kg/min

Step 1:   Convert to like units (mg to mcg, lb to kg).

Step 2:   Calculate desired dosage per minute: **mg/kg/min × kg = mg/min**

Step 3:   Calculate the dosage flow rate in mL/min: $\dfrac{\text{Dosage on hand}}{\text{Amount of solution on hand}} = \dfrac{\text{Dosage desired/min}}{\text{X Amount desired/min}}$

Step 4:   Calculate the flow rate in mL/h of the volume to administer per minute:

$$\frac{\text{Volume on hand}}{\text{Min to be infused}} = \frac{\text{X volume to be infused/h}}{\text{60 min/h}}$$

Or, **mL/min × 60 min/h = mL/h**

Calculation of Flow Rate for IV Medications Ordered Over a Specific Time Period (mg/min)

Step 1:   Calculate mg/mL.
Step 2:   Calculate mL/h.

Steps to Verify Safe Dosage of IV Medications Recommended in mg/min and Ordered in mL/h

Step 1:   Calculate mg/h.
Step 2:   Calculate mg/min.
Step 3:   Compare recommended dosage and ordered dosage to decide if the dosage is safe.

Steps to Verify Safe Dosage of IV Medications Recommended in mg/kg/min and Ordered in mL/h

Step 1:   Convert to like units.
Step 2:   Calculate recommended mg/min.
Step 3:   Calculate ordered mg/h.
Step 4:   Calculate ordered mg/min.
Step 5:   Compare ordered and recommended dosages to decide if the dosage is safe.

Calculation of Flow Rate for IV Medications That Include IV Piggyback

Step 1:	IV PB flow rate	$\frac{V}{T} \times C = R$
Step 2:	Total IV PB time	**Time for 1 dose × # of doses in 24 h**
Step 3:	Total IV PB volume	**Volume of 1 dose × # of doses in 24 h**
Step 4:	Total regular IV volume	**Total volume − IV PB volume = Regular IV volume**
Step 5:	Total regular IV time	**Total time − IV PB time = Regular IV time**
Step 6:	Regular IV flow rate	$\frac{V}{T} \times C = R$

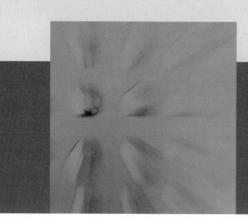

Appendix B: Apothecary System

The apothecary system was introduced in Chapter 3. The following units, abbreviations, symbols, and equivalents describe the remnants of this ancient method of measuring medication dosages. Because it is less accurate than the metric system, it is no longer recommended for safe practice. The basic units are the weight measure *grain (15 grains is approximately equivalent to 1 gram)* and the liquid volume measures of *dram* (similar to a teaspoon and still found on some medicine cups), *ounce* (same as household *fluid ounce*), and *minim* (approximately a drop). You can compare apothecary and metric measures with the following tables and figure.

Apothecary Units

Measure	Apothecary Unit	Abbreviation	Symbol
Weight	grain	gr	N/A
Volume	ounce	oz	ʒ
Volume	dram	dr	ȝ
Volume	minim	min	℥

Apothecary-Metric Approximate Equivalents

Volume		Weight	
oz mL	**min mL**	**gr mg**	**gr mg**
$1 = 30$	$45 = 3$	$15 = 1{,}000$	$\frac{1}{4} = 15$
$\frac{1}{2} = 15$	$30 = 2$	$10 = 600$	$\frac{1}{6} = 10$
	$15 = 1$	$7\frac{1}{2} = 500$	$\frac{1}{8} = 7.5$
dr mL	$12 = 0.75$	$5 = 300$	$\frac{1}{10} = 6$
$2\frac{1}{2} = 10$	$10 = 0.6$	$4 = 250$	$\frac{1}{15} = 4$
$2 = 8$	$8 = 0.5$	$3 = 200$	$\frac{1}{20} = 3$
$1\frac{1}{4} = 5$	$5 = 0.3$	$2\frac{1}{2} = 150$	$\frac{1}{30} = 2$
$1 = 5$	$4 = 0.25$	$2 = 120$	$\frac{1}{40} = 1.5$
	$3 = 0.2$	$1\frac{1}{2} = 100$	$\frac{1}{60} = 1$
1 **minim** = 1 **gtt**	$1\frac{1}{2} = 0.1$	$1 = 60$	$\frac{1}{100} = 0.6$
	$1 = 0.06$	$\frac{3}{4} = 45$	$\frac{1}{120} = 0.5$
	$\frac{3}{4} = 0.05$	$\frac{1}{2} = 30$	$\frac{1}{150} = 0.4$
	$\frac{1}{2} = 0.03$	$\frac{1}{3} = 20$	$\frac{1}{200} = 0.3$
			$\frac{1}{250} = 0.25$

Apothecary-Metric Approximate Equivalent "Conversion Clock"

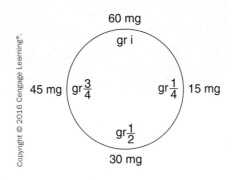

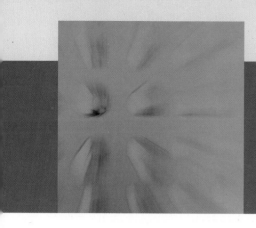

Index

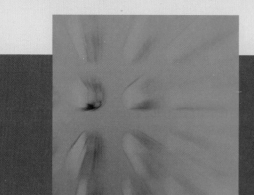

Drug Label Index

Boldface indicates generic drug name